AGING WELL

GERONTOLOGICAL EDUCATION
for Nurses and Other Health Professionals

Edited by

May L. Wykle, PhD, RN, FAAN, FGSA, FAGHE
Dean and Marvin E. and Ruth Durr Denekas Professor of Nursing
Frances Payne Bolton School of Nursing
Case Western Reserve University
Cleveland, Ohio

Sarah H. Gueldner, PhD, RN, FAAN, FNAP, FGSA, FAGHE
Arline H. and Curtis F. Garvin Professor of Nursing
Frances Payne Bolton School of Nursing
Case Western Reserve University
Cleveland, Ohio

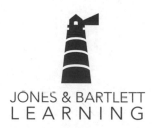

JONES & BARTLETT
LEARNING

World Headquarters

Jones & Bartlett Learning
40 Tall Pine Drive
Sudbury, MA 01776
978-443-5000
info@jblearning.com
www.jblearning.com

Jones & Bartlett Learning Canada
6339 Ormindale Way
Mississauga, Ontario L5V 1J2
Canada

Jones & Bartlett Learning International
Barb House, Barb Mews
London W6 7PA
United Kingdom

Jones & Bartlett Learning books and products are available through most bookstores and online booksellers. To contact Jones & Bartlett Learning directly, call 800-832-0034, fax 978-443-8000, or visit our website, www.jblearning.com.

Substantial discounts on bulk quantities of Jones & Bartlett Learning publications are available to corporations, professional associations, and other qualified organizations. For details and specific discount information, contact the special sales department at Jones & Bartlett Learning via the above contact information or send an email to specialsales@jblearning.com.

Production Credits

Publisher: Kevin Sullivan
Acquisitions Editor: Amy Sibley
Associate Editor: Patricia Donnelly
Editorial Assistant: Rachel Shuster
Production Editor: Amanda Clerkin
Associate Marketing Manager: Katie Hennessy

V.P., Manufacturing and Inventory Control: Therese Connell
Composition: Shepherd, Inc.
Cover Design: Scott Moden
Cover Image: © Monkey Business Images/ShutterStock, Inc.
Printing and Binding: Malloy, Inc.
Cover Printing: Malloy, Inc.

Library of Congress Cataloging-in-Publication Data

Aging well : gerontological education for nurses and other health professionals / [edited by] May L. Wykle and Sarah H. Gueldner
    p. ; cm.
  Includes bibliographical references and index.
  ISBN-13: 978-0-7637-7937-5
  ISBN-10: 0-7637-7937-7
  1. Gerontology—Study and teaching. 2. Geriatric nursing. 3. Older people—Health and hygiene. I. Gueldner, Sarah Hall. II. Wykle, May L.
  [DNLM: 1. Geriatric Nursing—education. 2. Aged—psychology. 3. Aging. 4. Geriatric Nursing—methods. WY 18 A267 2011]
  HQ1061.A4847 2011
  305.26—dc22
                              2010013291
6048
Printed in the United States of America
14 13 12 11 10   10 9 8 7 6 5 4 3 2 1

Contents

Foreword

What makes this excellent book by Wykle and Gueldner stand out is its conceptual and philosophical framework, which is rooted in holistic and positive views of aging and transcends disciplinary boundaries. The book calls for a client-centered approach focused on the personhood of the older individual and the possibilities of growth and expression in the later years of the lifecourse. The editors reframe aging to focus on the possibilities that aging brings, despite increasing functional limitations, with a focus on practical and easy-to-implement activities that enable elders to express their personhood and remain active in their social networks and communities. The book is a must-read for gerontological and geriatric educators in nursing and other disciplines because of its collection of learning strategies to engage students to be lifelong professionals in the field of aging.

There is indeed a real need for gerontology textbooks such as *Aging Well: Gerontological Education for Nurses and Other Health Professionals*. There is an urgent need to engage students in aging studies and a career in gerontology and geriatrics. For instance, a recent New York State survey of institutions of higher learning found that there were very few gerontology programs, with most having fewer than 10 students. Even more disturbing, almost 60% of the schools offered no courses at all on aging, and only 4% of the schools had a major in aging studies. Nationally, the number of programs focusing on gerontology has also declined precipitously over the last decade. This apparent lack of interest is found across all professional disciplines and is contributing to widespread shortages in the workforce, particularly when considering the projected demand over the next 20 years. With approximately 8,000 baby boomers in the United States turning 65 every day, almost 20% of the nation's population will be 65 and older in 2030.

One intractable issue in the field has been how to engage students and professionals in the field of aging given the prevalence of stereotypes and myths about older persons, the aging process, and careers in gerontology and geriatrics. The fact is that not much has changed since I was a young graduate student and many of my peers and professors tried to dissuade me from entering the field because they thought it to be "depressing" and "unrewarding." That we as gerontological educators have still not figured out effective means of engaging students and young professionals in the field of aging is indeed worrisome. This book is a step in the right direction. It is a very engaging book with 45 chapters written by almost 80 highly qualified authors drawn from a range of disciplines, including nurses, gerontologists, social workers, physicians, and other fields of specialization. The fact that Wykle and Gueldner have included many doctoral students and recent graduates as authors testifies to their commitment to fresh ideas, new perspectives, and "passing the torch" to the next generation of gerontologists.

Aging Well: Gerontological Education for Nurses and Other Health Professionals is aimed at engaging the reader as a potential change agent in promoting aging as a positive circumstance that people of all ages can relate to. The volume is organized into seven sections. The first section is a call to action by Binstock, who lays out the ethical, moral, and policy challenges of an aging society. The second section focuses on central issues in gerontological education. Poon and Isales speak to the need for structured mentoring programs to allay the hesitation of the younger generation to enter the field by debunking stereotypes about aging and highlighting the potential for innovation and creativity within the field. Brown, Hagedorn, and McMullen, two of whom are doctoral students, propose that a gerontological distance learning department can be most effective when it maintains open and constant communication with students and encourages community service and multicultural interaction. The third section focuses on innovative learning activities and includes an excellent chapter by Gugliucci outlining how she offers her students the opportunity to earn course credit by assuming the diagnosis and persona of an older person and living in a nursing home for 2 weeks. In the fourth section on social issues related to gerontology, there are excellent chapters on health disparities, manpower shortages in underserved areas, and engagement of elders in community events. Toner, for instance, describes a successful program in rural New York State that provides continuing education to providers in geriatrics and geriatric mental health. In the fifth section, the authors discuss practice imperatives in gerontology, including methods for preventing functional decline in hospitalized elderly people, poetry for caregivers of older adults, and cognitive rehabilitation for older people with dementia. For instance, Hill, who is a doctoral student, and Kolanowski discuss the use of cognitive rehabilitation for persons with dementia. The sixth section of the book includes chapters identifying methods for promoting personhood and quality of life in older persons, including programs on storytelling, therapeutic cooking, companion animals, and reminiscence. Quinn, Kolomer, and Burden describe an interdisciplinary place-based reminiscence intervention model. In the final section on cultural dimensions of aging, the authors present culturally sensitive interventions that engage older adults, including telenovelas for Latina women, self-health measures for African-American elders passed down over the ages, and life storybooks for older Irish Americans. Day and her colleagues describe a life story intervention for nursing home residents that promotes a holistic view of the older adult and promotes person-centered care.

This is a must-read book for both seasoned gerontologists and novice learners and will have wide applicability in both undergraduate and graduate classrooms. It is brimming with innovative ideas that are rooted in interdisciplinary and holistic practice and highlight the many possibilities of old age.

Judith L. Howe, PhD

Preface

The purpose of this book is to highlight the need for and provide commentary and exemplars of vibrant and relevant programs of gerontological education, with the goal of attracting students at all levels and from across disciplines to careers in the field of gerontology. The content of the book is organized into seven sections that address key aspects of gerontological education, beginning with a call to action offered by respected gerontologist Robert Binstock, who highlights important ethical, moral, and policy challenges in our aging society.

The chapters in Section II address issues central to gerontological education, including the urgent need for mentoring to recruit and develop the next generation of gerontologists. Toward this goal, chapters are offered by seasoned gerontologists as well as students and recent graduates. Novel programs involving student participation in interdisciplinary community-based projects are also featured.

Section III is a collection of chapters that describe innovative learning activities that are relevant for any type or level of gerontological education, including continuing education programs at nursing homes and other community-based care facilities. One professor invites her students to live for 2 weeks as a wheelchair-bound resident in a nursing home, assisted with their baths and toileting, enabling them to experience the diminished feelings associated with dependence on others. A young AmeriCorps worker who is assigned with the Office of Aging while she waits to start medical school conveys the unexpected regard she has found for elders in the senior centers, and notes that this experience has prompted her to consider gerontology as her field of practice. A new, doctorally prepared teacher describes service learning in the community for graduate gerontology students as the intercept of pedagogy and practice.

Section IV focuses on social issues that are detrimental to the field of gerontology and aging, particularly in regard to the effect of disparities in health services for minority elders and other underrepresented segments of the population. Manpower shortages and service gaps in medically underserved areas are also addressed, within the context of social capital, vulnerability, and accessibility to events in the community. One vocal professor who is also a nurse practitioner issues the charge that "we must get the home in nursing homes."

Section V addresses practice imperatives, including one physician's mandate to create a new philosophy for elder care. This section is not intended as a procedural guide, but is rather a collection of philosophical and concept-based essays about how to be with elders in a therapeutic way, with thoughtful discussions that address common practice issues, including:

- The management of pain
- Continued interface with the community
- Assessing and preventing the functional decline associated with hospitalization
- Special care needs of elders in the emergency department
- Helping elders to prepare in advance for life changes
- End-of-life care
- Morale upon admission to a nursing home
- Elders' often neglected need for dental care

Several authors also describe research-based interventions to connect with and enrich life for persons with dementia. A nurse who recently received her doctorate discusses her dissertation work of writing poetry using the words of caregivers, to give voice to and ease the burden of caregiving. A long-time physician speaks to the importance of end-of-life care, and a geriatric nurse practitioner who specializes in home care reminds us that "home is where the heart is."

Section VI features a number of activities based within the arts and humanities (i.e., storytelling, music, poetry, and painting) to preserve personhood and help elders and their family caregivers to increase their sense of vitality and find meaningful connections. One professor paints verbal portraits of elders who retained their sense of personhood by continuing to engage in the activities that they were good at, including quilting, painting, playing the piano, and plowing straight rows in the garden. A young drama therapist describes her work of "Making Moments That Matter" as a songwriter and poet in a nursing home. A certified recreational therapist and her colleagues describe their experience with cooking groups to help persons with dementia to tap into the pleasant times in their lives when they prepared food and ate together around the table.

A now-retired nurse educator and avid gardener reminds readers that growing plants is fulfilling, and that it can be a legacy that has meaning for future generations. An animal activist discusses the importance of companion animals for some elders, and outlines safety measures for both the elder and the animals. Virtually all of the interventions described brought a smile and a twinkle to the eyes of the elders and those around them.

Section VII reflects on the cultural aspects of aging, including caregiving traditions, as told by nurses and others in the United States as well as professionals in Japan, Africa, Korea, and Ireland. Authors also discuss novel educational ways of reaching minorities, including the use of *telenovelas* and *cafecitos* (i.e., similar to soap operas) for Latino populations. The still-widespread use of alternative therapies passed down through the ages by African-American, rural dwelling, and other elders is also discussed.

It is the purpose of this book to attract people of all ages, but particularly young people, to the betterment of elders. The authors remind us that as healthcare professionals we must expand our dated repertoire of care to include creative approaches that embrace the continuing expression of personhood in elders, even in the presence of limitations associated with aging. And as gerontologists from across disciplines we must join in addressing the daunting challenge of recruiting minority segments of the population to the field of gerontology. Finally, it is the hope of the editors and authors that the innovative thinking put forward in this book will generate additional novel ideas among the readers that will change the experience of aging around the world.

May L. Wykle, PhD, RN, FAAN, FGSA, FAGHE
Dean and Marvin E. and Ruth Durr Denekas Professor in Nursing

Sarah H. Gueldner, DSN, RN, FAAN, FSGA, FAGHE
Arline H. and Curtis F. Garvin Professor in Nursing

Frances Payne Bolton School of Nursing
Case Western Reserve University
Cleveland, Ohio

Contributors

Susan Allen, PhD
Brown University
Providence, Rhode Island

Beth E. Barba, PhD, RN, FAGHE, FAAN
School of Nursing
University of North Carolina–Greensboro
Greensboro, North Carolina

Michelle M. Berry, MBA
Broome County Community Alternative
  Systems Agency (CASA)
New York

Robert H. Binstock, PhD
Professor of Aging, Health, and Society
Schools of Medicine and Nursing
Case Western Reserve University
Cleveland, Ohio

Candy Blevins
Nursing Student
University of North Carolina–Charlotte
Charlotte, North Carolina

Marie P. Boltz, PhD, RN
Practice Director, NICHE
New York University School of Nursing
New York, New York

Martha H. Bramlett, PhD, RN
School of Nursing
University of North Carolina–Charlotte
Charlotte, North Carolina

Geraldine R. Britton, PhD, RN
Decker School of Nursing
Binghamton University
Binghamton, New York

Candace Brown, MAG, MEd
School of Allied Health Professions
Virginia Commonwealth University
Richmond, Virginia

Jane A. Brown, PhD
Department of Sociology
Case Western Reserve University
Cleveland, Ohio

Linda L. Buettner, PhD, LRT, CTRS
University of North Carolina–Greensboro
Greensboro, North Carolina

Kathleen Bunnell, RD
Director, Broome County Office of Aging
Binghamton, New York

Jeffrey Burden, PhD
Architectural Historian
National Trust for Historic Preservation
Charleston, South Carolina

Kimberly Campbell
Baccalaureate Nursing Student
Binghamton University
Binghamton, New York

Michael Carter, RN, DNSc, FAAN
University of Tennessee–Memphis
Memphis, Tennessee

Shelli Cordisco, MA
Action for Older Persons, Inc.
Binghamton, New York

Janice D. Crist, PhD, RN
University of Arizona College of Nursing
Tucson, Arizona

Maureen Daws, RN, MSN, PhD Student
Decker School of Nursing
Binghamton University
Binghamton, New York

Mary Rose Day, MA, HDip PHN, BSc,
    Dip. Manag., RPHN, RM, RGN
Catherine McAuley School of Nursing
    and Midwifery
Brookfield Health Science Complex
University College
Cork, Ireland

Evelyn G. Duffy, DNP, A/GNP-BC, FAANP
Bolton School of Nursing
Case Western Reserve University
Cleveland, Ohio

Lisa A. Ferretti, LMSW
State University of New York in Albany
Albany, New York

Joyce J. Fitzpatrick, PhD, RN, MBA, FAAN
Bolton School of Nursing
Case Western Reserve University
Cleveland, Ohio

Suzanne Fitzsimmons, RN, MS, ARNP
Sunset Hills Aging & Wellness
Greensboro, North Carolina

Sarah H. Gueldner, PhD, RN, FAAN,
    FNAP, FGSA, FAGHE
Garvin Professor in Nursing
Bolton School of Nursing
Case Western Reserve University
Cleveland, Ohio

Marilyn R. Cogliucci, PhD, MA, FAGHE,
    FSAG, AGSF
Director, Geriatrics Education and Research
College of Osteopathic Medicine
University of New England
Biddeford, Maine

Aaron Hagedorn, PhD
Director of Internship Training
University of Southern California
Los Angeles, California

John B. Haradon, MED, MSHP
Freelance Journalist and Researcher
Tucson, Arizona

Neil Hall, MD
Cary, North Carolina

Nikki L. Hill
Hartford Foundation PhD Nursing Student
The Pennsylvania State University

Yong Hae Hong, PhD, RN
Choonhae College of Health Sciences
Department of Nursing
Ulsan, Korea

Maria C. Isales
Graduate Student
University of Georgia Center for Aging
Athens, Georgia

Katherine R. Jones, PhD, RN
Bolton School of Nursing
Case Western Reserve University
Cleveland, Ohio

Evanne Juratovac, PhD, RN
Bolton School of Nursing
Case Western Reserve University
Cleveland, Ohio

Boaz Kahana, PhD
Case Western Reserve University
Cleveland, Ohio

Eva Kahana, PhD
Case Western Reserve University
Cleveland, Ohio

Lori Kidd, PhD, RN
Bolton School of Nursing
Case Western Reserve University
Cleveland, Ohio

Cheryl M. Killion, PhD, RN
Bolton School of Nursing
Case Western Reserve University
Cleveland, Ohio

Soo-kyung Kim, PhD, MD
Department of Pharmacology
Keimyung University School of Medicine
Daegu, Korea

Kareen M. King, MS, RDT, JD
Registered Drama Therapist
Osage City, Kansas

Evelyn Kintner, MS, MSW
State University of New York in Albany
Albany, New York

Stacey Kolomer, PhD
School of Social work
University of Georgia
Athens, Georgia

Ann M. Kolonowski, PhD, RN, FAAN
The Pennsylvania State University

Gee-youn Kwon, PhD
Department of Pharmacology
Keimyung University School of Medicine
Daegu, South Korea

Lynne B. Lacey, Dental Hygienist
SUNY Empire State College
Saratoga Springs, New York

Frederick J. Lacey, DMD, FACD
Binghamton, New York

Gail Mathieson-Devereaux, RN, MSN, FNP
Binghamton University
Binghamton, New York

Philip McCallion, PhD, ACSW
State University of New York in Albany
Albany, New York

Geraldine McCarthy, PhD, MSN, MEd,
    DIPN, RNT, RGN
Catherine McAuley School of Nursing
    and Midwifery
Brookfield health Sciences Complex
University College
Cork, Ireland

Ditsepelo M. McFarland, RN, PhD
Adelphi University
Garden City, New York

Tara McMullen, MPH
University of Maryland
College Park, Maryland

Jessica Kelley-Moore, PhD
Case Western Reserve University
Cleveland, Ohio

Mary Muscari, PhD, RN, CPNP, APRN-BC
Decker School of Nursing
Binghamton University
Binghamton, New York

Martha Neff-Smith, PhD, RN, FAAN
Global Consultants
Gordonsville, Virginia

Eric D. Newman, MD
Director, Dept of Rheumatology
Vice Chairman for Innovations, Division
    of Medicine
Geisinger Medical Center
Danville, Pennsylvania

Robert Paeglow, MD
State University of New York in Albany
Albany, New York

Carolyn Pierce, RN, DSN
Decker School of Nursing
Binghamton University
Binghamton, New York

Leonard W. Poon, PhD, FGSA, FAGHE
Director, Univ of Georgia Center for Aging
Principle Investigator, Georgia Centenarian
    Study
Athens, Georgia

William J. Puentes, PhD, RN, PMHCNS-BC
Nell Hodgson Woodruff School of Nursing
Emory University
Atlanta, Georgia

Mary Ellen Quinn, PhD, RN
Medical College of Georgia School of
    Nursing, Athens
Athens, Georgia

Barbara Resnick, PhD, RN, FAAN
University of Maryland School of Nursing
College Park, Maryland

Nancy Richeson, PhD, RN, CTRS
University of Southern Maine
Portland, Maine

Meredith Rowe, PhD, RN, FAAN
University of Florida School of Nursing
Gainesville, Florida

Susan Seibold-Simpson, PhD, RN
Decker School of Nursing
Binghamton University
Binghamton, New York

Amy Shaver, PhD, RN
The Sage Colleges, Nursing Department
Troy, New York

Yeonghee Shin, PhD, RN
Keimyung University College of Nursing
Daegu, Korea

Samantha Sterns, PhD
Brown University
Providence, Rhode Island

Laura Sutton PhD, RN, ACNS-BC,
    GNEC, SRC
University of Florida School of Nursing
Gainesville, Florida

Ryutaro Takahashi, MD, PhD
Vice-Director
Tokyo Metropolitan Institute of Gerontology
Tokyo, Japan

Susan Terwilliger, EdD, RN, PNP-BC
Decker School of Nursing
Binghamton University
Binghamton, New York

Anita S. Tesh, PhD, RN, CEA-l, CNE
School of Nursing
University of North Carolina–Greensboro
Greensboro, North Carolina

John A. Toner, MD, PhD
Associate Clinical Professor and Director,
    Geriatric Residency and Fellowship
    Programs
Columbia University Stroud Center
Senior Research Scientist
New York State Psychiatric Institute
New York, New York

Sally Venugopalans
New York State Veterans Home
    Administrator
Oxford, New York

Teresa Wills, MSc, PDipTLHED,
    BNS(Hons), RGN, RM
Catherine McAuley School of Nursing
    and Midwifery
Brookfield Health Sciences Complex
University College
Cork, Ireland

May L. Wykle, PhD, RN, FAAN, FGSA,
    FAGHE
Dean and Marvin E. & Ruth Durr Denekes
    Professor of Nursing
Bolton School of Nursing
Case Western Reserve University
Cleveland, Ohio

Jocelyn C. Young
AmeriCorps/Broome County Office
    of Aging
Binghamton, New York

Acknowledgments

The editors would like to acknowledge the many individuals and organizations that have provided the energy, expertise, and resources to make this endeavor possible. In particular, we would thank Jones & Bartlett Learning and their editorial staff for their interest in this important topic and their skillful guidance in bringing this book to print. Our sincere appreciation is extended to Amy Sibley (Acquisitions Editor, Nursing), Rachel Shuster (Editorial Assistant, Nursing), Rebecca Wasley (Marketing Manager), and Amanda Clerkin (Production Editor) for their support of this project, and to Mary Grivetti (Project Manager) and Kevin Campbell (Copyeditor) at Shepherd, Inc. for their production and copyediting. We also acknowledge and appreciate the assistance of Dr. Carolyn Pierce for her dogged persistence in retrieving elusive references. We express our deepest appreciation to our 75 wonderful colleagues from nursing and other disciplines, including students, who authored the chapters that brought this book to fruition. Collectively, they represent the finest group of colleagues one could ever hope to meet, and they bring a rich and dynamic perspective to the discussion of gerontological education.

We would also like to thank our colleagues from nursing and other disciplines at the Frances Payne Bolton School of Nursing and from across campus at Case Western Reserve University, who have supported us in every way toward the completion of this book. In particular, we thank Mandisa Molton for her long hours spent in retrieving references and reformatting the manuscripts for publication as chapters, despite her heavy course load as a second degree nursing student in the accelerated undergraduate nursing program. We also thank Samira Hussney, Director of the WHO Collaborating Center, and her assistant Wariya Muensa for their support of the book, doctoral student Eunsuk Lee for serving as the conduit for the international manuscripts, and dual degree undergraduate nursing student Kayla Tran for providing technical support and other assistance for the project. Finally, we thank Caron Baldwin and her team at the nursing help desk for the technical support that they provided to the project, and thanks to Toiya Benford, Pamela Collins, and Cookie Jones for their assistance in many ways.

Section I

A Call to Action: Policy Implications

Chapter 1

Ethical, Moral, and Policy Challenges in Our Aging Society

Robert H. Binstock

Developed nations throughout the world are experiencing population aging that is producing unprecedented proportions of older persons which, in turn, pose significant ethical, moral, and policy challenges. This chapter focuses on some of those challenges that affect the health and health care of older people.

In some countries population aging is due to an exceptionally large number of births in the years following World War II. In the United States, for example, 76 million people were born between 1946 and 1964; this population bulge has been described as the *baby boom*. The boomers have had distinctive impacts on American society for decades, such as a demand for more schools and educators, a large influx into the labor force, and a huge demand for housing. These boomers are now beginning to enter the ranks of old age, with the consequence that the number of Americans aged 65 and older will increase from 40 million in 2010 to 72 million in 2030. At that point nearly 20 percent of the US population—one in five persons—will be aged 65 and older (U.S. Census Bureau, 2008). This phenomenon will sharply escalate the aggregate demand for acute and long-term care in the United States and will require a retooling of the health care workforce (Institute of Medicine of the National Academies, 2009).

In European and some Asian nations *low fertility rates* are the major factor in population aging. Instead of baby booms, they have been experiencing baby *"busts."* The fertility rate that is needed to maintain a stable population size—known as the "population replacement rate"—is 2.3 children per woman. As can be seen in Table 1-1, however, Japan's fertility rate was only 1.54 in 1990 and dropped to 1.32 by 2006. Germany's fertility rate dropped from 1.46 to 1.33 during the same period, and Italy's fertility rate climbed from a very low 1.33 to 1.35. In contrast, the rate for the United States rose from 2.08 to 2.10.

Table 1-2 makes clear that the consequences of years of low fertility rates for the age structure of populations are already being felt in these (as well as other low-fertility) nations. About 1 in 5 Germans and Italians are aged 65 and older, and the proportion is

TABLE 1-1   Fertility Rate (Children per Woman), 1990 and 2006

	1990	2006
Germany	1.46	1.33
Italy	1.33	1.35
Japan	1.54	1.32
United States	2.08	2.10

Source: Berghammer et al. (2006) and Lutz et al. (2008).

TABLE 1-2   Percent of the Population Aged 65+ in 2007 and 2030

	2007	2030
Germany	19.8%	28.2%
Italy	19.9	27.9
Japan	21.5	31.8
United States	12.5	19.3

Source: Lutz et al. (2008).

slightly higher in Japan. The baby boomers will not have a comparable impact on the US population structure until 2030. By then, however, if their low fertility rates continue, more than 1 in 4 Germans and Italians will be aged 65 and older, and more than 3 out of 10 Japanese will be in that age range.

Regardless of whether population aging in specific nations is due to a baby boom or a baby bust, some of its public policy consequences—such as strains on public funding of pensions and healthcare costs—are frequently lamented by politicians, policy pundits, academicians, and journalists in aging societies throughout the world. For instance, a former US Secretary of Commerce, Peter Peterson, has written a number of articles and books that present apocalyptic visions of aging societies. One of his books is titled *Gray Dawn: How the Coming Age Wave Will Transform America—and the World*. The jacket and the title page immediately convey his distressing interpretation of the worldwide consequences of population aging by displaying the following call to arms:

> There's an iceberg dead ahead. It's called global aging, and it threatens to bankrupt the great powers. As the populations of the world's leading economies age and shrink, we will face unprecedented political, economic, and moral challenges. But we are woefully unprepared. Now is the time to ring the alarm bell. (Peterson, 1999)

Among the many challenges faced by our aging societies, three ethical, moral, and policy issues are especially relevant for the healthcare arena—for health professionals, their patients, and health policy:

- How aggressive should medical treatment be for individuals who have advanced Alzheimer's disease and other dementias?

- What is the appropriate division of public and private responsibility for long-term care of the functionally dependent elderly?

- Should health care for elderly persons be rationed?

Aggressive Treatment for Severely Demented Patients

Perhaps advances in pharmaceutical and other forms of biomedical research may eventually lead to effective prevention of, or treatments for, Alzheimer's disease and other forms of dementia. But current projections of the number of patients who will be afflicted by dementia are not optimistic. The national Alzheimer's Association in the United States, for instance, estimates that the number of *new* cases of Alzheimer's disease *each year* is likely to increase from 454,000 per year in 2010 to 615,000 per year by 2030, and nearly 1 million by 2050 (Alzheimer's Association, 2009). In the context of concerns about rising health care costs, will those with substantial cognitive impairments receive the same care for other medical conditions that their age peers receive? Should they?

In his book *The Moral Challenge of Alzheimer Disease*, bioethicist Stephen Post expresses the view that society places too much weight on the cognitive capacities of individuals in assigning worth to them. Consequently, he says, "I hold the belief that persons who lack certain empowering cognitive capacities have become the weakest among us and, due to their needfulness, are worthy of care" (Post, 2000, p. 128).

I certainly agree with the general principle articulated by Post, as applied to patients with severe dementia. But how aggressive should that care be? Clearly, there are no *scientific* answers to such a question. This is an issue that is resolved through myriad individual decisions (by health professionals and family members), institutional predilections, and societal policies.

The term *care*, of course, encompasses many types of endeavors and goals, at least including palliative care, care that provides direct support in activities of daily living, preventive care, chronic care (to prevent a deterioration in condition), rehabilitative care, and care that attempts to achieve a cure or a remission of a disease or condition. In my view, it is only within the last category—in instances when very aggressive interventions to achieve cures or remissions for severely demented patients are contemplated—that we find difficult dilemmas.

Such a case was that of my mother when she lived in a nursing home from age 96 to 100. Although she retained her cheerful and sociable personality, she was severely demented throughout this period. When I visited her she would ask who I was about five or six times an hour. The good news was that each time, when I told her, "I'm your son, Bob," she was absolutely thrilled.

After my mother had been in the nursing home for about a year, she began to experience episodes of internal bleeding, which were manifested through her rectum. In response to the first episode, the staff physician transferred her to a nearby hospital where he arranged for her to be transfused with several pints of blood. When the second episode of hospitalization and transfusions occurred some six months later, I asked the physician what was causing this now apparently chronic problem. He didn't have an opinion. I said, "Can't we do some diagnostic tests to find out?" He replied, "Yes, we could. But whatever we might find would probably require a major operation to deal with it. And frankly, I seriously doubt if she would survive such surgery. The alternative is to give her transfusions as needed." I reflected painfully, for some time, on what he said. As a son, I wanted my mother to *get well*. Yet the longer I reflected, the more I leaned toward the alternative of transfusions as needed, rather than invasive gastrointestinal diagnostic testing. I actively endorsed the transfusions alternative, which the physician implemented over the next few years.

Eventually, the doctor telephoned me one evening to say that my mother's organ systems were failing. He said, "I could transfer her to the hospital. But I could also leave her here in the nursing home, and do everything I can for her." Again, I took time to reflect. Soon, I called him back and told him to do everything he could for her in the nursing home. She died just a few hours later.

Perhaps I made "bad" or "wrong" individual decisions in these instances. Yet in our aging societies these decisions will become more frequent, and they may become collective decisions that are expressed through institutional and governmental policies because of the potential costs of aggressive care for patients such as my mother. It is important for our nations to undertake thoughtful deliberations regarding our ethical, moral, and pragmatic responsibilities in such cases. Health professionals should be heavily involved in promoting and participating in such deliberations.

Responsibility for Financing Long-Term Care

How to finance long-term care (LTC) is another dilemma confronting aging societies. The challenge is already substantial. Over the next two decades it will become even greater as more people will live to advanced old ages at which the percentage of persons needing long-term care supportive services—whether in institutional or community-based settings—increases markedly. In the United States, for instance, only 3.3% of persons aged 65 to 74 need assistance with their basic activities of daily living (ADLs); but 7.7% of those aged 75 to 84 need ADL supports, and 21.5% of those age 85 and older need them (Freedman, in press). Between now and 2030 aging societies will have a great many more persons in the elderly age range where help with ADLs is required. Over the next 20 years, for instance, the percentage of the population aged 80 and older will grow by 143% in Japan, 84% in Germany, 77% in Italy, and 46% in the United States (see Table 1-3).

TABLE 1-3   Percent of the Population Aged 80+ in 2007 and 2030

	2007	2030
Germany	4.5%	8.3%
Italy	5.3	9.4
Japan	5.6	13.6
United States	3.7	5.4

Source: Lutz et al. (2008).

To be sure, a substantial amount of long-term care is now provided on an unpaid, informal basis. A national survey in the United States found that more than seven million Americans (mostly family members) provided 120 million hours of unpaid care to elders that year (Stone, 2006). And various studies estimate that close to 80% of long-term care in home settings is provided by family members (Brody, 2004).

Yet family care giving may very well decline in the years ahead because of other, broader developments in the social structure of US family life. There have been steady declines in the rate of marriage, increases in the proportion of marriages that end in divorce, and reductions in remarriage by divorced persons (Harrington Meyer & Parker, in press). In analyzing these trends, demographer Douglas Wolf (2001) has predicted a significant shrinkage in the supply of informal eldercare in relation to the growing demand in the decades ahead. He concludes, therefore, that there needs to be a formal effort to address what is likely to be a growing national problem—the declining availability of relatives to provide unpaid assistance and care in our aging society.

A number of industrialized nations—e.g., Austria, Belgium, Germany, Italy, Japan, Luxembourg, and the Netherlands—have instituted government programs that address this problem through provision of help to individuals and families in financing long-term care. For a discussion of some of these programs—their origins, characteristics, strengths, and weaknesses—see Wiener (in press). But aside from nursing home coverage through the Medicaid program, confined to impoverished older persons (and several other categories of the poor), the United States has yet to do so.

The Costs of LTC in the United States

According to a 2009 survey by the MetLife Mature Market Institute (2009), the US national average annual cost of a private room in a nursing home was $80,000. Rates ranged from an average low of $50,000 in Baton Rouge, Louisiana, and Rochester, Minnesota, to a high of $213,000 in Alaska. The highest average for a private room in the continental United States was $138,000 in New York City, where the most expensive home charged $201,000. The national average for a semiprivate room was $72,000.

Staying at home does not significantly reduce costs unless the bulk of hands-on care is provided on an unpaid basis by family or friends. In fact, many national demonstration studies (see Weissert, 1990) have shown that paid round-the-clock long-term care in a home setting—in effect, a one-person nursing home—costs just as much as a nursing home. In the case of my mother, it actually cost more when she was in home care (including the costs of the home, food, and other basic expenses of daily living) than when she became a private-pay nursing home resident.

Long-term care costs are rising at a rate much faster than inflation. If the trend continues, these costs will quickly use up the savings of all but the wealthiest older persons needing such care, and they may often create substantial financial burdens for their adult children.

"Spending Down"

So how is an older person to cope financially with the need for long-term care? Even individuals with a decent amount of savings, theirs or those of their family, find that the expenses and consequences are daunting. Savings, and even home ownership, can easily be wiped out.

Again, let us consider the rather typical case of my mother, Ruth, a middle-class widow in the Chicago area. Due to Alzheimer's and other chronic conditions, she became unable to do several of the basic activities of daily living (ADLs) without help from someone else. When she began to employ round-the-clock home care in 1994 she had an annual income of about $40,000. Social Security and a private pension provided her with $30,000. She had roughly $250,000 invested in stocks that yielded another $10,000 in dividend income annually, and she also owned her home. However, her not insignificant income ($3333 a month) was insufficient to meet her total expenses when her 24-hour care began.

In this situation Ruth quickly began to "spend down" her assets. Each month, using the financial power of attorney she had granted to me, I had to sell off some of her stocks in order to raise cash to meet her bills. But the stocks I sold off had been sources of dividend income that now would no longer be available. So every month the gap between my mother's total income and her bills widened more than the last, and larger and larger amounts of stock had to be sold off.

Eventually, the progressively larger monthly sell-off of stocks meant that her savings were completely gone. So now, in order to keep paying the long-term care bills, I had to arrange for a "reverse mortgage" line of credit from a bank, with the $220,000 value of her condominium as collateral.

Some months later, Ruth experienced a stroke. After inpatient rehabilitation efforts, the effects on her left arm and leg were such that it was no longer possible for just one person to assist her in the activities of daily living. So her physician transferred her to a nursing home.

Welfare

Now that my mother was no longer living at home (and clearly would never be able to resume residence there), I sold her home and paid off the debt incurred from the bank's line of credit. The sale still left a sufficient amount of funds to help finance the full costs of her nursing home care for more than two years. Finally, when the home sale funds were used up, she was eligible for Medicaid, a government welfare program for the poor elderly, who have no assets to speak of and whose income is insufficient to pay all the costs of nursing home care. In effect, she became a pauper—a ward of the state—and Medicaid (together with her Social Security and pension income) paid her long-term bills until she died.

This case is typical of what happens to middle-class older people in the United States when they need long-term care. My mother's spending down of assets is such a common experience among older Americans that Medicaid pays 35% of overall long-term care expenses nationally for older adults and 40% of nursing home costs (Stone, 2006).

Federal government and state government officials regard the growth of Medicaid expenditures for long-term care as a critical policy problem, and they have been developing ways to cut back on them in recent years. Moreover, the estimated expenditures by Medicaid when members of the baby boom cohort need long-term care are especially alarming. The Congressional Budget Office projects that the 1.5% of gross domestic product (GDP) spent on Medicaid in 2006 could quadruple to 5.9% of GDP by 2050 when all baby boomers will be in the advanced old age ranges at which high rates of long-term care are necessary (Marron, 2006).

Private Insurance

Both government and individual expenditures on long-term care would be substantially reduced if persons of advancing old age purchased private long-term care insurance policies that pay daily cash benefits for long-term care at home, in nursing homes, or in other residential settings such as assisted living complexes. If my mother had purchased such a policy, she might have held on longer to some or all of her savings, as well as her home, and she might not have required support from governmental welfare. Yet, relatively few people buy such policies. As a consequence, for example, private insurance pays only 4% of all US long-term expenses (Congressional Budget Office, 2004).

Why haven't more people bought long-term care insurance? One reason may be widespread psychological denial of the eventual need for long-term care and the expenses involved. Another is that some people who apply for policies are excluded from coverage because the insurance company learns from medical records that they have a "pre-existing condition" that is likely to lead to the need for long-term care fairly soon, and continue for a relatively long time.

Still another barrier for many potential customers is the high cost of purchasing a policy. A 65-year-old in the United States who purchases 36 months of benefits at $150 a day, with 5% annual inflation protection, will likely have to pay nearly $3000 a year in premiums. The older the customer, the higher the initial price; with advancing age, of course, the odds are much higher that the insurance company will need to pay out benefits for long-term care. Young customers get a relatively low premium price but, of course, they are likely to pay the premium for many, many years. (Although insurance companies advertise that individuals will not be singled out for premium increases, they can raise premiums for all policy holders in certain government-approved circumstances.)

There is much debate about whether private insurance will play a larger future role in paying for long-term care. As long-term care policy analyst Robyn Stone has observed, some argue that there will be a substantial growth in this market as our nations undergo greater population aging, but others argue that long-term care insurance will never be more than a "niche" market for the relatively prosperous "young-old" (Stone, 2000).

Expanded Public Financial Support

From 1989 through 1994, there were major political efforts to create a US approach to financing long-term care that would help the middle class. During that period a number of legislative bills—including President Bill Clinton's failed proposal for healthcare reform (White House Domestic Policy Council, 2003)—were introduced to provide some governmental support for long-term care to individuals not poor enough to qualify for Medicaid. None became law.

After the failure of the Clinton health care plan in 1994 there were no significant efforts to address this issue until 2009. In 2005, the President's Council on Bioethics published a report calling for the establishment of a Presidential Commission on Aging, Dementia, and Long-Term Care. But its charge to this new commission was very timid. It specifically precluded the option of significant expansion of government financial support for long-term care, and said that the primary aim of this commission should be "to improve the capacity of families to care for their loved ones" and to recommend measures to assist family caregivers in their tasks (President's Council on Bioethics, 2005, p. 220). This report, reflecting the bias of President Bush's bioethics commission against government activism, did nothing to advance the United States toward emulating many of the world's industrialized nations that have come to grips with the issue of greater public responsibility for financing long-term care.

Five years later, however, with Democrats in control of the presidency and both houses of Congress, a new, though limited, mechanism for financing long-term care did emerge as part of broader legislation developed to reform health care. The Patient Protection and Affordable Care Act (2010) created a new, voluntary, public long-term care insurance program to help purchase services and supports for people with functional limitations. Premiums are to be paid into this program through payroll deductions by employers (with employees having the ability to opt out of this arrangement). Premium levels set by the U.S. Secretary of Health and Human Services are expected to range between $85 and $100 a month. The Secretary will also determine if the level of inability to perform ADLs that would qualify individuals for benefits would be set at two or three ADL deficiencies; equivalent cognitive impairment would also qualify a person for benefits. An additional eligibility requirement in the bill is that an individual must have contributed monthly premiums for at least five years. Eligible beneficiaries will receive a cash benefit, based on degree of disability or impairment, averaging no less than $50 a day.

The daily benefits paid through this program will be relatively small, but they are aimed at helping disabled persons remain at home or in another community-based residential setting of their choice, rather than being institutionalized with Medicaid support. Moreover, private long-term care insurance carriers can offer "wrap-around" complementary coverage (much like Medigap policies help to fill the gaps in Medicare coverage), which will presumably be cheaper to purchase than fuller coverage.

Rationing Health Care of Older People

For more than 25 years, constantly escalating costs of health care have become a matter of concern in the United States. Medicare costs in particular have received a great deal of attention, even though the program is far more administratively efficient than private sector programs and population aging has not been a major cause of increased healthcare costs (Binstock, 1999; Reinhardt, 2003) and may not be in the future (Aaron, 2009) as boomers join the ranks of old age. One reason for this focus on Medicare is that because it is a government program, controlling its costs is a far more feasible task than trying to rein in the expenses of the private-sector aspects of the system, which are fragmented and not amenable to central control. A second reason is a sense among some that spending on health care for elders, who have already had their "fair share" of life, should be a low priority compared with spending on health care for younger persons and for other worthy social causes (e.g., see Sawhill & Monea, 2008).

Informal Ageism in Health Care

Informally, lower priority has been given to the health care of older patients for many decades, both in the United States and abroad. In his Pulitzer Prize–winning book published in the mid-1970s, *Why Survive? Growing Older in America*, Robert Butler (1975) pointed out that ageism in cultural attitudes manifests itself in discrimination against older persons within the healthcare arena and other societal institutions. Butler's observations about ageist attitudes toward older patients in US healthcare settings were vividly reflected a few years later in a best-selling autobiographical novel about a recent medical school graduate who was interning at a first-tier hospital in Boston, Massachusetts (Shem, 1978). Among other things, the novel highlighted the annoyance that physicians expressed toward elderly patients who arrived for service at the emergency room, where effort, time, and other resources were scarce. Such a patient was referred to as a "GOMER," standing for "Get Out of My Emergency Room."

Informal ageism in health care is hardly confined to the United States. Ageist attitudes and practices reflecting them have also been manifest, for instance, in the British National Health Service (NHS), which is funded by a fixed governmental budget. As long ago as 1980, cardiologists in the NHS who were frustrated by a high demand for a limited number of hospital beds, in a complaint similar to that expressed about GOMERs, referred to patients aged 65 and older as "bed blockers" (Wilson, 1980). And in 2006, a joint report of England's Audit Commission, Healthcare Commission, and Commission for Social Care Inspection reported that standards of care for older people were "unacceptably poor" (Eaton, 2006).

Public Discussions of Limiting Care for Older Persons

However, suggestions that health care for elderly patients should be formally rationed as a matter of public policy are another matter. Such suggestions emerged in public discourse in the United States in the 1980s, and they dominated the news for a period of several months in 2009.

In a major public speech in 1983, the noted economist Alan Greenspan observed that 30% of Medicare funds were annually spent on Medicare enrollees who died within the year (Schulte, 1983). Although he was overstating this proportion by a few percentage points (see Lubitz & Riley, 1993), Greenspan pointedly asked his audience "whether it [the money we spend] is worth it" (Schulte, 1983, p. 1). About a year later, the governor of Colorado, Richard Lamm, was widely quoted as stating that "older persons have a duty to die and get out of the way" (Slater, 1984, p.1).

These widely disseminated quotes from Greenspan and Lamm were the opening shots in a campaign by some public figures, economists, and bioethicists to limit health care for older Americans, a campaign that has persisted to this day. Conferences and books have explicitly addressed the subject of limiting health care for the elderly, with titles such as *Should Medical Care Be Rationed By Age?* (Smeeding, 1987). Ethicists and philosophers began generating principles of equity to govern "justice between age groups" in the provision of health care, rather than, for instance, justice between rich and poor, or justice among ethnic and racial groups (Daniels, 1988; Menzel, 1990).

The most prominent proponent of old-age–based rationing has been biomedical ethicist Daniel Callahan, whose 1987 book *Setting Limits: Medical Goals in an Aging Society* received substantial popular attention. In it he characterized the older population as "a new social threat" and a "demographic, economic, and medical avalanche . . . one that could ultimately (and perhaps already) do [sic] great harm" (Callahan, 1987, p. 20). Arguing that healthcare spending on the elderly would pose an unsustainable fiscal burden, Callahan urged the use of "age as a specific criterion for the allocation and limitation of health care." This would be accomplished by denying life-extending health care—as a matter of public policy—to persons who are aged in their "late 70s or early 80s" and/or have "lived out a natural life span" (Callahan, 1987, p. 171). Specifically, he proposed that the Medicare program not pay for such care, and he hoped that other insurers would follow suit.

Although Callahan described "the natural life span" as a matter of biography (the personal details of one's life course experiences) rather than biology, he used chronological age as an arbitrary marker to designate when, from a biographical standpoint, the individual should have reached the end of a natural life. More recently, in an article in the prestigious *New England Journal of Medicine*, he expressed the view that the only deaths that are "premature" are those that occur before age 65 (Callahan, 2000).

Callahan's rationing proposal attracted a lot of attention. It provoked widespread and ongoing discussion in the media and directly inspired a number of books and scores of articles published in national magazines and academic journals (e.g., Barry & Bradley, 1991; Binstock & Post, 1991). Although many of these books and articles strongly criticized the idea of old-age–based rationing, the idea has stayed alive and has even been advocated recently by physicians in prestigious forums. For instance, in the spring of 2009, the Institute of Medicine and the National Academy of Science (of the US National Academies) organized and hosted a symposium on "The Grand Challenges of Our Aging Society." In a speech entitled "Judicious Use of Resources," a noted geriatrician argued that healthcare resources are scarce and that we need to think seriously about principles for rationing some of our healthcare efforts for elderly patients (Reuben, 2009).

Healthcare Reform, "Death Panels," and "Pulling the Plug"

The theme of healthcare rationing for older Americans became especially prominent in the summer of 2009. The health reform bill in the House of Representatives contained a provision that expanded Medicare to cover the costs of a voluntary consultation with a physician, every five years, concerning end-of-life planning through living wills and healthcare durable power of attorney documents (see Blumenauer, 2009). Moreover, from the outset of the healthcare reform effort, an overarching message from President Obama was that the costs of reform would be substantially offset by savings in the Medicare program (see White House, 2009). A number of prominent Republican politicians and broadcasters transformed these two themes—end-of-life planning and savings from Medicare—into the specters of "death panels" and efforts to "pull the plug on granny," and when members of Congress returned to their districts during the summer recess to hold town hall–style meetings, they faced rowdy crowds that expressed concern about rationing in the Medicare program (Blumenauer, 2009).

A few weeks later, the themes of "death panels" and "pulling the plug on granny" were culturally ratified by the cover of *Newsweek* magazine (*Newsweek*, 2009). It featured a big, bold headline saying, "The Case for Killing Granny," accompanied by a picture of a "pulled" electrical plug, to draw attention to a lead article in that issue (Thomas, 2009). Subsequently, the 40-million-member AARP (formerly the American Association of Retired Persons) acknowledged that it faced a challenge of explaining to its members why it endorsed healthcare reform (Calmes, 2009).

From a societal point of view, the emergence of a widespread rationing discussion in the context of national healthcare reform efforts by the president and Congress is an important development. It explicitly introduced to most Americans the idea that the power of government might be used to limit the health care of older persons. As implied previously, it has been long acknowledged by medical care experts that informal rationing does occur. Physicians do this, especially with regard to the health care of older persons, through day-to-day, case-by-case decisions in various types of circumstances. But these practices are not official policy. Is it possible that they might become official in some form? Perhaps a harbinger of such a development is a recent governmental report that discusses strategies for identifying which Medicare enrollees are likely to be "future high-cost beneficiaries" (Congressional Budget Office, 2006)—possibly a preliminary step toward identifying those whose care might be rationed.

The Social and Moral Costs of Rationing

If the intent of old-age–based rationing is to spend less on the Medicare program, some have suggested that the economic "savings" from such a policy or policies would be insignificant in the overall scheme of things (e.g., Binstock, 2002; Pan, Chai, & Farber, 2007). More important, there are substantial social and moral costs involved in policies that would ration health care on the basis of old age.

One possible consequence of denying health care to elderly persons is what it might do to the quality of life for all of us as we approach the "too old for health care" category. Acceptance of the notion that elderly people are unworthy of having their lives saved could markedly shape our general outlook toward the meaning and value of our lives in old age. At the least, it might engender the unnecessarily gloomy prospect that old age should be anticipated and experienced as a stage in which the quality of life is low. The specter of morbidity and decline could be pervasive and overwhelming.

Another cost lies in the potential contributions that will be lost to all of us. Many older persons who benefit from lifesaving interventions will live for a decade or more and, perhaps, will make a number of contributions to society, their communities, and their families and friends during this "extra" time. Human beings often are at their best as they face mortality, investing themselves in the completion of artistic, cultural, communal, familial, and personal expressions that will carry forward the meaning of their lives for generations to come.

Perhaps the foremost potential cost of any old-age–based rationing policy would be that it could start our aging societies down a moral "slippery slope." If elderly persons can be denied access to health care categorically, officially designated as unworthy of lifesaving care, then what group of us could not? Members of a particular race, religion, or ethnic group, or those of us who are disabled? Any of us is vulnerable to social constructions that portray us as unworthy. Rationing health care on the basis of old age could destroy the fragile moral barriers against placing any group of human beings in a category apart from humanity in general. To me, this is the most critical of the ethical, moral, and policy issues confronting our aging society.

References

Aaron, H.J. (2009). What drives health care spending? Can we know whether population aging is a "red herring"? Working Paper 2009-18, Center for Retirement Research at Boston College, Chestnut Hill, MA.

Alzheimer's Association. (2009). *2009 Alzheimer's disease facts and figures: Executive summary.* Retrieved from http://www.alz.org/national/documents/summary_alzfactsfigures2009.pdf

Barry, R.L., & Bradley, G.V. (Eds.). (1991.) *Set no limits: A rebuttal to Daniel Callahan's proposal to limit health care for the elderly.* Urbana, IL: University of Illinois Press.

Berghammer, C., Gisser, R., Lutz, W., Mamolo, M., Phillipov, D., Scherbov, S., & Sobotka, T. (2006). *European demographic data sheet: 2006.* Vienna: Austrian Academy of Sciences; Washington, DC: Population Reference Bureau.

Binstock, R.H. (1999). Older persons and health care costs. In R.N. Butler, L.K. Grossman, & M.R. Oberlink (Eds.), *Life in an older America* (pp. 75–95). New York: Century Foundation Press.

Binstock, R.H. (2002). Age-based rationing of health care. In D.J. Ekerdt (Ed.), *Encyclopedia of aging* (pp. 24–28). New York: Macmillan Reference USA.

Binstock, R.H., & Post, S.G. (Eds.). (1991). *Too old for health care: Controversies in medicine, law, economics, and ethics.* Baltimore, MD: The Johns Hopkins University Press.

Blumenauer, E. (2009, November 15). My near death panel experience. *New York Times.* Retrieved from http://www.nytimes.com/2009/11/15/opinion/15blumenauer.html

Brody, E.M. (2004). *Women in the middle: Their parent care years* (2nd ed.). New York: Springer Publishing Company.

Butler, R.N. (1975). *Why survive: Being old in America.* New York: Harper and Row.

Callahan, D. (1987). *Setting limits: Medical goals in an aging society.* New York: Simon and Schuster.

Callahan, D. (2000). Death and the research imperative. *New England Journal of Medicine, 342,* 654–656.

Calmes, J. (2009, October 14). AARP says its chore is educating members on bill's benefits. *New York Times.* Retrieved from http://prescriptions.blogs.nytimes.com/2009/1014/aarp-says-its-chore-is-educating-elderly-on-bills-benefits/

Congressional Budget Office. (2004). *Financing long-term care for the elderly.* Washington, DC: Congressional Budget Office.

Congressional Budget Office. (2006). *High-cost Medicare beneficiaries.* Retrieved from http://cbo.gov/showdoc.cfm?index=6332&sequence=0

Daniels, N. (1988). *Am I my parents' keeper?* New York: Oxford University Press.

Eaton, L. (2006). Care of England's older people still "unacceptably poor." *British Medical Journal, 332,* 746.

Freedman, V.A. (in press). Disability, functioning, and aging. In R.H. Binstock & L.K. George (Eds.), *Handbook of aging and the social sciences* (7th ed.). San Diego: Academic Press.

Harrington Meyer, M., & Parker, W.M. (in press). Gender, aging, and social policy. In R.H. Binstock & L.K. George (Eds.), *Handbook of aging and the social sciences* (7th ed.). San Diego: Academic Press.

Institute of Medicine of the National Academies. (2009). *Retooling for an aging America: Building the health care work force.* Washington, DC: The National Academies Press.

Lubitz, J.S., & Riley, G.F. (1993). Trends in Medicare payments in the last year of life. *New England Journal of Medicine, 328,* 1092–1096.

Lutz, W., Mamolo, M., Potancokov, M., Scherbov, S., & Sobotka, T. (2008). *European demographic data sheet: 2008.* Vienna: Austrian Academy of Sciences, and Washington, DC: Population Reference Bureau.

Marron, D.B. (2006, July 13). Medicaid spending growth and options for controlling costs. Testimony by the Congressional Budget Office before the U.S. Senate Special Committee on Aging, Washington, DC

Menzel, P.T. (1990). *Strong medicine: The ethical rationing of health care.* New York: Oxford University Press.

MetLife Mature Market Institute. (2009). *The 2009 MetLife market survey of nursing home, assisted living, adult day services, and home care costs.* Retrieved from http://www.metlife.com/assets/cao/mmi/publications/studies/mmi-market-s

Newsweek. (2009). Cover. September, 21.

Pan, C.X., Chai, E., & Farber, J. (2007). *Myths of the high medical cost of old age and dying.* New York: International Longevity Center-USA.

Patient Protection and Affordable Health Care Act. (2010). Public Law Number 111-148 (H.R. 3950).

Peterson, P.G. (1999). *Gray dawn: How the coming age wave will transform America—and the world.* New York: Times Books.

Post, S.G. (2000). *The moral challenge of Alzheimer disease* (2nd ed.). Baltimore, MD: The Johns Hopkins University Press.

President's Council on Bioethics. (2005). *Taking care: Ethical caregiving in our aging society.* Washington, DC: President's Council on Bioethics.

Reinhardt, U.E. (2003). Does the aging of the population really drive the demand for health care? *Health Affairs, 22*(6), 27–39.

Reuben, D.B. (2009, May 28). Judicious use of resources. Speech delivered at the National Academies in Washington, DC. Documentation of program retrieved from http://www.iom.edu/Activities/Workforce/agingamerica/2009-May-28.aspz

Sawhill, I., & Monea, E. (2008). Old news. *Democracy: A Journal of Ideas, 9*(Summer), 20–21.

Schulte, J. (1983, April 26). Terminal patients deplete Medicare, Greenspan says. *Dallas Morning News,* p. 1.

Shem, S. (1978). *The house of God: The classic novel of life and death in an American hospital.* New York: Marek.

Slater, W. (1984, March 29). Latest Lamm remark angers the elderly. *Arizona Daily Star,* p. 1.

Smeeding, T.M. (Ed.). (1987). *Should medical care be rationed by age?* Totowa, NJ: Rowman & Littlefield.

Stone, R.I. (2000). *Long-term care for the elderly with disabilities.* New York: Milbank Memorial Fund.

Stone, R.I. (2006). Emerging issues in long-term care. In R.H. Binstock & L.K. George (Eds.), *Handbook of aging and the social sciences* (6th ed., pp. 397–448). San Diego: Academic Press.

Thomas, E. (2009, September 21). The case for killing granny: Rethinking end-of-life care. *Newsweek,* pp. 34–35, 38–40.

U.S. Census Bureau. (2008). *National population projections. Projections of the population by selected age groups and sex for the United States: 2010–2050.* Retrieved from http://www.census.gov/population/www/projections/summarytables.html

Weissert, W.G. (1990). Strategies for reducing home care expenditures. *Generations, 14*(2), 42–44.

White House Domestic Policy Council. (2003). *The President's health security plan: The Clinton blueprint.* New York: Times Books.

White House. (2009). *America's seniors and health insurance reform: Protecting coverage and strengthening Medicare.* Retrieved from http://www.healthreform.gov/reports/seniors/index.htm

Wiener, J. (in press). Cross-national perspectives on long-term care. In R.H. Binstock & L.K. George (Eds.), *Handbook of aging and the social sciences* (7th ed.). San Diego: Academic Press.

Wilson, L.A. (1980). Blocked beds. *The Lancet, 316,* 1013.

Wolf, D.A. (2001). Population change: Friend or foe of the chronic care system? *Health Affairs, 20*(6), 28–42.

Section II

Issues Central to Gerontological Education

Chapter 2

The Art of Mentoring: Developing the Next Generations of Gerontologists

Leonard W. Poon and Maria C. Isales

This chapter begins with a review of the literature on mentoring with particular focus on gerontology. Next, the voices of faculty and students are summarized in a survey regarding the mechanics, meaning, and outcomes of mentoring. The chapter concludes by outlining our understanding of the objective and subjective findings and experiences, gaps and pitfalls, and by sharing the reflections of a mentor and a mentee who is about to begin a new career.

A Parable

One sunny day a rabbit came out of her hole in the ground to enjoy the fine weather. The day was so nice that she became careless and a fox snuck up behind her and caught her.

"I am going to eat you for lunch," said the fox.

"Wait," replied the rabbit, "you should at least wait a few days."

"Oh yeah? Why should I wait?"

"Well, I am just finishing my thesis on 'The Superiority of Rabbits Over Foxes and Wolves.'"

"Are you crazy? I should eat you right now! Everybody knows that a fox will always win over a rabbit."

"Not really, not according to my research. If you like, you can come into my hole and read it for yourself. If you are not convinced, you can go ahead and have me for lunch."

"You really are crazy!" But since the fox was curious and had nothing to lose, it went with the rabbit. The fox never came out.

A few days later the rabbit was again taking a break from writing and sure enough, a wolf came out of the bushes and was ready to set upon her.

"Wait," yelled the rabbit, "you can't eat me right now."

"And why might that be, my furry appetizer?"

19

"I am almost finished writing my thesis on 'The Superiority of Rabbits Over Foxes and Wolves.' "

The wolf laughed so hard that it almost lost its grip on the rabbit. "Maybe I shouldn't eat you. You really are sick . . . in the head. You might give me something contagious."

"Come and read it for yourself. You can eat me afterward if you disagree with my conclusions."

So the wolf went down into the rabbit's hole . . . and never came out.

The rabbit finished her thesis and was out celebrating in the local lettuce patch. Another rabbit came along and asked, "What's up? You seem very happy."

"Yep, I just finished my thesis."

"Congratulations. What's it about?"

" 'The Superiority of Rabbits Over Foxes and Wolves.' "

"Are you sure? That doesn't sound right."

"Oh, yes. Come and read it for yourself."

So together they went down into the rabbit's hole. To the right there was a pile of fox bones, to the left a pile of wolf bones. And in the middle was a large, well-fed lion.

The moral of the story: The title of your thesis doesn't matter. The subject doesn't matter. The research doesn't matter. All that matters is who your mentor is. (Original author unknown)

Introduction

To extend the preceding parable a bit further, many rabbits are eaten by foxes and wolves. Many rabbits escape capture by their own wits. And yes, some rabbits might have recruited or learned from stronger or more experienced allies to survive and flourish.

The successful transmission of knowledge by more experienced teachers is called mentoring. Much has been written about mentoring regarding the imparting of "wisdom" from one generation or cohort to another. Based on these writings and our own experiences, it is our belief that mentoring is not for everyone. Some sage persons are not meant to be teachers or mentors. Some individuals, such as Einstein, Freud, and Socrates, have no need of mentors. However, it is generally acknowledged that mentors can provide positive influences on the development of the mentees, and research has revealed characteristics of productive mentor-mentee pairs. Mentoring takes on many different forms. There are short- and long-term, formal and informal mentoring relationships. Individual differences in personality, temperament, motivation, and intrinsic and extrinsic environmental circumstances make it almost impossible to identify all factors relating to successful mentoring. Therefore we posit that successful mentoring is an art form subject to mutual respect and motivation.

We begin this chapter with an outline of what we know and don't know about mentoring. Next, we survey faculty and students who attended a mentoring conference series in gerontology and geriatrics and report their personal experiences. Then we share our own respective reflections and introspections about mentoring as a mentor and a mentee. Finally, we summarize our findings and conclusions. To be expedient, we focus our review and comments on mentoring that is associated with academic programs in the United States in general and gerontology in particular; however, we integrate relevant knowledge from other disciplines to reflect the movement toward an interdisciplinary approach to mentoring (Eby & Allen, 2008).

What Do We Know About Mentoring?

We performed a comprehensive, computerized bibliographic search of peer-reviewed articles from AARP Ageline (Ovid) and PsycINFO using the terms *university, mentor, gerontology, mentoring, mentorship, and protégé*. A total of 2351 articles were retrieved. Articles with relevance to university-based mentoring were identified. We reviewed the reference list of each article to identify additional citations that were not revealed by other search means.

Mentoring literature spans nearly three decades of intensive research and includes over 1500 published articles from the social science and education databases in the last 20 years (Colley, 2001). We observed that researchers find mentoring difficult to quantify; this is underlined by a rapid increase of publications on the one hand and a lack of new information and models of mentoring on the other. We noted that the majority of articles published in the 2000s on mentoring cited Kram's (1985) research on organizational mentoring as being the most up-to-date information available. Another observation is that mentoring literature gained popularity with Levinson et al.'s (1978) publication, *The Seasons of a Man's Life*; however, the negative aspects of mentoring were largely ignored until 1998 with Scandura's article, "Dysfunctional mentoring relationships and outcomes" (Scandura, 1998). The vast number of published articles begs the question: What do we *think* we know about mentoring?

In our review of the literature, recent publications on mentoring can be summarized in five clusters:

1. **Formal vs informal relationships.** There is a misconception in the literature that the majority of academic mentoring relationships develop formally through research and teaching assistantships (Sedlacek et al., 2007). Formal relationships have a specified duration with specific goals in mind. Faculty members in higher education are increasingly called upon to mentor students through formal mentoring programs. Unfortunately, the literature noted that formal mentoring can ultimately lead to discontentment on both sides. Naturally occurring relationships that are spontaneous and gradual are described as informal. Though they are often not sanctioned by the university, the duration of informal mentoring relationships tends to be significantly longer than other relationships. In graduate school, these relationships are considered deeper and more effective than formal relationships (Johnson & Ridley, 2004).The bottom line is that if a student wants a mentor, he or she should not wait to be assigned one.

2. **Mentored vs nonmentored students.** There is an intuitive belief, linked to its positive connotation, that mentoring produces positive outcomes. The belief that mentoring in doctoral education is critical for a student's development is well substantiated (Hall & Burns, 2009; Cronon, 2006; Stacy, 2006; Wilson, 2006). Without a knowledgeable mentor, it is more difficult for a student to adequately prepare for research and publishing. It can be argued that mentoring is even more critical in gerontology than in other fields because of the variety of disciplines that are involved (Peyton, Morton, Perkins, & Dougherty, 2001). Favorable mentoring outcomes include behavioral, attitudinal, health-related, interpersonal, motivational, and career outcomes (Eby et al., 2008). The literature noted that poor mentoring can be destructive (Scandura, 1998). Individuals in dissatisfying or marginally effective mentoring relationships reported satisfaction levels that were equivalent to those of nonmentored individuals (Ragins, Cotton, & Miller, 2000).

   An unexpected finding from the literature is that the proportion of students who are mentored in graduate school settings is smaller than one might assume (Wright & Wright, 1987). The increased ratio of students to faculty is one explanation. One study found that in a sample of 90 psychology doctoral students in a university only 53% reported having a mentor (Cronan-Hillix, Gensheimer, Cronan-Hillix, & Davidson, 1986). A national survey found that only two-thirds of clinical psychology doctorate students had a faculty mentor during graduate school. Approximately half of these relationships were initiated by the student (Clark, Harden, & Johnson, 2000). In situations where no formal mentoring is available, students must develop their own resources (Johnson & Huwe, 2003). This point is illustrated by an anecdote about the world-famous cellist, Pablo Casals. At the age of 80, Casals was asked by a young student why he continued to work so hard. "Why?" Casals answered. "This is simple. Because I want to get better!" Self-motivation can be far stronger than anything a mentor has to offer.

3. **Mentor-mentee power differential.** Mentors derive their status from their position and contacts, their knowledge and information. A favored mentee often receives rewards in the form of opportunities for greater and more extensive research as well as the development of critical professional skills (Hall & Burns, 2009). These technical, social, and political skills are certainly useful, but they may not further character development. It would be impractical to believe that a mentor could pass on the cardinal virtues of courage, justice, wisdom, and temperance in a four-year time period (Carr, 1998). However, living in the post–"Enron and Madoff" era requires that mentors stimulate their mentees and challenge them to consider the intricate world of ethics and morality (Moberg, 2008). Mentoring is an unequal power relationship that can foster opportunities for abuse of power, such as applying unjustified pressure (Weinreich, 2004). A mentee's autonomy needs to be preserved. It is imperative that mentors be attentive to their moral obligations to a mentee rather than simply focusing on purely career-related outcomes.

4. **Mentor-mentee attraction.** Mentors are attracted to mentees with high potential and a need for assistance, and mentees are attracted to mentors whom they perceive as being powerful (Allen, Poteet, & Russell, 2000). This belief has been longitudinally tested. The findings indicate that mentors tend to choose "rising stars," or someone with a strong promotional history, advancement expectations, and engagement in proactive career behaviors (Singh, Ragins, & Tharenou, 2009). However, mentors also often choose mentees who are similar to them (Allen, 2007). From the mentee's perspective, knowledge of a professor's academic record does not necessarily lead to selection of an adequate mentor. In a recent study (Bennouna, 2003), only 10% of doctoral graduates chose their chair based on knowledge of the mentor's record. Eighty-six percent chose their advisors based on personal interest in their topic.

   An internal and individual priority scale (Turban & Dougherty, 1994) could be used to determine the type of mentee a mentor would choose. For example, some mentors may be looking for power and prestige from the relationship, while others are looking for friendship and a self-esteem boost. Mentors and mentees in the latter category are looking for individuals with similar personalities and interests rather than remarkable innate talent (Lankau, Riordan, & Thomas, 2005). It should be noted that gender differences exist. Female doctoral students were more likely than male doctoral students to identify acceptance and confirmation as qualities that were desirable in a mentor (Bell-Ellison & Dedrick, 2008). Attraction and attachment play a critical role in both parties' devoting time and energy to the relationship. The dynamics of the mentoring relationship can contribute heavily to the happiness and professional success of the pair (Zey, 1991). In addition, the majority of mentors look for a mentee who appreciates their investment in the mentee's growth (Johnson & Huwe, 2003). In conclusion, pinpointing the attraction in a mentor-mentee interaction is as difficult as explaining the chemistry of any relationship.

5. **The final phase of mentoring: redefinition.** There is a widely held belief that a mentee may achieve at a higher level than a mentor. Outgrowing a mentor seems to be an archaic concept, as it can be equated to outgrowing one's parents. The final stage in the mentoring process, known as the redefinition phase (Kram, 1983), has on average been found to yield equal levels of career and psychosocial development for mentees and their mentors (Chao, 1997). This finding supports the belief that we never stop learning, particularly from our mentors.

Definitions

Perhaps the most controversial feature of mentoring is its definition. The literature shows significant disagreement over the basic functions of the mentor and mentee and disagreement over the most productive outcomes based on the age difference between the mentoring pair and the duration of the relationship (Eby, Rhodes, & Allen, 2007). Jacobi's (1991) review of mentoring yielded 15 definitions in the educational, psychological, and management spheres; and this number has since increased to 50 (Crisp & Cruz, 2009). Definitions of mentoring range from general to specific. While the *Oxford English Dictionary* (2009) defines a mentor as an "experienced and trusted counselor or friend," Berk et al. (2005) define a mentor as "one that may vary along a continuum from informal/short-term to formal/long-term in which faculty with useful experience, knowledge, skills, and/or wisdom offers advice, information, guidance, support, or opportunity to another faculty member or student for that individual's professional development." Despite all the deliberation on the topic, the literature shows there is no universal agreement on the definitions, characteristics, and outcomes of mentoring owing to individual differences in expectations and preferences of the dyads (Merriam, 1983).

The lack of consensus in the operational definition of mentoring in the literature is problematic as different conclusions were made on the review of the literature with different definitions. Though it is clear that mentoring is perceived to be important by the majority of papers in the literature, evidence-based recommendations require studies using more rigorous methods than are currently present in the literature. For example, studies were conducted with unmatched samples of mentors and mentees, small and non-representative samples, and the seminal and most cited work on mentoring has a sample size of no more than 18 mentor-mentee pairs working for a single organization, which is difficult to generalize to other situations (Waldeck et al., 1997).

The current literature contains gaps that researchers have been trying to fill, such as dysfunctional relationships and mentoring from the vantage point of the mentor. More study is needed to further explore and describe these areas as well as how interactions with the mentee modify the relationship. An example of such a study shows that mentors derive a sense of satisfaction and fulfillment from the mentoring experience (Ragins & Scandura, 1999); however, opportunistic mentees and the toll on time and energy can lead a mentor to modify the perception of mentoring and therefore the outcome behavior. Other interesting questions should explore the cyclical nature of mentoring, including how mentors and mentees shape each other's behaviors and how different types of positive and negative reinforcements on both sides influence the relationship and level of development in the short and long term.

Finding Out for Ourselves

Given the variability of the literature in attempting to define and study the phenomenon of mentoring and the lack of meaningful advances in studying the relationship, we decided to survey the opinions on mentoring from faculty and students who had attended the Southeastern Student Mentoring Conference on Gerontology and Geriatrics over the 20-year life span of this conference (see Christie & Shovali, 2010). This conference seeks to provide students with practical experiences associated with academic and applied gerontology. The conference was conceived as a vehicle for students to network with key professionals in aging and to gain first-hand experiences in all aspects of organizing and hosting a conference, including postconvention monographs and publications. Further, the convention is used to promote student professional development, share important student work in the fields of gerontology and geriatrics, and teach faculty/student mentoring. Attendance at the conference is open to all persons interested in gerontology and geriatrics, including the general public.

Brief Methodology

We attempted to contact and survey previous participants in the conference by e-mail in late spring of 2009. The survey was conducted anonymously using the web-page mechanism of "Survey Monkey," and the survey was approved by the University of Georgia Institutional Review Board. Fifty-one individuals agreed to be surveyed: 17 faculty members and 34 students, 19.6% male and 80.4% female. Approximately 50% of the faculty members had held their positions for over 20 years and were over 50 years old. All faculty members had PhDs, and 41.2% of the students were between 26 and 30 years old. Over 60% of the students were currently pursuing a PhD. One hundred percent of the survey participants said that they had had a mentoring experience at some point in their careers. It is noted that our survey obtained a convenient, and not representative, sample with which caution must be exercised in the generalization of conclusions. However, some faculty and student respondents spent significant time and effort in sharing their mentoring experiences with us. The following are some of the themes from the survey.

Overall Impressions

Although the survey was conducted in an anonymous manner using the mass survey mechanism of Survey Monkey in which no personal identifying characteristics were detectable, the impressions of mentors on mentees, and vice versa, were overall very positive. The majority of the survey required qualitative responses; approximately 10% of the questions were quantitative. For example, the mentees were asked to rate their mentors on a variety of attributes in role modeling, intellectual development, career development, and personal communication skills. The mentees rated their mentors' attributes along these dimensions on the average of greater than 4.0 on a 5-point scale. Similarly, the mentors also rated their mentees highly (greater than 4.0 on a 5-point scale) on work habits, teamwork skills, meeting expectations, high ethical standards for research, and personal communication skills.

Mentors' Input

The question of how one chooses the field of gerontology was one of the first questions for both mentors and mentees. A paradox exists in that the number of health professionals is insufficient to care for the growing needs of the aging population; however, among all the health-related specialties, aged care is ranked among the lowest. The lack of interest is due in part to the perception that gerontology/geriatrics is "unglamorous" and lacks excitement (Wray & McCall, 2007). Examining the path toward choosing a career in gerontology is an important first step in attracting students to the profession.

As would be expected in a multidisciplinary/interdisciplinary field, the primary disciplines of the faculty respondents were varied and included sociology, physiology, psychology, adult education, and gerontology. Over half of the survey's faculty respondents chose gerontology as a career because they had a general interest in older persons. The remainder of the faculty chose gerontology as a result of a personal life connection, career opportunity, or serendipity. This supports the findings in the literature that most gerontology students report an emotional attachment to an older adult, and the primary factor for choosing gerontology as a career is having been taken care of by an older person during childhood (Robert & Mosher-Ashley, 2000). Motivation to stay in the gerontology field was split equally between "pure enjoyment" and "a commitment to advocacy for older adults."

The majority of faculty defined a mentor as someone who was willing to share knowledge. Other mentor attributes included being caring and providing guidance. An interesting finding is that none of the faculty respondents' definitions for a mentor mention a reciprocal relationship. Though there is no general consensus on a definition for mentoring, the reciprocity of mentoring is an attribute that has been noted and identified as important (Eby, Rhodes, & Allen, 2007).

Another interesting outcome of faculty surveys that was noted in the literature was the lack of consensus on the degree of career and psychosocial mentoring that should be provided. Career-related mentoring includes coaching and challenging assignments, while psychosocial mentoring is provided through friendship and counseling (Welsh & Wanberg, 2008). The literature shows that the greatest level of combined vocational and psychosocial functioning is provided by older mentors and mentors who spend more time with their protégés (Mullen, 1998). One participant, a female faculty member with a PhD and over 20 years of experience, is a strong proponent of career and psychosocial mentoring. She states: "In addition to sharing experiences with my mentees, I become their personal advocate." Her definition of a mentor is "someone who gives a damn about students and is willing to go the extra mile to help them succeed." Because her own best experiences with mentors occurred during social interactions, she ensures that her mentees can reach her with personal and professional issues.

The literature supports the notion that there is a continuum of effectiveness in mentoring rather than an all-or-none situation (Ragins, Cotton, & Miller, 2000). Negative relationships can be characterized as marginally effective, ineffective, or dysfunctional. Marginal mentors may not provide the degree of mentoring that the mentee expected or hoped for. Mentees in marginal mentoring relationships do not differ in level of satisfaction from nonmentored individuals (Ragins, Cotton, & Miller, 2000). At the lowest end of the mentoring continuum, dysfunction occurs when "one or both parties' needs are not being met in the relationship or one or both of the parties is suffering distress as a result of being in the relationship" (Scandura, 1998). Of those faculty members who had negative experiences with a mentee, 50% described the relationship as marginally effective, 25% as ineffective, and 25% as dysfunctional. The finding that dysfunctional mentoring relationships are likely to come to an end could explain the lower reported numbers of ineffective and dysfunctional relationships (Ragins & Scandura, 1997). An example of a dysfunctional relationship was described by one faculty member as: "There was dishonesty and vindictiveness on the part of the student. I tried to get them to do more than was in their range of capacity and stuck to my rigidly high standards that they were incapable of meeting." This experience with an "imbalanced" mentee appeared to negatively impact her perception of future mentees, as evidenced by a rating of 2.8 out of 5. Nonetheless, it appears that in general these negative experiences were minimal, as the average overall rating of mentees was 4.2 out of 5. The lowest ratings were in personal communication between the mentor and mentee, specifically in listening carefully to the concerns of the mentor, and the highest ratings were in conveying high ethical standards for research.

Mentee's Input

Compared to the varied disciplines of the mentors, the student respondents' dominant disciplines were in psychology and social work. Students' decisions to choose gerontology as a career were split between a general interest in aging and hands-on experience working with older adults. Less frequently cited reasons were connections with grandparents and serendipity. Motivations to continue in the gerontological field were fueled primarily by interest in the content and the opportunity to work with older adults.

An individual's mentoring perspective and expectations are changes based on his/her experiences. One graduate student compares her experiences with different mentors. She describes how a previous mentor was disorganized, did not prepare for meetings, and did not provide timely feedback. Although the mentor was very knowledgeable, it was not a good working relationship. Given this student's experience with multiple mentors, her perspective on mentoring was changed. At first, this student perceived mentoring as a formal academic relationship, but a later interaction with another mentor furthered her expectations: "I now realize it encompasses so much more than that. I really expect my mentor to not only teach me research and writing, but also to lead as an example in my professional development."

Though most dysfunctional relationships terminate, there are exceptions (Ragins & Scandura, 1997). Some students are independently passionate about a field despite poor direction. One student described her graduate school mentor as "dominating, passive-aggressive, and a micromanager." Nonetheless, she believes strongly in the importance of mentoring and tells her fellow PhD students to "choose your mentor very carefully because they can make or break your graduate and life-long career."

The degree of reciprocity and role modeling received from a mentor predicted mentee satisfaction with the mentor (Ensher, Thomas, & Murphy, 2001). This belief is also substantiated by the surveys. One student in her first year of graduate school has only had positive mentoring experiences. She stresses the importance of mentoring as a give-and-take relationship. The respondent's relationship with mentors has led her to believe that mentoring "requires active participation and an understanding of where a person is at in their academic career. It also takes a lot of experience in order to best understand how to get a person where they need to be without carrying them along too much."

A Brief Synthesis

The voices of a limited and convenient sample of mentors and mentees reflected the findings from the literature. That is, mentors and mentees are subject to the many dimensions of positives and negatives in human nature and relationships. There were significant individual differences in definitions and expectations as well as degree of mentor involvement from the perspective of mentees. This may be the very basis of confusion as well as stagnation in the literature in attempts to define mentoring. Given the overall mutual positive ratings from mentors on mentees and vice versa in this survey, we had not expected too much dissatisfaction in the mentoring relationships. And yet, meaningful and interesting complaints were voiced by both sides in the survey. These negative relationships are underreported in the literature, and it may be instructive to both potential mentors and mentees to illustrate how some negative experiences could run counter to their educational goals and career development.

Our Personal Reflections

Personal Experiences From a Mentee

I am currently a research assistant at the University of Georgia, and I will be applying to medical school for the 2010 entering class. I received a bachelor's degree in Latin American Studies from Yale University, a master of public health degree, and a graduate certificate of gerontology from the University of Georgia.

> "Treat a man as he is, he will remain so. Treat a man the way he can be and ought to be, and he will become as he can be and should be."—Goethe

The concept of mentoring originated circa eighth century BC with a character in *The Odyssey*. When Odysseus left to fight in the Trojan War, he entrusted his household to Mentor, who served as a teacher to Odysseus's son, Telemachus. Years later, Odysseus returned to a ravaged household. Though the short-term outcome was negative, Mentor had the wisdom to abstain from repairing the household himself; instead Mentor illuminated ways for his *mentee* to right the wrong, which Telemachus eventually did. This story could have unfolded disastrously if Telemachus had not heeded or grasped Mentor's advice. Present-day mentors face similar dilemmas in over- or undercompensating for their mentees' lack of experience.

The world of academia is constantly in flux due to changes in language, theories, laws, faculty, and above all changing opinions. I believe that the exchange between a mentor and a mentee is largely a result of specific cultural and core values that guide each individual. Stated another way, the attitude of a mentor toward a mentee and vice versa originates from the unique environment that each experiences. In addition to innate characteristics, minute changes in one's daily life can dramatically impact the interaction between a mentor and a mentee. Following are four key virtues that, in my opinion, a mentee should possess, not simply to avoid calamity but to excel. I chose to focus on the following virtues as they encompass issues that affect the present cohort of graduate students in their interactions with previous generations.

The first virtue is perseverance. Many people are looking for shortcuts to success. It is my perception that some graduate students believe that networking can substitute for hard work. Without question, networks facilitate access to information and resources that can jump-start a career; however if they are not linked with hard work and a bit of luck, they are useless. I experienced the importance of perseverance and chance while attempting to obtain an internship at the Centers for Disease Control and Prevention (CDC). Using the contact information available on the CDC website, I began a process of repeated calls and e-mails. After five months, I secured an internship. I worked intensively at the CDC, and I would use my breaks and leisure time to help people in other departments. By the end of the summer, I had a job offer. It has been my experience that students should view mentors as reinforcements in their endeavors rather than infrastructure, and focus inward to achieve their utmost potential. As Louis Pasteur said, "chance favors the prepared mind."

The second virtue is humility. Humility can be difficult to acquire because you must acknowledge two truths: that your knowledge is limited and that someone else's is more extensive. Some mentees are not willing to accept the advice of a mentor regardless of its apparent value. Students' curiosity inspires them to challenge old ideas and chase after innovation. In doing this, it may be tempting to eschew the wisdom of elders. My first mentor was my high school English teacher, intimidating to 11th graders at a small Southern school not only because he hailed from Connecticut but also because he had served a number of years in the army. His use of the Socratic Method was daunting not only to our class but also to his colleagues. Through either "tough love" or very slow torture, he drew me out of my shell over the course of a year. He did this primarily by challenging me to always offer an opinion on the material that he presented in class. It is tempting to cite "generational differences" as a reason for discordance in a mentoring relationship, particularly since a mentor's experiences may not correlate with those of a mentee. However, there is a strong likelihood that, given the opportunity, similar themes will emerge in a discussion between a mentor and a mentee's beliefs and practices.

The third virtue is responsibility. Many people assume that seniority follows competency and ultimately results in the acceptance of responsibility. There is no better place to see the dissolution of this notion than in the examples of excess and abuse that pervade the news reports. Financial titans, who not long ago flew on private jets, are bankrupt, athletes unabashedly confess to the long-term use of steroids, and politicians have moved beyond logrolling to delve into influence peddling. Responsibility often resides mainly with those in senior positions; however, it is important to learn to handle responsibility as a student in order to prevent the tendency to avoid difficult situations. Reciprocity is one of the most important responsibilities for individuals in any relationship. I have had a mentor who has boosted my confidence by showing continual encouragement and belief in my ability. One of the ways in which he has done this is by seeking my opinion or advice on matters where *he* is acknowledged as a worldwide expert. However, as a mentee, my responsibility is to fulfill the goals and expectations that we have agreed upon. Living without regard to the interdependency of human interactions can be considered imprudent.

The fourth, and perhaps most important, virtue is self-understanding. Knowing oneself allows decisions to be based on personal preferences. On the other hand, a lack of self-understanding opens the individual to yielding control of his or her destiny to outside influences. I believe that the only way to achieve self-understanding is through a process of trial and error. The dynamic universe forces us to be in a constant state of redefinition. Being exposed and open-minded to the wisdom of our mentors facilitates this process. However, it is important to realize that there are, as previously explored in the literature review, bad mentors. There is a distinction between being wise and having answers. Wisdom, often associated with mentors, is much more difficult to acquire than the literature would lead you to believe. Unfortunately, it does not always come with age. Some mentors, self-assured in how their most recent curriculum vitae reads, will be certain that you are seeking their guidance because you want to follow their path exactly. This hubris will ensure that you are either led through his/her exact steps to reach the desired endpoint or thrown by the wayside. This is the point where the student's true character surfaces. It is easier to succeed under an encouraging mentor; however, the real challenge comes when facing an abrasive mentor.

I have had a handful of mentors who have appeared serendipitously. These individuals have *taken time* from their schedules, *listened* to my goals, *trusted* my ability to succeed, and through these actions, *empowered* me with the confidence to believe in my competence. My mentoring experiences have varied enormously with regard to time spent, personality, and expectations from both parties. Despite their differences, each individual made a deep impact upon my personal and work life. I would like to end with some advice. First, gain self-understanding by questioning widely held beliefs. Later, gather as many mentors as you can because in this constantly changing, tenuous world, you are going to need it. I am left wondering if Homer could have imagined the complex issues that mentors are now confronted with!

—*MCI*

Personal Experiences From a Mentor

I have been a full professor at the University of Georgia since 1985. Prior to 1985, I was an assistant professor at Harvard University Medical School and the VA Medical Research Service. My teaching experiences have focused primarily on postdoctoral training with some experience at the graduate level.

I initiated an annual Southeastern student mentoring conference on gerontology and geriatrics some 20 years ago. Each year, nine research or teaching universities participate as sponsors and about 100 faculty and students attend. Hence, once a year I spend time with colleagues organizing a conference program and thinking about how to instill the essence of mentoring from both the faculty and students' perspectives. I have noted that the goal of the conference is to train graduate students on how to be successful assistant professors and beyond. We have a tradition of inviting noted gerontologists and academicians as faculty keynoters to talk about teaching, mentoring, and career development. We invite exceptional students from previous conferences to present their work as student keynoters. Sometimes students are commissioned to present review papers, and at other times alumni of this conference are invited to share their experiences after graduation. Students are encouraged to form networks with fellow students and faculty members. However, the heart of this conference is the "poster-discussion" sessions in which each presenter produces a poster and orally presents the work in a supportive and nonthreatening environment. Students learn by being presented with models of successful career development as well as practices in the art of writing, presentation, networking, and editing of an annual published monograph.

After thinking about and working with mentoring issues over the years, I often asked myself and colleagues these questions: what is mentoring, how should we teach and expose mentoring in our conferences, and what attributes should be practiced in the mentoring processes? I was not surprised that answers to the questions were often vague, nonspecific, and varied among my colleagues. Although a primary focus of a college professor is to teach, few have been trained to teach in a formal manner at graduate school or while practicing as a professor. I put myself in this category, as teaching has been a trial-and-error process for me over the years. It is important to note that most universities are beginning to offer formal teaching institutes, and the number of faculty members who take advantage of these programs is increasing, particularly junior faculty.

While professors teach hundreds of students in the formal classrooms, the number of students that we mentor is significantly smaller. It is my view that mentoring is a mutual selection process. Many students do not have the time or inclination to take advantage of the office hours or seek additional help beyond the classroom. Graduate students are required to interact more frequently with their professors and advisors; however, there is a continuum of contact and collaboration, from just doing the minimum to an active pursuit of learning in preparation for an independent career.

Does being mentored improve academic performance and levels of career development? The answer to this question is dependent on the quality and motivation of the mentor and mentee. Based on my experience, motivated students will find a way to excel with or without the help of the professor or advisor. Having a successful, informed, experienced, and willing mentor could most likely be helpful to motivated students to develop faster and at a higher level. For example, my advisors introduced me to their networks of colleagues when I was a graduate student and postdoctoral fellow. I was able to communicate on a first-name basis with these individuals when I became an independent researcher, and these contacts definitely accelerated my career development in terms of paper and grant consultation and job possibilities, as well as increased opportunities for journal paper review, inclusion in conferences and grant review study sections, book publications and special journal projects, and committee assignments in professional societies. I follow the same practices with my mentees. Not every graduate student, postdoctoral fellow, or junior professor takes advantage of opportunities that come along. People must make their own decisions, follow their own tempo, and develop their careers at levels and directions of their own choosing. From this perspective, diversity is good. If everyone became an Einstein, then there would be leaders with no followers!

Looking back at my career development, the advice from my mentors at graduate school and postdoctoral training was invaluable and critical to my level of success. Without the support of my mentors, I would not be able to efficiently navigate the many academic demands of coursework, teaching, and research in addition to balancing a family life. When I was a junior independent investigator, I was grateful for advice and mentorship from senior investigators who had taken an interest in my career development.

Three incidents occurred when I was a graduate student and a junior professor that shaped my philosophy and approaches to my mentoring. The first was when my advisor gave me a chance to matriculate in graduate school when I clearly was not qualified. My undergraduate training and professional experience was in engineering in the aerospace industry. My undergraduate grade point average was too poor to matriculate in graduate school for experimental psychology, yet my advisor gave me a chance. My advisor reviewed my work accomplishments in engineering and believed my undergraduate record did not reflect my capacity to succeed in graduate school. At the end of my first year of graduate school I published with my advisor a monograph containing seven experiments in a top-tier journal. I graduated with a master's and a PhD degree in two and three-quarter years. I have since provided opportunities to marginal students and hoped that they would excel given a second chance. Unfortunately, my record of success has not been impressive so far. A second formative incident for me occurred when I was a postdoctoral fellow. I was not informed that I was expected to work in one laboratory under the supervision of one mentor. I chose to work in three laboratories because the topic areas interested me. Although there was some discussion about whether I would be able to handle the work, I published work in all three laboratories at the end of my two-year tenure. My students can take on as much or as little work as they desire, and I let their record of achievements lead them to the next steps. The third formative experience came when I was a junior professor. A pioneer in gerontology took an interest in my work. He was a professor and a don at Cambridge University, England, and he travelled to the United States on an annual basis. He made it a habit of visiting me annually to discuss my work on a more social than academic basis. He is my model on how a senior professor can mentor junior professors in a friendly and constructive manner. This has been my approach in advising students and junior investigators worldwide.

It has been said that we stand on the shoulders of those who have gone before us. Many had journeyed on their own, and stood tall as giants (or midgets as the case may be). After about 40 years in the academy, I have noted that not everyone is suited to be a mentor or mentee, and not every mentor-mentee pair has a successful relationship or is appropriately suited to each other. Mentoring is not about helping students get by with the minimal in order to get a desired grade. On the contrary, mentoring is about nurturing, caring, and advancing the next generations of potential contributors to one's field of expertise. Mentoring is about providing the necessary and sufficient experience, practice, and modeling in what is required to be continually successful as well as the resources, strategies, and armaments to meet the inevitable adversities that are part of career development. I am most grateful to have received the "love of learning" award by faculty and students at the University of Georgia. To summarize, a mentor should inculcate the love of learning as well as the desire to persistently pursue excellence and achieve inner potential in the mentee.

—*LWP*

The Art of Mentoring

As in any relationship, mentoring requires give-and-take between a pair within dyads. Mentoring dyads generally involve a senior and a junior member. The relationship is not equal, and sometimes this results in dissatisfaction and mismatch. The success of the relationship depends on the sensitivity of both parties to personality, style, preferences, temperament, and expectations. Hence, successful mentoring is an art, as there are too many variables to manipulate in the matching of two individuals who vary in experience and accomplishments. It should be noted that a mentor was once a mentee, and a mentee expects to be a mentor one day. It stands to reason that the quality of mentoring will impact the quality and style of this mentee when he or she becomes a mentor (Ragins, Cotton, & Miller, 2000).

In the next few decades, the aging population will likely overburden the US healthcare system. An increase in the number of gerontology and geriatric professionals will be crucial to adequately meet the needs of the older adult population. Originally derived from business and general education, mentoring has been shown to be an extremely effective method of cultivating the future leaders of gerontology. As explored previously, the study of older adults is not an automatic career choice for the younger cohort. Senior mentors have a responsibility to ease the hesitancy of students entering into gerontology by debunking stereotypes about aging and highlighting the potential for innovation and creativity within the field.

Acknowledgments

The authors of this chapter dedicate our work to our mentors and colleagues who have contributed to our development. The work is supported by a grant, "Distance Learning Partnership in Gerontology Special Initiative," from the Board of Regents of the University System of Georgia to the senior author. This manuscript would not have been possible without the wisdom of both faculty and students who have attended the 20 Student

Mentoring Conferences since 1989. We especially acknowledge those who contributed to the sharing and discussion about mentoring, including senior colleagues in gerontology and geriatrics as well as faculty and students from the nine sponsoring institutions. They are: Armstrong Atlantic State University, North Georgia College and State University, Georgia Southern University, Medical College of Georgia, Georgia State University, University of Kentucky, University of Alabama, University of South Florida, and the University of Georgia. We are indebted to their dedication and special efforts in the mentoring of their students over the years.

References

Allen, T.D., Poteet, M.L., & Russell, J.E. (2000). Protégé selection by mentors: What makes the difference? *Journal of Organizational Behavior, 21*(3), 271–282.

Allen, T.D. (2007). Mentoring relationships from the perspective of a mentor. In B.R. Ragins & K.E. Kram (Eds.), *The handbook of mentoring at work: Research, theory, and practice* (pp. 123–148). Thousand Oaks, CA: Sage Publications.

Bell-Ellison, B.A., & Dedrick, R.F. (2008). What do doctoral students value in their ideal mentor? *Research in Higher Education, 49*(6), 555–567.

Bennouna, S. (2003). *Mentors' emotional intelligence and performance of mentoring functions in doctoral education.* Unpublished doctoral dissertation, University of South Florida, Tampa, FL.

Berk, R.A., Berg, J., Mortimer, R., Walton-Moss, B., & Yeo, T. (2005). Measuring the effectiveness of faculty mentoring relationships. *Journal of Medical Education, 80*(1), 66–71.

Carr, D. (1998). After Kohlberg post-postscript: A response to Agnes Tellings. *Studies in Philosophy and Education, 17,* 185–192.

Chao, G.T. (1997). Mentoring phases and outcomes. *Journal of Vocational Behavior, 51*(1), 15–28.

Christie, J., & Shovali, T. (2010). 20 years of gerontology: Past, present, and future. Athens, GA: University of Georgia.

Clark, R.A., Harden, S.L., & Johnson, W.B. (2000). Mentor relationships in clinical psychology doctoral training: Results of a national survey. *Teaching of Psychology, 27*(4), 262.

Colley, H. (2001). Righting re-writings of the myth of Mentor: A critical perspective on career guidance mentoring. *British Journal of Guidance and Counseling, 29*(2), 177–198.

Crisp, G. & Cruz, I. (2009). Mentoring college students: A critical review of the literature between 1990–2007. *Research in Higher Education, 50,* 525–545.

Cronan-Hillix, T., Gensheimer, L.K., Cronan-Hillix, W.A., & Davidson, W.S. (1986). Students' view of mentors in psychology graduate training. *Teaching of Psychology, 13*(3), 123–127.

Cronon, W. (2006). Getting ready to do history. In C.M. Golde & G.E. Walker (Eds.), *Envisioning the future of doctoral education* (pp. 327–350). San Francisco: Jossey-Bass.

Eby, L. T., & Allen, T.D. (2008). Moving toward interdisciplinary dialogue in mentoring scholarship: An introduction to the Special Issue. *Journal of Vocational Behavior, 72,* 159–167.

Eby, L.T., Allen, T.D., Evans, S.C., Ng, T., & DuBois, D.L. (2008). Does mentoring matter? A multidisciplinary meta-analysis comparing mentored and non-mentored individuals. *Journal of Vocational Behavior, 72,* 254–267.

Eby, L.T., Rhodes, J.E. & Allen, T.D. (2007). Definition and evolution of mentoring. In T.D. Allen & L.T. Eby (Eds.), *The Blackwell handbook of mentoring: A multiple perspectives approach* (pp. 7–20). Oxford: Blackwell Publishing.

Ensher, E.A., Thomas, C., & Murphy, S. (2001). Comparison of traditional, step-ahead, and peer mentoring on protégés's support, satisfaction, and perceptions of career success: A social exchange perspective. *Journal of Business and Psychology, 15*(3), 419–438.

Hall, L.A., & Burns, L.D. (2009). Identity development and mentoring in doctoral education. *Harvard Educational Review, 79*(1), 49–70.

Jacobi, M. (1991). Mentoring and undergraduate academic success: A literature review. *Review of Educational Research, 61(*4), 505–532.

Johnson, W.B., & Huwe, J.M. (2003). *Getting mentored in graduate school.* Washington, DC: American Psychological Association.

Johnson, W.B., & Ridley, C.R. (2004). *The Elements of Mentoring,* New York: Palgrave, MacMillan.

Kram, K.E. (1983). Phases of the mentoring relationship. *Academy of Management Journal, 26,* 608–625.

Kram, K.E. (1985). *Mentoring at work: Developmental relationships in organizational life.* Glenview, IL: Scott, Foresman.

Lankau, M.J., Riordan, C.M., & Thomas, C.H. (2005). The effects of similarity and liking in formal relationships between mentors and protégés. *Journal of Vocational Behavior, 67*(2), 252–265.

Levinson, D.J., Darrow, C., Klein, E., Levinson, M., & McKee, B. (1978). *The seasons of a man's life.* New York: Knopf.

Merriam, S. (1983). Mentors and protégés: A critical review of the literature. *Adult Education Quarterly, 33,* 161–173.

Moberg, D.J. (2008). Mentoring for protégé character development. *Mentoring & Tutoring: Partnership in Learning, 16*(1), 91–103.

Mullen, E.J. (1998). Vocational and psychosocial mentoring functions: Identifying mentors who serve both. *Human Resource Development Quarterly, 9*(4), 319–331.

The Oxford English Dictionary. (2009). "mentor, *n.*" *OED Online.* Oxford University Press. 22 Jul. 2009 @ http://dictionary.oed.com/cgi/entry/00306010

Peyton, A.L., Morton, M., Perkins, M.M., & Dougherty, L.M. (2001). Mentoring in gerontology education: New graduate student perspectives. *Educational Gerontology, 27,* 347–359.

Ragins, B.R., Cotton, J.L., & Miller, J.S. (2000). Marginal mentoring: The effects of type of mentor, quality of relationship, and program design on work and career attitudes. *Academy of Management Journal, 43,* 1177–1194.

Ragins, B.R., & Scandura, T.A. (1997). The way we were: Gender and the termination of mentoring relationships. *Journal of Applied Psychology, 82,* 945–953.

Ragins, B.R., & Scandura, T.A. (1999). Burden or blessing? Expected costs and benefits of being a mentor. *Journal of Organizational Behavior, 20,* 493–509.

Robert, R., & Mosher-Ashley, P.M. (2000). Factors influencing college students to choose careers working with elderly persons. *Educational Gerontology, 26,* 725–736.

Scandura, T. (1998). Dysfunctional mentoring relationships and outcomes. *Journal of Management, 24*(3), 449–67.

Sedlacek, W.E., Benjamin, E., Schlosser, L.Z., & Sheu, H.B. (2007). Mentoring in academic: Considerations for diverse populations. In T. D. Allen & L.T. Eby (Eds.), *The Blackwell handbook of mentoring: A multiple perspectives approach* (pp. 259–280). Oxford: Blackwell Publishing.

Singh, R., Ragins, B.R., & Tharenou, P. (2009). Who gets a mentor? A longitudinal assessment of the rising star hypothesis. *Journal of Vocational Behavior, 74,* 11–17.

Stacy, A. M. (2006). Training future leaders. In C.M. Golde & G.E. Walker (Eds.), *Envisioning the future of doctoral education* (pp. 187–206). San Francisco: Jossey-Bass.

Turban, D.B., & Dougherty, T.W. (1994). Role of protégé personality in receipt of mentoring and career success. *Academy of Management Journal, 37*(3), 688–702.

Waldeck, J.H., Orrego, V.O., Plax, T.G., & Kearney, P. (1997). Graduate student/faculty mentoring relationships: Who gets mentored, how it happens, and to what end. *Communication Quarterly, 45*(3), 93–109.

Weinreich, D.M. (2004). Interdisciplinary teams, mentorship, and intergenerational service-learning. *Educational Gerontology, 30,* 143–157.

Welsh, E.T., & Wanberg, C.R. (2008). Launching the post-college career: A study of mentoring antecedents. *Journal of Vocational Behavior, 74,* 257–263.

Wilson, S. (2006). Finding a canon and a core: Meditations on the preparation of teacher educator-researchers. *Journal of Teacher Education, 57,* 315–325.

Wray, N., & McCall, L. (2007). Plotting careers in aged care: Perspectives of medical, nursing, allied health students, and new graduates. *Educational Gerontology, 33,* 939–954.

Wright, C.A., & Wright, S.D. (1987). The role of mentors in the career development of young professionals. *Family Relations, 36,* 204–208.

Zey, M. (1991). *The mentor connection: Strategic alliances in corporate life.* New Brunswick, NJ: Transaction Publishers.

Chapter 3

The Necessity of Mentorship Among Gerontologists: The Student and Emerging Professional Perspective

Tara McMullen and Candace Brown

The Mentor

Since the formalization of the word "mentor" in the classic piece *The Odyssey*, the term has been linked to aiding those who are less experienced (Mueller, 2004). Additionally, "mentor" can be defined as an individual who is an expert on a specific subject, and who guides another (mentee) in his/her area of expertise. However, this developmental partnership between the mentor and mentee is not explicitly defined by a specific age. Gerontologists, among other professionals who study aging, anticipate that the growing number of students, mentees, or protégés will not necessarily fall within the 18 to 21 years range. In addition, mentors may have various backgrounds and various levels of relationships with their students.

Mueller (2004) recognized that mentoring programs became commonplace in the 1970s with the development of human resource centers. One of the first publications to demonstrate mentoring was the 1978 title, *The Seasons of a Man's Life* (Barondess, 2005). Author Daniel Levinson, and researchers from Yale, found that transitions are a cause for continuous development throughout the life span, elucidating the importance of mentorship through these transitions. According to Levinson, "the realization of the dream," is a mentor's most critical function in supporting and facilitating a student's transitional development (Barondess, 2005); specifically for the gerontology student, early educational mentorship can be beneficial for future academic success (Peyton, Morton, Perkins, & Dougherty, 2001). This academic mentorship has a positive effect on the transition from an individual's academic tenure to the beginning of their professional career. Recent surveys among business professionals and academic faculty have associated career satisfaction and accomplishment with mentoring guidance (Barondess, 2005).

Eight Aspects to Mentorship

For the student and emerging professional, a mentor can be helpful in various ways. Farren (2006) identified eight categories of mentorship: (1) professional or trade; (2) industry; (3) organization; (4) work processor; (5) customer; (6) technology; (7) work/life integration; and (8) career development. Due to the field's multidisciplinary nature, each of these mentoring categories can be utilized in the field of gerontology. Mentors exist within each area, enabling students to receive guidance and excel in their area(s) of interest (Brown, 2009). The mentor may also provide guidance outside of their specific mentorship category, thus minimizing the need for multiple mentors (Brown, 2009).

Farren (2006) states that a professional or trade mentor stays current on changes in the field, teaches how to apply new practices, and ensures that competencies are mastered. An example of a professional or trade mentor in gerontology could be someone in the field of health (e.g. public health practitioner). Industry mentors give insight into trends, are knowledgeable about studies and research development, and suggest associations to join for the purpose of networking. Both organization and work processor mentors introduce the conventional wisdom of the field, keep abreast of the surrounding politics, and advise on how a workplace position can contribute to the mission of an organization. An example of this type of mentor would be a professional who maintains a position in an organization (e.g., Gerontological Society of America). Consumer mentors communicate knowledge of key players, expectations, and successes and failures of a specific demographic group. A gerontology consumer mentor might be involved with aging policy or governmental issues.

Further, Farren (2006) defines the technology mentor as one who advises on technological systems and integration of these systems. A technology mentor is a person who uses their marketing knowledge to enhance innovative ideas for the aging population. The work/life and career development mentorship is most well recognized by gerontologists (Farren, 2006), due to these mentors serving as advisors, confidants, and leaders, both professionally and personally. These mentors aid mentees in establishing their life's priorities, and support their personal and professional development. Most students recognize their professors as work/life, or career mentors. All of the categories of mentorship can be utilized by gerontology students; however, the foundation discipline, research, and professional interests of both parties need to match for a mentoring relationship to succeed (Peyton et al., 2001).

Why We Need Mentors

There are a variety of reasons why students may need mentoring. Peyton, Morton, Perkins, and Doughtery (2001) identify three major reasons for mentoring: (1) students need clarification of academic and professional responsibilities across the discipline; (2) students need guidance for advancement toward their career goals; and (3) students need to remain informed of available opportunities.

In the study of gerontology, the academic curriculum is typically standardized, whereas professional responsibilities may vary by specialization (Peyton et al., 2001). Pelham (2008) indicates that a gerontology student's coursework in other disciplines is valuable and the participation of interdisciplinary faculty is favored. However, Pelham's (2008) contention that gerontological knowledge can be adequately conveyed to students through traditional courses in science, health, and social services may not encompass the dynamic nature of the field. Rather, the interdisciplinary nature of gerontology incorporates the study of sociology, psychology, political science, biology, economics, and anthropology (Bass & Ferraro, 2000), all of which are disciplines that stem beyond the scope of science, health, and social services. Further, the study of gerontology has become a part of preparation for nursing, law, public health, social work, and business (Bass & Ferraro, 2000). However, despite the value of outside faculty and coursework, a gerontology student primarily requires a mentor well versed in the study of gerontology (Peyton et al., 2001).

Mentors in gerontology provide guidance regarding professional responsibilities throughout their mentee's academic and professional development (Peyton et al., 2001); further, gerontological professors present the multifaceted nature of aging as a life course event (Peyton et al., 2001). Ideally, by means of a mentorship with a gerontologically trained professor, students can apply the general knowledge they obtain to focus their academic exploration and interests (Peyton et al., 2001). Having a mentor and building strong networks of colleagues helps promote the growth and development of a student's research interests (Brown, 2009). As one gerontology student stated, "Building a gerontology network is vital to promoting cross pollination of ideas and research within the field" (A. Tripp, personal communication, January 2, 2009).

Interprofessional Education

Interdisciplinary gerontological education focuses on the multifaceted nature of aging across the life span (Achenbaum, 1995). It has been suggested that understanding the study of gerontology is similar to understanding the impact that society, environment, political environments, and biological circumstances have on human interaction and education outcomes. The importance of an interdisciplinary approach has recently gained attention in the professional world. The American Geriatrics Society (2005) coined the term "interprofessional" as a way to describe the integration of educational teams to assimilate knowledge from collective academic and professional backgrounds. This coalescence provides knowledge on how to effectively address various issues in the field of geriatrics. Unfortunately, there is a gap in the literature on a "unified theory across the social sciences that bridges the components of individuals, context, epoch, community, economy, policy, and society" (Bass, 2009).

It has been suggested that interprofessional concepts are important in theory but difficult to integrate into a mentorship. Even though interprofessional concepts within the field of gerontology are difficult to integrate, it is still important that interprofessional mentorship be made available to provide the mentee an opportunity to achieve multidisciplinary training.

Professional Development Toolbox

Mentors guide students along the most appropriate route for the advancement of their career goals (Peyton et al., 2001). Mentorship may be specialized based on a student's academic interest. Thus, having a mentor who will utilize an interdisciplinary development "toolbox" is essential (Brown & McMullen, 2009). This "toolbox" is known as the "4 P's of professional development."

The 4 P's of Professional Development

Developed by Brown and McMullen (2009), the "4 P's of professional development" are essential for a student's academic success. The 4 P's are: projects, presentations, practicum, and published. This toolbox enhances the academic experience for the student by preparing the student for a career after graduation and by providing support in the development of academic and professional skills (Brown & McMullen, 2009).

Projects are research ideas that supplement classroom studies. Following projects, presentations build a foundation essential for effective classroom demonstrations and exhibition at national conferences. Practicums, also known as internships, are offered to students to prepare them for teaching or career development. Finally, published materials (e.g., research, chapters in a book) demonstrate knowledge of the field, applied research skills, writing proficiency, and provide an avenue for the exchange of new ideas. In academia, the 4 P's are particularly important as they enhance the student's curriculum vitae or resumé (Brown & McMullen, 2009). A mentor should inform a student of these opportunities in order to prepare him or her for each facet of professional development within the field of gerontology. Each academic discipline features various professional development techniques. Therefore, each mentor/mentee relationship must focus on the most appropriate techniques in their specific area.

Organizations and Mentorship

The discipline of gerontology is supported by various organizations with either a specific or a nonspecific focus on the study of aging. The Gerontological Society of America (GSA), the Association for Gerontology in Higher Education (AGHE), and the American Society on Aging (ASA) are organizations that hold annual national conferences. Students, professors, and professionals attend these conferences to network and foster their research skills in the field of gerontology. In order to further develop the discipline, mentoring will need the ongoing support of these organizations and their members. Programs within these organizations are evolving to address the gap in mentoring among gerontologists.

The Gerontological Society of America (GSA) recently completed a two-year pilot mentoring initiative through its Social Research, Policy, and Practice (SRPP) group section. SRPP committee members are practitioners, educators, researchers, and policy makers with varying backgrounds in nursing, medicine, sociology, social work, counseling, political science, policy, and economics. This SRPP initiative explored the effectiveness of mentoring among GSA members. The fourteen participants who served in the SRPP two-year initiative were available for mentoring to all association members, as announced through the GSA website. Additional information, including their personal research interests and mentoring specializations, was listed on the GSA website. This information served as a guide for students attempting to find the appropriate mentor for their research interests. Mentoring was available to students and emerging professionals through electronic mail and telephone contact (www.geron.org/Students/mentoring/srpp-section). Results of the SRPP initiative led the section to continue utilizing mentoring roundtables at the annual Gerontological Society of America national conference (R. Newcomer, personal communication, January 2, 2010). Students who attend future GSA meetings may take part in these mentoring roundtable meetings.

As the educational arm of GSA, the Association for Gerontology in Higher Education (AGHE) has incorporated mentoring as part of its primary mission (Association for Gerontology in Higher Education, 2009). At the annual AGHE meeting, mentoring is made available to students and emerging professionals, by means of sessions and workshops (N. Silverstein, personal communication, January 2, 2010). "I found these sessions [of GSA and AGHE] extremely valuable because I strongly believe it's important for students to have wide and varied (potential) mentoring influences," stated gerontology professor Eric Goedereis (personal communication, January 6, 2010) about his time as a student who received mentoring.

Within the American Society on Aging (American Society on Aging), the New Ventures in Leadership (NVL) interest group promotes the leadership by professionals of color and supports their involvement in the national aging arena. NVL participants develop and enhance their skills in areas aligned with their career objectives, such as community building and advocacy, leadership development, applied research techniques, grant writing, and fundraising. The mentoring program empowers the participants to assume leadership roles within their organizations and communities (American Society on Aging, 2009).

As the number of elders around the world increases, so does the demand for qualified gerontologists. The proper preparation of students to serve the aging population is the responsibility of the students themselves, their professors, and professionals involved within the field of aging. Mentorship prepares students to understand the needs and demands of a growing aging population. Professors and students must harness the opportunity to better understand how an academic collaboration could benefit the field of gerontology. "Mentoring requires a relationship, the building of trust, and for mentees, a sense that the potential mentor is actually willing to play that role" (T. Fox-Wetle, personal communication, January 2, 2010).

However, the responsibility for obtaining a mentorship relies heavily on the student. Mentorship in gerontology can be difficult to acquire, given the relatively small number of gerontology programs that are available. An internet word search produced a listing of over 100 gerontology programs available for undergraduate degrees, and over 50 graduate programs in gerontology (gradschools.com, 2010). Many of these degrees are derived from onsite campus programs. However, the expansion of distance learning is influencing how gerontologists are educated (Brown, 2009). Currently, nine onsite doctoral gerontology institutions exist within the United States, three of which are specific to social gerontology (Brown, 2009). The lower number of gerontological doctoral programs gives value to one-on-one mentorship between a student and a professor. Undergraduate students should be encouraged to research potential mentors willing to guide their future endeavors as graduate students.

The Outcome of Mentorship

Examples of Mentorship

Research suggests that academic mentorship programs aid in helping students achieve their academic and career goals (Detsky & Baerlocher, 2007). However, research findings vary about what types of mentorship programs are advantageous to specific student cohorts. In a review of mentoring programs that were offered to medical students and physicians, Sambunjak, Straus, and Marusic (2006) explained that mentorship influences a student's personal growth, career selection, research output, and grant attainment. How these variables are influenced can solely be dependent on the form of mentorship each student receives.

As mentorship programs evolve, a new perspective on the mentor-mentee relationship is emerging. Brown University's ADVANCE Program (2010) is an innovative initiative whose purpose is to increase the retention of female faculty in science and engineering using the "personal approach" to mentorship (Brown University, 2010). Funded by a grant from the National Science Foundation, ADVANCE utilizes the concept of personal mentorship to support student development and research collaboration, while also providing financial support. The face-to-face, personal support that the students receive supplements the core program objectives of gender sensitivity, promotion processes of mentoring, and networking across academic disciplines.

A collaborative effort between the Brown University Office of the Dean of the Faculty, Office of the Dean of Medicine and Biological Sciences, and the ADVANCE program provides a formal mechanism for tenure-track faculty members to connect with a mentor outside their current departments and to mentor students within their departments (Brown University, 2010). The peer mentor relationship allows tenure track and tenured faculty members to be "matched" based on responses to a questionnaire. Mentors assist junior faculty members with professional development by providing information about university resources, policies, and culture, thereby establishing direction for balancing commitments and strategies for attaining both national and international recognition in their fields (Brown University, 2010).

Face-to-face mentoring appears to be the most effective type of mentoring (T. Fox-Wetle, personal communication, January 2, 2010). However, the use of electronic mentoring is becoming popular within many educational settings. Electronic mentoring, also referred to as cybermentoring, utilizes the Internet as a means to connect with individuals who live in rural areas (Mueller, 2004). The effectiveness of this form of mentorship program stems from the cost-effectiveness of the online communication, coupled with flexibility of online communication, an open forum to express thoughts and concerns freely, and the timeliness of correspondence (D. Yee-Melichar, personal communication, January 2, 2010); however, the difficulty with this type of mentoring program lies in the lack of interpersonal communication between mentors and mentees (Mueller, 2004). Without face-to-face communication, mentors and mentees may not be able to establish and sustain an academic "bond."

Group and peer mentoring using Listserve (electronic mailing list), and online forums are seen as an innovative approach to increase a student's academic development (D. Yee-Melichar, personal communication, January 2, 2010). Modifying the existing student-mentorship model by adding a component of accessibility can be seen as an inventive way to expand student mentorship (McMullen, 2009). In order to make mentorship a viable option for students who depend on support and guidance, an online aging support network that is accessible to students and mentors should be developed. In this online network, students could pose questions and discuss concerns in an interactive aging online forum (McMullen, 2009). In order for this mentorship program to be successful, professors and mentors are needed to address student inquiry. This online community may present an opportunity to enhance the current mentorship model and could potentially create a sustainable online aging network that will keep students, professors, and professionals informed and in contact with one another (McMullen, 2009). Further, an online gerontology network could connect students with professors so that they can receive multidimensional input and perspectives (D.Yee-Melichar, personal communication, January 2, 2010). Students may also be able to learn from one another in this virtual forum, thereby enabling them to network with students who share similar interests (D. Yee-Melichar, personal communication, January 2, 2010).

The Realization of the Dream

Mentorship is not a new idea for increasing student academic achievement. However, new models of mentorship are increasing the likelihood that students will be able to expand their knowledge within in their field(s) of interest, while still being able to market their degrees in a workforce setting. Mentorship should be perceived as a group effort rather than an individual (student) effort. Academic disciplines must recognize that creating a student-first culture takes a team of professors who are willing to expand beyond the current curriculum. As long as mentorship is seen as an undesired side project, fulfilling it for the purpose of student achievement may not be entirely possible. Academic institutions must join together using interprofessional methods beyond the classroom, and the institution, in order to create an atmosphere that promotes growth from the inside out, as well as, from the outside in.

Acknowledgments

The authors would like to graciously thank Drs. Sarah Gueldner, May Mykle, Terrie Fox-Wetle, Eric Goedereis, Nina Silverstein, and Darlene Yee-Melichar. The authors would also like to thank Courtney Brown, Thomas Taber, and Aaron Tripp.

References

Achenbaum, W.A. (1995). *Crossing frontiers: Gerontology emerges as a science.* New York: Cambridge University Press.

American Geriatrics Society. (2005). *Improving the quality of transitional care for persons with complex care needs.* Retrieved (2009) from http://www.americangeriatrics.org

American Society on Aging. (2009). *A Leadership Program for Professionals of Color in Aging.* New Ventures in *Leadership.* Retrieved (2009) from www.asaging.org/nvl

Association for Gerontology in Higher Education. (2009). Welcome to AGHE. *AGHE Website.* Retrieved (2009) from www.aghe.org

Barondess, J. (2005). *A brief history of mentoring.* New York: New York Academy of Medicine.

Bass, S.A. (2009). Toward an Integrative Theory of Social Gerontology. In Bengtson, V.L., Gans, D., Putney, N.M., & Silverstein, M. (Second Ed.), *Handbook of Theories of Aging* (pp. 347–373). New York, NY: Springer Publishing Company, LLC.

Bass, S.A., & Ferraro, K. (2000). Gerontology education in transition: Considering disciplinary and paradigmatic evolution. *The Gerontologist, 40,* 96–106.

Brown, C. (2009). *Mentors in gerontology: The case of the distance learning student.* Unpublished manuscript.

Brown, C., & McMullen, T. (2009). *The 4 P's of professional development in gerontology.* Unpublished manuscript.

Brown University (2010). Advance Program at Brown University. *ADVANCE at Brown.* Retrieved from (2009) http://www.brown.edu/Administration/Provost/Advance/

Detsky, A.S., & Baerlocher, M.O. (2007). Academic mentoring—How to give it and how to get it. *The Journal of the American Medical Association, 297,* 2134–2136.

Ewen, H., Carr, D., & Kunkel, S. (2008). Professional growth of students in gerontology doctoral education: Influence of program dynamics and faculty mentoring. *The Gerontologist, 48,* 45.

Farren, C. (2006). Eight types of mentors: Which ones do you need? *Mastery Works, Inc.* Retrieved (2009) from http://www.masteryworks.com/newsite/downloads/Article3_EightTypesofMentors-WhichOnesdoyouNeed.pdf

Gerontological Society of America. (2009). Mentoring: Social, research, policy and practice. Retrieved from www.geron.org/Students/mentoring/srpp-section

GradSchools.com (2010). Gerontology Graduate School Programs—Masters and PhD Degrees. *Gradschools.com: Find a Program.* Retrieved (2009) from www.gradschools.com/Subject/Gerontology/177.html

McMullen, T. (2009). *New models of mentoring.* Unpublished manuscript.

Mueller, S. (2004). Electronic mentoring as an example for the use of information and communications technology in engineering education. *European Journal of Engineering Education, 29*(1), 53–63.

Pelham, A. (2008). Can academic gerontology keep from becoming irrelevant? *Aging Today,* 3–4.

Peyton, A., Morton, M., Perkins, M., & Dougherty, L. (2001). Mentoring in gerontology education: New graduate student perspectives. *Educational Gerontology, 27,* 347–359.

Sambunjak, D., Straus, S.E., & Marusic, A. (2006). Mentoring in academic medicine: A systematic review. *The Journal of the American Medical Association, 296,* 1103–1115.

Chapter 4

Enhancing the Graduate Student Experience: Student Engagement and the Internship Survey

Candace Brown, Aaron Hagedorn, and Tara McMullen

"Distance education provides a needed fresh perspective. It forces our thinking beyond the confines of campus and out into the changing world about which we are supposed to be teaching and preparing our students." (Ohler, 1991, p. 23)

Introduction

This quote supports the notion that access to distance education has the potential to be influential both onsite and offsite the campus environment. Distance education is the chosen route of education for many learners (Ohler, 1991). Distant learners share a similar trait: a distant feeling or sense of exclusion from the educational system which may be physical, cultural or psychological (Ohler, 1991). This chapter offers a fresh look at alternatives to reverse the sense of exclusion by means of innovative methods to increase student engagement among distance students.

The feeling of exclusion experienced by distance students may be due to a lack of engagement. This is important because engagement theory posits that learning best occurs when students are meaningfully engaged in learning activities through tasks and personal interaction with others (Kearsley & Shneiderman, 1999). Thus, there is more to the student's school experience than classroom instruction and completing individual course requirements. A well-rounded student is one who demonstrates academic excellence, and who is involved in extracurricular activities involving community support (Brown, 2008).

Creating well-rounded students is the responsibility of the university, teachers, and the students, themselves (Brown, 2008). Universities that actively attempt to enhance students' academic and social engagement (Vontius & Harper, 2006) often do so by encouraging teachers to promote extracurricular activities for students. Students can choose to be involved through leadership groups, award programs, volunteer activities, competitions and membership in national organizations. Most of these opportunities need not be limited to those who are on campus, but can apply to distance learners as well (Brown, 2008).

Thus, the challenges associated with creating well-rounded distance learning students include student engagement, internship capability, and thorough information about career choices. Extensive review of engagement in distance education research reveals there are gaps in case studies detailing university commitment to promoting student engagement, which is vital to the enhancement of individual experiences for the distance learner. Universities that offer internship opportunities for distance students assist students through exposure to a variety of career opportunities and internship reviews, useful tools for distance learners. Further studies may increase an understanding of the impact of the aforementioned challenges.

In this study, an individual participant purposely engages in professional activities, incorporates short term internships, and creates the idea of an internship review to enhance the distant learning experience. In this chapter, the following words will represent various subgroups of types of students. A "campus student/learner" will indicate a full-time student who lives on campus. "Distance student/learner" will refer to students who commute to campus and/or take classes solely through the Internet. The word "student," used alone, will describe all previously mentioned.

Background

For more than 50 years, educational institutions have sought ways to expand their learning environments. Courses taught via correspondence or through telecommunication devices, including tapes, television, Internet, live or asynchronous interactive have contributed to the education of students who are unable to attend the traditional classroom setting. Distance education, now provided almost exclusively through the World Wide Web, continues to evolve. The current techniques most often used include electronic mail, recorded or live-streamed video, and cyber classrooms (also referred to as discussion boards) to make instruction more interactive (Hannay & Newvine, 2006).

There are several advantages to distance education. Programs are especially designed to meet the education needs of off-campus populations; thus students have the choice of "attending" class and completing coursework at their convenience. This feature is particularly important when demographic factors such as age and proximity to campus are considered. In addition, communication among instructors and other students from different facets of life brings exposure to rich knowledge that cannot be learned from a book or research journal (Coleman, 2005).

Conversely, drawbacks to distance learning include attaining the proper skills to navigate within and beyond the browser. Many distance learners have full-time careers, marital and/or parental responsibilities, as well as other extracurricular activities in their lives. Inefficient time management could cause cognitive overload (Hannay & Newvine, 2006). It has also been found that if course expectations are unclear, problems are often more difficult to resolve, due to the physical separation between student and teacher (Hannay & Newvine, 2006).

The expansion of education beyond the confines of a campus classroom fosters many opportunities for research related to student engagement. Research has presented insights into the engagement of campus-based students who use online systems (Coates, 2006). For instance, it has been observed that students are more likely to continue a program if their educational experience is personalized through engaging activities (Betts, 2008). However, supporting literature on personalized studies of distance learner engagement was not found.

Purpose and Participant Description

A lack of student engagement among distance learning students was observed (Brown, 2008). In this case study, the personal experience of one distant learner was examined to allow for observation and knowledge gained from the individual perspective (Yin, 2003). The approach of this case study focused on the participant; exploring the individual motives and actions of the subject. The primary objective was to understand the variety of activities a distance learner engaged in. The secondary objective was to explore several career choices before graduation by means of a series of short-term internships. A tertiary objective was to develop a written internship review or evaluation form. This compiled list of internship experiences would serve as a reference guide for students who may be unaware of job opportunities within the field of gerontology. The observation of the lack of student engagement among distance learners led to the following research questions:

1. What is the reason behind the lack of student engagement? If students are afforded an opportunity to be involved, would it be taken?

2. If distance learners are not currently working in the field, could a rotating internship assist in narrowing their career choices? If distance learners are not aware of career choices, would a gerontological internship review be a useful resource tool for students?

Description of Participant

This chapter presents a 15-month personal case study design using qualitative data. The participant is a married, 32-year-old, full-time mother of three living in Denver, CO. She is actively involved in her community through several organizations, while pursuing her master's degree part-time at the University of Southern California through distance learning. In an attempt to understand the distance learning paradigm, it was deemed appropriate for this study to represent a smaller population (distance learners) within the field of gerontology and education. The research questions guided an in-depth exploration into the participant's personal attitudes about distance education engagement and university response to distance learners' engagement (Brown, 2008). The results of this study reflect the idea of new engagement practices and behaviors for distance learners and internship programming modifications for universities (Ambert, Adler, & Detzner, 1995).

Opportunities taken by traditional campus students compared to those not available to a distance learner was examined to better understand the options for an engaging graduate experience. However, the student engagement experience cannot be achieved alone. Within the realm of student engagement are components that may need special consideration. For instance, if a university has not established engaging opportunities for its campus students, encouraging distance learning students to participate will prove difficult (Council of Graduate Schools, 2008).

To begin, the participant in this case study completed the National Survey of Student Engagement, which has a web version (http://nsse.iub.edu). A weekly blog of opportunities pursued as well as those not chosen was written. The following open-ended questions were used as directional guides to specify needed answers within the blog: How did you engage in activities beyond the virtual classroom? Have you actively made an effort to prepare for your future in gerontology? What impact did you make in your community? How will your experience be beneficial to another student?

Institutions recognize the need for improving student engagement. Case Western Reserve University integrated the findings of a survey as a basis for improving their graduate and professional student engagement. The Student Engagement Task Force at the school then formed to address this issue by acknowledging the importance of educating the total person. For a more effective learning experience among their graduate students, financial support, faculty mentoring and advising, and diversity were influences cited for further improvement. (Case Western Reserve University, 2008).

Using Chickering and Garrison's "Seven Principles for Good Practice in Undergraduate Education" (1987) as a framework for institutional improvement, Vontius and Harper (2006) offer a set of philosophical principles as a guide to enhance graduate student engagement. The authors offer the following principles for universities to apply to distance learning students. Following a review of these principles, we maintain that a gerontological distance learning department can be most effective when it addresses these efforts:

1. *Continually strives to abate marginalization among underrepresented populations.* On most campuses, distance learning enrollments are relatively low and represent fewer than 5% of all students (Organisation for Economic Co-Operation and Development, 2005). The provision of support groups and mentoring programs in departments that lack technological diversity (campus versus distance students)

creates a safe place where feelings of disconnect and isolation may otherwise characterize the distance learning student experience.

2. *Maintains open and constant communication with students.* Timely distribution and updated materials, including teacher/class surveys, newsletters, and websites are necessary for student engagement. Information about out-of-class events and leadership opportunities should also be disseminated. Departments should also be responsible for ensuring representation of voting members on relevant campus committees (Vontius & Harper, 2006).

3. *Encourages community service and multicultural interaction.* Students can most effectively understand community purpose (Pestello, Saxton, Miller, & Donnelly, 1996) and cross-cultural interaction (Vontius & Harper, 2006) through personal interaction. The elderly in the next several decades will have more members from diverse populations (Torres-Gil, 1992), and students will need more than electronic or textbook knowledge about these populations to be effective in their communities.

Student Engagement

When a university establishes opportunity for engaging experiences, the choice to participate is the students'. For example, all students with an interest in gerontology are encouraged to join the Student Gerontology Association (SGA) at the University of Southern California. SGA is an organization for undergraduate, graduate, and doctoral students who pursue educational, philanthropic and social activities. Students are committed to the promotion of gerontological issues on campus and in the community through annual participation in activities such as the Alzheimer's Association Memory Walk and Fall Prevention Awareness Week (www-scf.usc.edu/~sga).

The Assistant Dean of the Davis School of Gerontology and president of SGA were welcoming when questioned about distance students joining the organization (M. Henke & C. Wise, personal communication, March 25, 2007). State of residence did not deter this organization from accepting members. In the original application to join SGA, the participant wrote, "I noticed that Denver (the participants' place of residence) is also hosting an Alzheimer's Association Memory Walk in the city. This could provide additional exposure for the distance program that USC offers, and show that the SGA is not limited to those that reside in Los Angeles" (C. Brown, personal communication, March 25, 2007). The participant represented the SGA of USC in two consecutive, annual, local Alzheimer's Association Memory Walks. To further expand communication between on-site and distance learners, the participant was elected to hold a new SGA position on their board as online representative for the 2008–2009 school year.

The participant recognized that distance student involvement is not limited to university or local community activities. Distance learning students can be members of national organizations, which can be used as networks to many other persons in the gerontological community. The participant in this study was appointed to a two-year Student Committee position with the Association for Gerontology in Higher Education and a position on the board of the American Society on Aging (ASA) Student Interest Group.

Professional Development

Professional development among graduate students prepares them for future roles (Vontius & Harper, 2006). In times past, interning in the healthcare industry was often the established route for careers with elder populations. Yet, as the elder population increases, so will the demand for an extension of gerontology-related fields. The United States Bureau of Labor Statistics (2008) estimates that the need for workers in gerontological fields will increase by more than 50% by the year 2016. Workplace sectors expanding to fit the needs of an aging population include: financial and legal services, fitness and wellness, and housing and home modification (Wiener, 2004). With these statistics, an expansion of preparation for graduate students through outreach, workshops, counseling, career fairs and internships is essential for effective, professional development (Vontius & Harper, 2006).

The completed education of a campus-based graduate student often includes an internship. However, distance learners are not always required or encouraged to complete an internship during their academic program. Those who do not complete an internship may stifle their opportunity to acquire more knowledge of the varying careers in the field of gerontology, or lack professional contacts to serve as references for future employment. The transition from being a student at a university to being a valuable asset to an employer is eased through pre-professional work experiences (Valo, 2000). Concerns about preparation for the working world should not be limited to campus students only, especially if universities pride themselves on their distance education programs. Efforts to promote student engagement and create a specialized internship program that meets the needs of distance learning students should be incorporated into this transition.

Internship directors play a vital role in this transition (A. Hagedorn, personal communication, November 24, 2008). For graduate students in academia, professional development is most often recognized by projects, presentations, practicums, and publishings, also known as "The 4 P's of Professional Development" (Brown & McMullen, 2009). Accordingly, the second part of this study involved the participant's role in several small internships. The first internship developed after the participant embraced the opportunity to volunteer as a monitor at the American Society on Aging (ASA) West Coast Conference in San Francisco. The registration fee was covered for volunteer services, and the opportunity to meet others in the field was invaluable for professional development in gerontology. During one session, the participant met Brian Berchtold, CEO of ALCiS. Then over the next several months, the participant developed skills to market a topical cream designed to provide immediate relief for arthritis, joint, and muscle pain to aging active adults and athletes. The experience led to a professional poster presentation at the AGHE Educational Leadership Conference the following semester.

After graduation, the participant completed a four-day training course to learn how to effectively help seniors successfully manage and maintain their health. The Consortium of Older Adult Awareness, in Colorado, bases its Wellness Leader program on the evidenced-based program *Healthier Living, Managing Your Ongoing Chronic Conditions,* which has resulted in an excellent way to help seniors in the community (www.coaw.org). After successful completion of the training, the participant led a six-week course that ran 2.5 hours each week for seniors in a retirement community near where she lived.

Rotating Internships

Rotating internships have been an effective means for learning in various for academic fields. For example, the practice of rotating internships had been favored over traditional internships since the 1950s, as it enabled students to have practical experience where they could mature and have in-depth perspectives before choosing a specialty. However, the American Medical Association discontinued rotating internships in the 1970s, and replaced post-education accreditation with residencies. This change forced students to choose a specialty immediately, without the chance of gaining differing perspectives (Rothstein, 1987).

In the book, *Life After Medical School*, one medical doctor explains his regret over the dissolution of the rotating internship. "It gave a good opportunity to pick and choose among medical fields because one could almost design one's own curriculum" (Laster, 1996). While attending veterinary school, Dr. Janelle Davis, DVM, wished to specialize in large sea mammals. After spending a clerkship at the Miami Sea Aquarium, however, she no longer wanted to specialize in large sea mammals. She was thankful that programs were set up around the country for veterinary students so they could have hands-on experience and choose a career track that best suited their personal interests and aspirations (J. Davis, personal communication, November 20, 2008).

Recognizing the inability for some distant learners to complete a full time internship, the participant thought of a rotating internship and short term internship as viable alternative options. The purpose of a short term internship is to expose a distance student to various opportunities in the field. An example of a short term internship is what the study participant completed with ALCiS. The length of a short term internship can vary from 2 to 9 weeks and can be less than 20 hours per week (Brown, 2008). Distance students are not required to complete an internship at USC; however, it has been noted that students who intern at more than one site have an opportunity to "gain new and valuable job skills" (A. Hagedorn, personal communication, September 11, 2008).

Internship Review Options

After completing an internship, students' perceptions on the intern position, time at internship, facility and resources, leadership and professional development and overall experience are observed (http://kantell.org). Internships also provide a way for students to receive information about available career tracks (Brown, 2008) and job sites before interviewing or accepting a position (www.interneval.com). Completing an internship may be difficult for a distance student due to full-time work, or an internship may not be required by an institution for graduation. The creation of an internship review may assist distance students in their quest in securing a job in gerontology after graduation.

The participant described the premise behind the review and its benefits: students who previously completed internships would complete the survey, providing an account of their experiences and views of interning in a certain area of gerontology. Dr. Hagedorn mentioned his knowledge of "Angie's List" (2008), a website dedicated to thousands of unbiased reviews by members about service companies (www.angieslist.com). However, he had not previously considered applying the same function to intern students at USC. After discussing how the review could be accomplished, Dr. Hagedorn agreed that the review would be a useful asset and implemented it into the internship program immediately (A. Hagedorn, personal communication, November 24, 2008). The first draft of the survey was adapted from the 2008 Kansas Teaching, Learning and Leadership Survey (see Figure 4-1).

After modifications, the survey has since been used to measure internship satisfaction for three consecutive semesters at USC, assessing more than 50 internship experiences for campus students. The preliminary findings of the review are shown in Figures 4-2, 4-3, and 4-4.

The survey was administered at the end of each semester, and is completed with a mentor's evaluation and letter of reference. Because the survey is relatively short and quick to complete, it has been very well received by students and has enjoyed a 100% response rate. The survey has provided significant information concerning weaknesses in career exposure and skill-gaining experiences at some sites, as well as the mismatched expectations and outcomes of students and mentor supervisors. The survey has inspired longer-term tracking of graduates and further investigation of how the internship experience related to later career opportunities. As more data is gathered it will become easier to establish patterns about which experiences are most valuable, and could potentially be useful in better informing mentors of intern needs and expectations a priori.

Most questions utilized a 5 point Likert scale, making data analysis fairly simple. The graphs display average responses from survey respondents, and demonstrate general satisfaction with internship experiences. Results showed that improvement by greater involvement by the internship coordinator in sharing network contacts, and improved communication about unmet expectations over the semester, is feasible. Use of the survey at mid-term, in addition to the end of the semester, might be especially valuable to the internship coordinator in exploring whether experiences fluctuated as a result of increased awareness of internship experience goals.

Figure 4-1 Internship Survey.

Name (optional) _____

School Affiliation _____

Date of Internship _____

Name of Site _____

Address _____

Position Description _____

TIME

Rate how strongly you agree or disagree with the following statements about the use of your time during your internship.

	Strongly Disagree	Somewhat Disagree	Neutral	Somewhat Agree	Strongly Agree
Training was appropriate and completed in a timely fashion.	_____	_____	_____	_____	_____
The skills I learned would be useful in the real world.	_____	_____	_____	_____	_____
I can get a letter of recommendation from my mentor.	_____	_____	_____	_____	_____
If I had concerns, I was given appropriate time to consult with my supervisor.	_____	_____	_____	_____	_____
The number of work hours was sufficient to meet expected responsibilities.	_____	_____	_____	_____	_____
Efforts were made to minimize the amount of non-essential work not pertaining to my position.	_____	_____	_____	_____	_____
I feel like I could get a better job as a result of this experience.	_____	_____	_____	_____	_____
I know the key people in the management of this organization.	_____	_____	_____	_____	_____

(continues)

Figure 4-1 Internship Survey (continued).

	Strongly Disagree	Somewhat Disagree	Neutral	Somewhat Agree	Strongly Agree
I know key people at related organizations (beyond the staff of the organization I worked for).	_____	_____	_____	_____	_____
I have a chance of a getting job at the company where I did my internship.	_____	_____	_____	_____	_____
My experience at this organization is likely to be recognized as valuable to other related companies.	_____	_____	_____	_____	_____
I feel that I was a good fit at the organization.	_____	_____	_____	_____	_____
I adapted to the organizational culture of the organization.	_____	_____	_____	_____	_____

FACILITIES AND RESOURCES

Please mark "Yes" or "No"

	Yes	No
Did the site create a safe work environment?	____	____
Did your site offer necessary communication tools (telephone, email, printer)?	____	____
Were resources available to gain further understanding of your position?	____	____
Was the facility well-kept in a manner that would not violate any regulation codes?	____	____
Did the facility offer parking?	____	____
Was the facility in a convenient location?	____	____
Were you given adequate workspace?	____	____

LEADERSHIP AND PROFESSIONAL DEVELOPMENT

a. Who provided mentoring to you in your professional development?

_____

b. What new knowledge, skills and abilities did you learn?

_____

Figure 4-1 Internship Survey (continued).

Rate how strongly you agree or disagree with the following statements about leadership and professional development.

	Strongly Disagree	Somewhat Disagree	Neutral	Somewhat Agree	Strongly Agree
This site created an atmosphere of trust and respect.	_____	_____	_____	_____	_____
My internship gave me an opportunity to network.	_____	_____	_____	_____	_____
The administration communicates clear expectations to all the workers within the site.	_____	_____	_____	_____	_____
Evaluations given were fair and honest.	_____	_____	_____	_____	_____

OVERALL

What best describes your future intentions for your professional career?

____ Build on this experience and apply for a higher ranking job.

____ Continue working at my current internship position after graduating.

____ Work a similar position at a different location.

____ Would not consider working my internship job at any site.

On a scale of 1 to 5, please rate the following with 1 = low and 5 = high.

a. Adequate facilities/resources   _____

b. Adequate leadership   _____

c. Adequate professional development   _____

d. Congenial atmosphere among staff   _____

e. Sufficient time for duties   _____

f. Explanation of duties suffice   _____

g. Overall experience   _____

This survey was adapted from the 2008 Kansas Teaching, Learning and Leadership Survey. Written by Candace S. Brown, MAG, M.Ed. Revised by Dr. Aaron Hagedorn, Director of Internship Training, University of Southern California.

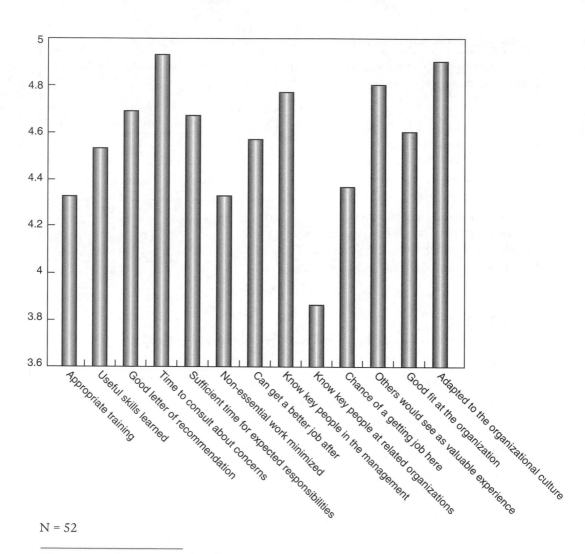

N = 52

Figure 4-2 Description of students' positions of time spent, during internships.

Source: Authors' calculation from the Internship Survey, 2009.

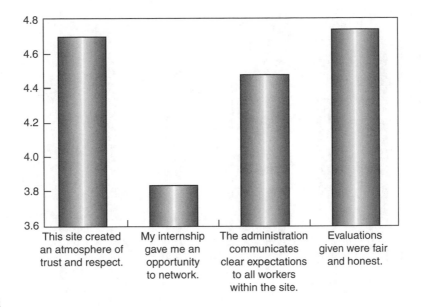

N = 52

Figure 4-3   Students' perceptions of the facilities and resources during internship.

Source: Authors' calculation from the Internship Survey, 2009.

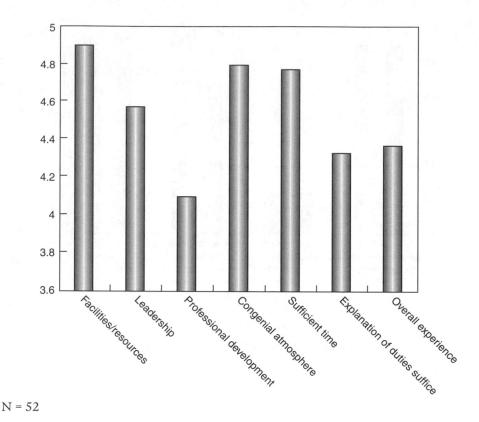

N = 52

Figure 4-4   Overall student ratings of internships conducted.

Source: Authors' calculation from the Internship Survey, 2009.

Conclusion

In 2008, the National Survey of Student Engagement (NSSE) found that benchmarks of effective educational practices with the greatest impact on students in colleges and universities include level of academic challenge, active and collaborative learning, enriching educational experiences, and a supportive campus environment. Setting high expectations for performance challenges students' intellectual and creative work for achievement (NSSE, 2008). These challenges lead to active learning in various settings which may require collaborating with others. Mastery of solving difficult material and problems are preparatory tools of professional development for unexpected life situations during and after college. Diverse learning opportunities such as internships and community service are invaluable for students as they make learning more meaningful and useful for life after college. Finally, students are more satisfied at colleges which are committed to cultivating their success through positive working and social relations on campus (NSSE, 2008).

Although the results of these benchmarks were based on undergraduate student engagement, the participant's graduate engagement has positively impacted her institution and local community, and has led to the application of knowledge in the outside world (Brown, 2008). The shifting of education from classroom-based instruction to technology-enhanced modes of distance learning needs further exploration. It is recommended that the current pilot survey at USC be expanded to include distance students in the future.

Engagement by distance learners is often described in terms of technological tools, such as Blackboard. As technology-enhanced learning becomes part of mainstream education, engagement for students living in physically disparate areas will become a salient issue for teachers to be concerned about. Student engagement likely varies based on gender, age, socioeconomic status, cultural background, and ethnicity. Therefore, future research should be expanded to include those variables.

Student engagement can promote networking with others who are actively engaged and well connected in the field of gerontology. Networking often leads to real jobs and opportunities for career advancement. The distance student should also be able to tap into these opportunities and to benefit from internships. Rotating internships help to increase one's knowledge of the many careers in gerontology. They may make the difference between choosing a career one loves versus doing a job as a necessity. For those who can complete an internship, the gerontological internship review is offered as a resource to direct students toward more suitable opportunities.

The case study described in this chapter has led to a pilot study, but it can also lead to many avenues for further research. Our aging society will create a demand for students who are properly prepared for roles in the gerontological community. Student engagement, placement of internships, and choosing a career are essential to the advancement of the graduates of gerontology programs, whether they are campus or distance students.

References

Ambert, A., Adler, P., & Detzner, D. (1995). Understanding and evaluating qualitative research. *Journal of Marriage and the Family, 57*(4), 879–893.

Angie's List. (2008). *Frequently asked questions: "What is Angie's List?"* Retrieved from http://angieslist.com/Angieslist/Visitor/Faq.aspx#whatis

Betts, K. (2008). Online human touch (OHT) instruction and programming: A conceptual framework to increase student engagement and retention in online education, Part 1. *MERLOT Journal of Online Learning and Teaching, 4*(3), Retrieved from http://jolt.merlot.org/vol3no2/panke.htm

Brown, C. (2008). *Enhancing the student experience: Outside involvement and the rotating internship review.* Unpublished manuscript.

Brown, C., & McMullen, T. (2009). *Mentoring: A student and emerging professional's perspective.* Unpublished manuscript.

Case Western Reserve University. (2008). *Student engagement task force: preliminary report.* Retrieved from http://www.case.edu/provost/uplan/Documents/StudentEngagementTaskForce.pdf

Chickering, A., & Garrison, Z. (1987). Seven principles for good practice in undergraduate education. *American Association for Higher Education Bulletin, 39*(7), 3–7.

Coates, H. (2006). *Student engagement in campus-based and on-line education: University connections.* New York: Routledge.

Coleman, S. (2005). Compelling arguments for attending a cyberclassroom: Why do students like online learning? *World Wide Learn.* Retrieved from http://www.worldwidelearn.com/education-articles/benefits-of-online-learning.htm

Council of Graduate Schools. (2008). *PhD completion and attrition: Policy, numbers, leadership and next steps.* Washington D.C.: Author.

Hannay, M., & Newvine, T. (2006). Perceptions of distance learning: A comparison of online and traditional learning. *Journal of Online Learning and Teaching, 2*(1), 1–11.

Kearsley, G., & Shneiderman, B. (1999). Engagement theory: A framework for technology-based teaching and learning. Naval Sea Systems Command. Retrieved from http://home.sprynet.com/~gkearsley/engage.htm

Laster, L. (1996). *Life after medical school: 32 doctors describe how they shaped their medical careers.* New York: WW Norton & Company Inc.

National Survey of Student Engagement: Promoting Engagement for all Students Imperative to Look Within, 2008 Results. Retrieved November 15, 2008 from http://nsse.iub.edu/NSSE_2008_Results/docs/withhold/NSSE2008_Results_revised_11-14-2008.pdf

Ohler, J. (1991). Why distance education? *Annals for the American Academy of Political and Social Science, 514*(1), 22–34.

Organisation for Economic Co-Operation and Development. (2005). *E-learning in tertiary education: Where do we stand?* Paris, France: OECD Publishing.

Pestello, F., Saxton, S., Miller, D., & Donnelly, P. (1996). Community and the practice of sociology. *Teaching Sociology, 24*(2), 148–156.

Rothstein, W. (1987). *American medical schools and the practice of medicine: A history.* New York: Oxford University Press.

Torres-Gil, F. (1992). *The new aging: Politics and change in America.* Westport, CT: Auburn House.

United States Bureau of Labor Statistics. (2008). *Average annual job openings due to growth and total replacement needs, 2006-2016.* Retrieved from http://data.bls.gov/oep/servlet/oep.noeted.servlet.ActionServlet?Actim=empoccp

University Southern California Student Gerontology Association. (2007). *About SGA 2007–2008.* Retrieved from http://www-scf.usc.edu/%7Esga/about_gsa.htm

Valo, M. (2000). Experiencing work as a communications professional: Students' reflections on their off-campus work practice. *Higher Education, 39*(2), 151–179.

Vontius, J., & Harper, S. (2006). Principles for good practice in graduate and professional student engagement. *New Directions for Student Services, 115,* 47–58.

Wiener, L. (2004). *Exploring Careers in Aging.* (2nd ed.). Vancouver, WA: Linda Weiner Publishings.

Yin, R. (2003). *Case study research: Design and method* (3rd ed.). Newbury Park, CA: Sage Publications.

Chapter 5

Interdisciplinary Community Practice: Patient Activation in a Community Context

Lisa A. Ferretti, Philip McCallion, Robert Paeglow, and Evelyn Kintner

A host of factors are associated with health and health behaviors, and influencing those factors presents opportunities for health professionals to improve health and health outcomes for the people they work with. Motivation, self-efficacy, access to health care, nutritious foods, and safe places to be physically active; race and ethnicity; gender; socio-economic status and even neighborhood makeup have all been suggested as important influences on health and health behaviors (Elder et al., 2010; Feldman & Steptoe, 2004; Hibbard, et al., 2008; Stange, 2010). Research on these influences has already resulted in greater understanding and is helping practitioners to reduce morbidity and increase healthcare savings and positive health outcomes for individuals and communities. There is the promise in the years ahead of even greater opportunities to successfully apply such knowledge.

While much has been learned, many practitioners in medicine, nursing, and social work continue to manage practice roles where the link between individual and environmental factors is sometimes murky, even if clearly influential. This individual–environment disconnect is of particular concern in communities that experience a disparate burden of health care (Elder et al., 2010; Feldman & Steptoe, 2004), and is especially pertinent to persons with chronic health problems, including adults over age 65, 84% of whom have one or more chronic health conditions. One estimate places the 2007 annual costs of care for the six most prevalent chronic illnesses at $196 billion (Van Houtven et al., 2008), further highlighting how critical more successful management of such conditions is today.

Change does begin with the person, but practitioners increasingly recognize that individual behavior change does not happen in isolation from family, friends, community, and environment. Even when individuals are personally motivated to change and have the knowledge they need to improve their health, moving from motivation to action requires skills (Hibbard et al., 2007a, 2007b). The way in which we perceive self and environment and our ability to control and change either is critical to attempting and/or sustaining changes in behavior (Bandura, 1993). Long-term change requires support from others, including support from within one's community (Elder et al., 2010; Feldman & Steptoe, 2004).

These data suggest a need for movement from patient education focused upon helping people to understand their disease condition and needs, to patient activation that offers skill development to build capability and willingness to manage one's own health (Hibbard et al., 2008), including the building of a more supportive environment where activation is possible. Literature describing successful patient activation efforts illustrate a four-stage behavior change process where patients move from passive knowledge that they can or should be involved in managing their own health, to demonstrating that they are fully competent managers of their own health needs and can overcome barriers in a maintenance phase (Hibbard et al., 2007a, 2007b). The context in which individual behavior changes occur and are maintained is embedded within these stages, and activation levels are predicted by the socio-environmental context (Hibbard et al., 2008). Similarly, literature on Stages of Change Theory describes a behavior change process that relies on individual-level knowledge and skills but also recognizes the need for attention to the context for these changes, as well as the value of relapse prevention education and skills to assist in maintaining patient-level changes when personal and/or environmental factors interfere with successful attainment or maintenance (Prochaska, Redding, & Evers, 1997).

Healthcare professionals in medicine, nursing and social work have an opportunity, perhaps even an imperative, to promote the development of skills and linkages that will benefit their patients. A professional view that sees behavior change only as an individual responsibility turns a blind eye to an environment that is at times harsh; such a view discounts cultural, family, and community access influences, and blames the patient for failing to follow professional recommendations without acknowledging the context within which the person must change (Feldman & Steptoe, 2004). If we persist with this perspective, will we ever reach a point where communities become healthier and support their members in changing, and more importantly maintaining, lifelong health habits? There is an interest in individual and community change, but with a recognition that the skills training and evaluation approaches needed are different. Training for the health professions increasingly, therefore, includes community-based internships and training as integral rather than ancillary, and the orientation of new practitioners includes a focus on neighborhood and cultural as well as individual characteristics.

Yet it must be acknowledged that at a time when professional roles in health care are changing rapidly, interventions and practices that simultaneously engage individuals and their communities in health-related behavior change are still rare, although they are getting more attention as healthcare reform efforts increase. The work involved is labor intensive, particularly in communities where daily challenges such as unemployment, violence, poor access to food, and substandard housing are rampant—and where individual health, while a major concern, is outflanked by these more pressing and immediate needs (Elder et al., 2010; Feldman & Steptoe, 2004).

The Healthy Hearts on the Hill Coalition

To better understand the synergies that are created when health professionals engage with individuals in their communities to connect them with making healthier choices, a small group of practitioners in medicine and social work founded a local community-based coalition, known as the Healthy Hearts on the Hill Coalition. The coalition was built with the support of local health and social service providers, retired professionals, community residents, local business and faith-based organizations, and students in social work and medicine. The effort included a community-wide health contest, *The Biggest Winner*, that engaged more than 200 local residents in making healthier choices in nutrition, physical activity, and preventive health management, and in building a community where needed supports for change could develop. As a result of this community initiative, hundreds of pounds (in weight) were lost, many miles walked, and healthy foods purchased and consumed; and the lives of individuals and the community changed.

The coalition continues its work today and is now 40-plus members strong. It has received additional funds to target specific behavior change efforts, and it provides a forum for advocacy for this small upstate New York neighborhood.

A description of this community-wide effort to activate patients and their community to make and sustain healthier behaviors is provided in the following paragraphs. The description is adapted from several reports, including the *Healthy Hearts Coalition Final Project Report* (Ferretti, 2009) and the *Biggest Winner Project Final Report* (Ferretti & Kintner, 2010).

The Healthy Hearts on the Hill Coalition was cofounded in 2007 by the Center for Excellence in Aging Services (now the Center for Excellence in Aging Services & Community Wellness) at the State University of New York at Albany (CEACW), and Koinonia Primary Care, a nonprofit faith-based healthcare provider. The Coalition initially formed to promote efforts to transcend the deficit lens through which most people view the West Hill area, but it now offers hope to the community by increasing access to services and improving health practices by building capacity that begins with the community's strengths (instead of its weaknesses). In the absence of mainstream services reaching out effectively to this health disparity community, the Healthy Hearts on the Hill (HHH) Coalition provides leadership and advocacy and builds awareness and access to the means for sustainable behavior change. Further, participation in events by county and city legislators, the police department, and the state legislature helps the coalition to influence policy and systems change.

A Health Disparities Neighborhood

West Hill, the home of the Coalition, is a 60-block neighborhood located on the west side of the city of Albany in upstate New York. Today more than 60% of the population in West Hill is black, non-Hispanic, and almost 7% is Hispanic. More than 20% of the adult population has not completed high school and 35% of individuals live below the poverty line, with 63% of those below 200% of the poverty line. Over 20% of the population is over age 65 (Ferretti, 2009). West Hill has been the entry point for immigrants to Albany for over a century, offering low rents but few amenities, and it remains one of the most disadvantaged areas in New York's Capital Region.

West Hill is a relatively high-crime neighborhood; most housing is multistory, rented, older, in a dilapidated state, and not easily made more accessible. Community surveys have indicated that both large numbers of at-risk children and many shut-in elderly people live there, and that this is a neighborhood with a high turnover in population with high levels of obesity, diabetes, and heart disease. Violence has discouraged employers, businesses, and health services from locating there.

Health Challenges

Coalition-organized interviews with local hospitals, service agencies, and faith communities confirmed the following characteristics:

1. High levels of service use, repeat hospitalizations and emergency room use;

2. Low levels of individual knowledge of risk factors and prevention strategies;

3. Lack of community awareness regarding the extent and consequences of disease, and that there are prevention strategies that will successfully reduce incidence;

4. Few transportation options to access services outside the community for a population who rarely have their own reliable transportation.

Additional interviews with community leaders in West Hill further confirmed a paucity of local healthcare options and follow-up, few local or culturally specific diabetes and cardiovascular education efforts, and a lack of access to pharmacies and grocery stores carrying healthy, reasonably priced foods compounding these problems. Information gathered confirmed that previous outreach, education, and screening programs in West Hill were highly fragmented. It was confirmed that providers were often not located in the neighborhood, and that there was little to no consistency in outreach efforts; little tailoring of efforts to the community; assumptions of high levels of literacy; and no resources to support recommended nutritional and exercise changes (Ferretti, 2009). In short, this was a community in need of strategies to mitigate poor health behaviors and outcomes, but lacking the resources needed to support and sustain these efforts.

Building the Needed Resources

The Coalition and its projects were funded initially by a Practice Change Fellow's award to the first author, and it has since attracted a Centers for Disease Control and Prevention–funded Legacy Award through Bronx Health REACH, and an Active Living by Design Program grant from the New York State Department of Health. Private donations, member items from legislators, and donations from businesses, health insurers, and providers have all added to the resources, as have hundreds of hours of volunteer time donated by community residents, students in medicine and social work, and retired professionals.

Four Coalition-endorsed principles have influenced resource procurement:

1. The project should rely upon local low-cost resources to the greatest extent possible. For this reason there is a heavy reliance on volunteers and contributions from local businesses, faith communities, and providers.

2. Data on behavior changes and health outcomes valued by insurers and health networks are used to support requests for external funding.

3. The use of evidence-based approaches will increase access to external funding.

4. Potential and actual funding partners should be at the Coalition table rather than funding from afar.

Using Data to Measure Outcomes and Improve the Approach

An evaluation approach was co-developed with the project partners, consistent with the principles of action research, an approach that encourages respectful relationships and communication with, and active participation and inclusion of the people and community being researched (Stringer, 2007). Many researchers talk about involving the community and being respectful of the wishes of participants, but action research goes much farther, building genuine partnerships between researchers, universities, practitioners, and community members, and community members are recognized as active participants with an ownership stake rather than passive recipients in a project. The design and management of the evaluation therefore occurred within the Coalition rather than being presented and managed at arm's length by a research partner.

After examination of a number of approaches, the specific performance measures were guided by the RE-AIM Framework (**R**each, **E**ffectiveness, **A**doption, **I**mplementation, and **M**aintenance) (Glasgow, 2006), designed to identify the translatability and public health impact of health promotion interventions. In this framework the interest is as much in contextual, organizational, and policy issues as in individual outcomes. Traditionally, evaluation frameworks have targeted the effectiveness of interventions. However, an intervention proven effective in one community, often through a tightly controlled randomized control trial, is often found to be of limited use when applied in other communities or with participants facing greater challenges than the original study participants. Equally, if local agencies are unable or unwilling to try the intervention or find it difficult to deliver the intervention as originally described, then that intervention is unlikely to be adopted or continued, regardless of the original study results. Finally, adoption by agencies and continuation of an intervention often require that there be a mechanism to fund its use, a point which is rarely addressed in research studies (Fortune, McCallion & Briar-Lawson, in press). The RE-AIM Framework seeks to address these issues by focusing on the concepts put forward in its title (**R**each, **E**ffectiveness, **A**doption, **I**mplementation, and **M**aintenance), all issues that the Coalition saw as relevant to its work. Specific measures were therefore adopted to address individual knowledge, evidence-based intervention participation, provider education, partnerships and networks, organizational practices, and policy context.

Individual Knowledge and Skills

Baseline knowledge of diabetes risk, preventive strategies, exercise and nutrition recommendations, and **effectiveness** were assessed by measuring changes in both level of knowledge and application of that knowledge over time. The ***Biggest Winner*** report card was a key data collection tool.

Evidence-Based Intervention Participation

Success was assessed using input from participants and leaders, review of the report cards, and data on numbers of people **reach**ed compared with population with potential to benefit. Observation of **implementation** helped to determine if programs are being delivered with fidelity.

To Assess Partnerships and Networks, and Organizational Practices

A baseline measurement was completed of identified health needs, level of collaboration between "within neighborhood" providers and external healthcare providers, and healthy food practices of local corner stores (bodegas). Annually, semi structured interviews were conducted with all key stakeholders, illustrative case studies were developed, and data related to frequency, density, and types of interactions between stakeholders and readiness to **maintain**/sustain new approaches were gathered.

Changing Organizational Practices

Via interviews with key stakeholders, organizational and other barriers to changing the health profile and health practices of the community were identified. Over time the success of efforts to address these barriers and increase the **adoption** of new practices was assessed.

Policy Context

Policy happens at the federal, state, county, and local levels, and includes organizational as well as public policy. Policy-level barriers identified by the Coalition included eligibility and application practices for health insurance, both public and private; requirements for the delivery and reimbursement of needed health-related education and services; and policies and practices in policing, street management, code enforcement, and accessing of public buildings and other resources. All of these policy issues were seen as critical concerns for **adoption, implementation,** and **maintenance** and, if addressed, increased the potential for **reach**. Engagement with federal and state funders, including the welcoming of these and local funders to the Coalition's meetings and events, and presentations at state and national conferences are examples of steps taken to influence policy issues at multiple levels. Periodic interviews with stakeholders and reviews of Coalition meeting minutes helped to identify the issues of concern and progress over time in their being addressed.

Sharing Findings

Findings were regularly shared at Coalition meetings, and they proved to be useful tools in improving the Coalition's activities and in establishing priorities and critical next steps. Statistical and summary reports were provided to funders, and presentations and posters at local, regional, and statewide conferences helped highlight findings from the project and engage assistance and new partnerships.

The Work of the Coalition

The HHH Coalition envisions a time when all of our neighbors in the West Hill and surrounding communities will have the means and access to live heart-healthy lifestyles within and supported by the community. Long-term goals of the Coalition include changing attitudes and behaviors around nutrition, physical activity, and health care by creating opportunities for the people of West Hill to try different and healthier foods and food preparations, engage in regular physical activity programs, and become aware of and able to access affordable local health care with a focus on self-management strategies for persons with chronic conditions.

The Coalition anchored its work in a unique approach that targeted individual community members and the broader community simultaneously in developing, planning, and implementation of the change effort. Faith community leaders, local advocates, food pantry staff, and local providers were the initial planning group, and community surveys carried out by community members provided much of the data on which planning was based. As the project grew, the core group of Coalition members expanded. From word-of-mouth beginnings, new partners have sought out the Coalition, including many who were initially skeptical of what was proposed. Monthly meetings of the

Coalition are supplemented by newsletters, Listservs, mailings, events, and almost daily contact between Coalition members and project staff.

The HHH Coalition Strategy

The HHH Coalition has positioned itself to serve the broadest community in West Hill and adjacent neighborhoods, through a two-step process:

First, the building of an infrastructure for sustained health promotion to include:

- Biweekly screenings for glucose, cholesterol, and blood pressure
- Referral to physicians and nurses at a local health clinic without concern for ability to pay
- Access to health and wellness information
- Evidence-based physical activity/exercise, nutrition, and other health promotion programs
- Initiation of the evidence-based Diabetes Self-Management Program and other diabetes self-management educational approaches
- Healthy eating instruction and demonstration
- A walking club utilizing current resources and/or restructuring resources for this purpose
- Contacts with local grocery stores (bodegas) to improve healthy food choices and initiation of a small matching grants program to support stocking of healthy food options
- Engagement of food pantries in increasing healthy food choices and related cooking demonstrations
- A matching grants program to establish safe indoor exercise space in community organizations
- Development of a Health Promotion Buddy System to increase participation by individuals

There is a heavy reliance on evidence-based programs and approaches drawn from CEACW's prior and current work with caregivers and with persons with chronic illness, and from the best or proven practices recommendations of Coalition members.

Second, the **Biggest Winner** contest united, motivated, and activated community members over a nine-month period as they took steps toward making healthy choices: engaging in healthy behaviors, seeking health care, increasing participation in healthy food tastings and community dinners, purchasing healthy foods, physical activity/exercise, and reducing glucose and cholesterol levels and blood pressure (where indicated). The contest provided opportunities for participants to earn points for engaging in these healthy behaviors, and it culminated with a prize drawing from a pool of participants who demonstrated sustained effort throughout the contest period.

The *Biggest Winner* Contest

The *Biggest Winner* contest encouraged adult residents of the West Hill and surrounding neighborhoods to join in creating heart-healthy communities, and it created an incentive to learn more about health, to seek routine and preventive health care, to engage in physical activity, and to eat right. The original idea for this *Biggest Winner* project was developed by HHH coalition members, influenced by the "Biggest Loser" television program. However, community members were not interested in a single focus on weight loss; instead they helped develop a project that targeted the three major means of health-related behavioral change: nutrition, physical activity, and healthcare monitoring/management. The contest was designed to reward changes made in each of these areas, with higher awards when more than one area was targeted by the participant.

Local media from a large regional newspaper to neighborhood and faith community newsletters and radio and television stations were engaged to publicize the program and to help build both motivation and momentum for the project. The Coalition also worked with local businesses to obtain many of the prizes.

A combination of paid and volunteer staff supported the initiative. CEACW provided paid staff and student interns to handle logistical issues, to manage screenings and delivery of evidence-based programs, and to oversee data collection and evaluation. Similarly, Koinonia Primary Care provided a medical director to the project and physicians and nurses to support screening and physician referrals. Staff from several health plans, other medical centers, social services providers, and local businesses provided support, helped underwrite many activities, and provided prizes and other incentives. Over time, a cadre emerged of retired nurses, community health advocates, faith community leaders, and other volunteers who helped extend the offering of screenings, delivery of classes, and recruitment of participants. Social work and medical students worked in the project as volunteers and as part of internships. A noteworthy development was the number of students who agreed to be trained as leaders in evidence-based health promotion programs, greatly extending the reach in the community of these programs. Students were also critical in staffing large-scale screening and health education efforts at community fairs and festivals.

Participants aged 18 and older who were identified through screening as being at risk for heart disease or diabetes, and others with a diagnosis of hypertension, heart disease, diabetes, or obesity were invited to participate in the program and received a scorecard to record achievements. Many participants were recruited at community screening events, and others by their physicians, and more than 40 local agencies and faith communities agreed to be community portal sites providing information and often recruiting the most hard to reach as participants. Again, volunteers and students were critical in staffing these efforts.

The opportunity to earn points was key to participant retention, with points awarded for activities like visiting the doctor; going to health screenings; regular participation in walking clubs; attendance at educational health promotion and physical activity classes, healthy taste testing events and healthy community dinners; and purchasing healthy foods. A prime focus was to encourage at least 100 participants to stay with the program for 9 months, but others were encouraged to join at any time and were also eligible for the interim prizes. Only those participating for at least 4 months were eligible for the grand prize.

A public event to award the grand prize resulted in considerable media attention, and the city's mayor drew the name of the winning participant. Among the finalists were individuals who had lost over 100 pounds and/or had so reduced their blood glucose that they were no longer considered diabetic. Many others were found to have brought elevated blood glucose or cholesterol under better control, increased the amount of exercise they completed each day, ended a cycle of repeat hospitalizations, and/or dramatically changed eating and food purchase habits.

A Health Careers Perspective

For many of the students who participated, the experience was their first in a health disparities community, and many reported a better appreciation of the challenges faced by the people they were working with. However, the biggest contribution of the project to their preparation as future practitioners lay in helping the students to see themselves as facilitators and partners in building health management capacity, rather than solving problems for their patients/clients. On the one hand, students were able to see the many challenges people in West Hill face—to better understand the reasons for nonadherence to treatment plans and how the environment contributes to symptoms and the multiplication of chronic conditions. On the other hand, over time the students also came to see the strengths in individual community members, grassroots organizations, and storefront churches dedicated to the West Hill community; the interest among patients/clients in better managing their health conditions; and the potential for greater success when they actively worked with community partners and volunteers to build screening opportunities, increase access to physician care, and promote self-management. Finally, they were inspired by the people they met and their success stories, often despite incredible adversity.

Inspiration should always be a part of educational experiences, but theoretical understanding, skills training, and preparation for future professional practice are equally critical. The "why" of the internship experience was emphasized by improving the interns' understanding of the challenges of health disparities communities, grounding in participatory practice, direct involvement in recruitment, screening, and follow-up activities, and engagement as evidence-based program leaders. Particular attention was drawn to the health impacts of transportation, insurance, and physician access barriers, as well as to the lack of attention to self-management, and to the physician's or social worker's role in lowering these barriers. There was also encouragement of more collaborative and interdisciplinary practice, "partnering with" rather than "caring for" the patient/client, and there was an increased emphasis on advocacy. Most importantly, the experiences were designed to recast older, infirm, low-income individuals from passive recipients of what health services have to offer (if we choose to offer) into resilient community members who, despite many barriers, may be actively engaged in the long term in the management of their own health and in the health of their community.

It should be noted that there were some challenges related to student involvement. For instance, most medical, nursing, and social work internship experiences are clinic or facility based, and the competencies targeted are more frequently around the successful demonstration of clinical skills; participatory or empowerment practice and collaboration are rarely measured, and activities to overcome policy and access barriers are not often highly valued. Again, the engagement by Coalition members of field staff from local professional schools, the willingness of staff at CEACW and Koinonia to serve as field instructors and supervisors, and the co-designing of field and internship placements to meet required standards while being engaged in the Coalition's activities proved critical. However, in the spirit of participatory action, the welcoming of students by community members and the interest by many students in participating in the full range of the Coalition's activities was equally essential.

Conclusion

The decades ahead will be both challenging and exciting for health care. Burgeoning population growth among the elderly and ethnic minorities, the sustaining of longevity among those with chronic illness, the political imperative to control healthcare costs, and concern for equality and the promotion of quality of life will increase attention to chronic disease management issues in health disparity communities. The danger is that interventions will continue to be done *to* or *for* individuals and their communities, rather than in partnership with them, perpetuating dated methods and power differentials that have ill proven their ability to support change in the most challenging patients. As one of the authors frequently says of his community, "We are sick and tired of being sick and tired." Health disparity communities are not interested in being passive—they wish to be active. The HHH Coalition is one example of the new approaches to disease management being investigated, including the recasting of patient activation and self-management, and the new relationships being forged. Interesting and compelling opportunities await students entering nursing, social work, and medicine that can further advance such cooperative work in the future.

References

Bandura, A. (1993). Perceived self-efficacy in cognitive development and functioning. *Educational Psychologist*, 28(2), 117–148.

Elder, J.P., Arredondo, E.M., Campbell, N., Baquero, B., Duerksen, S., Ayala, G., Crespo, N.C., Slyman, D., & McKensie, T. (2010). Individual, family and community environmental correlates of obesity in Latino elementary school children. *Journal of School Health*, 80(1), 20–30.

Feldman, P.J., & Steptoe, A. (2004). How neighborhoods and physical functioning are related: The role of neighborhood socioeconomic status, perceived neighborhood strain and individual health risk factors. *Annals of Behavioral Medicine*, 27(2), 91–99

Ferretti, L.A. (2009). *Healthy Hearts on the Hill Coalition final project report*. Albany, NY: Center for Excellence in Aging & Community Wellness.

Ferretti, L.A., & Kintner, E. (2010). *Biggest Winner Project final report*. Albany, NY: Center for Excellence in Aging & Community Wellness.

Fortune, E., McCallion, P., & Briar-Lawson, K. (in press). Building evidence-based intervention models. In E. Fortune, P. McCallion, & K. Briar-Lawson (Eds.), *Practice research for the 21st century*. New York: Columbia University Press.

Glasgow, R.E. (2006). RE-AIMing research for application: Ways to improve evidence for family practice. *Journal of the American Board of Family Practice*, 19(1), 11–19.

Hibbard, J.H., Greene, J., Becker, E.R., Roblin, D., Painter, M.W., Perez, D.J., Burbank-Schmitt, E., & Tusler, M. (2008). Racial/ethnic disparities and consumer activation in health. *Health Affairs*, 27(5), 1442–1453.

Hibbard, J.H., Mahoney, E.R., Stock, R., & Tusler, M. (2007a). Self-management and health care utilization: Do increases in patient activation result in improved self-management behaviors? *Health Research and Educational Trust*, 42(4), 1443–1463.

Hibbard, J.H., Mahoney, E.R., Stock, R., & Tusler, M. (2007b). Development and testing of a short form of the Patient Activation Measure. *Health Services Research*, 40(6), 1918–1930.

Prochaska, J.O., Redding, C.A., & Evers, K.E. (1997). The transtheoretical model and stages of change. In K. Glanz, F.M. Lewis, & B.K. Rimer (Eds.), *Health behavior and health education*. San Francisco: Jossey-Bass.

Stange, K.C. (2010). Actionable ideas to improve health and health care. *Annals of Family Medicine*, 8, 82–84.

Stringer, E. (2007). *Action research*. London: Sage

Van Houtven, G., Honeycutt, A., Gilman, B., McCall, N., Throneburg, W., & Sykes, K. (2008). *Costs of illness among older adults: An analysis of six major health conditions with significant environmental risk factors*. RTI Press publication No. RR-0002-0809. Research Triangle Park, NC: RTI International. Retrieved [Feb 18 2010] from http://www.rti.org/rtipress.

Chapter 6

The Changing Face of Aging: New Challenges, New Opportunities

Shelli Cordisco and Michelle M. Berry

The famous ad slogan of the late 1980s, "It's not your father's Oldsmobile," was all about reinventing the car's outdated image to better appeal to a newer generation of drivers. Stoic (aka stodgy) respectability was moved aside to make way for sleek, cool sophistication. Much the same can be said about today's generation of elders and the changes they're evoking in the field of aging services. As the healthiest and wealthiest group of seniors in the history of mankind, elders today are redefining what it means to age successfully. Outward appearances may look the same, but beneath the gray is a whole new set of challenges and opportunities.

With significant advances in medicine, health care, and information technologies, it is no surprise that Americans are now living longer than in previous generations. Babies born in 1900 were generally expected to live about 45 years. Today, life expectancy at birth is closer to 78 years (Lichtenberg, 2007). People are now living so long, in fact, that aging services providers refer to three distinct groups over the age of 65 years: 65 to 74 years, 75 to 84 years, and 85 plus years. When viewed together, these groups present a continuum of vastly different needs.

Moreover, a reduction in the poverty levels among adults over the age of 65 years. The U.S Census found poverty levels in 1965 for persons over 65 years of age to be at 30% (U.S. Census bureau, 2009a), while recent data indicates that number has fallen to 13% (Henry J. Kaiser Family Foundation, 2008). This translates into one of the greatest social changes of the last quarter of the last century and can be related to a combination of public policy and corporate stewardship. The enactment of Social Security in 1935 and Medicare/Medicaid legislation in 1965, coupled with employer-sponsored pension and health plans, created steady retirement incomes for the first time in US history. And across the nation, adults born in 1940 have witnessed, on average, more than a sevenfold increase in their standard of living as real gross domestic product (GDP) has increased over 862% during this time (Summer, Friedland, Mack, & Mathieu, 2004).

Yet the tide continues to turn as the nation's "baby boomers"[1] move onto the aging scene. Less than one year from now (2011), more than 78 million baby boomers will begin turning 65. While this newest cohort of older adults is expected to move into their golden years with unprecedented discretionary incomes and even healthier lifestyles than their parents, it is inevitable that they too will move toward their own brand of dependency. For instance, an editorial from *The Journal News* (2006) asserted that new and soon-to-be retirees in both the private and public sectors are now facing shrinking pension plans and entitlement programs that are being threatened simply by the weight of demand. This editorial's stark forecast regarding the social and public policy challenges of the elder boom acknowledges the difficulties in maintaining the pensions, Social Security checks, Medicare for all seniors, and Medicaid for the poorest that the American society has come to expect. By all accounts, it appears the days of stable, reliable retirement incomes—as enjoyed by baby boomers' parents—are numbered. Add to this the likelihood that boomers' parents may still be living, and/or that boomers may have young children at home or adult children who they are supporting financially. All of this means that at a relatively advanced stage of their own lives, boomers may have a full plate of family responsibilities (Pew Research Center, 2005).

With the coming of old age for baby boomers, American society has entered an historic transition period where service providers and consumers alike must learn to balance long-standing attitudes with new expectations, and longstanding service models with new ways to offer and finance aging services and long-term care. In short, it really isn't our fathers' Oldsmobile anymore.

Public Policy Drives Elder Services

By signing the original Social Security Act of 1935 into law as part of the New Deal,[2] President Franklin D. Roosevelt became the first US president to advocate for the protection of older adults. In addition to several general welfare provisions, this act created a retirement benefit meant to provide continued income to workers who retired at age 65 or older. Forty years later (1965) under President Lyndon B. Johnson's administration, Medicare and Medicaid[3] were added as health coverage amendments to the Social Security legislation. Also in 1965, Congress passed the Older Americans Act (OAA) to address a growing awareness among policy makers of the need for community social services targeting older adults. Both the Medicare and Medicaid amendments contained in the Social

---

[1]Baby Boomer—defined by the US Census Bureau as someone born between 1946 and 1964.
[2]The New Deal refers to the economic programs passed by Congress during the Roosevelt administration in response to the Great Depression.
[3]Medicare is an entitlement program funded entirely by the federal government that provides health insurance coverage primarily to people who are age 65 and over. Medicaid is a joint federal-state program that provides health insurance coverage primarily to individuals of low income who meet certain eligibility requirements.

Security Act of 1965, as well as the new OAA legislation, were part of President Johnson's Great Society[4] reforms.

Under the auspices of the OAA, the Administration on Aging (AoA) was established to oversee grants awarded to states and to act as the federal liaison on matters regarding older adults. Typically, the OAA must be reauthorized by Congress every 5 years. In advance of the most recent reauthorization of the OAA, a White House Conference on Aging (WHCoA) was held in December 2005 in Washington, DC. It was the fifth WHCoA in history, and like its predecessors, its purpose was to make recommendations to the president and Congress to help guide national aging policies for the next 10 years and beyond.[5] The top two resolutions adopted by the 1200 delegates attending the WHCoA were the reauthorization of the OAA and the development of a coordinated and comprehensive long-term care strategy. Subsequently, the Act was reauthorized in 2006, with provisions that support the development of a national long-term care strategy. The Act is scheduled to be reviewed and updated again in 2011.

Today, the OAA continues to drive the AoA's service delivery of social and nutrition initiatives for adults who are primarily age 60 years and older. According to the AoA's website:

> [The Older Americans Act] authorizes a wide array of service programs through a national network of 56 State agencies on aging, 629 area agencies on aging, nearly 20,000 service providers, 244 Tribal organizations, and 2 Native Hawaiian organizations representing 400 Tribes. The OAA also includes community service employment for low-income older Americans; training, research, and demonstration activities in the field of aging; and vulnerable elder rights protection activities. (U.S. Department of Health & Human Services, 2009)

Home- and community-based long-term care has been a consistent focus of the OAA since 1965 (O'Shaughnessy, 2009). Currently, twelve AoA-sponsored initiatives fall under this core program category, which is intended to help older adults maintain their independence in their own homes and communities. The OAA is rather prescriptive when it comes

---

[4]The Great Society refers to the largest national reform movement since the New Deal. In addition to Medicare, Medicaid and OAA legislation, the Great Society's "war on poverty" social welfare agenda included initiatives such as: Head Start preschool education and health programs; Job Corps teen job training; and Volunteers in Service to America (VISTA) assistance for poor neighborhoods.
[5]The 2005 WHCoA theme, "The Booming Dynamics of Aging: From Awareness to Action," focused on the aging of today and tomorrow, including the 78 million baby boomers who began to turn 60 in January 2006. The WHCoA hosted approximately 1200 delegates selected by governors, members of Congress, the National Congress of Americans Indians (NCAI), and the WHCoA Policy Committee. Delegates voted on 50 resolutions they considered priorities and worked together to recommend innovative solutions reflecting actions that might be taken by federal, state and local governments, tribal organizations, business and industry, communities and individuals to prepare for the challenges and opportunities of an aging nation. http://www.whcoa.gov/

to some of these initiatives, such as Nutrition Services;[6] however, the Act offers broader leeway in service provision for other initiatives. One such example is the Aging and Disabled Resource Center Program (ADRC). Since 2003, this collaborative effort between AoA and the Centers for Medicare and Medicaid Services has made grants available to 47 states to support the development of local Aging and Disabled Resource Centers. The purpose of these centers is to provide "one stop shopping" for anyone, regardless of age or income, in need of information on long-term care and other related services.

Like these centers, most area agencies on aging (nonprofit entities or regional, county, or city government; also referred to as "AAAs") support the development and promotion of the AoA-sponsored National Family Caregiver Support Program, another of the 12 Home and Community Based Long Term Care initiatives. The specific set of supports available locally under this program, however, is designed to meet the particular needs of residents living in the area being served. Thus, a caregiver support program in Vermont might look quite different from one in Arizona. The same holds true for other AoA initiatives that fall under the core program categories of Health, Prevention and Wellness, and Elder Rights Protection.

The questions local providers ask when designing services are varied, yet the area's demography provides a basic blueprint from which to launch programming: Is the service intended for rural or urban seniors, or both? What transportation systems exist? What assistance is available from other community agencies to support service delivery? Does the service target frail, vulnerable oldest elders or healthy, active new retirees? What is the percentage of home ownership among older adults in the community? What education levels did these older adults attain? How do they receive their information?

Moving forward, it will be especially important to differentiate between the needs of our nation's oldest elders born during the Depression and who served in World War II, versus our youngest elders—the baby boomers—born between 1946 and 1964. While reluctant to identify themselves as "old," baby boomers are more likely than previous generations to embrace, use, and seek out innovative technologies to enhance their lifestyles. Likewise, senior housing trends are beginning to favor efficient, functional designs that emphasize efficiency rather than spaciousness. In addition, civic engagement and volunteerism are increasingly sharing the stage with travel, second careers, and lifelong learning opportunities. These trends all attest to the need to create a mix of services and products that is capable of evolving to meet the changing needs of a rapidly aging population.

In the words of Dr. Paul Hodge, JD, MBA, MPA, chairperson, Global Generations Policy Institute and Director, Harvard Generations Policy Program, when he addressed the Policy Committee in 2004:

> While many experts, popular pundits and the press have made predictions about how
> the aging of the baby boomers will affect the United States, in actuality, no one really

---

[6]Nutrition Services includes Congregate Nutrition Services, such as those served in senior community centers, and Home-Delivered Nutrition Services such as Meals on Wheels.

knows with any certainty what will happen. What is clear is that the policy implications and ramifications are unprecedented in history. America's graying will transform politics, retirement systems, health care systems, welfare systems, labor markets, banking and stock markets. It will force a re-thinking of social mores and prejudices, from issues of age/gender discrimination in the job market to end-of-life care. Whether that transformation is positive or negative will depend on planning and preparation that must begin today. (White House Conference on Aging, 2005, p. 1)

Aging Demography Drives Elder Services

As one of the greatest feats of the last century, increasing longevity in the United States is now making way for dramatic growth in older populations through the first half of the twenty-first century. Since 1900, the percentage of Americans age 65 years and older has tripled (from 4.1% in 1900 to 12.8% in 2008), with the number of these older adults having increased from 3.1 million to 38.9 million (Figure 6-1). By 2040, it is projected that this number will reach 80 million. This means that for the first time in our nation's history, one out of every five Americans will be age 65 or older. These demographic shifts carry profound implications for our society.

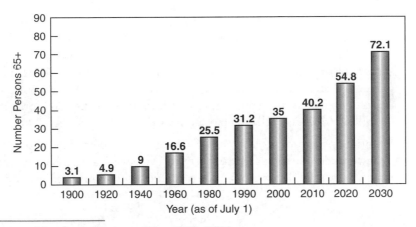

Figure 6-1   Number of Persons 65+, 1900–2030

Projections for 2010 through 2050 are from: Table 12. Projections of the Population by Age and Sex for the United States: 2010 to 2050 (NP2008-T12), Population Division, U.S. Census Bureau; Release Date: August 14, 2008.
The source of the data for 1900 to 2000 is: Table 5. Population by Age and Sex for the United States: 1900 to 2000, Part A. Number, Hobbs, Frank and Nicole Stoops, U.S. Census Bureau, Census 2000 Special Reports, Series CENSR-4, Demographic Trends in the 20th Century. This table was compiled by the U.S. Administration on Aging using the Census data noted.

It is further expected that as people live longer, the rate of growth of our nation's oldest elders will exceed that of any other age group. Should mortality rates continue to decline as expected, the 5.5 million Americans age 85 and older in 2007 could experience a nearly fourfold increase by 2040. It was noted in the final report of the 2005 White House Conference on Aging that such a trend would have a significant influence on both health and long-term care because use of formal and informal healthcare services increases with age (White House Conference on Aging, 2005).

Additional aging demographic highlights as reported in the AoA's *A Profile of Older Americans: 2009*,[7] along with some potential implications of the statistics for the future of elder services design and delivery, are (see also Figure 6-2):

- About 31% of noninstitutionalized older persons live alone (8.3 million women, 2.9 million men); with 50% of women age 75 and over living alone.
  - Potential Implications: With nearly one-third of community-based older adults living alone, providers of healthcare and support services are challenged to develop and implement strategies to reduce the risks of isolation (e.g., depression and other mental illnesses, self-neglect, poor nutrition, lack of physical and mental stimulation) and to promote social engagement among growing numbers of homebound elders. Key solutions will focus on innovative technologies that bridge the distance between home and community.
  - About 471,000 grandparents aged 65 or more had the primary responsibility for their grandchildren who lived with them in 2008. Taking this finding one step further, the total number of grandparents at any age who had the primary responsibility for their grandchildren who lived with them in 2008 was more than 2.5 million, with the majority falling into the age 50-to-64-year-old range. This total represents a 4% increase over the 2000 total of 2.4 million (U.S. Census Bureau, American Community Survey, 2008).
  - Potential Implications: The trend of increasing numbers of grandparents raising grandchildren has led to emerging evidence that this caregiving role poses several specific areas of concern, including unfamiliarity with updated

[7]A Profile of Older Americans: 2009 was developed by the Administration on Aging (AoA), U.S. Department of Health and Human Services. The annual Profile of Older Americans was originally developed and researched by Donald G. Fowles, AoA. Saadia Greenberg, AoA, developed the 2009 edition.

educational policies and services that can look much different from the grandparent's parenting days. Key solutions will involve moving beyond basic information and referral services to a comprehensive system of supports that connect grandparents and their grandchildren to programs, assistance, and services that decrease risks for school failure and other social consequences that could diminish positive life outcomes (Whitely & Kelly, 2007).

- Minority populations are projected to increase from 16.3% of the elderly population in 2000 (5.7 million) to 20.1% in 2010 (8.0 million) and then to 23.6% in 2020 (12.9 million). These figures translate into an anticipated 126% increase in the older minority population in only 20 years, versus a 56% increase in the older white population.

  - Potential Implications: As recognized by the AoA and the nation's network of aging services providers, older minority populations are especially at risk of chronic health conditions, social isolation, and poverty. An increasingly diverse (both racially and ethnically) aging population emphasizes the need for culturally competent and linguistically appropriate services that are easily accessible. Key solutions will require "increasing access to practical, nontraditional, community-based interventions for reaching older individuals and their family caregivers who experience barriers to home and community-based services due to language and low literacy as well as other barriers directly related to cultural diversity" (U.S. Administration on Aging, 2009, p. 6).

- From 2007 to 2008, only 3.7% of older persons moved, as opposed to 13.1% of the under-65 population; and of those who did move, only 20.1% moved out of state. Moreover, in 2008, about half (51.2%) of persons 65 and over lived in nine states: California, 4.1 million; Florida, 3.2 million; New York, 2.6 million; Texas, 2.5 million; Pennsylvania, 1.9 million; and Illinois, Ohio, Michigan, and New Jersey each had well over 1 million (Figure 6-2).

  - Being less likely than any other age group to change their residence, older adults prefer to age in place. In addition, the proportion of older persons in the population varies considerably by state, with some states experiencing much greater growth in their older populations. While most older people live in adequate, affordable housing, several health and social services have been identified as critical to maintaining independence and successfully aging in place. Key solutions include care management, health promotion services, education, socialization, recreation, and civic engagement opportunities (U.S. Health & Human Services, Community Innovations for Aging in Place, 2010).

Numbers	Number of Persons 65 and Older	Percent of All Ages	Percent Increase from 1998 to 2008
US Total (50 States + DC)	38,869,716	12.8%	13.0%
Alabama	641,667	13.8%	12.9%
Alaska	50,277	7.3%	49.8%
Arizona	862,573	13.3%	39.7%
Arkansas	407,205	14.3%	12.1%
California	4,114,496	11.2%	13.8%
Colorado	511,094	10.3%	27.2%
Connecticut	478,007	13.7%	1.9%
Delaware	121,688	13.9%	26.3%
District of Columbia	70,648	11.9%	–2.8%
Florida	3,187,797	17.4%	16.6%
Georgia	981,024	10.1%	29.9%
Hawaii	190,067	14.8%	20.1%
Idaho	182,150	12.0%	30.9%
Illinois	1,575,308	12.2%	5.3%
Indiana	813,839	12.8%	10.0%
Iowa	444,554	14.8%	3.1%
Kansas	366,706	13.1%	3.6%
Kentucky	565,867	13.3%	14.8%
Louisiana	540,314	12.2%	7.3%
Maine	199,187	15.1%	13.9%
Maryland	679,565	12.1%	14.9%
Massachusetts	871,098	13.4%	1.2%
Michigan	1,304,322	13.0%	6.6%
Minnesota	650,519	12.5%	11.6%
Mississippi	371,598	12.6%	10.5%

Figure 6-2   The 65+ Population by State, 2008

Source: Population data is from Census Bureau 2008 Population Estimates. State level poverty data is from the Census 2008 American Community Survey. National level poverty data is from the 2009 Current Population Survey/American Social and Economic Supplement.

Numbers	Number of Persons 65 and Older	Percent of All Ages	Percent Increase from 1998 to 2008
Missouri	805,235	13.6%	8.0%
Montana	137,312	14.2%	17.3%
Nebraska	240,847	13.5%	5.3%
Nevada	296,717	11.4%	48.1%
New Hampshire	169,978	12.9%	19.5%
New Jersey	1,150,941	13.3%	4.1%
New Mexico	260,051	13.1%	31.3%
New York	2,607,672	13.4%	7.6%
North Carolina	1,139,052	12.4%	20.3%
North Dakota	94,276	14.7%	2.5%
Ohio	1,570,837	13.7%	4.7%
Oklahoma	490,637	13.5%	9.4%
Oregon	503,998	13.3%	16.5%
Pennsylvania	1,910,571	15.3%	0.3%
Rhode Island	147,646	14.1%	−4.3%
South Carolina	596,295	13.3%	27.3%
South Dakota	116,100	14.4%	9.8%
Tennessee	819,626	13.2%	20.7%
Texas	2,472,223	10.2%	23.6%
Utah	246,202	9.0%	33.7%
Vermont	86,649	13.9%	19.4%
Virginia	940,577	12.1%	22.6%
Washington	783,877	12.0%	20.2%
West Virginia	285,067	15.7%	3.8%
Wisconsin	750,146	13.3%	8.6%
Wyoming	65,614	12.3%	18.2%
Puerto Rico	540,006	13.7%	

Figure 6-2 (Continued)

Needs of an Aging Population Drive Elder Services

The future needs of our nation's rapidly aging population will be as diverse and varied as the population itself. A popular, albeit unfortunate belief among Americans of all ages is that being old means being infirm. This mindset leads many students to think that career opportunities serving older adults are limited to healthcare positions in nursing, medicine, or therapies. As this chapter illustrates, however, older adults are increasingly in need of a broad range of services and supports to address a myriad of changing needs at different periods in their lives. This broader range of aging services runs the gamut from financial planning, travel arranging, and career counseling, to demography, urban planning, and home maintenance. More and more, demand is also growing for senior-targeted computer/technology maintenance and education, and niche sales and marketing, as well as social and intergenerational program development and management.

New services are already beginning to evolve in these areas. For instance, as previously stated, most older adults prefer to remain in their own homes as long as possible. And contrary to popular belief, older adults do not tend to move out of states—or even out of the counties—they have resided in for years. In testimony about the Older Americans Act, Secretary Carbonell described how seniors have an overwhelming preference to receive support at home even if they need 24-hour care. Indeed, many elders would prefer to die than move to institutional care. She ended by reiterating the need to provide more home and community-based services (Carbonell, 2005).

In response, the Remodeler's Council of the National Association of Home Builders (NAHB), in collaboration with the NAHB Research Center, the NAHB 50+ Housing Council, and AARP, has developed the Certified Aging-in-Place Specialist (CAPS) program to help consumers live comfortably and safely in their own homes as their needs and abilities change (American Association of Retired Persons, 2009a). A CAPS professional assesses an older person's home and identifies and/or makes home modifications that include widening doorways, installing outlets that are within reach, and/or positioning countertops at a convenient height for a wheelchair to roll under.

In addition, because they have most likely lived in their homes for years or decades, many older adults have accumulated a lot of "stuff" which poses a potential falling hazard as well as a stressor. Helping people de-clutter or prepare to move from their homes has become big business; and in many communities around the country professional organizers are available to assist people (for a fee, of course) with this oftentimes daunting chore.

Maintaining independence at home also involves socialization, recreation, and civic engagement opportunities. At every age of our lives it is important to maintain social connections for both our mental and physical well-being, but it is especially important that older adults stay active. The older a person becomes, the more at risk he/she is to experience the negative effects of loss and potential isolation due to the death of a spouse or a late life divorce, having children grow up and move away, retiring from work, and/or the passing of family members and friends. Despite these losses, however, the later phases of life can also bring positive changes, as illustrated in the two case scenarios that follow:

Case Scenario 1

While retirement often means leaving one set of daily contacts behind, it presents opportunities to pursue interests that have long been "on hold." Here is Janet's story:

> *Janet enjoyed her job as a casework supervisor for the local social services agency. She also had an interest in food preparation and service. On weekends, she catered meals for special events and became well known in the area for her innovative menus. After 30 years working in human services, Janet decided to retire at the age of 60.*
>
> *When a nearby country club heard she was retiring, they approached her about a seasonal position as an events planner. This would involve meeting with people who were planning weddings and other galas, developing the menus, and coordinating the events. Janet liked the fact that the job was not full-time, yet it was a reflection of an interest and expertise she had developed over many years. In this instance, she was leaving one set of daily contacts behind to cultivate a new set of colleagues and friends. At age 60, she was not yet ready for total retirement and wanted to stay actively engaged in the community.*
>
> *To enhance her skills at her new job, Janet might want to take advantage of educational opportunities to learn about event planning. She might also need guidance in menu planning, how to take advantage of buying local produce year round, or bulk purchasing perishable items. As a result, the needs she faces at this stage of her life are much different from traditional services that are available to older adults.*

Janet is a "young" elder. She is making a major life change, yet staying socially connected. What about elders in the later phase of the retirement years? What types of changes might affect their ability to stay connected, and what types of services might they need?

Case Scenario 2

Increasing life expectancies combined with declining rates of functional limitations among our nation's oldest elders means major life changes are likely to continue well beyond initial retirement years. Consider Helen and John's story:

> *Helen and John are in their early 80s. They have lived in the same home, in the same community, for over 50 years. Their three children are grown. Robert lives locally, but Marge and Linda have moved away.*

Robert has noticed that his parents are slowing down and that the big house they live in has become difficult for them to manage. His father is also in need of assistance with his physical care, and the situation is getting increasingly difficult for his mother to handle. Robert read in the local newspaper that a new senior housing complex is being built in his parents' neighborhood. He convinced them to apply for this housing, and their application was accepted.

Now Helen and John had to get the house ready to sell. They decided to engage a professional organizer to assist them in sorting through their belongings and weeding out a lifetime of accumulated possessions. They also needed to engage a contractor to make simple repairs that would increase the value of their home, as well as a decorator who could assist them in updating their décor.

Helen and John were making a major life change in giving up the home that they had lived in their entire adult lives. But by moving to a senior housing complex, they would have many opportunities to meet new people. Their new home included a clubhouse and planned activities. It was also wired to provide high-speed Internet access. Helen and John are interested in taking classes on Facebook and the Internet, and they need someone to come to their new home to network their laptop, printer, and fax machine. Helen is also thinking about taking a class on how to use Photoshop to scan the many years' worth of photographs she has in boxes.

Helen and John are "older" elders. Like Janet, they too are making major life changes while staying socially connected. In what ways do these scenarios reflect the values of consumer choice, control, and independence? How do the needs for service delivery differ between these scenarios? What age-related challenges are Helen and John likely to face next?

The Value of Social Connections Drives Local Initiatives in Broome County, New York

A primary function of local Area Agencies on Aging (AAAs) is community assessment and planning. In New York State, most AAAs are known as Offices for Aging and are operated by county governments. Offices for Aging operating within New York City are administered by the city government.

Broome County, New York, presents a glimpse of what's in store for the rest of the nation.[8] According to the Broome County 2000 Census, the percentage of residents age 60 years or older is 20.7%, which is substantially higher than both the state and national percentages of 16.8% and 16.2%, respectively. More recently, Binghamton University's

---

[8]Broome County, NY, is a mixed urban (with the city of Binghamton at its core) and rural county bordering Pennsylvania.

Geography Department estimated that 43,633 adults over age 60 (within the total population of 196,000 residents) would reside in Broome County in 2008. This projection represents a 5% increase since the 2000 US Census. Other recent trends show a 19% growth rate in the county's age 60 to 64 cohort, and an increase of almost 40% in the age 85 and over population (Broome County Office for Aging, 2007).

Since 1973, the Broome County Office for Aging has led the local aging services network to stay one step ahead of the aging boom by spearheading comprehensive, systemic planning and community-wide program development. To this end, the agency was instrumental in convening a group of 20 organizations and individuals to form the *Aging Futures Partnership* in 1989.

Today, the Partnership has grown and diversified to include more than 65 agencies representing consumers, municipal planners, private and public businesses, builders and real estate representatives, economic development specialists, educators, transportation planners and providers, and key decision makers in the fields of health care and human and aging services. The Partnership's vision is to realize an integrated long-term care delivery system that improves the quality of life for frail older adults, and that evolves to meet the changing needs and preferences of all older adults. Toward this end, the Partnership provides ongoing assessment of services and supports needed by seniors and their caregivers, in order to ensure that the community-based long-term care system responds to those needs. The initial needs assessment completed by the Partnership in the mid 1990s resulted in securing grants to build three senior centers, expanded chronic disease management and home repair programs, and gave us clear directions and goals for several years.

In 2002, the Partnership's success resulted in the award of a prestigious *Community Partnerships for Older Adults Program* grant from the Robert Wood Johnson Foundation. A key pursuit of this funding was to find and implement ways to promote social connections and thereby reduce the isolation of older adults. To focus planning efforts, the Partnership's core leadership group developed the Social Connections–Reducing Isolation Assessment Tool shown in Figure 6-3.

Tools such as this one assist planners when they are developing new programs and strategies for interventions by focusing their efforts on the target group in mind, rather than on an entire population.

Application of the Social Connections–Reducing Isolation Assessment Tool

Because the older adult population is as diverse as its needs, a person's ability to engage the system and take care of his or her own needs is identified by "Tiers." This designation indicates that people who fall into "Tier 1" are capable of using existing community "Supports and Services" to obtain the information they need. This triggers the design and

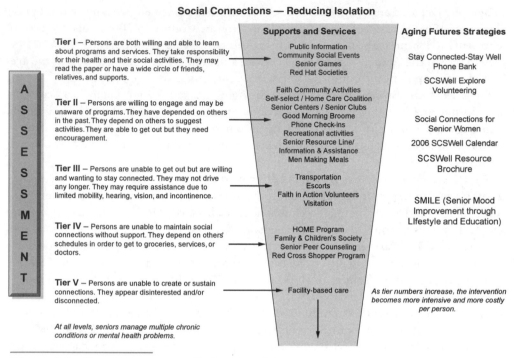

Figure 6-3 Social connections: Reducing isolation.
Designed by Aging Futures Partnership, Core Committee.

implementation of Aging Futures strategies that ensure that public information resources are up-to-date. People's ability to engage the system independently becomes increasingly limited as they move from Tier 1 to Tier V. As a result, the corresponding support systems and Aging Futures strategies designed to meet their needs become more detailed and intense.

Use of this planning tool led to the Partnership's development and/or implementation of several successful strategies to promote positive health and socialization practices among older adults. These include the Strike-Out Stroke, Powerful Tools for Caregivers, SMILE (Senior Mood Improvement through Lifestyle and Education), and Livable Communities initiatives.

Of special note, "**Social Connections for Senior Women . . . Women Sharing, Women Caring**" was launched in June 2005. This program promotes friendship building and the development of informal support networks among its female members. The program's goal is to enhance and empower the lives of older women via the sharing of ideas, experiences, and concerns related to aging and beyond. The Broome County Council of

Churches[9] coordinates the program and uses trained peer volunteers to lead weekly group meetings. An undergraduate student intern from Binghamton University recruits group members and trains the peer volunteer facilitators. Currently, six groups of 10 to 14 members are spread throughout the county; they meet in churches, the public library, senior centers, and even long-term care facilities.

The weekly group meetings are meant to foster new friendships that will eventually guide each group in a unique direction that meets the specific needs of its members. One group, for instance, has evolved into a weekly song fest. Sheet music is passed around, and the group sings songs they enjoyed from the big band era. Some friends have gone on bus trips together and meet outside the weekly meetings for lunch. A high degree of flexibility in how each group functions has helped ensure the program's success.

Another unique and prestigious opportunity came earlier to the Partnership in the summer of 2003 when the Community Foundation for South Central New York and the Stewart W. and Willma C. Hoyt Foundation jointly issued a special Request for Proposals (RFP). This opportunity allowed agencies in a five-county region to explain some of the most important needs they face and to propose projects that would make a significant impact on those needs. Of two awards totaling $150,000 that the foundations ultimately granted, one was proposed by Action for Older Persons, Inc. on behalf of the Aging Futures Partnership: **"A Multi-Media Public Awareness Campaign for Broome County's Older Adults and Their Caregivers."**

The proposal for this campaign was in direct response to newly collected Aging Futures data indicating that Broome County has a wealth of services for its growing population of older adults, yet too often the people who need those services most are unaware that they exist. This need to increase awareness of local aging services, combined with the need to provide simplified, educational messages to our older adults at the individual, caregiver, and community levels, had become an overarching and recurring theme throughout the Aging Futures Partnership's 18-month planning process.[10] Clearly, the community needed a better way to link older adults with organizations that were waiting to serve them.

With a $77,500 grant from the Community Foundation and Hoyt Foundation, in-kind dollars from WBNG-TV and Time Warner, and additional financial support from the Community Partnerships for Older Adults initiative of the Robert Wood Johnson Foundation, the Campaign was launched in February 2004 and ran through May 2005. Its primary accomplishments relate directly back to the original objectives outlined in the grant

---

[9]The Broome County Council of Churches, founded in 1941, connects volunteers from local faith communities, businesses, and organizations with tangible needs in the greater Binghamton area.
[10]The Aging Futures Partnership planning process was funded by a grant from the Community Partnerships for Older Adults Initiative of the Robert Wood Johnson Foundation for the period August 1, 2002 through January 31, 2004.

proposal. Specifically, the campaign was successful in meeting all of the following deliverables:

- A total of sixteen 30-second spot announcements were produced and televised.
- A total of 52 weekly *Senior Connections* interviews were coordinated and posted as video clips on WBNG-TV's *Senior Connections* webpage.
- A total of two phone banks were coordinated and televised.
- A total of four *Community Corner* programs were produced and televised.
- Outreach was conducted and printed education materials related to the Senior Resource Line and Broome County Elder Services Guide were distributed through a variety of methods.
- A documentary video was produced and duplicated, and is now being distributed to providers and consumers. This deliverable has the potential to be used as a building block for more targeted media messages in the future, and is perhaps the most tangible, unique, and replicable product to result from the campaign.
- Various secondary print media efforts were implemented.
- Multiple project evaluation measures were implemented, leading to the compilation of a comprehensive Outcomes *Report*.

An assessment of data obtained during the completion of campaign objectives indicates the following consumer-oriented outcomes and findings:

- Use of multiple and far-reaching media messages was an effective strategy to impact the campaign's target audiences. As expected, residents living within Broome County's urban core were reached most often and most consistently; however, consumer responses were also generated throughout other outlying counties (Tioga, Tompkins, Sullivan, Chenango, Cortland, Delaware, and Otsego) as well as the neighboring town of Susquehanna, PA.
- Consumer response trends demonstrated a dramatic immediacy of demand that tends to taper off and return to normal levels within a day or two of the service's on-air publicity. However, a more sustained level of demand was created when consistent messages were aired continuously over longer periods of time.
- Among the top anticipated needs of older adults (as self-reported by consumers), transportation was cited most (22%), followed by financial help and caregiver assistance (both at 19%), then help around the house (18%). And while consumers were willing to share their thoughts on potential needs in the future, they were much less eager to admit if they personally had any immediate and/or past need for services.

The campaign also affected the professional community in several significant ways; for instance, those participating agencies that incorporated action messages into their media announcements were better able to track an increase in demand for services. Ongoing education and media exposure, increased referrals, and new collaborative outreach opportunities were positive benefits reported consistently among participating agencies. Another positive factor to surface during the campaign was the Aging Future Partnership's ability to use newly established business relationships with media partners for other collaborative ventures. One overwhelmingly successful example was Aging Futures' and WBNG-TV's co-sponsorship of *Health Expo 2004.*

The last deliverable to be rolled out in April 2005 was the caregiver support video, *Now That Your Loved One Is Home: What Do You Do?* With more than 100 copies of this video released for viewing by families, friends, and caregivers of older adults as well as aging service providers, the campaign's positive influence on these populations is expected to continue well into the future.

Integral to the success of this campaign was the reliance on project staff who had solid backgrounds and experience working with similar media campaign models in the past. The original proposal, in fact, was modeled after two local multimedia campaigns that the Action for Older Persons' executive director had developed back in the early 1990s: *Success By Six*™ and the subsequent *Connecting with Kids*™ campaigns.

Likewise, AOP was fortunate to recruit a project intern who was soon to graduate from Binghamton University with a bachelor's degree in dual majors: cinema and human development. This intern's technical knowledge of video productions, combined with a sincere interest in the field of human services, made him an invaluable resource to this project. The agency's ability to shift this project internship to a paid communications specialist position further ensured the success of the campaign through its end date, since the original proposal underestimated the labor-intensive and time-consuming nature of the campaign once all of its strategies were up and running at the same time. The bottom line is that the whole community benefits when older adults remain tuned-in and connected. To this end, it behooves all of us to continue finding creative ways to support the social engagement of adults throughout all stages of the aging process.

Brain Fitness and Social Connections Drive the Use of Innovative Technologies

A daunting, negative effect of greater longevity is the prevalence of dementia in later life. According to MetLife Mature Market Institute's three-year study, *Boomers: The Next 20 Years,* currently Alzheimer's and the other types of cognitive impairment affect up to 50% of all adults age 85 and older. A greater likelihood of social isolation and/or experiences of loss in later life can also lead to depression, anxiety, and mental decline. In fact, studies suggest that people with the most limited social connections are twice as likely to die over a given period as those with the widest social networks, and many experts believe that social isolation may create a chronically stressful condition that accelerates aging (American Association of Retired Persons, 2009b.)

The good news is that a new generation of technology-based resources is offering the prospect of building general cognitive fitness based on the ability of the brain to generate

Box 6-1

"E-training" programs utilize technology to open new vistas for engagement with family and other significant members of one's social network, including physicians. Teaching older adults to use word processing and internet navigation systems can empower them to remain, and even become contributing members of society. Many opportunities exist for e-literate older adults to engage in paid work, volunteer activities and to provide informal help to others from the safety and comfort of their homes.

(Pew and Van Hamel, 2003)

new capabilities in response to mental stimulation. A recent study provided evidence that even video games hold some promise for improving late-life cognition (Marsiske, 2009). Other studies indicate that maintaining social connections in later life is key to preventing depression and related mental disorders. For example, the American Association of Retired Person's publication called *Taking Control of Brain Health* (2009b) cited several recent studies finding that people who engaged in leisure activities such as learning to play a musical instrument or dancing were less likely to develop dementia. Similarly, this publication cited that people with strong relationships had less mental decline and lived more active, pain-free lives without physical limitations.

These encouraging research results are coming at the same time that more and more older adults are taking active steps with physical exercise regimens to promote healthy aging and prevent disease. This desire to take control of one's physical health in later life now extends to wanting to maintain—and improve—one's mental fitness as well. In January 2006, 38% of Americans age 65 and older were going online (Pew Internet & American Life Project, 2010). Moreover, growing numbers of older adults are becoming attracted to online social networks like Facebook,[11] online communities focused on specific interests or life issues such as health, and video gaming systems like the Wii. These findings suggest there's no better time than the present to guide and encourage older adults' enthusiasm to participate in a technology-rich life (Box 6-1).

The 2010 debut of Action for Older Persons, Inc.[12] (AOP) TechSmart Cyber Center program is a prime example of how one local aging services agency located in Binghamton,

---

[11]On January 4, 2010, istrategylabs.com reported that the 55 and older audience on Facebook grew a whopping 922.7% in 2009. In January 2009 this population on FB consisted of 954,580 registrants. By January of 2010 this population had grown to 9,763,900 registrants.

[12]Action for Older Persons, Inc. (AOP) is a private, nonprofit agency that was established in 1967 to assist individuals by providing timely, accurate, and unbiased information in preparation for aging. AOP educates and collaborates to promote quality of life through the aging process for older adults, their families and caregivers.

New York, is taking full advantage of this current market boom of seniors seeking out "brain fitness" activities to expand on proven teaching modalities that have been used in the agency's computer education program since 2000. Full-capacity classes and waiting lists, along with students' wish list topics for future classes, attest to the critical need for upgraded computers and the availability of the latest technologies if the agency is to continue meeting the demands of these students. By striving to make technology available in its infinite variety (i.e., e-mail, webcams, games, shopping, downloading music, information seeking, scanning, web building, blogging, digital photography and editing), the TechSmart Cyber Center positions itself as a local forerunner in promoting cognitive fitness in later life.

A significant feature of the TechSmart program is that it weaves together several existing areas of expertise in one exciting initiative. Since 2000, AOP's Edward Zola, Jr. Computer Lab has offered introductory computer classes designed to fit the learning styles of older adults. In 2002, the excellence of AOP's computer education program was recognized by the New York State Coalition for the Aging, Inc., which awarded the program a 1st Place Senior Service Achievement Award. While most computer instruction at local senior centers is done by volunteers who may or may not have access to a set curriculum, AOP's recipe for success relies on a consistent, expert presence of paid staff instructors who teach from standardized, pilot-tested curricula, a model that directly carries over to TechSmart.

A related venture is AOP's partnership with New York State Senator Thomas Libous's BOOKS program that helped move the agency into intergenerational programming and takes advantage of innovative technologies to build connections across generations. AOP spearheaded the *Celebrity Read-Along* feature on the BOOKS website by recording and adding sound effects to the voices of local community leaders reading from children's books that relate to their life experiences (http://www.booksprogram.com/readalong). AOP also produced the interactive interviews that let children learn about the reader and his connection to the book while providing a unique way for older generations to share local history with our youth. This use of technology to build bridges between the ages is integral to TechSmart.

In short, the primary purpose of TechSmart is to enhance the quality of life among older adults with normal brain function, as well as those with mild cognitive impairment, by designing and offering technology-based education, services, and special events that help preserve and build upon the critical skills of reasoning, memory, and speed of processing within a socially supportive setting. Rather than simply focusing on learning computers as an end goal, TechSmart offerings seek to engage seniors in myriad ways whereby computer/technology use translates into broader lifestyle goals related to healthy living and healthy aging.

Clearly, the rapid rate of technological advancements mirrors the nation's rapidly aging population. How best to harness and expand the energies on both sides of this mirror is, indeed, an exciting challenge for consumers and professionals alike. It is the authors' belief that we must learn to balance best practices from existing programs with a liberal dose of risk-taking by investing in groundbreaking new strategies that push those existing programs toward modern solutions for the changing needs of tomorrow's elders.

In Conclusion

Aptly, the theme for Older Americans Month 2010,[13] *Age Strong! Live Long!* recognizes the diversity and vitality of today's older Americans who span three generations. As stated in the AoA's promotional materials about this annual recognition of the contributions of our nation's older citizens:

> [Today's older Americans] have lived through wars and hard times, as well as periods of unprecedented prosperity. They pioneered new technologies in medicine, communications, and industry while spearheading a cultural revolution that won equal rights for minorities, women, and disabled Americans.
>
> These remarkable achievements demonstrate the strength and character of older Americans, and underscore the debt of gratitude we owe to the generations that have given our society so much. But the contributions of older Americans are not only in the past.
>
> Older Americans are living longer and are more active than ever before. And with the aging of the baby boomer generation—the largest in our nation's history—America's senior population is expected to number 71.5 million by 2030.
>
> While keeping the growing population of older Americans healthy and active will increase the demand for senior services, what is remarkable is the extent to which older Americans themselves are supporting each other. As the new generations of seniors become better educated and more financially secure than their predecessors, they are spending more time making significant contributions in their communities through civic and volunteer opportunities.
>
> In fact, older Americans are a core component of service delivery to seniors—embodying and modeling the drive to *Age Strong! Live Long!* They volunteer at group meal sites and deliver food to homebound seniors; they act as escorts and provide transportation for older adults who cannot drive; they help seniors with home repair, shopping, and errands; and they provide vital counseling, information, and referral services. Their energy and commitment remind all Americans—not just senior citizens and their caregivers—to do their part to enhance the quality of life for older generations. (U.S. Department of Health and Human Services, May is older Americans month, 2010)

Perhaps more so now than at any other time in history, older adults are redefining what it means to be "old." As a nation, we would be wise to embrace the innovative, determined attitude of this *Age Strong! Live Long!* theme as we settle into our new image of aging.

---

[13]Historically, Older Americans Month has been a time to acknowledge the contributions of past and current older persons to our country, in particular those who defended our country. Every president since John F. Kennedy has issued a formal proclamation during or before the month of May asking that the entire nation pay tribute in some way to older persons in their communities. Older Americans Month is celebrated across the country through ceremonies, events, fairs and other such activities. http://www.aoa.gov/AoARoot/Press_Room/Observances/oam/oam.aspx

References

American Association of Retired Persons. (2009a). Certified aging-in-place specialists. Retrieved from: http://www.aarp.org/family/housing/articles/caps.html

American Association of Retired Persons. (2009b). Taking control of brain health. Retrieved from: http://www.aarp.org/health/brain/takingcontrol/engage_your_brain.html

Broome County Office for Aging. (2007). . . . bringing senior and services together. Plan for services 2009–2012. Retrieved from: http://www.gobroomecounty.com/files/senior/pdfs/completed%20plan%202009.pdf

Cabonell, J. (2005). Reauthorization of the Older Americans Act. Retrieved from: http://www.hhs.gov/asl/testify/t050517a.html

Henry J. Kaiser Foundation. (2008). Poverty rates by Age, States (2007-2008). U.S. Retrieved from: http://www.statehealthfacts.org/comparebar.jsp?ind=10&cat=1

Lichtenbeg, F. R. (2007). Why has longevity increased more in some state than in others? The role of medical innovation and other factors. *Medical Progress Report,* (No. 4). Manhattan Institute of Policy Research.

Marsiske, M. (2009). Intervening with late-life cognition: Lessons from the ACTIVE study. Retrieved from: http://www.agingconference.org/asav2/mindalert/pdfs/booklet_2008.pdf

O'Shaughnessy, C. (2009). The basics: Older Americans Act of 1965. National Health Policy Forum. Retrieved from: http://www.nhpf.org/library/the-basics/Basics_OlderAmericansAct_10-08-09.pdf

O'Shaughnessy, C. (2008). The aging services network: Broad mandate and increasing responsibilities. *Public Policy & Aging Report. 18* (3), 1.

Pew Internet and American Life Project. (2010). Demographics of internet users. Retrieved from: http://www.pewinternet.org/Static-Pages/Trend-Data/Whos-Online.aspx

Pew Research Center. (2005). *Baby boomers approach age 60: From the age of Aquarius to the age of responsibility*. Retrieved from http://pewresearch.org/pubs/306/baby-boomers-from-the-age-of-aquarius-to-the-age-of-responsibility

Summer, L., Friedland, R., Mack, K., & Mathieu, S. (2004). Measuring the years: State aging trends and indicators. Washington, DC: National Governors Center for Best Practices.

The Journal News. (2006, January 3). Attention, baby-boomers. Westchester, NY: Gannett News, Inc.

U.S. Census Bureau. (2008). *Projections of the Population by Age and Sex for the United States: 2010 to 2050 (NP2008-T12)*. Retrieved from http://www.census.gov/population/www/projections/summary tables.html

U.S. Census Bureau. (2008). *Census 2008. American community survey*. Retrieved from: http://factfinder.census.gov/servlet/DatasetMainPageServlet?_program=ACS&_submenu Id=&_lang=en&_ds_name=ACS_2008_1YR_G00_&ts=

U.S. Census Bureau. (2009). Historical poverty tables. (2009a). *2009 Current Population Survey/American Social and Economic Supplement*. Retrieved from: http://www.census.gov/hhes/www/poverty/histpov/hstpov3.html

U.S. Department of Health and Human Services. Administration on Aging. (2009). *A profile of older Americans: 2009*. Retrieved from http://www.aoa.gov/AoAroot/Aging_Statistics/Profile/2009/index.aspx

U.S. Department of Health and Human Services, Administration on Aging. (2009). *Community innovations for aging in place*. Retrieved from http://www.aoa.gov/AoARoot/AoA_Programs/HCLTC/CIAIP/Index.aspx

U.S. Department of Health and Human Services. Administration on Aging. (2010). *May is older Americans month*. Retrieved from http://www.aoa.gov/AoARoot/Press_Room/Observances/oam/oam.aspx

U.S. Department of Health and Human Services. Administration on Aging. (2009). Program announcement and grant application instructions. National Minority Aging Populations. Technical Assistance Centers. OMB Approval No. 0985-0018.

U.S. Department of Health and Human Services. (2009). *Older Americans act*. Retrieved from: http://www.aoa.gov/AoARoot/AoA_Programs/OAA/index.aspx

White House Conference on Aging. (2005). *The booming dynamics of aging: From awareness to action*. Executive Summary. Retrieved from: http://www.whcoa.gov/Final_Report_June_14nowater.pdf

Whitely, D. & Kelly, S. (2007). Grandparents raising grandchildren: A call to action. Retrieved from: http://chhs.gsu.edu/nationalcenter/docs/Grandparentsbroch2-8.pdf

Section III
Innovative Learning Activities

Chapter 7

Learning by Living ©: Living the Life of a Nursing Home Resident

Marilyn R. Cogliucci

> *Above all I learned that life is not perfect, but it does have its rewards if you listen and learn before it is too late.*
>
> —Edward, 81, Chelsea, MA

Introduction

America has a new demography. Life expectancy nearly doubled during the twentieth century, realizing a 10-fold increase in the number of Americans age 65 and older. The latest census estimated that 35 million people in the United States are over the age of 65 (Administration on Aging, 2002). This constitutes 12.4% of the total population, and it is estimated to increase to 20% by 2030 (US Census Bureau, 2005). Older people of today have the opportunity to live longer and, if fortunate enough, healthier lives. For those older adults in need of nursing home care, I contend it is far too easy for our society to dismiss them rather than embracing them as the wisdom keepers for future generations regardless of physical or cognitive ability. Although it is reported that 5% of America's older adults reside in nursing homes, the finer details reveal the following delineation of age categories for people living in nursing homes: 5% of 65- to 74-year-olds; 10% of 75- to 84-year-olds, and 15% of those 85 and older (US Census Bureau, 2005). The truth is that the reporting of data is inadequate in presenting details of life lived in a nursing home, or in conveying the opportunities and challenges associated with nursing home living. Additionally, those aged 65 years and older use more than 50% of healthcare resources. As the older population increases and lives longer, their healthcare utilization is predicted to increase dramatically (Lee, Wilkerson, Reuben, & Ferrell, 2004). Despite the growing elderly population, the number of geriatricians fell by a third between 1998 and 2004. It is estimated that by 2030 there will be only one geriatrician for every 7665 older adults (American Geriatrics Society [AGS], 2006), or a shortage of 28,000 geriatricians (Association of Directors of Geriatric Academic Programs [ADGAP], 2007; Alliance for Aging Research, 2002). Clearly, we are challenged in replacing the geriatricians going into retirement, let alone providing care for the country's growing elderly population. Also troubling is the decline in the number of applications to adult primary care training programs, while certain specialties such as plastic surgery and radiology receive a record number of applications (Gawande, 2007). One authority noted, "Whether we admit it or not, most doctors don't like taking care of the elderly" (Gawande, 2007, p. 4). As a result, the challenge for many of us who teach in the field of aging is to determine how best to motivate students, especially those in the health professions, to recognize the value of providing care to older adults.

In 2005, at the completion of my lecture on aging, a female student came to my office and stated, "Dr. G, I want to learn how to speak to institutionalized elders." Upon hearing this, my mind instantly engaged in a variety of ways. It was curious to me that she used the term "institutionalized" when this is a word I never use. My initial thought regarding her question was, "you speak to them as you would any adult." However, there was something in that moment that made me realize this response would neither be satisfying nor motivating for learning. Instead, I answered, "Would you live in a nursing home for 2 weeks as if you are an elder resident in order to find out?" There was a pregnant pause, her eyes grew wide, and then a choked "yes" was expressed. This was the beginning of the Learning by Living© project.

The Learning by Living Project, piloted in 2005, was designed and implemented at the University of New England College of Osteopathic Medicine, and since its inception medical and other health professions students have been "admitted" into nursing homes to live the life of an elder nursing home resident for a period of 2 weeks—24 hours a day, 7 days a week—complete with a medical diagnosis and "standard" procedures of care. Until this project, long-term care education in nursing homes was accomplished through traditional medical education methods; short visits to the nursing home with quick exits. However, according to White (2008), "Long-term care services represent a growing aspect of our medical system that receives little attention in medical education" (p. 75). Furthermore, medical student training and experiences in nursing homes are often viewed as negative, which mirrors the views expressed by the general public (White, 2008). The truth is, in our society, nursing homes receive negative attention. Learning by Living is therefore based on two premises for medical education in nursing homes: (1) older adults residing in nursing homes are human beings deserving of good care, respect, and "community" connection; and (2) medical students can attain medical care skills, including advanced relationship-building skills, with older adults from living the life of an older nursing home resident.

This project utilizes a qualitative ethnographic and autobiographic research design, whereby a "culture" is observed and reported by the researcher (student) living within an environment (in this case a nursing home). This chapter first presents three contributing perspectives that provided the impetus for the Learning by Living Project: (1) the author's personal views on aging; (2) western social constructs of aging; and (3) role of interpretive science in capturing the life lived experience that is the foundation of Learning by Living.

Contributing Issues

Personal Views of Aging

I was socialized to believe that aging was a positive occurrence. Throughout my childhood and adolescence my maternal grandparents were regarded with respect. The changes that evolved as they "aged" were not significant enough for me to categorize them as old. For example, even though my grandfather's hair had turned white, it happened at the age of 25, hardly an indicator of old age. My grandparents maintained their status of role models and mentors throughout my younger years. When my grandfather died at the age of 72 and my grandmother at the age of 79, it wasn't old age that *got them;* they got sick. It happened to my brother when he was 6, an uncle at the age of 45, a friend at 17. Old age was not associated with death or decline.

My grandparents had optimistic, inquisitive, and refreshing perspectives until the day they died, irrespective of their physical health. In retrospect I realized, from my memories of them, that there was much more to becoming old than chronological age. The model for aging that my grandparents imparted included involvement, fun, knowledge, growth, productivity, independence, health, and most importantly choice. During wellness or illness, their voices and choices were meaningful in our family. I realize there are others who may not be able to relate to my experiences. My family was fortunate to avoid the devastation that dementia, stroke, or other diseases and challenges associated with older age may bring; but we have also missed the gifts my colleagues share when caring for a loved one.

I never had the opportunity to ask my grandparents about their aging process, so I'll never know what it was like for them. What I have been able to do is read about the theories of aging that were prevalent in their time. As a gerontologist, I feel there was a discrepancy between the lives of my grandparents and the theories of aging that were applied to them. This variance has led me to search for elders' perspectives of aging through books written by older adults, videos of older peoples' lives, and most importantly, listening to their experiences and stories. I want to know what it means to grow old from the very people who are doing it rather than through the academic lenses of theory, research, and/or didactics.

Social Constructs of Aging

Age is simply a number. Numbers have the meaning that we assign to them. If age were the determinant of health, all people of the same age would be exactly alike by all health standards. But we know that is not true.

—Nancy, 72, Tucson, AZ

Old age is a difficult concept to describe precisely. Temporal definitions tend to define old age in relation to a certain number of birthdays one has had. Most commonly, in contemporary society, having reached the age of 65 a person is considered to be in the young-old category.[1] Defining age in this way may be artificial and not an applicable or accurate measure of old age. Although the possibility exists to determine when old age ends—since death, in the western culture, is considered to be terminal—it is difficult to establish when old age begins.

Role transformations undergone by older adults through the years in our society reveal a rise and fall pattern that may repeat itself. During colonial times older adults were revered, during the Industrial Revolution they were devalued, and now, as the pendulum swings once more, we are moving into a fraternity of young and old (Fischer, 1978). There is much to do to balance the pendulum. Ageism (Butler, 1975) and societal structures such as health care, Social Security, politics, and policies designed to address the needs of our older society are wedded to the disease-and-decline model typically associated with older age in our society. Tindell (1998) underscores this commonly held belief:

> I wondered if many people relate to others simply on the basis of their age and physical appearance. If that is true, then I believe those who do are really missing out on something, especially as they deal with older persons. If they look at the elderly and see only gray hair or wrinkly skin—if they notice nothing other than their use of walkers or canes or that they are in wheelchairs or that they can't see or hear very well—if that is the only way they see and relate to them, then unfortunately, everyone misses an enriching human encounter. (Tindell, 1998, p. 39)

Tindell, an older man at the time this quote was published, brings to the forefront that older people are clearly more than their physical attributes. Cole (1984), a cultural historian, has pointed out that the spectacular gains in longevity through scientific and technological advances have been accompanied by "widespread spiritual malaise . . . and confusion over the meaning and purpose of human life, particularly in old age" (p. 329). It is important to the spirit and generativity of America to gain knowledge and understanding of what growing old means to the people who are experiencing it. Reker and Wong (1988) suggest that "by learning more about how other people have lived their lives, one gains some understanding of how to live one's own life" (Reker & Wong, 1988, p. 215). I contend that in order to provide better care to older adults it is essential for practitioners to become aware of stereotypes and to increase their understanding of aging from multiple perspectives. The challenge before us, especially in health care, is to release stereotypes, ascertain *who* each older adult is, and provide care that honors aging as defined by the person. Economics of care often forces "institutionalization" where accommodations and staffing may be viewed as minimalist. In such settings our society has made up the story that the provision of health care is not particularly provided to individuals, although one would assume so. The intent then is to initiate more meaningful

---

[1]The young-old are 65 to 74; the old-old are 75 to 84; and the oldest-old are 85 years of age and older (Rieske and Holstege, 1996).

models of "practice" in the future for older people. The Learning by Living Project raises consciousness about assumptions and stereotypes associated with aged individuals who reside in a nursing home by providing an intense experiential education event that requires the student to be the ethnographic researcher.

There is a never-ending flow between society, science, and practice, and back again. If we don't begin to think outside the proverbial box for the preparation of our future health care practitioners, we are at risk of proliferating cookie cutter medical education.

Learning By Living©

Interpretive Science

Always remember that we get old outside but inside we have the same feelings, hopes, and beliefs as we did when we were young.

—Anne, 82, Kent, WA

As a gerontologist in a medical school, I feel challenged to spark the interest of future practitioners to care for older adults. By transforming conventional approaches to teaching it is possible to achieve an enhanced understanding of aging and what it means to be older. Living with older adults for an extended period of time stimulates learning by making it dynamic and personal, two components of interpretive science. My goal is to integrate theory, experience, and practice through reflection and action—praxis. It is the students' interpretations of their life lived as an elder in a nursing home that empowers the other residents and raises consciousness of the nursing home staff, administration, and family members of older residents. In the positivist world of traditional science, the physical world is the only reality that can be quantified. For example, traditional theories of aging created an image of aging based on younger persons' concepts of pathology. Older people were compartmentalized in the positivist world. An approach such as this limits the occasion to look beyond the empirical box that is devoid of individual experience and to interpret findings outside the lines of convention. The antithesis of the positivist paradigm is the social interpretive model.

Interpretive science is not limited to only one reality, the physical world. In fact, it acknowledges the existence of several realities. The symbolic realities of meanings, feelings, images, experiences, and knowing are in some ways more important than physical reality "because symbols have a much more direct and pervasive influence on human behavior" (Reker & Wong, 1988, p. 217).

These symbols constitute a reality that is self-evident both to the individual and to others who share the same reality of everyday life, and with whom one communicates and interacts (Berger & Luckmann, 1966). This multidimensional construct has the following related components: *cognitive*—making sense of one's experiences in life; *motivational*—the value system constructed by each individual that guides living and what goals we pursue, which is determined by our needs, beliefs, and societal norms; and *affective*—feelings of satisfaction and fulfillment to the pursuer accompany the realization of personal meaning (Reker & Wong, 1988).

True to the tradition, the interpretive approach should be devoid of underlying assumptions or should at least identify them to acknowledge their existence (the first step in consciousness raising). Observations are made, and qualitative data are collected. This method of research leads to the emergence of themes and developing patterns that generate explanations or theories (Glaser & Strauss, 1987). In Learning by Living, qualitative methods, phenomenological approaches to nursing home events, and behaviors and reactions of students who live as older adults are critical in representing the life of an older adult nursing home resident. This approach connotes gaining practical knowledge or wisdom through what one has encountered or undergone. This broadens the students' ability to interpret and understand how to communicate and work with older adults.

Methods

Learning by Living utilizes qualitative ethnographic and autobiographic research methodologies. Ethnography is a form of research whereby the researcher participates in people's daily lives for an extended period of time to: (a) watch what happens; (b) listen to what is said; (c) ask questions; and (d) collect information that increases understanding of the culture without purposefully altering the culture. These components focus on answering the questions: *What is it like to live in a nursing home; what does it mean to be a nursing home resident?*

There are three stages of the Learning by Living ethnographic immersion: (1) pre-fieldwork—Getting ready for the experience; (2) fieldwork—Living in the environment, which includes a diagnosis, "medication" regimen, group and solitary meals, and engaging in relationship building; and (3) post-fieldwork—Reflection on what occurred during fieldwork (Denzin & Lincoln, 1994). Qualitative note taking or journaling begins with the pre-fieldwork stage, usually 1 to 3 days prior to admission. These notes taken throughout the three stages of the research are the key data source for Learning by Living.

Students volunteer for this immersion research experience (since its inception, Learning by Living has been a volunteer project for all involved). A registration form is completed that collects demographic data as well as the student's assumptions about older adults and nursing homes, which is necessary for augmenting consciousness or what one believes to be true. An orientation is conducted prior to "admission" that provides information on how to prepare as a researcher and considerations for the affective domain of the research experience. The nursing home that volunteers to "admit" a student for 2 weeks also participates in an orientation that includes discussion of the parameters regarding what it means to have a student living in the environment for an extended period, staff preparation, and possible communication with residents and families.

Qualitative note taking involves presenting a descriptive and detailed account of the student's experiences, thoughts, and actions. Each entry requires day, date, and time accountability, as each student tends to write at varying times of the day or when presented with a significant event. Notes include subjective accounts—"my" feelings as a younger person living in a nursing home—and objective accounts—"my" thoughts as a medical student. While the student is living in the nursing home, his or her notes are reviewed daily, and I maintain periodic contact with the student during the stay—as a dutiful daughter might for an elder parent. Constant review of the student's field notes is critical to ensure that data collection is effective and meets qualitative research standards. This process also monitors each student's well-being as s/he experiences a new culture. Based on past developments in qualitative ethnographic research and in this project in particular, the 10- to 14-day period assists with: (1) allowing the culture to get desensitized (approximately 4 days) to the new member (the student) so that daily activities fall into routine again; (2) providing the student with the feeling that he or she is part of the culture; (3) allowing the student to experience the changes in shifts from weekdays to weekends; and (4) permitting time to build relationships with residents in the nursing home.

To date, nursing homes have provided a bed and meals at no cost, and they design a medical condition for the student to "live" with. Students are required to be proficient note takers since these are the basis for all data. Other key issues to attend to prior to admission are the contract with the nursing home, determination of dates, services, rules, and preferred debriefing for the staff with the student at the close of the project experience.

Data Analysis

Data (students' notes) were analyzed and categorized into themes revealing key impressions and experiences of life lived as an elder nursing home resident, relationships formed, and lessons learned. Analysis involved: (1) reading through the text, making margin notes, forming initial codes; (2) formatting transcripts and downloading into QSR NVivo computer software; (3) conducting axial coding—causal condition, context, intervening conditions, strategies, consequences; (4) conducting open coding—categories, properties, dimensionalized properties; and (5) conducting selective coding and development of student's perspectives that entails identifying and listing statements of meaning in relation to "what it means to live the life of an elder nursing home resident."

QSR NUD*IST Vivo (Non-numerical Unstructured Data*Indexing, Searching, and Theorizing), also known as N-Vivo 2 (2004) software, is a qualitative data analysis program. Complete transcripts in addition to researcher comprehension, qualitative research ability, and interpretation are critical components to comprehensive data analysis. It is not the intention of this data analysis section to provide or explain the details of NVivo; however, some specific steps are necessary for qualitative data analysis with NVivo, including: (a) format data transcripts to import into NVivo; (b) code data through *node*[2] creation

---

[2]A "node" in NUD*IST is equivalent to a "code" or "theme" in manual methods of qualitative research.

techniques that are similar to the manual qualitative techniques of cut and paste; and (c) compare and contrast data with other concepts and/or nodes throughout the process. Project evaluation is ongoing as data are collected with each student "admission." Data are stored in NVivo files for continued and/or future analysis.

Results

> *What the qualitative researcher is interested in is not truth per se, but rather perspectives.*
> —Taylor and Bogdan, 1984, p. 98

For each student there were four stages of experiences: (1) arriving at the nursing home, (2) first days at the nursing home, (3) daily life at the nursing home, and (4) leaving the nursing home. Within the period of admittance and leaving, five themes were prevalent: (1) acclimation, (2) dependence, (3) daily life, (4) life as an elder resident, and (5) routine/change.

The following are sample quotes from each phase that are reflective of most students' experiences.

Pre-Admission Visit

I was unbelievably nervous, sick to my stomach actually. I dreaded every minute that I would be staying there. To me it felt like a prison, but I felt it was something I needed to do, especially to be the kind of doctor I wanted to be. Dr. G wanted me to visit with the nursing home before I actually moved in which I agreed would be a great idea. It may either make me even more nervous or ease my worries. It definitely eased me. [Female, 2006]

Author's Note: Some students are admitted into nursing homes without a pre-admission visit. There are nursing homes that have 70% or more of their admissions from hospitals. Students admitted without a prior visit are considered "hospital admits," which in reality means there is no opportunity to see the environment prior to admission.

First Day

I've been in a wheelchair now for about two hours. And my lower back is killing me. Only one of the past five people who have entered my room has sat down (on my bed) to look me in the eye, and not down to me. I never realized how much that mattered. Until today. [Male, 2008]

Author's Note: A longitudinal outcome of this research has been that students understand the importance of communication, including voice tone, personal appearance, body position, word cadence (how fast or slow a person speaks), and eye contact. And that these forms of communication may be even more important than words.

Daily Life—Day 4

I am homesick. I got hit with it very hard just now. I feel very alone. I am making great friends and it is wonderful here but I miss my old life. . . . But remembering my "old life" really makes it feel so far away. I don't remember driving my car here, I don't remember living in my house. I mentioned this to the ladies here and they asked me to think about how they feel and I couldn't fathom it. [Female, 2005]

Author's Note: In ethnographic research it takes about 3-4 days for the student, residents and staff to "settle in." After this period of time, the environment gets desensitized to the research that is going on and life in the nursing home reverts back to "normal." At this point, students begin to understand and feel that they are actually a resident in a nursing home.

Daily Life—Day 7

Wow. The things I've seen, experienced . . . the friends that I've gained. The understanding that I've received. The human connections I've made in times of stress, anxiety, fear, joy, happiness, and laughter. They all come together into this. This feeling I have right now, that if I ever needed it, I could come back here, not as a pretend patient, but as a family member. Who'd be my family? Everyone in here. Staff, veterans, all of them. [Male, 2008]

Author's Note: This quote illustrates that the student has now acclimated to the environment and feels a part of it. This is now "home."

Daily Life—Day 9

It's interesting how this research is designed not to alter the environment. Or at least to have as little impact as possible. It's difficult to not alter the environment when you are experiencing a very large impact on the residents' psyche. I have healed residents during my stay here and I have not held a stethoscope or a prescription pad. [Male, 2008]

Author's Note: Ethnographic research is designed so that the researcher becomes an integrated part of the environment. However the truth is that a twenty-something year old resident is unusual and s/he could have an effect on the older residents. For this student, he experiences how touch, compassion, laughter, being present with the people he lived had healing qualities.

Routine/Change

I was woken up by an assistant who was not my normal staff member and it was a very interesting experience. She asked if I wanted to sleep in or if I normally got up this early. But I had no idea what time it was. I didn't ask, because I figured it was close to 8:00 AM, since that is when my usual assistant wakes me. After I got a little settled and I found a clock, it was 7:00 AM. It's interesting, I got used to a certain routine, a certain group of caretakers and this new person naturally did things just a little different. It threw me off. Not for the whole day, but just as I was starting to get into a routine, used to certain things, used to the schedule, it threw me for a loop. And I'm not compromised in any real, discernable way. [Male, 2008]

Author's Note: We all have routines in our lives, it is part of living, we look for the familiar whether we realize or not. In the nursing home, staff change, systems may change, but above all the resident's are cared for and safe. This quote raised the awareness of nursing home administrators, in that good care models are only part of the equation in this environment.

Leaving

It was very hard saying bye to everyone. It was like they were my family that was all I really remembered because I felt like I was there forever; it made me really sad to leave them. As stressful, depressing and exhausting as these 2 weeks were, I am so thankful that I learned so much. I learned more in 2 weeks than I ever did in my first year of medical school, and the knowledge is more useful. I am thankful for all the wonderful people I met, especially the residents who taught me so much. [Female, 2005]

> So today is the last full day that I have here. I never thought I would say that and have it affect me so much. I really do not wish to leave my friends, my family. So much has happened . . . So many days of personal growth. I started learning the first minute I was here and have not stopped since. I have touched the lives of patients, just because I was there to listen. I have helped the staff, just because I was younger and challenged elder stereotypes. I have helped the medical profession, just by wheeling a mile in the shoes of elders and making strides towards better medical education. [Male, 2008]

Re-entry

> So I got back onto campus after I was dropped off. My car is here. I can drive home. . . . "home" . . . "drive" . . . Things I haven't thought of for the past two weeks. I walk through the medical school and see faces of young people everywhere. . . . They're all self-absorbed into whatever they are there for. Unaware of the humanity not 15 minutes down the road. Ignorant of the deep human connections possible with those elders. Here they are, living their lives. . . . I was once like that too. I've lived . . . lived . . . more in the past 2 weeks than I have through many days of my life. I've seen what is important. People. Not stuff. [Male, 2008]

Authors' Note: The quotes from "Leaving" and "Re-entry" illustrate that the students integrated within the environment. Heart to heart connections were established that transcended age, ability, frailty, and disease. When these students become physicians they will have had the benefit of living as an older adult and hopefully remember that it is what's in a person's heart (his or her essence) that matters.

These quotes are representative of students' experiences. Overall, students' living as an elder precipitated such issues as time disorientation, dependence, lack of touch and/or sleep and periods of what felt like endless waiting. Students reported telling time by staff shift changes and noted the differences from midweek living to weekend living. It is no wonder they felt the weight of dependence. They experienced being brought to the dinner table and waiting for their meal of pureed foods, being fed, toileted, and bathed. One student got her wheelchair stuck in her bathroom, which only happened to her once! Students also learned about the importance of nonverbal as well as verbal communication, both with those who had good cognition and those who didn't. By living in the environment, students faced their fears about communicating with older adults regardless of their cognitive abilities. Students reported the ability to adjust and gain skills that will better serve them in their future role as physicians. They learned by living and experiencing day-to-day life, watching staff, embracing repetition, and accepting immersion.

Benefits were bountiful; students developed "heart to heart" connections and friendships with residents and staff they had no idea were even possible. They gained insights into caring and what personhood means, including the role of individuality and the ways a person residing in a nursing home approaches the homogenization that is often foisted upon them by visitors, and at times, by the staff. Attainment of better physician skills was high on the students' list of outcomes. All medical students felt the extended period of time offered breadth and depth in learning far beyond what they could learn in the classroom. The longitudinal data thus far confirm that those students who have resided in a nursing home continue to apply their learning from this ethnographic experience in their current practice. Specifically, they employ the purposeful use of touch and eye contact, enhanced and intentional communication utilizing voice tone, body language, and word usage. They report maintaining their consciousness of treating the person rather than the disease or condition. The increased awareness of the role of routine and/or change is significant, creating pathways toward a better understanding of this dynamic from the person's perspective.

Discussion

To date, the program has had a 100% success rate, and follow-up data after 4 years have shown that the students and medical school graduates practice medicine differently, with all ages, because of their experience of living in a nursing home. An outcome that one could only dream of attaining was actually achieved with each student admittance—that of connecting heart-to-heart with residents so that chronological age, frailty, and disease states were shed as barriers or issues. In every case student assumptions about nursing homes and older adult residents such as nursing homes are terrible places to live or older nursing home residents are lonely, were disproven. Students report newfound skills in patient care such as the: (1) importance of physical touch; (2) enhancement of communication by being at eye level regardless of whether the person is in a bed, a wheelchair, or on a treatment table; (3) communication with authenticity and sincerity that comes from being comfortable with oneself; and (4) connection with and awareness of the person rather than merely treating the diseases or frailties. These are remarkable lessons learned within a 2-week span of time, and they have been shown to be maintained as students continue their clinical training in medical education.

Although Learning by Living focuses on the students, nursing home administrators expressed that the staff learning that results from this experience works better than many of their in-service training sessions on the care of elder residents. Having a student live the life of an elder resident raises consciousness for all involved and has resulted in nursing home environment enhancements for residents and increased staff sensitivity.

Future Goals for Learning by Living

It appears that the University of New England College of Osteopathic Medicine is the only medical school in the country and quite possibly in the world to be admitting medical students into nursing homes for extended periods to live the life of an elder resident. The plan is to attain funding to nationalize this learning experience as a Medical Student Trainee Research Fellowship Program. Students in their predoctoral education years as well as interns and residents would be eligible to apply.

In 2010, Learning by Living at Home will be piloted. Medical students will live for 2 weeks with an informal caregiver, meeting the needs of an older spouse or family member with Parkinson's disease and/or dementia in their home. The Maine Parkinson's Association and Maine Alzheimer's Association are assisting with project development. Both Learning by Living Projects would eventually be developed to include nurses and other health professions students.

Conclusion

In looking back on my life of 87 years, I can appreciate how many more educational opportunities are available today than when I was young. Look for diverse experiences, ask questions, listen to all people, young and old, develop a passion for reading, and always keep an open mind. I believe that education is knowledge and knowledge is power.

—Lillian, 87, Wellesley, MA

The only "truth" of old age that we can know is what elders tell us, and this knowing may be devoid of understanding. This project illustrates the breadth, depth, and diversity of information and enduring learning that can be attained by "wheeling a mile" in a nursing home resident's wheelchair for an extended period. The Learning by Living Project provides a framework for ensuring students' immersion in the phenomenology of nursing home living by: (1) making learning relevant and anchoring their medical knowledge with personal experiences; (2) increasing experiences with older adults and the staff who care for them; (3) providing opportunities to test, challenge, and evaluate personal and professional attitudes and assumptions related to older adults; (4) illuminating the lived experiences of students with those of older people; (5) critically examining societal constructs and principles of "institutionalized" older adults with students' experiences; and (6) providing opportunities for reflection and action.

Older adults hold the reality-driven content of aging—a dynamic "truth" that textbooks are unable to impart. So, as a result, the most important component of gerontology/

geriatric medical education is the provision of opportunities, structural and contextual, for gaining a better understanding of aging through closer and extended contact with older persons. My goal in teaching is to integrate theory, experience, and practice through reflection and action—praxis. Students' that live the life of an older nursing home resident express that they are better able to provide care to older adults. Anecdotally, Learning by Living empowers nursing home residents and raises consciousness of the nursing home staff, administrators, and family members of older residents.

The time has come to apply lived experiences within our geriatrics educational curricula. The expected outcome is that those who work with older adults will become acquainted with the self-determination, individuality, purpose, and choices exercised by older adults. Those working with older adults need to comprehend that they have value, meaning, and influence regardless of physical ability or frailty. The Learning by Living© Project has offered a new approach for teaching medical students. Admitting students into nursing facilities for extended and experiential learning will increase our chances for improved care models in the future.

References

Association of Directors of Geriatric Academic Programs. (2007). Fellows in geriatric medicine and geriatric psychiatry programs. *Training & Practice Update, 5*(2), 1–7.

Administration on Aging. (2002). *A profile of older Americans: 2008; The older population*. Retrieved from http://www.aoa.gov/prof/Statistics/profile/1.asp

Alliance for Aging Research. (2002). *Medical never-never land: Ten reasons why America is not ready for the coming age boom*. Washington, DC: Alliance for Aging Research.

American Geriatrics Society. (2006). Fact sheet: The American Geriatrics Society. Retrieved from http://www.americangeriatrics.org/news/ags_fact_sheet.shtml

Berger, P.L., & Luckmann, T. (1966). *The social construction of reality: A treatise in the sociology of knowledge*. New York: Doubleday and Company.

Butler, R. (1975). *Why survive? Being old in America*. New York: Harper & Row.

Cole, T.R. (1984). Aging, meaning, and well-being: Musings of a cultural historian. *International Journal of Aging and Human Development, 19*, 329–336.

Denzin, N.K., & Lincoln Y.S. (1994). *Handbook of qualitative research*. Thousand Oaks, CA: Sage Publications.

Fischer, D.H. (1978). *Growing old in America*. Oxford, England: Oxford University Press.

Gawande, Atul. (2007, April 30). Annals of medicine: The way we age now. *The New Yorker*. Retrieved from http://www.newyorker.com/reporting/2007/04/30/070430fa_fact_gawande/

Glaser, B.G., & Strauss, A.L. (1987). *The discovery of grounded theory: Strategies of qualitative research*. New York: Aldine.

Lee, M., Wilkerson, L., Reuben, D.B., & Ferrell, B.A. (2004). Development and validation of a geriatric knowledge test for medical students. *Journal of the American Geriatrics Society 52*, 983–988.

NVivo 2 (2004) QSR International Pty Ltd. Cambridge, MA 02140.

Reker, G.T., & Wong, P.T.P. (1988). Aging as an individual process: Toward a theory of personal meaning. In J.E. Birren & V.L. Bengston (Eds.), *Emergent theories of aging* (pp. 214–246). New York: Springer Publishing.

Riekse, R.J., & Holstege, H. (1996). *Growing old in america*. New York: McGraw-Hill.

Taylor, S.J., & Bogdan, R. (1984). *Introduction to qualitative research methods: The search for meanings.* New York: John Wiley & Sons.

Tindell, C. (1998). *Seeing beyond the wrinkles.* Northridge, CA: Studio 4 Productions.

US Census Bureau. 2005. Dramatic changes in US aging highlighted in new census, NIH report. http://www.census.gov/Press-Release/www/releases/archives/aging_population/006544.html. Accessed August 27, 2009.

White, H.K. (2008). The nursing home in long-term care education. *Journal of the American Directors Association, 9,* 75–81.

Chapter 8

Rural Geriatric Education and Mental Health

A Multidisciplinary Clinical Immersion Experience

Sarah H. Gueldner, John Toner, Sally Venugopalan, Kathleen Bunnell, Gail Mathieson-Devereaux, and Maureen Daws

Introduction

Urban and rural areas alike are experiencing serious shortages of healthcare professionals with expertise in geriatric care. By the year 2015, the population of older Americans will grow rapidly as an increasing proportion of the baby boom generation turns 65, exacerbating an already serious situation of workforce shortages. The situation is severe in rural areas where it is more difficult to attract and retain health professionals. The problems that accompany these workforce shortages are even more acute in medically underserved areas (MUAs), especially those MUAs in rural areas. Government estimates indicate that at least 20 million of an estimated 70 million rural Americans have inadequate access to health care (US Department of Health and Human Services, 2003).

Older people are at increased risk for serious mental illness, particularly depression and anxiety, in the face of declining physical health and inadequate access to health care, which are intensified in rural areas, especially MUAs (Schoevers, Beekman, Deeg, Jonker, & van Tilburg, 2003; Schoevers, Beekman, Deeg, Geerlings, Jonker, & van Tilburg, 2000). These issues are especially relevant in New York State, where the rate of growth is the third lowest and the proportion of older people in the population is one of the highest in the country (Roberts, 2006).

Overview

Specialized training of healthcare professionals and allied healthcare providers in mental health is therefore essential to meet the increasing mental health needs of this growing elderly population in medically underserved areas of upstate New York. In 2005, the US Department of Health and Human Services awarded a grant to three co-applicants: Columbia University Stroud Center, New York University (NYU) Division of Nursing, and Utica College, as part of the DHHS Quentin N. Burdick Program for Rural Interdisciplinary Training. The program became known as the Geriatric Education in Mental Health Program, or GEM. The purpose of GEM was to develop, implement, evaluate, and sustain a program of interdisciplinary rural training for students in the healthcare professions, with the goal of improving access to mental health services for the geriatric population of three medically underserved counties located in central New York State (Herkimer, Oneida, and Madison). The program co-applicants were also joined by the following five partners: Binghamton University Decker School of Nursing, the Bronx VA GRECC, the Oneida Indian Nation, and Masonic Care Community and Heritage Health Care Center in Utica, New York.

GEM integrated the interdisciplinary, geriatric, and mental health expertise and resources of the coapplicant academic institutions from New York City with: (1) educational institutions in upstate central New York with interested learners; (2) supervised training opportunities at rural clinical sites, and (3) the programmatic support of local community organizations. A core faculty employed innovative strategies, including distance learning, to train learners from five different disciplines—nursing, occupational therapy, physical therapy, psychology, and rehabilitation—in the knowledge and skills required to provide interdisciplinary geriatric mental health services for elderly patients in rural areas of central New York State.

GEM recruited three different groups of learners: (1) interdisciplinary undergraduate students and medical residents, (2) local and regional healthcare professionals who wished to earn CME/CEU credit, and (3) selected healthcare professionals who were trained as project faculty using a "teach the teacher" model, which was developed at the Columbia University Stroud Center (see Table 8-1). The clinical and didactic components of the GEM training program explicitly focused on **interdisciplinary** teamwork (Toner, 2002; Toner, 1994a; Toner, 1994b; Toner, Miller, & Gurland, 1994). The didactic curriculum aimed to prepare future and present healthcare professionals to work on interdisciplinary healthcare teams. In the clinical practicums, GEM trainees were integrated onto the existing interdisciplinary healthcare teams at the clinical sites, which were affiliated with the partnering institutions. The GEM trainees experienced interdisciplinary teamwork in action in several ways: participation on interdisciplinary teams, membership on trainee teams with team projects, interdisciplinary seminars, workshops, and interactive exercises which were led by interdisciplinary faculty who taught the GEM trainees to model interdisciplinary collaboration.

The primary goal of the project was to use new and innovative methods to train healthcare practitioners to provide mental health services in rural underserved areas through a partnership of academic faculty, rural healthcare providers, community organizations, and local educational institutions to provide a collaborative rural learning experience for students, faculty, and practitioners in rural areas.

TABLE 8-1   **Characteristics of Learners**

Discipline	
Nursing	14
Psychology	4
OT/PT	7
Recreational Therapy	1
Other	1
Total	27
Gender	
Female	24
Male	3
Age	
Range	19–48 years
Mean Age	23 years

(continues)

TABLE 8-1 (Continued)

Ethnic Background	
White	23
African American	2
Black (non AA)	1
Asian/Pacific Islander	1

Educational Level	
Freshman	3
Sophomore	1
Junior	6
Senior	13
Masters	1
PhD	2
Other	1

Training Sites (Some participated at more than one site)	
Heritage Healthcare	4
Masonic Home	3
Oneida Indian Nation	3
Rome Memorial Hospital	1
Utica College	3
New York State Veterans Home	6
Broome County Senior Centers	8

Clinical Immersion Experience

A prominent feature of the program of education for undergraduate and graduate students was an intensive interdisciplinary rural immersion experience based within one of the collaborating clinical facilities. The remainder of this chapter describes a model component of GEM, the GEM interdisciplinary training at the New York State Veterans Home in Oxford, NY.

Exemplar

Binghamton University Nursing Student Clinical and Research Immersion Experiences

This section highlights the exceptional 140-hour immersion experience of six Binghamton University nursing students (three women and three men) with residents and clinical staff at the New York State Veterans Home in Oxford, New York. The purpose of the experience was to develop, implement, evaluate, and sustain a program of interdisciplinary rural training for health professions students (in this case baccalaureate and masters level nursing students), with the goal of improving access to health services for the diverse geriatric populations who reside in rural upstate New York. Activities were designed to meet the following objectives:

> Develop linkages among rural healthcare providers, academic faculty, and interdisciplinary healthcare professionals to provide collaborative learning experiences for students and practitioners in rural areas.
>
> Provide opportunities for healthcare students (i.e., baccalaureate and masters level nursing students in this case) to participate in the delivery of evidence-based best practices within an interdisciplinary climate that increases the students' likelihood of choosing to work with rural-dwelling elders.

Five senior level baccalaureate nursing students and one masters student at the Decker School of Nursing, Binghamton University (located in upstate New York), were offered and chose the option to complete their final 14-week (140-hour) clinical leadership intensive at the New York State Veterans Home, located at Oxford, New York, a rural area of upstate New York about an hour's drive northeast of Binghamton. The students went there for 6 hours, 2 days each week, throughout the semester. The goal of the experience was to provide the students with the opportunity to develop their clinical leadership skills in a state-based skilled nursing facility that is known for providing exceptional care for elders who have served in the military services (and in some instances their spouses or parents).

The students were assigned to work as partners with nurse leaders in the facility, including nurse practitioners, as well as physicians' assistants, the optometrist, professionals in social and psychological services, the dietary department, recreational therapy, physical therapy, occupational therapy, the wound care team, and transport services, to plan and manage the care of the residents. In addition, students often accompanied the residents to special music programs and other scheduled activities.

Supervised by their teacher or clinical staff, students had the opportunity to start intravenous infusions (IVs) in the fragile veins of elders, to reinsert and manage complex urinary catheter care, to change dressings, and to take care of PIC lines, feeding tubes, and colostomies, as well as many other daily care procedures. Each student also spent time with residents in the innovative "cottage" for residents who had dementia.

Another key aspect of the experience was every student's participation in the daily report, where an interdisciplinary team met to review any problems, including falls or other mishaps, that had occurred within the past 24 hours. Skin problems were always a concern, as well. It was very enlightening for the students to be a part of the interdisciplinary team working together to address the problems that had occurred each day, in the effort to prevent them from happening again.

Special Moments

The 14 weeks were also marked with many special individual and group moments; a few are highlighted in the paragraphs that follow.

One student rode in the ambulance with a woman resident who developed an acute problem and had to be transported to the hospital an hour's drive away. The woman passed out during the ride, and due to the distance, the woman's family was not there to meet them when they arrived at the hospital. The student told her classmates that it was one of the most poignant experiences of her time in school, because she felt she was able to make a crucial difference in reducing the woman's fear.

A very touching moment for us all came as we attended the 99th birthday celebration of the oldest veteran in Broome County. He was clear mentally, and he offered a few inspirational comments before the cake was cut. The students asked to have their picture taken with him.

Another group highlight came on the last day, when the students prepared and presented their evidence-based quality management project, which was an hour-long inservice program on urinary incontinence for about 25 professional staff from across disciplines. The students were extraordinarily creative and resourceful, drawing rave reviews from their audience. They even administered a pre and post quiz to evaluate the learning of their attendees!

But then the students broke away from their PowerPoint presentation and performed four informal but poignant "improv" skits depicting the personal problems, including embarrassment and difficulty getting to the bathroom in time, commonly associated with urinary incontinence. Prior to the first skit they distributed a disposable baby-sized diaper to each staff member who was sitting in the audience. Then the students moved around the circle with pitchers of water, pouring ¼ to ½ cup of water into each diaper, and instructed each person to tape the wet diaper to their wrist or elbow for the duration of the presentation, simulating the experience of incontinence as they watched the skits.

Then, as the audience sat wearing their wet diapers taped to their arms, the students took turns being the patient and the staff in their clever situational improvisations of the problems that nursing home residents with urinary incontinence encounter. They did a wonderful job of leading the audience of professionals in a realistic simulated experience of incontinence. The activity was both entertaining and sensitivity raising, and very effective. Many of the staff in attendance lingered to talk with the students after the program, and one attendee suggested that they do it again for the nurse aides and auxiliary staff. The facility taped their presentation and skits and planned to show it to those working closest with the residents. Working as a group, the students submitted a final paper on evidenced-based care for persons with urinary incontinence.

Eden Alternative

On the last day of the semester, the five undergraduate nursing students and the masters' geriatric nurse practitioner student drove together with their teachers to the 80-bed Chase Memorial Nursing Home in New Berlin, New York, which is the birthplace of the innovative and internationally known *Eden Alternative* movement, founded and promoted by Dr. William Thomas, author of *What Are Old People For?* The administrator of the facility explained that the concept is based on the goal of bringing life into the facility, rather than isolating the residents from the sights, smells, and sounds of the life they knew before coming there. The facility has always had a child day care center on the grounds, and the babies and toddlers are brought to visit with the elders each morning. It was a delightful experience, seeing the babies sitting on elders' laps, and every baby, toddler, and elder had big smiles on their faces. There is also a playground on the premises of the facility, positioned so that the elders can sit outside nearby and watch and listen to the children play, or watch them through the large windows. Several hundred live plants, more than 40 songbirds, two retired greyhounds, and three cats also live *inside* the facility.

Involvement in Research

Working with the faculty, and with formal approval and consent from the facility's board of directors, the six students assigned to the New York State Veterans' Home also participated as research assistants in a larger research project to measure depression and well-being among willing residents who had scored in the top "0" and "1" (i.e., most independent) categories of the Minimum Data Set evaluation that is routinely administered to each resident at the time of admission and at regular intervals thereafter. Each student participated both in recruiting participants and in administering the *Geriatric Depression Scale* and the *Well-Being Picture Scale*. In addition, the students, working in pairs, scored the completed instruments, and some assisted in entering and analyzing the data. The study was conducted as part of a community project, in conjunction with a local Robert Wood Johnson Aging Futures community grant. The students' course evaluations indicated that they had a very positive experience with the more than 70 elders they tested. (Simultaneously, another group of eight nursing students from Binghamton University administered the *Well-Being Picture Scale* and the *Geriatric Depression Scale* to 215 community-dwelling elders who had gathered for lunch at six senior centers operated under the auspices of the Broome County Office of Aging and Aging Futures Committee.)

The students, faculty, and community-based healthcare providers who collaborated on these research projects testing the correlation between the *Well-Being Picture Scale* and the *Geriatric Depression Scale* presented their findings as a poster session at a regional interdisciplinary research conference cosponsored by Binghamton University and the Binghamton Clinical Campus of the SUNY Upstate Medical Center, and at the 2007 meeting of the Gerontological Society of America.

Evaluation

The students met with their teachers over breakfast on the morning after the last day of the immersion experience, and they unanimously agreed that the experience was exceptional, noting that the 14-week experience was marked with many special individual and group moments. But perhaps the best evaluation of the experience is that upon graduation, at least four of the six nursing students interviewed for and obtained positions in elder care. One of the students took a job at a long-term care facility in Binghamton, one applied for a position at the VA Hospital in Syracuse, one accepted a position in an adult care facility in the downstate area, and another took a position in home care rehabilitation for elders in another state.

Acknowledgments

This educational project was supported by the Quentin N. Burdick Rural Program for Interdisciplinary Training (DHHS HRSA Grant Number 5D361-02-00), and was conducted through the Partnership of the Consortium of New York Geriatric Education Centers; School of Nursing, New York University; Columbia University Stroud Center; Utica College; Bronx–New York Harbor VAMC GRECC; Mount Sinai School of Medicine; Binghamton Clinical Campus; Oneida Indian Nation; and Decker School of Nursing, Binghamton University. The authors would like to express appreciation to these groups for their exceptional support, which culminated in the success of this important student immersion experience. We also extend our gratitude to the administration, staff, and residents of the New York State Veterans Home; to the Broome County Office of Aging and Aging Futures Committee; and to other community partners who provided support for the program; their collaborative spirit gave vibrancy to this educational endeavor. Finally, we would thank the students who self-selected to participate in this project, including Jackie Brass, Autumn Tokos, Allison Pinney, Jay Mahler, Karen Sidi, Kacee Conrad, Kristen Byrnes, and others.

References

Roberts, S. (2006). Flight of young adults is causing alarm upstate. *New York Times*, June 13, 2006, pp. A1, B4.

Schoevers, R.A., Beekman, A.T., Deeg, D.J., Geerlings, M.I., Jonker, C., & van Tilburg, W. (2000, August). Risk factors for depression in later life; Results of a prospective community based study (AMSTEL). *Journal of Affective Disorders*, 59(2):127–137.

Schoevers, R.A., Beekman, A.T., Deeg, D.J., Jonker, C., & van Tilburg, W. (2003). Comorbidity and risk-patterns of depression, generalised anxiety disorder and mixed anxiety-depression in later life: Results from the AMSTEL study. *International Journal of Geriatric Psychiatry, 18,* 994–1001.

Toner, J. (2002). Developing and maintaining links between service disciplines (POISE). In J.R.M. Copeland, M.T. Abou-Saleh, & D.G. Blazer (Eds.), *Principles and practice of geriatric psychiatry* (2nd ed.,795-798). New York: John Wiley & Sons.

Toner, J. (1994a). Developing and maintaining links between service disciplines. In J.R.M. Copeland, M.T. Abou-Saleh, & D.G. Blazer (Eds.), *Principles and practice of geriatric psychiatry* (1021-1026). New York: John Wiley & Sons.

Toner, J. (1994b). Interdisciplinary treatment team training in geriatric psychiatry: A model of university-state-public hospital collaboration. *Gerontology and Geriatrics Education, 14*(3), 25–38.

Toner, J., Miller, P., & Gurland, B. (1994). Conceptual, theoretical and practical approaches to the development of interdisciplinary teams: A transactional model. *Educational Gerontology, 20*(1), 53–69.

US Department of Health and Human Services. (2003). *Rural mental health outreach: Promising practices in rural areas.* Rockville, MD: US Department of Health and Human Services, Substance Abuse and Mental Health Services Administration, Center for Mental Health Services.

Chapter 9

Using Reminiscence as a Teaching Tool

William J. Puentes

Introduction

Memories play a powerful role in our lives. Preliterate societies relied heavily on stories and memories to develop and sustain culture. Social mores, events that significantly affected the direction of societal development, and the sense of social and individual continuity are all aspects of our humanity that are intimately associated with the use of memories. More recently, healthcare providers have begun to recognize that memories play an important role in our conception of who we are and how we fit into and relate to the world around us.

Nursing, medicine, and other healthcare professions have recognized the importance of using life narratives to develop practitioners' empathy with their clients, to enhance provider-client communication, and to encourage a holistic approach to delivering healthcare services. Charon (2001) proposed that the effective practice of medicine requires narrative competence. Narrative competence is defined as "the competence that human beings use to absorb, interpret, and respond to stories" (p. 1897). She argues that scientific competence alone does not prepare the healthcare provider to effectively partner with clients in the management of their health. Others have also argued for a broadening of educational approaches to more adequately prepare healthcare providers to function effectively within the evolving healthcare system of the twenty-first century.

For instance, Brown, Kirkpatrick, Mangum, and Avery (2008) discuss the importance of art, film, and literature as sources of information for reflective learning activities. Reflective learning helps nurses to develop new ways of knowing the worlds in which they exist, and helps them to recognize the importance of viewing their clients as more than the sum of factual data. These authors also identify storytelling as a powerful tool for transferring information. Similarly, Brown et al. note that "stories capture interest and attention, enable recall of details by association, and bring facts to life by putting them in personal scenarios" (p. 284). While discussing the importance of narrative, Richardson (1990) noted that,

> Narrative displays the goals and intentions of human actors; it makes individuals, cultures, societies and historical epochs comprehensible as wholes, it humanizes time, and allows us to contemplate the effects of our actions and to alter the directions of lives. (p. 120)

In her discussion of using narrative in research activities, Overcash (2004) noted that this methodology is extremely effective for gathering rich, multidimensional data.

One approach to incorporating life stories into the assessment and treatment aspects of the nursing process relies on the use of an activity known by the umbrella term *reminiscence*. The *Nursing Interventions Classification* document (Dochterman & Bulechek, 2004) refers to the activity as Reminiscence Therapy, which is defined as using the recall of past events, feelings, and thoughts to facilitate pleasure, quality of life, or adaptation to present circumstances. This definition represents a broad category that subsumes several distinct types of reminiscence. Each type is used for different purposes, and to accomplish different goals. The purpose of this paper is to describe each of the different types of reminiscence, to identify the circumstances under which each type should be used, and to discuss the expected outcomes. Finally, examples of the use of different types of reminiscence in nursing education will be presented.

Defining Reminiscence

Currently, in the field of reminiscence we find use of reminiscence activities from a wide variety of perspectives and settings, and by different types of practitioners. It is important, therefore, to explore the concept of reminiscence itself before proceeding to a discussion of its use as a tool to enhance teaching.

The concept of reminiscence encompasses a group of phenomena that are intuitively appealing to most people. These phenomena have diverse theoretical underpinnings, and have been explained from a variety of perspectives. Despite an intense interest in these phenomena, which can be traced to Butler's (1963) seminal article, they continue to be shrouded in an air of ambiguity. The term *reminiscence* itself continues to be used inconsistently. Webster and Haight (1995) noted "much of the discourse of the past 30 years might have been avoided if we had started with a taxonomy in 1963" (p. 282).

A number of researchers and theorists lend support to the idea that the term *reminiscence* is best thought of as an overall term that encompasses several more specific processes involving the use of memories to accomplish various biopsychosocial functions. Haight and Burnside (1993) described the differences between life review and reminiscence. And over the past 40 years, others (Beaton, 1980; Bluck & Alea, 2002; Cappeliez & O'Rourke, 2006; Coleman, 1974; Kovach, 1995; LoGerfo, 1980-81; Merriam, 1993; Romaniuk & Romaniuk, 1981; Watt & Wong, 1991; Webster, 1993) have offered taxonomies of reminiscence describing two to eight types. Taxonomies are knowledge structures that organize phenomena into ordered groups of categories based on predetermined criteria, and they are the basis for empirically distinguishing phenomena.

None of the several proposed reminiscence taxonomies has been generally accepted as a basis for practice or research. However, even though none of the taxonomies has been fully developed or tested, reminiscence-type activities are often implemented as therapeutic interventions, especially for older adult clients, without a sound understanding of the underlying dynamics of the interventions. One factor that may be contributing to the dearth of consensus regarding reminiscence phenomena is the lack of criteria by which to compare the proffered taxonomies.

This discussion proposes criteria that can be used to distinguish among various reminiscence phenomena. The development of a clear set of distinguishing criteria will contribute to taxonomy development and acceptance by standardizing the terminology and definitions surrounding these phenomena. It is hoped that this clarification will help researchers to conceptually and operationally define the concept of reminiscence in research studies as a basis for empirical investigation of the phenomena. It will also provide beginning guidelines for practitioners (1) to understand the circumstances under which it is appropriate to use the different kinds of reminiscence as interventions, (2) to have some understanding of the underlying psychodynamic process associated with each kind of reminiscence, (3) to have some basis to identify expected outcomes, and (4) to recognize both positive and negative responses to reminiscence interventions. Finally, it will provide educators with criteria to design and implement educational activities involving the use of reminiscence in a consistent manner with clear learning outcomes.

Taxonomy Classification Criteria

A review of the literature published between 1950 and 2009 from multiple disciplines using multiple electronic databases indicates that there are several criteria that are important to consider when comparing suggested taxonomies and distinguishing the different types of reminiscence. These criteria include: (1) the theoretical perspective underlying the reminiscence process, (2) the level of insight required to utilize the particular type of reminiscence, and the (3) locus, (4) stimulus, and (5) expected outcomes of the reminiscence process. The theoretical perspective underlying the reminiscence process directly drives the interpretation of the remaining criteria.

Theoretical Perspective

The research base of the nursing profession is built on an eclectic mix of theoretical perspectives that have been adapted and synthesized to describe the concepts central to the nursing process, including nursing, person, health, and environment. A similar process needs to begin to occur in the field of reminiscence. This effort will be challenging, due to the multidisciplinary nature of the field. However, it is not an impossible task.

It has been suggested that perspectives might be best viewed as models. Theoretical models articulate assumptions about a phenomenon. In addition, they discuss how these assumptions are related. Models help us to give meaning to the things we experience as human beings. No one particular theoretical model provides an absolute explanation of a phenomenon. Rather, theoretical models help us to understand a phenomenon through the lens of a particular worldview. Different worldviews result in different assumptions, relationships and, ultimately, understandings of a phenomenon.

Fawcett (1984) posited that ". . . theories may be characterized as sets of concepts, definitions, and propositions that address the metaparadigm phenomena . . ." (p. 22). At least one description of reminiscence phenomena at the metaparadigmatic level has been alluded to. Bluck and Alea (2002) suggested that all reminiscence activity may ultimately represent forms of adaptation while acknowledging that there are different types of reminiscence that are used to accomplish different biopsychosocial functions. The umbrella term of reminiscence itself, defined as the use of memories to accomplish a biopsychosocial task, may adequately express the metaparadigm of the field.

Recognition of the theoretical perspective or models underlying the suggested types of reminiscence is the first step in coherently organizing our knowledge regarding reminiscence phenomena, a prerequisite to sound taxonomy development and utilization of reminiscence techniques in research, practice, and education. The theoretical perspective affects how the remaining criteria are interpreted. These criteria are insight, locus, stimulus and, outcome.

Insight

Insight has been defined in several different ways. Sadock and Sadock (2007), for instance, take a problem-oriented approach and define insight as "the conscious awareness and understanding of one's own psychodynamics and symptoms of maladaptive behavior" (p. 279). Stuart and Laraia (1998) look at the concept of insight from a broader perspective and define it as "the patient's development of new emotional and cognitive understandings" (p. 186).

For the purposes of this discussion, insight refers to the abilities to accurately perceive or recall memories, interpret or analyze the information, and incorporate the results of the analysis into the personal worldview. Level of insight is best thought of in terms of a continuum ranging from no insight to a high degree of insight. Insight cannot be viewed dichotomously. Descriptions of various uses of reminiscence in the literature suggest that different types of reminiscence appear to require different levels of insight to be used effectively.

Locus

Even though the various types of reminiscence are processes that can be facilitated (read "made easier") by "reminiscence professionals," it is important to remember that these are processes that are being experienced by the reminiscer. The locus of the process, which again is best viewed in terms of a continuum, ranges from a strong internal locus to a strong external locus. As with insight, the characteristic of locus cannot be looked at dichotomously. The locus of the process refers to the psychodynamic orientation of the experience of reminiscence for the reminiscer. For instance, issues related to the resolution of the integrity versus self-despair conflict, as described by Erikson's (1959) work in developmental psychology, are internally focused in nature. On the other hand, the psychodynamics associated with a sociological theoretical perspective primarily focus on relationships with other individuals, groups, communities, and the environment. Some descriptions of reminiscence processes in the literature suggest that internal and external factors may play equally important roles.

Stimulus and Outcome

The stimuli and outcomes of the various types of reminiscence are directly related to the theoretical structures. A developmental perspective suggests that the reminiscence process occurs in response to some unmet developmental need, for instance the need to resolve the developmental conflict of integrity versus self-despair. The most successful outcome in this situation would be the attainment of a sense of integrity. A stress-adaptation theoretical perspective would support the concept of a stimulus as a perceived psychological or physical threat, and a successful outcome of the process is accommodation or adaptation to the perceived threat. Finally, the perceived need for knowledge transmission may be one stimulus associated with a sociological perspective of reminiscence. The success of the reminiscence process would be determined by the extent to which that knowledge is transmitted.

When each of the different suggested types of reminiscence are evaluated according to these criteria, similarities and differences between suggested taxonomies will become clearer, and movement toward a unified perspective of reminiscence will occur.

Types of Reminiscence

Based on the criteria described above, three distinct types of reminiscence are apparent. These are Life Review, Simple Reminiscence, and Social Reminiscence (Puentes, 2005).

Life Review

The theoretical and empirical literature, as well as clinical practice, suggest the phenomenon of Life Review is best interpreted from a developmental perspective. Life Review was first described by Butler (1963). According to Butler:

> . . . Life Review is a naturally occurring, universal mental process characterized by the progressive return to consciousness of past experiences, and, particularly, the resurgence of unresolved conflicts; simultaneously, and, normally, these revived

> experiences and conflicts can be surveyed and reintegrated. Presumably this process
> is prompted by the realization of approaching dissolution and death, and the inabil-
> ity to maintain one's sense of personal invulnerability. It is further shaped by con-
> temporaneous experiences and its nature and outcome are affected by the lifelong
> unfolding of character. (p. 68)

Most past work done in the area of Life Review, as well as the broader category of reminiscence, utilizes the theoretical description proposed by Butler.

Butler's (1963) references to dealing with issues associated with being confronted by
one's own mortality are consistent with the developmental tasks associated with older
adulthood as described by Erikson (1959). Erikson describes the primary psychological
task of old age as the resolution of the conflict of ego integrity with self-despair. Successful resolution of this conflict involves evaluation of both positive and negative life experiences and integration of the results of this evaluation process into the individual's
perception of self. Hopefully, the outcome of this self-evaluation process will result in a
sense of ego integrity and an enhancement of self-esteem. But, as implied by Erikson's
description of the psychological conflict and overtly discussed by Butler, the Life Review
may not have a positive outcome. In fact, the outcome may be psychologically devastating.

Another important aspect of Butler's description of Life Review is the implication that
the process, at least to some degree, requires a certain amount of insightful analysis on the
part of the reminiscer/life reviewer.

It is important to remember that Butler's description of Life Review was an effort to
quantify observations of clinical phenomena on a theoretical level. In the 45 years since it
was first presented, there have been some efforts to empirically test the theory of Life
Review. These efforts have been hampered by inconsistent identification of the phenomenon as well as methodological issues. Butler's description of the phenomenon of Life
Review is intuitively appealing to practitioners. A number of practitioners have published
anecdotal and pre-experimental observations praising the utility of the phenomenon as a
therapeutic intervention.

For the purposes of this taxonomy, Life Review is identified by the following
characteristics:

- The client exhibits the need to complete the developmental tasks associated
  with Erikson's ego integrity versus self-despair stage. This need includes issues
  of coming to terms with the events of one's life.
- A thoughtful analysis requiring a high degree of insight is exhibited.
- Both positive and negative aspects of the reviewer's life are evaluated.

Simple Reminiscence

In this taxonomy of the phenomena of reminiscence, Simple Reminiscence is defined as
an adaptive mechanism that an individual resorts to in time of stress (Puentes, 1998).

We perceive and evaluate the world around us from a time perspective that includes past, present, and future spheres. Under normal circumstances, one evaluates present situations in terms of past experiences and consequently makes judgments regarding the future. Typically, the individual has a tendency to look at past experiences that are perceived as positive or meaningful to find support for present functioning and decisions regarding the future. This time perception process is an adaptive function, especially in middle-aged and older adults who possess a wealth of past experience from which to draw.

In times of stress, such as psychological or physical illness, people may become so overwhelmed that they cannot expend the energy required to look back or ahead and become "stuck" in the present. The adaptive functions provided by the ability to move between the spheres of time orientation is lost, and an important coping strategy is disrupted. Simple Reminiscence may be one intervention that the registered nurse can use to help the client move toward reintegration of past, present, and future spheres of time orientation and regain this adaptive function.

In this taxonomy, Simple Reminiscence is identified by the following characteristics:

- The client exhibits signs of a stress response.
- The client identifies past situations in which similar stressors were experienced.
- The recalled events are typically positive in nature.

Social Reminiscence

Social Reminiscence is best understood within the broader context of sociological theory. Atchley (1978) discussed aging from a sociological perspective. He notes that in preindustrial times, there were many different views of aging. Some societies honored older people as sages and leaders. Others left their old to die. In modern industrial societies, the question of the role of older people assumes critical importance. Because of the large numbers of people who are living into old age due to technological and healthcare advances, there is ambiguity regarding this group's place within modern American society. He notes that society's designation of a circumstance as a "social problem" requires the subjective definition of a condition as undesirable. In the United States, material productivity is highly valued. When social conditions such as temporally defined social roles impair the older adult's ability to remain materially productive and do not replace it with an equally highly valued role, the parameters for "social problem" designation are set. Social Reminiscence is a role that, historically, has had important cultural implications.

Knowledge transmission is a crucial component in the development and maintenance of a culture. In preliterate societies, oral transmission of culture was an essential factor in the survival of the culture. Individuals with the resources to pass on the culture, primarily older adults with significant life experience, were highly valued and respected.

For the purposes of this taxonomy, Social Reminiscence is defined as the oral or written transmission of previous life experience, the purpose of which is to provide an historical context, moral and ethical guidelines, or identification of relational commonal-ties with a specific group. The process of Social Reminiscence requires a lower degree of insight than the other types of reminiscence. Intense, insightful analysis is not required. The process is externally motivated by social circumstances. The stimulus of the process is the perceived need for cultural transmission, and the determination of a successful out-come of the process would be adequate transmission of knowledge.

Reminiscence as a Nursing Intervention

Anecdotal accounts and pre-experimental studies appear to support the proposition that the various types of reminiscence are useful nursing interventions. Despite the fact that further testing is needed to develop a better understanding of the psychodynamic charac-teristics and processes of the various types of reminiscence, the existing literature does suggest some guidelines for using reminiscence-type techniques as nursing interventions.

Identifying the Type

The initial step in the process of implementing reminiscence techniques is to determine which type of reminiscence is most appropriate to the clinical needs of the client. This is accomplished by identifying the overall themes of the initial client interviews. For instance, existential themes are indicative of the conflicts associated with the develop-mental tasks of old age. In this case, the Life Review would be the intervention of choice. However, a client who focuses on coping difficulties or stress-related issues would benefit from a Simple Reminiscence intervention. Relational themes are best approached from the perspective of Social Reminiscence.

A Priori Assumptions

Once the clinical needs of the client and the most appropriate therapeutic approach are determined, it is important to test several assumptions prior to implementing the inter-vention. The assumptions revolve around the issues of insight, client resources, and nursing/system resources.

Insight

In order for either of the reminiscence interventions to be effective, it is imperative that the client exhibit a degree of insight adequate to pursue the specific reminiscence process. In this taxonomy, Life Review is conceptualized as a fairly complex process requiring a high degree of insight. Researchers (Merriam, 1993) have questioned Butler's proposition that Life Review is a universal process experienced by all older adults. It may, in fact, be a process that is only pursued by those individuals with the psychological and emotional resources, including a fairly high degree of insight, necessary to complete the process. The essence of Life Review is the insightful analysis of life experiences, both positive and negative. Without the degree of insight necessary to pursue this analysis, Life Review is not possible.

It is important at this point to remember that, as mentioned earlier, insight is best thought of in terms of a continuum. It is not a question of having insight or not having insight. Rather, someone may be high enough along the continuum to pursue a Life Review regarding some issues. But they may not be at the same level as a peer with a much higher degree of insight and who, therefore, is in a better position to pursue the Life Review in a much greater depth about a broader number of issues.

The other types of reminiscence, though still requiring a degree of insight, do not require it at the same depth as Life Review. Typically in Simple Reminiscence, the recalled memories are positive. In this type of reminiscence, the client is searching for an example of adaptive coping. Judgments are not made about the goodness and badness or rightness or wrongness of the recalled memories. The goal is to determine past behaviors that worked or did not work in dealing with stressful situations. These recalled memories are used as a basis for making decisions, as opposed to judgments, on how to respond to current stressors.

Social Reminiscence requires the least amount of insight. Frequently, the recalled memories are based on what the audience perceives as important rather than what the reminiscer perceives as important. Decisions are made about which memories are appropriate to the specific social situation. But, again, judgments with the potential to affect the underlying cognitive schema are not made. In fact, the opposite may be true, and one role of Social Reminiscence may be to reinforce the underlying cognitive schema.

Other Client Resources

In addition to insight, it is important to evaluate the client's cognitive abilities and motivation. Again, it is important to think of both characteristics in terms of a continuum rather than a dichotomy. As with insight, Life Review requires a fairly high degree of cognitive functioning and motivation on the part of the Life Reviewer. Life Review involves multiple cognitive processes including memory (immediate-recent-remote), recall, analytic ability, judgment, and an understanding of underlying ethical principles. The other types of reminiscence do not require the same degree of cognitive functioning. In one study, for instance, Woods and McKiernan (1995) were testing the effects of participation in reminiscence activity on clients diagnosed with dementia. The type of reminiscence used in this study can be categorized as Social Reminiscence. By definition, a diagnosis of dementia involves impaired cognitive functioning. In this study, the effects of the reminiscence activity on the older adult participants were ambiguous. However, these authors pointed out the serendipitous finding that the staff in the setting where the study took place were positively affected by the reminiscence activity of their clients. This study demonstrates that the expected outcomes of Social Reminiscence can occur despite a very low level of cognitive functioning on the part of the reminiscer.

In this taxonomy, the locus of the reminiscence process is described on a continuum ranging from internal for Life Review to external for Social Reminiscence. The external locus associated with Social Reminiscence suggests that the motivating factors for participating in the reminiscence process are external in nature and the decision to pursue the Social Reminiscence process does not require a great amount of psychological energy on the part of the reminiscer. Participation in Life Review, on the other hand, requires a willingness to question the underlying cognitive schema, which requires a much higher degree of motivation on the part of the reminiscer.

In addition to psychological resources, there are some pragmatic issues to consider. Does the client have the time to participate in the reminiscence process? Are they physically capable of participating in the process? Past research has looked at single sessions versus multiple sessions and individual versus group processes. Though no definitive conclusions have been reached, it does seem reasonable to assume that an investment of time and expenditure of physical resources are necessary to participate adequately in any of the reminiscence processes.

Nursing/System Resources

There are also several important nursing/system resources that must be taken into account when considering the use of reminiscence. The skill level of the practitioner and the availability of time and follow-up resources are all crucial to the successful implementation of any of the reminiscence interventions.

As implied in the taxonomy, there is an increasing level of complexity in the structure and dynamics of the process as we move from Social Reminiscence through Simple Reminiscence and on to Life Review. To be most effective in facilitating the Life Review process, the nurse must be skilled in dealing with a variety of psychodynamic issues. Recognition of changes at the psychodynamic level, the ability to move from one type of intervention to another (and to understand the rationale for doing so) and experience in facilitating psychotherapeutic interventions are all essential skills. This level of skill is typically associated with nurses prepared as clinical specialists or nurse practitioners. Simple Reminiscence and Social Reminiscence, in contrast, rely on skills that are within the realm of the competent general practitioner. Stuart and Laraia (1998), for instance, articulate a model known as the Stuart Stress Adaptation Model that describes the general practitioner's role in helping clients deal with stress response issues. And the psychosocial perspective, which fits well with the concept of Social Reminiscence, is generally accepted as a hallmark of basic nursing practice.

In addition to having a skill level appropriate to the intervention, it is important to consider more pragmatic issues, such as having the time and follow-up resources necessary to support the reminiscence process once it is begun. The literature suggests that Simple Reminiscence and Social Reminiscence can be fairly discrete, time-limited interventions. Both interventions have very specific stimuli and the processes are very focused in nature. Life Review, on the other hand, is stimulated by more intrinsic, fundamental triggers, and the process appears to require a more significant amount of time and energy. The practitioner who utilizes Life Review techniques must be prepared to follow through with multiple visits and work within a system that supports the development of an ongoing therapeutic relationship.

Examples of the Use of Reminiscence in Nursing Education

Shellman (2006) examined the impact of participating in a Reminiscence Education Program on students' perception of reminiscence experiences involving themselves and older adults clients. Forty-one baccalaureate registered nurse students participated in the program. The reminiscence experience was based on the incorporation of integrative reminiscence techniques, a type of reminiscence that is analogous to life review (Cohen & Taylor, 1998; Watt & Cappeliez, 2000), into students' interactions with older adult clients over a 13-week community health nursing clinical experience. Prior to beginning the clinical experience, each student received a reminiscence booklet developed by the investigator and participated in a structured learning experience that focused on learning how to incorporate integrative reminiscence techniques into their interactions with older clients. The program employed a variety of teaching techniques including lectures, handouts, group discussions, and role-playing activities.

Program evaluation occurred within a qualitative framework and relied on data obtained from surveys completed by the students at the end of the clinical experience (Shellman, 2006). An editing analysis style (Crabtree & Miller, 1999) was used to extract meaningful segments from the data, and these were merged to identify patterns and themes in student responses. Three major themes emerged from the data. The students felt like the reminiscence experience allowed them to make a connection with their older adult clients. In addition, they developed a better understanding of the older adults' life experiences because they felt they could see the world through the older adults' eyes. Students were also able to identify the benefits to themselves and older adults of participating in reminiscence activities.

In another study, Shellman (2007) discussed the importance of preparing baccalaureate registered nurse students who are competent in the areas of older adult nursing and cultural sensitivity. Using a quasi-experimental, multiple-time series with a nonequivalent control group design, she explored the impact of a reminiscence education program on these areas in a convenience sample of 64 baccalaureate registered nurse students. Integrative reminiscence was again used as the basis of the educational experience. Students participated in a 2-hour educational program about using integrative reminiscence techniques while interacting with older adults. The program employed a variety of teaching techniques, including lecture supplemented with handouts and a reminiscence booklet, group discussion, and role-playing. Students had the opportunity to apply the knowledge and skills gained from the 2-hour program during a 13-week follow-up period in their community health nursing course.

A modified version of the cultural self-efficacy scale (Bernal & Froman, 1987, 1993) was used to collect data at four points during the reminiscence education program. The modified scale, the Eldercare Cultural Self-Efficacy Scale (ECSES), measured students' self-efficacy and confidence for performing gerontological nursing skills when caring for older adults. A repeated measures analysis of variance showed statistically significant differences in ECSES scores for students who participated in the reminiscence-based learning program versus those who did not (Shellman, 2007). The results suggest that engaging students in reminiscence activities can positively influence their development as professional registered nurses. Perese, Simon, and Ryan (2008) pointed out that the number of older adults who will need mental health services is expected to rise dramatically over the next 20 years. At the same time, gerontological mental health nursing, as well as mental health nursing in general, are among the least desirable specialty practice areas for registered nurse students. The authors point out that positive undergraduate clinical experiences have been shown to increase students' interest in these areas. They described the development and evaluation of a clinical learning activity based on the integration of support group and reminiscence techniques. The type of reminiscence they described appears to represent social reminiscence. The goal of the experience was to provide a positive clinical experience for the students as well as a useful clinical nursing intervention for the older adult participants.

The nursing intervention developed for this learning activity took place in a geriatric psychiatric day treatment program. It involved one 30-minute group meeting that focused on a different theme each week for a total of 11 weeks. Themes were chosen prior to the implementation of the activity and were based on activities that would be common to all older adult group members (i.e., music, food and cooking, seasons of the year, etc.). A total of 11 weekly sessions were planned. Students facilitated this group activity using techniques derived from the support group and reminiscence literature. The group members and agency staff both reported very positive feelings about the experience in the follow-up evaluations. In addition, students had the opportunity to develop and participate in an activity that positively impacted their perceptions about this patient population (Perese, Simon, & Ryan, 2008).

Effective communication skills are essential in today's healthcare environment. To develop these skills, registered nurse students need to master a fundamental set of competencies, the most important of which is the ability to effectively listen. Using Social Reminiscence is one effective teaching strategy for developing listening skills (Puentes, 2000). Forty-three registered nurse students enrolled in a gerontological nursing course with both didactic and clinical components were provided with a list of questions adapted from Haight's Life Review and Experiencing Form (Haight, Coleman, & Lord, 1995) to guide their conversations with older adult nursing home residents during a 3-week clinical experience. At the end of the 3-week experience, students turned in a one-page typewritten paper that briefly summarized their client's life. They identified at least three significant life events from at least two life stages that were meaningful to the client. They also identified the topics they were most and least comfortable discussing with the client.

Experience outcomes were measured through a structured, faculty-developed survey tool. Students identified that they were most comfortable discussing situations that they perceived as having something in common with the client. Students' overall perception of the assignment was positive, and they noted that the assignment helped them to understand the humanity of their client. In addition, they found listening to their client's story enjoyable.

Puentes (1999) also found that engagement in Social Reminiscence activities was beneficial to practicing registered nurses. A continuing education program for registered nurses that focused on enhancing acute care nursing practice with older adults was developed to examine the effects of this type of activity on RNs' attitudes toward and empathy with their older adult clients. The study employed a post-test-only control group design with random assignment to treatment (*n* = 49) and control (*n* = 49) groups. The Reminiscence Learning Experience (RLE) comprised two components. The first was a 1-hour didactic program developed by the investigator that included a variety of learning techniques: lecture, overhead projections, group discussion, and group participation in a social reminiscence activity. This was followed by a 3-week period during which the participants independently implemented the reviewed techniques in their clinical practice. Both groups completed the Kogan's Attitudes Toward Old People Scale (Kogan, 1961) and the Hogan's Empathy Scale (Hogan, 1969) after the 3-week practice period. Scores on both measures were significantly higher for treatment group subjects than for control group subjects. The results of this study supported the hypothesis that a carefully developed continuing education with both didactic and clinical components can positively impact the nurse-client relationship.

The "Make a Difference" project (MADP) (Kirkpatrick & Brown, 2004) was a component of a gerontological nursing course that employed life story work as an integral aspect of the experience. The course was developed within the narrative pedagogy framework. Students were involved in viewing films with themes relevant to older adults and aging (e.g., *Fried Green Tomatoes*) and engaged in critical and reflective thinking assignments about these films. Another component of this course involved having the students spend 12 hours with an older adult and listen to their client's life stories. Through reflective and critical thinking activities, faculty worked with students to help them to draw moral insights and guiding principles from the information gathered from these conversations for both themselves and their clients. Program evaluation suggested that students found these activities to be fun, meaningful, and a way to enhance their understanding of multiple psychosocial issues.

Puentes and Cayer (2001) developed a modified version of Feeley's (1991) "Campus Wellness Vacation" as the framework for a gerontological nursing course for baccalaureate registered nurse students. Students spent one 40-hour week in the theory component of the course being exposed to gerontological nursing theory, including the use of social reminiscence in interactions with older adults. The second component of the course involved participating in a week-long series of seminars regarding issues of importance to older adults that were run by invited community experts. A group of invited community-residing older adults participated in this experience with the students. Topics included accessing services, Medicare and Social Security updates, Exercise, Home Safety, Legal Issues, and Spiritual Issues. In addition to the formal seminars, the opportunity for the students to interact socially with older adults at meals and break times was built into the program. Students were encouraged to ask the older adults to share their perceptions of the seminars, personal experiences with the issues discussed, and life stories through the use of social reminiscence techniques.

Students completed the Palmore's Facts on Aging Quiz (1998) and Kogan's Attitudes Toward Old People Scale (1961) prior to the beginning of the theory component of the course and at the end of the week-long series of seminar (Puentes, & Cayer, 2001). One-tailed t-tests for dependent groups showed significantly positive changes in knowledge of ($t = -4.4.567$, df = 32, p = .000) and attitudes toward ($t = -3.862$, df = 32, p = .001) older adults. Students also reported an increased respect for the humanity of their older adult colearners, and many students maintained ongoing relationships with their older adult community partners.

Schwartz and Abbott (2007) noted:

> Storytelling benefits patients, nurses and students. The patient is able to express who they are, relieve tensions, and resolve conflicts. It also provides the chance to reflect and reminisce, which can be therapeutic in helping patients cope with current conditions and illness. As a result, patients may develop an increased sense of accomplishment and self-awareness. . . . The nurse benefits from storytelling by deriving information from the story that may not have been collected from a basic health history and physical assessment. Stories have much to offer as a way of understanding. (p. 182)

Based on these ideas, Schwartz and Abbott worked on the development of a project to design and implement a model for teaching healthcare management in community-based settings that relied heavily on a variety of storytelling projects. Evaluation data from their project suggests that the use of storytelling in interactions with clients enhances listening skills and practitioner-client partnerships. In addition, it facilitates the development of common bonds leading to mutuality in practitioner-client relationships.

Conclusion

Reminiscence as a form of narrative pedagogy has been shown to be an effective approach to facilitate knowledge development, positive changes in attitudes, and empathy toward clients, and a better understanding of the humanity of the individuals for whom registered nurses provide care (Brown, Kirkpatrick, Mangum, & Avery, 2008; DasGupta & Charon, 2004; Gleeson-Krieg, Sayward, & Condon, 2006). Educators must move beyond old paradigms that focus exclusively on knowledge development and skill acquisition, toward educational paradigms that prepare registered nurses to effectively partner with clients to achieve the highest level of health and well-being possible. When utilizing reminiscence and other forms of narrative as teaching techniques, educators must understand the underlying dynamics of each of these teaching strategies. They must clearly articulate the goals of the learning experience and identify the professional development trajectory needed to prepare safe, effective, and knowledgeable practitioners who will be able to function effectively within an increasingly complex healthcare system. Reminiscence and narrative pedagogical techniques represent powerful teaching tools for accomplishing these goals.

References

Atchley, R.C. (1978). Aging as a social problem: An overview. In M.M. Seltzer, S.L. Corbett, & R.C. Atchley (Eds.), *Social problems of the aging: Readings* (pp. 4–21). Belmont, CA: Wadsworth Publishing.

Beaton, S.R. (1980). Reminiscence in old age. *Nursing Forum, 19*, 271–283.

Bernal, H., & Froman, R. (1987). The confidence of community health nurses in caring for ethnically diverse populations. *Image: Journal of Nursing Scholarship, 19*(4), 201–203.

Bernal, H., & Froman, R. (1993). Influences on the cultural self-efficacy of community health nurses. *Journal of Transcultural Nursing, 4*(2), 24–31.

Bluck, S., & Alea, N. (2002). Exploring the functions of autobiographical memory: Why do I remember the autumn? In J.D. Webster & B.K. Haight (Eds.), *Critical advances in reminiscence work: From theory to application* (pp. 61–75). New York: Springer Publishing.

Brown, S.T., Kirkpatrick, M.K., Mangum, D., & Avery, J. (2008). A review of narrative pedagogy strategies to transform traditional nursing education. *Journal of Nursing Education, 47*(6), 283–286.

Butler, R.N. (1963). The life review: An interpretation of reminiscence in the aged. *Psychiatry, 26*, 65–76.

Cappeliez, P., & O'Rourke, N. (2006). Empirical validation of a model of reminiscence and health in later life. *Journal of Gerontology: Psychological Sciences, 61B*(4), P237–P244.

Charon, R. (2001). Narrative medicine: A model for empathy, reflection, profession, and trust. *JAMA, 286*(15), 1897–1902.

Cohen, G., & Taylor, S. (1998). Reminiscence and ageing. *Ageing & Society, 18*, 601–610.

Coleman, P.G. (1974). Measuring reminiscence characteristics from conversation as adaptive features of old age. *International Journal of Aging and Human Development, 5*, 281–294.

Crabtree, B.F., & Miller, W.L. (Eds.). (1999). *Doing qualitative research*. Newbury Park, CA: Sage.

DasGupta, S., & Charon, R. (2004). Personal illness narratives: Using reflective writing to teach empathy. *Academic Medicine, 79*(4), 351–356.

Dochterman, J.M., & Bulechek, G.M. (Eds.). (2004). *Nursing interventions classification (NIC)* (4th ed.). St. Louis, MO: Mosby.

Erikson, E. (1959). Identity and the life cycle. *Psychological Issues, 1*, 101–164.

Fawcett, J. (1984). *Analysis and evaluation of conceptual models of nursing*. Philadelphia: Davis.

Feeley, E.M. (1991). Campus wellness vacation: A creative clinical experience with the elderly. *Nurse Educator, 16*(1), 16–21.

Gleeson-Krieg, J., Sayward, W.R., & Condon, M. (2006, July). Using narrative pedagogy to create evidence seekers. In A. Bongiorno (Symposium Organizer), *Empowering future nurses to use evidence-based practice through educational strategies.* Symposium conducted at the 17th International Nursing Research Congress Focusing on Evidence-Based Practice, Montreal, Canada.

Haight, B.K., & Burnside, I. (1993). Reminiscence and life review: Explaining the differences. *Archives of Psychiatric Nursing, 7,* 91–98.

Haight, B.K., Coleman, P., & Lord, K. (1995). The linchpins of a successful life review: Structure, evaluation, and individuality. In B.K. Haight & J.D. Webster (Eds.), *The art and science of reminiscence: Theory, research, methods, and applications* (pp. 179–192). Washington, DC: Taylor & Francis.

Hogan, R. (1969). Development of an empathy scale. *Journal of Counseling and Clinical Psychology, 33*(3), 307–316.

Kirkpatrick, M.K., & Brown, S. (2004). Teaching geriatric content with stories and the "Make a Difference" project (MADP). *Nursing Education Perspectives, 25*(4), 183–187.

Kogan, N. (1961). Attitudes toward old people: The development of a scale and an examination of correlates. *Journal of Abnormal and Social Psychology, 62,* 44–54.

Kovach, C.R. (1995). A qualitative look at reminiscing: Using the autobiographical memory coding tool. In B.K. Haight & J.D. Webster (Eds.), *The art and science of reminiscing: Theory, research, methods, and applications* (pp. 103–122). Washington, DC: Taylor & Francis.

LoGerfo, M. (1980-81). Three ways of reminiscence in theory and practice. *International Journal of Aging and Human Development, 12*(1), 39–48.

Merriam, S.B. (1993). Butler's life review: How universal is it? *International Journal of Aging and Human Development, 37,* 163–175.

Overcash, J.A. (2004). Narrative research: A viable methodology for clinical nursing. *Nursing Forum, 39*(1), 15–22.

Palmore, E.B. (1998). *The facts on aging quiz: A handbook of uses and results* (2nd ed.). New York: Springer Publishing.

Perese, E.F., Simon, M.R., & Ryan, E. (2008). Promoting positive student clinical experiences with older adults through use of group reminiscence therapy. *Journal of Gerontological Nursing, 34*(12), 46–51.

Puentes, W.J. (1998). Incorporating Simple Reminiscence techniques into acute care nursing practice. *Journal of Gerontological Nursing, 24*(2), 14–20.

Puentes, W.J. (1999). Effects of reminiscence learning on nurses' attitudes and empathy with older adults. *Image: Journal of Nursing Scholarship, 31*(1), 94.

Puentes, W.J. (2000). Using Social Reminiscence to teach therapeutic communication skills. *Geriatric Nursing, 21*(6), 315–318.

Puentes, W.J. (2005, November). Toward a unified perspective of reminiscence. In S. Melia (Chair), *Fifty Years of Life Review: Where is it at now? Where has it been? and Where is it going?* Opening plenary symposium conducted at the International Reminiscence and Life Review Conference 2005, Orlando, FL.

Puentes, W.J., & Cayer, C.A. (2001). Effects of a modified version of Feeley's campus wellness vacation on baccalaureate registered nurse students' knowledge of and attitudes toward older adults. *Journal of Nursing Education, 40*(2), 86–89.

Richardson, L. (1990). Narrative and sociology. *Journal of Contemporary Ethnography, 19*(1), 116–136.

Romaniuk, M., & Romaniuk, J.G. (1981). Looking back: An analysis of reminiscence functions and triggers. *Experimental Aging Research, 7,* 477–489.

Sadock, B.J., & Sadock, V.A. (2007). *Kaplan & Sadock's synopsis of psychiatry: Behavioral sciences/clinical psychiatry.* Philadelphia, PA: Lippincott, Williams, & Wilkins.

Schwartz, M., & Abbott, A. (2007). Storytelling: A clinical application for undergraduate nursing students. *Nurse Education in Practice, 7,* 181–186.

Shellman, J. (2006). "Making a Connection": BSN students' perceptions of their reminiscence experiences with older adults. *Journal of Nursing Education, 45*(12), 497–503.

Shellman, J. (2007). The effects of a reminiscence education program on baccalaureate nursing students' cultural self-efficacy in care for elders. *Nurse Education Today, 27,* 43–51.

Stuart, G.W., & Laraia, M.T. (1998). *Stuart & Sundeen's principles and practice of psychiatric nursing* (6th ed.). St. Louis, MO: Mosby.

Watt, L.M., & Cappeliez, P. (2000). Integrative and instrumental reminiscence therapies for depression in older adults: Intervention strategies and treatment effectiveness. *Aging & Mental Health, 4*(2), 166–177.

Watt, L., & Wong, P. (1991). A taxonomy of reminiscence and therapeutic implications. *Journal of Mental Health Counseling, 12,* 270–278.

Webster, J.D. (1993). Construction and validation of the Reminiscence Functions Scale. *Journal of Gerontology, 48,* 256–262.

Webster, J.D., & Haight, B.K. (1995). Memory lane milestones: Progress in reminiscence definition and classification. In B.K. Haight & J.D. Webster (Eds.), *The art and science of reminiscing: Theory, research, methods, and applications* (pp. 273–285). Washington, DC: Taylor & Francis.

Woods, B., & McKiernan, F. (1995). Evaluating the impact of reminiscence on older people with dementia. In B.K. Haight & J.D. Webster (Eds.), *The art and science of reminiscing: Theory, research, methods, and applications* (pp. 233–242). Washington, DC: Taylor & Francis.

Chapter 10

My Eye-Opening AmeriCorps Assignment at Senior Centers

Jocelyn C. Young

Becoming a full-time service corps member seemed to be my best option coming out of college. I was not ready to start medical school right away, and I did not want to start a full-time job that I would only hold for one year. So I applied to join AmeriCorps. When the program manager for the Rural Health Service Corps contacted me, we discussed my future plans. Since I knew I had a specific timeline for when I needed to be available to return to school, the only option was for me to interview for a position with the Office for Aging, in Broome County, in upstate New York.

It was not until after my first interview with the program manager that I was given a copy of the position description and began to question what I had gotten myself into. There were several classes that I would be expected to teach, volunteers needed to be recruited, and events were to be planned. I had no idea what the Office for Aging did exactly, and having the position description in my hands did little to answer that question. My second interview was at the agency itself with my soon-to-be supervisors. I was curious to see what went on there. However, it seemed to be a relatively generic office.

My interviewers did not ask many questions regarding my interest in working with seniors, which was good because I had none. Their focus was on my office skills, leadership abilities, and my willingness to speak in front of groups of people. After the interview I was under the impression that it was a desk job that I could easily handle for a year. That it might not be particularly stimulating, but for 10 months, it would do. When I received the phone call in which I was offered the position at the Office for Aging, I felt mostly relief to have a plan for the coming year.

The first few days on the job were how I imagined them to be, meeting the seemingly endless new faces, learning protocol, and getting my security badge. But then it came time to visit the 11 senior centers managed under the auspices of the Broome County Office of Aging. I was under the impression that the term *senior center* was synonymous with nursing home. Walking into the first center changed my perception completely. Rather than the dark and too-warm building I was expecting, it was open and well lit. There was a computer class going on where the "students" were learning to use the Internet. An adaptive yoga class was in session in the exercise room, puzzles were being worked, and cards were being played. It seemed every room in the center was buzzing with activity.

From that day on my perspective of what it meant to age and to be a senior was altered. When I began running events for the Senior Games, a sporting competition, I discovered just how active some older adults are. The competition level in some of the sports was extremely high. On the day of the competitive volleyball tournament, my mom and sister stopped by to see exactly what my job entailed. My sister's first comment was, "I didn't know old people could make skidding sounds with their feet." It struck me then how biased I was when I first started my service year; like my sister, I had no idea that there were throngs of active and vibrant seniors in the community. (I later learned that during the regular men's Wednesday morning practice sessions, other volunteers such as myself (i.e., two female nursing students) had been invited to actually join them in the volleyball practice games—one nursing student on each team—and word has it that they cut the students no slack! They played serious competitive volleyball, even at their regular practice sessions, and the students were impressed with their ability to keep the ball in the air until they had a chance to slam it into their opponents' faces! And everybody on both sides of the net cheered good naturedly each time a point was scored!)

As the events continued I discovered that 65 is not "old." Some of them were in better shape than me! A small reminder that while they were fit, their bodies were still aging, would come at the end of each event. I handed out a survey to the competitors, and I would often find myself reading the words to each person and filling in the answers because they did not have their glasses. When the Senior Games came to a close, I knew that I would miss being at all of the events, but I was already excited to see what would come next.

I began training to be a leader for two programs, A Matter of Balance and Chronic Disease Self-Management. It became apparent that I would be working with people at a much different fitness level when I began leading these classes. A Matter of Balance is best described as an educational support group for older adults who have a fear of falling. The issues that people in the class face on a daily basis are heartbreaking to hear. And I feel driven to help them brainstorm possible solutions and ways their lives can be more manageable.

The Chronic Disease class is eye opening in a different way; many of the participants are struggling with their health on a daily basis. Issues like shortness of breath, fatigue, and pain are common among those in the class. One of the major components of the course is problem solving, and I find it very interesting. Sometimes the solutions I come up with are not at all applicable to them, and the suggestions that other classmates give sometimes do not make sense to me. Both the differences and the similarities between our lifestyles become clear. While the participants in these classes are not the healthiest seniors I work with, it is very apparent that they want to be able to live an independent and fulfilled life.

An ongoing program I created takes place in the exercise room at one of the centers. It is equipped with a treadmill, stationary bikes, a gazelle, a rowing machine, "ab" machines, and free weights. A few days out of each month I set up a block of time to be in the exercise room to show people how to use the equipment. Since the program started four months ago I have given demonstrations to over 40 people. The number of seniors working out in the center has increased dramatically. Doing these demonstrations proved to us that many older adults want to exercise, but they are intimidated by the equipment. I enjoy working with everyone who comes into the exercise room because they are excited and really want to get in better shape.

Working with all of these different groups of seniors on a daily basis has opened my eyes to a generation that I did not know very much about. As I now understand my role at the Office for Aging, I am an educator and I provide opportunities for older adults to be active, to become more fit, to understand their bodies, and to improve their quality of life. While their ability levels vary widely, they all want information and opportunities to remain independent and social. When my year of service with AmeriCorps comes to an end in a few months, I will be beginning medical school. Based on the experiences I have had so far with the older generation, I am seriously considering gerontology to be my specialty. This is a group of people who have needs and desires unlike the other generations, and I look forward to serving them as a physician in the future.

Chapter 11

Where Pedagogy and Practice Converge

Engaging Graduate Gerontology Students in the Community Through Service Learning and Caregiver Education

Evanne Juratovac

This chapter provides illustrations of how blended service learning and gerontology-focused caregiver education promoted learning among both formal and informal caregivers for older adults.

Introduction and Background

One way to improve the health of older adults is to disseminate evidence-based information and to teach tips and strategies to caregivers. However, students who pursue a career path specializing in the care of older adults may not have an opportunity to teach the family (informal) caregivers and other agency (formal) caregivers of the older adult with whom they share the care. Facilitating this opportunity has been the mission of a Care Networks project administered through the nursing school and the community-responsive academic university gerontology center at Case Western Reserve University (CWRU).

The Care Networks project promotes interdisciplinary student involvement in the community through existing academic–community partnerships. While most of these gerontological experiences are offered as interdisciplinary experiences, the following examples largely involved graduate nursing students who were enrolled in an advanced practice Master of Science in Nursing (MSN) program. Through the Care Network project, the nursing students were offered an opportunity to participate in developing, presenting, and evaluating educational content for caregivers for older adults.

Opportunities for Students to Collaborate in the Community

At the host university (CWRU), a highly valued part of students' education has been community engagement through service learning (CETSL). Service learning as an educational method goes beyond mere service to the community to include strengthening students' learning and strengthening their attachment to the community (Corporation for National and Community Service, 2009).

Within the Care Networks, students participated in service learning activities to meet real needs of the community, rather than just fulfilling course requirements. Two points were reaffirmed throughout these experiences: First, that *service* learning seeks to serve the community by meeting an educational need that the community identifies, not merely a topic that the student wants to address; and second, that service *learning* creates an opportunity to increase the student's own learning outside of traditional didactic and clinical learning settings through educational encounters with family as well as formal caregivers.

Service learning may be an especially prominent experience in the academic trajectory that graduate nursing students pursue. A natural tendency for advanced practice nurses may be to focus on the needs of individuals, acquiring skills to both assess the individual's health status and intervene to promote health and maximize function. The potential exists, unfortunately, to de-emphasize family-focused and public health experiences in an already full academic curriculum. But an identified benefit of community–academic partnerships is that they strengthen the public health experience of advanced practice nurses through service learning projects at the university-affiliated nursing school (Narsavage, Lindell, Chen, Savrin, & Duffy, 2002). Thus graduate student-delivered education has the potential to be a springboard to greater quality improvement initiatives in the community (Bonner, MacColloch, Gardner, & Chase, 2007).

The community experiences described in the following paragraphs offered an opportunity for the students to teach the family and other care providers about recognizing and responding to health conditions and topics related to aging. Topics were requested by consumer and agency stakeholders in the region, including family caregivers, members of a community advisory board that represented partnering agencies, and the feedback of participants in previous educational sessions. The most commonly requested topics were related to mental health or behavioral care issues of older adults, such as depression or agitation, enhancing safety for older adults, and enhancing communication among formal and informal caregivers. This discussion features two commonly encountered exemplars: agitation and pressure prevention.

Defining Educational Need

The graduate students who engaged in service learning projects through the Care Networks had a variety of experiences. Typically, a way that students sought to meet the educational needs of caregivers was by helping to define and refine those needs, based on topics that had been requested by caregivers in the community. For example, when family caregivers expressed a need for education about problem behavior, their requests were clarified and member-checked with families and translated as a need for content about recognizing and managing agitation. In another example, formal caregivers wanted to learn how to decrease the incidence of stage one pressure ulcers in their care areas; their expression of this need was then embedded into relevant educational content related to the expert recognition of the risks, symptom presentations in vulnerable populations, and pressure prevention strategies.

Developing Educational Content

In the transition from defining need to developing content, students had an opportunity to co-develop educational content with the faculty member, a gerontological nursing expert. In response to abstract topics that were requested, such as "agitation" and "intimacy," the students participated in determining how to translate these requests into a finished educational product. Meeting this challenge involved several activities. One was to determine key words in order to search the literature and review the available evidence on a topic. Another early decision centered on how much time and detail could be allotted to various parts of the educational session, such as symptoms, risk factors, and management strategies. These activities were designed to encourage the students to use both critical thinking skills and time management skills to determine essential content and identify reasonable learner outcomes.

Presenting Educational Content

Several students had the opportunity to co-present educational content in the community that was both relevant and tailored to the audience. This was achieved in several ways. Some students presented content that they had co-developed with the faculty member, which afforded the students an opportunity to evaluate how the material was actually received in the live, iterative format of an educational session. Others modified content that had previously been developed for formal caregivers, giving them an opportunity to consider the specific content and approaches that were best suited to a family caregiver audience. For example, students had to consider the appropriateness of language that would be used in the session. Whereas words such as "patient" and "assessment" were common in the students' nursing lexicon, they were challenged to consider what terms might be more suitable for family caregivers who are managing health conditions and behaviors of loved ones (not "patients") in their homes. Other educational topics included "pain" and "exercise."

Other experiences of students in graduate programs at CWRU took the form of education as a foundation for process improvements in long-term care settings. For example, "pressure prevention" in older adult patients across settings, the educational session that was co-developed by the faculty member and a doctoral student, was prepared in response to a practice problem encountered by the staff of a skilled care facility. The agency leadership had determined that the early formation of pressure ulcers on the residents' heels represented a prominent vulnerability that needed to be addressed, both because the condition was being missed prior to admission and because the potential existed to improve the staff's recognition of risk factors and appropriate preventive interventions. Disseminating evidence-based information, including recommendations for standards of care, helped the formal caregivers who attended the educational session to improve their early recognition of a serious condition, and to take the first steps toward reducing the comorbidity associated with the condition.

Evaluating Educational Content

Finally, students had an opportunity to evaluate the impact of the educational content and process; an evaluation of the didactic content was disseminated to caregivers, and they were invited to offer their reflections on the process of a community-responsive teaching experience. A concrete example of an unplanned, though not unexpected, outcome for both students and families of older adults was the realization that a word such as "agitation" might actually be a multifactorial concept, with inconsistent methods of assessing and intervening. A more abstract outcome associated with this realization was an appreciation for the complexities and ambiguity often encountered in gerontological health care.

Almost to a person, students expressed an increase in their appreciation of the skill set and the sophistication of the family caregivers they encountered during the educational sessions. This theme suggested that the community gerontology experience clarified some misinformation about the capacity of families who provide care to older adults. Students also articulated an improved understanding of the role of the advanced practice nurse in recognizing and responding to these caregivers' most pressing educational needs.

Students' Evaluation of Their Community Caregiver Education Experience

Through the Care Networks, students participated in mentored individual and small group experiences; and they had opportunities to interact with other students across academic programs, undergraduate and graduate, as well as from across disciplines. For students who are pursuing careers in primary care and older adult care, these community-responsive, collaborative experiences have the potential to be positive formative experiences as they advance in their knowledge in collaborative practice with their future peers.

Importantly, community engagement as students experienced through their service learning fulfilled two of the competencies that the American Association of Colleges of Nursing (AACN) expects nurse practitioners and clinical nurse specialists in gerontological nursing to display. Specifically, students had an opportunity to "educate older adults, families, and caregivers about normal vs. abnormal events, physiological changes with aging, and myths of aging" (AACN, 2004, p. 8) and to "disseminate knowledge of skills required to care for older adults to other health care workers and caregivers through peer education, staff development, and preceptor experiences" (AACN, 2004, p. 8).

Several themes emerged as the students were immersed in community-based gerontological education. First, through their participation in community caregiver education, the nursing students had spontaneous engagement with informal caregivers, allowing them to better understand the role and sometimes heavy responsibilities that families have in the care of older family members. In addition, they gained an increased understanding of the impact of gerontological nurses in supporting this role. Secondly, students were exposed to the realities of community-responsive programming, where the role of the educator also includes attending to the group process and potentially managing unexpected emotional reactions to content. For both of these reasons, the faculty member, a gerontological specialist, was present with the students to provide supervision and support. Finally, and perhaps most importantly, students had the opportunity to observe faculty modeling the interdisciplinary and interagency collaborations that are at the core of gerontological practice and education. Community-based service learning and caregiver education is clearly a positive and meaningful experience for both the learners and the community.

Acknowledgment

I would like to thank my mentor, Diana L. Morris, PhD, RN, FAAN, FGSA, the project director of the Care Networks project, who encouraged my muse and skills to promote these community-based, interdisciplinary, gerontological experiences. On behalf of Dr. Morris and myself, I would also like to thank the Elisabeth Severance Prentiss Foundation, without whose generous funding these academic–community partnerships would not have been possible.

References

American Association of Colleges of Nursing (AACN). (2004). *Nurse practitioner and clinical nurse specialist competencies for older adult care.* Washington, DC: Author.

Bonner, A., MacCulloch, P., Gardner, T. & Chase, C.W. (2007). A student-led demonstration project on fall prevention in a long-term care facility. *Geriatric Nursing, 28*(5), 312–18.

Corporation for National and Community Service. (2009). *What is service learning?* Retrieved from http://servicelearning.org/what-service-learning

Narsavage, G., Lindell, D., Chen, Y., Savrin, C., & Duffy, E. (2002). A community engagement initiative: Service-learning in graduate nursing education. *The Journal of Nursing Education, 41*(10), 457–61.

Further Information

http://caregiving.case.edu/
http://fpb.case.edu/Community/CETSL.shtm

Section IV

Addressing Social Issues Related to Gerontology

Chapter 12

"Age Old" Health Disparities: Daunting Challenges in This Millennium

May L. Wykle

Minorities have poorer health and higher death rates than whites—at all age levels until very old age, when genetics are presumed to dominate longevity outcomes.

—Wykle & Kaskel, 1991, p. 24

The health challenge of growing old while confronting "age old" disparities in health care represents a major task for professionals in this millennium. According to the US Census Bureau, the minority population aged 65 and older is predicted to increase significantly over the next 40 years (Figure 12-1), including Blacks, Hispanics, Asians and Pacific Islanders, and American Indians. These groups are particularly affected by the process of aging and psychosocial circumstances that influence their health experiences and perception of control of their everyday lives.

Health Care for Minority Elders

In terms of receiving health care, minority elders are in jeopardy in a number of categories, including:

Age
Racial and /or ethnic discrimination
Income and poverty
Gender (i.e., women)
Dependence on government programs
Other barriers (language, culture, access to health care services, and mistrust of health-care providers)

Census data confirm beyond question that inadequate income is a significant factor in the disparities that are encountered by older minority members (Figure 12-2), and that older minority women are at particular risk for low income (Figure 12-3). In fact, African-American older women are likely to face multiple jeopardies, including ageism, culture, low income, and gender.

153

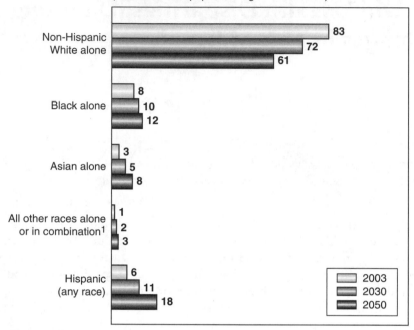

Population Aged 65 and Over by Race and Hispanic Origin: 2003, 2030, and 2050
(Percent of total population aged 65 and over)

[1]The race group "All other races alone or in combination" includes American Indian and Alaska Native alone, Native Hawaiian and Other Pacific Islander alone, and all people who reported two or more races.

Note: The reference population for these data is the resident population.

Figure 12-1 Population aged 65 and over by race and Hispanic origin: 2003, 2030, and 2050.

Source: US Census Bureau, 2004b.

It should also be noted that family care issues are compounded among minority family caregivers, who are most often unpaid for their services. In addition, minority family caregivers often work full time in low–decision-making-status jobs, and they can't take time off to care for their family members without losing their jobs. They often have to arrange for paid care during their work hours, but eventually money to pay helpers runs out. The burden for family caregivers is heavy, and there is little time for them to attend support groups that could help lower their stress. In addition, minority caregivers and the

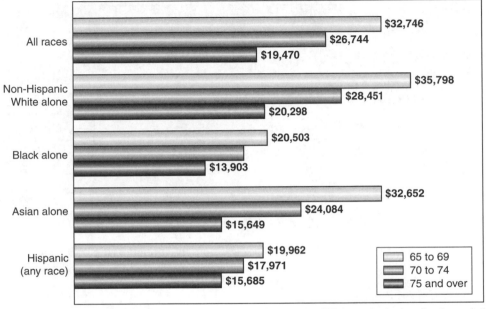

Median Household Money Income for Older Households by Age, Race, and Hispanic Origin of Householder: 2003
(Households with householder aged 65 and over)

Note: The reference population for these data is the civilian noninstitutionalized population.

Figure 12-2 Median income for older households by age, race, and Hispanic origin: 2003.

Source: US Census Bureau, 2004a.

care recipients are usually reluctant to place their loved ones in a nursing home, even when the caregivers' health is in jeopardy. Many express their values that focus on home as the best place to be, rather than a setting that may be foreign to the care recipients' cultural background. This is particularly true for Hispanic and Asian elders, who point to the language differences, their nutritional preferences and ADL needs, and cost.

But today's minority elders have faced more than merely financial problems. During their lifetimes they have experienced the impact of many crises in a disjointed healthcare system. They grew up when bias was legal and supported by discriminatory policies, and they experienced this bias not only in health care but in all aspects of their daily living. "The cumulative effects of poverty, segregation, discrimination, racism, official neglect, and exclusionary immigration laws, experienced over a lifetime, sometimes for generations, have left their mark on the older members of minority groups now living in the

Aged 65 to 74			
Male	**Poverty Rate (%)**	**Female**	**Poverty Rate (%)**
White	5.6	White	8.0
Black	18.1	Black	27.2
Hispanic origin	19.0	Hispanic origin	21.2
Total	7.7	Total	10.8
Aged 75 and Older			
Male	**Poverty Rate (%)**	**Female**	**Poverty Rate (%)**
White	6.0	White	12.2
Black	18.2	Black	27.7
Hispanic origin	19.8	Hispanic origin	25.6
Total	7.8	Total	14.1

Figure 12-3 Poverty status, measured by age, sex, household relationship, race, and Hispanic origin: 2003.

Source: US Census Bureau 2005.

United States. Generally poorer physical health and greater disability, compared to that of White persons of the same age and gender, give mute evidence of disadvantages endured" (Amasa B. Ford, cited in Wykle &Ford, 1999, p. 1). Dr. Ford, an expert geriatrician, was cofounder and senior member of the University Center for Aging at Case Western Reserve University, and was a geriatrician at the Eliza Simmons Bryant Nursing Home established for older Black women.

African Americans also face double jeopardy as they reach elder status because of the accumulation of specific disadvantages due to old age on the one hand and minority status on the other, compounded by the stress and poor health associated with the long history of racism, ageism, and lower income that this group has endured. (Kahana et al., 1999; Markides, Liang, & Jackson, 1990). Cultural traditions of minority elders, including their religious beliefs, may provide valuable coping skills; yet these traditional coping skills are often not effective when the elder also has developed serious chronic illnesses. These culturally based skills may also prevent them from seeking early healthcare interventions.

Minority elders are also at greater risk for certain diseases. For instance, African Americans are at greater risk for diabetes; 25% of African Americans between 65 and 74 have type 2 diabetes, and for every white American who gets diabetes, 1.6 African Americans will get diabetes. African-American women are at an even higher risk than African-American men for having diabetes. (National Institute of Diabetes and Digestive and Kidney Diseases, 1997; Harris et al., 1998) Likewise, African-American women appear to be at greater risk of developing more aggressive forms of breast cancer and are more likely to die from this disease than are white breast cancer victims. African-American women are also 3 to 4 times more likely to develop systemic lupus erythematosus (SLE), and are at 3 to 9 times higher risk for needing a hysterectomy than white women. African-American and Hispanic elders who suffer from arthritis are also significantly less likely to receive joint replacements (Markides & Black, 1996).

Another factor that greatly limits health care for minorities is the lack of caregivers from minority groups. For instance, only 7% of practicing physicians are African American, Hispanic, or American/Alaskan Native. The disproportions in nursing also continue to be a serious and lingering concern in terms of disparate health care. The underrepresentation of racial/ethnic groups and men in nursing education is perhaps the most important issue in this regard, and it compels leaders in nursing to renew their efforts to overcome barriers to the successful recruitment, retention, and graduation of male students and of students from racial/ethnic groups. The Council on Collegiate Education for Nursing of the Southern Regional Education Board (SREB) (2002), citing statistics beginning 30 years ago, notes that the barriers associated with too few minority healthcare providers are not new, and it urges university and school leaders to become actively involved in changing this statistic. The Council noted that African-American nursing students in baccalaureate, masters, and doctoral programs comprised only 16% of the total nursing students in the 16 states comprising the SREB, compared with 74% Caucasion students. The percentage of Latino nursing students within the SREB schools was 5%, Asian students comprised 3%, and American Indian students comprised only 1% of the total enrollment. The lack of success in recruiting minority students to nursing and other healthcare professions is a pressing problem that must be addressed if we are to improve the health of minority segments of the population, including elders, and create a healthier world. The health challenge of growing old while confronting "age old" disparities in health care is a major task for professionals in the new millennium. We need to identify minority elders' unique physical and mental health needs and examine the causes and effects of chronic illnesses and functional disability, keeping in mind that minority elders have experienced both social biases and ageism. We need research that addresses the ethical, spiritual and cultural issues in providing comprehensive models of eldercare.

But a related problem that must also be addressed in the effort to eliminate healthcare disparity is the even more prominent lack of nursing faculty and nursing education administrators who represent minority groups. According to the SREB report, 87.5% of the nursing faculty and administrators in the 16-state region were Caucasian, with the percentage of African-American faculty and administrators in nursing educational programs trailing at 9.2%. Latino and American Indian nursing faculty and administrators made up only 1.1% of this group, and Asian faculty and administrators were lowest in number, comprising only 0.7% of the total. The gender bias in nursing is also an issue, as male nursing students constituted only 9% of students in bachelor's programs, 9.5% in master's programs, and 6.1% in doctoral programs. (The survey did not include enrollment in associate degree programs.)

Twenty years ago Edmonds (1990) listed the following factors that influence minority health status and their use of health care:

Experience of racial segregation
Suspicion of dominant culture and its institutions
Reliance on kinship networks
Preference for traditional medicines and faith healing
Reliance on religious beliefs over the healthcare system
Lack of understanding and denial of illness symptoms
Unwillingness to adopt the "sick role"
Inadequate healthcare information
Unrealistic perception of health status
Poverty leading to inadequate health insurance, transportation, and nutrition
Insensitivity of healthcare planners and policy makers
Inadequate number of trustworthy healthcare practitioners, including minority
Perceived or real unequal treatment within the healthcare system

It is unfortunate that most of these limiting factors still prevail today, especially among older minorities. However, there is growing recognition about the impact of human potential and creativity in later life. But research in the past that pointed to possible directions for elder care has been inadequate.

Solutions

Whether due to insufficient finances or discrimination, inadequate access to health care negatively affects health promotion and the self-care practices of minority elders. It is therefore imperative that access to health care be available to everyone, including minority groups and those who do not have sufficient funds to pay for needed preventive health care services and treatment. As a society, and as healthcare providers, we can build culturally competent care into the education of nurses and other healthcare providers, and strive to insure that every elderly adult has access to the healthcare services that they need. And it is imperative that these changes begin immediately. Additional research is needed to shed light on the differing developmental needs of aging adults and their care givers, with particular focus on the cultural influences on aging adults from minority groups.

A great deal of emphasis is now placed on the physical health of elders and their limitations in being able to perform the activities of daily living. Because of this emphasis, the mental health of older adults is sometimes neglected. Poor mental health often affects older adults' ability to manage their self-care. Yet mental health interventions, including the treatment of the underlying causes of stress, are often given a low priority among health professionals and family caregivers. Depression and anxiety are two major mental health issues that are important to diagnose and assess, so that older adults can experience a sense of wholeness and well-being. Minority elders often neglect their emotional needs and fail to seek mental health intervention. Health disparity also affects the older minorities' opportunity for mental health treatment. We need health care for minority elders that is affordable, acceptable, and attainable.

The Frances Payne Bolton School of Nursing at Case Western Reserve University has a program of research that specifically addresses health disparities; you are invited to visit the website at http://www.case.edu/med/ccrhd/research/.

References

Council on Collegiate Education for Nursing (2002). *Racial/ethnic and gender diversity in nursing education.* Atlanta: Southern Regional Educational Board (SREB), 1–13.

Edmonds, M. (1990). The health of the black aged female. In Z. Harel, E. A. McKinney, & M. Williams (Eds.), Black aged (pp. 205.220). Newbury Park, CA: Sage.

Harris, M.I., Flegal, K.M., Cowie, C.C., Eberhardt, M.S., Goldstein, D.E., Little, R.R., et al. (1998). Prevalence of diabetes, impaired fasting glucose, and impaired glucose tolerance in US adults. The third national health and nutrition examination survey, 1988-1994. *Diabetes Care, 21*(4), 518–524.

Kahana, E., Kahana, B., Kercher, K., King, C., Lovegreen, L., & Chirayath, H. (1999). A model of successful aging. In M. Wykle & A. Ford (Eds.), *Serving minority elders in the 21st century* (pp. 287–322). New York: Springer Publishing Company.

Markides, K., Liang, J., & Jackson, J. (1990). Race, ethnicity and aging: Conceptual and methodological issues. In R. Binstock & L. George (Eds.), *Handbook of aging and the social sciences* (3rd ed., pp. 112–129). Boston, MA: Academic Press.

Markides, K.A., & Black, S.A. (1996). Aging and health behaviors in Mexican Americans. *Family and Community Health, 19*(2), 11–18.

National Institute of Diabetes and Digestive and Kidney Diseases, National Institutes of Health. (1997). National diabetes international clearinghouse. Retrieved from http://diabetes .niddk.nih.gov/

US Census Bureau. (2004a). Median income for older households by age, race, Hispanic origin: 2003. Retrieved from http://www.census.gov/

US Census Bureau. (2004b). Populations aged 65 and over by race and Hispanic origin: 2003, 2030, and 2050. Retrieved from http://www.census.gov/

US Census Bureau. (2005). Poverty status, measured by age, sex, household relationship, race, and Hispanic origin: 2003. Retrieved from http://www.census.gov/

Wykle, M., & Ford, A.B. (1999). Serving Minority Elders in the 21st Century. New York: Springer Publishing Company, p.1.

Wykle, M., & Kaskel, B. (1991). Increasing the longevity of minority older adults through improved health status. In *Minority elders: Longevity, economics, and health—building a public policy base* (special ed., pp. 24–31). Washington, DC: Gerontological Society of America.

Chapter 13

Addressing Health Sector Manpower Shortages and Service Gaps in Medically Underserved Areas: University-Facilitated Geriatric Continuing Education Collaborations

John A. Toner

Introduction[1]

The current manpower shortage of healthcare workers specializing in geriatric care is especially serious in rural and semirural communities. These communities, already stressed by the serious economic downturn, cannot adequately meet the healthcare needs of the expanding population of older persons. The older population, that is, those over the age of 65, is rapidly expanding as the baby boomer generation enters their retirement years. This mushrooming of the older population is exacerbating an already serious situation. The problems associated with the overall growth of the older population are more evident in medically underserved areas, particularly in rural regions of the country. According to the US Department of Health and Human Services (2003), 20 million of an estimated 70 million Americans living in rural areas do not have adequate access to health care. Complicating healthcare matters further is the fact that older persons with physical

[1]The author wishes to recognize with appreciation the POISE International Advisory Council, which sets the curriculum standards and annual continuing education course offerings, and the Columbia University Stroud Center (under the direction of Dr. Barry J. Gurland, Sidney Katz Professor of Psychiatry) for its ongoing support of aging research, policy development and education in medically underserved areas. The following members of the International Advisory Council are acknowledged: Othmane Alami, MD; Hugh Barr, PhD; Judith Blanding, PhD; Lenore Boris, JD, MS; Terri Bobal, CSW; Barbara Brozovic, GNP; Christine Decker; Della Ferguson, PhD; Sarah Gueldner, RN, PhD; Neil Hall, MD, MBA; Judith Howe, PhD, John Krout, PhD; William Luley, Lisa McMurray, MD; Mahfuzur Rahman, MD; Martha Nelson, RN, MS; Chaplain Betty Pomeroy; Scott Reeves, PhD; John Toner, EdD, PhD (Program Chair); Lori Webster, RN; Regina Sokal, RN, Paula Salinas, BS (Program Coordinator), and Tricia Carman, BA (Program Consultant).

health problems are at increased risk of serious mental illness. For example, older persons with declining physical health have more depression and anxiety, particularly if they are bereaved, live by themselves, have few and/or weak social supports, and suffer from physical problems and limitations of their activities of daily living (Schoevers, Beekman, Deeg, Jonker, & van Tilburg, 2003; Schoevers et al., 2000). All these conditions are more prevalent in rural areas, especially in medically underserved rural areas.

Rural older persons in New York State, for example, are more likely than the general population to have incomes below the poverty level, have poor health, lack access to public transportation, have fewer available services, and reside in inadequate housing, with few adequate housing alternatives available to them (Maiden, 2003; Krout & Maiden, 2000). The large proportion of older persons in the population of upstate New York, coupled with staggering rates of migration of younger healthcare professionals and allied healthcare workers who leave the upstate regions for job opportunities in the cities, present special challenges to healthcare planners and providers of care. Overall, the upstate New York population had the third-lowest rate of growth in the United States in 2005 due primarily to the exodus of the young from upstate rural counties. Consequently, the proportion of older persons in upstate New York is one of the highest nationally (Roberts, 2006). One approach to addressing this challenge has been to use continuing education in geriatrics and gerontology as a vehicle for retaining healthcare professionals, who frequently move from medically underserved areas for more lucrative professional opportunities elsewhere. Just as there is a special need for more services, there is also a special need for continuing education of health professionals and allied healthcare workers in rural medically underserved areas. The widening gaps between the healthcare needs of older persons, the treatment skills needed by the healthcare professionals who serve them, and the overall decrease in numbers of healthcare professionals in medically underserved areas has resulted in a dire need for creative recruitment and enhanced interprofessional and interdisciplinary education for healthcare workers in the field of geriatrics (York, 2007).

For the purposes of this discussion, the following definitions of terms apply: *Interprofessional education* refers to interactions during which two or more professions learn with, from and about each other to improve collaboration and quality of care (CAIPE, 2002). *Interdisciplinary education* emphasizes teamwork and collaborative engagement among professionals from diverse backgrounds and disciplines who share common goals and joint responsibility for treatment outcomes (Baldwin & Tsukuda, 1984; Miller & Toner, 1991). *Continuing interprofessional and interdisciplinary education* refers to ongoing, formal, post-qualification education incorporating interprofessional and interdisciplinary methods for the professional development of participants' knowledge, competence, and job performance (Barr, Koppel, Reeves, Hammick, & Freeth, 2005; Curran, Sargeant, & Hollett, 2007). The report from Health Canada's Initiative for Enhancing Interdisciplinary Collaboration in Primary Health Care indicates that although there is only limited empirical study of outcomes of interdisciplinary team collaboration, interdisciplinary team collaboration results in increased provider and patient satisfaction and access to care, and decreased hospitalization (Shaw, 2008). The aim of this chapter is to describe a program which: (1) has been developed for and successfully implemented with healthcare professionals serving older persons in medically underserved rural areas; (2) increases competency in geriatrics and geriatric mental health knowledge; and (3) includes interprofessional and interdisciplinary experiences. This is not primarily a research report of an empirical study. Although the results of evaluations are included, these results are included to demonstrate with preliminary data that the programs were viewed by participants as successful and as having achieved their stated objectives. The chapter aims to demonstrate how continuing interprofessional and interdisciplinary education in geriatrics and gerontology can be implemented in medically underserved rural areas to address health sector shortages and service gaps created by the exodus of healthcare professionals from these areas.

Program Description

In response to the challenges mentioned previously, and as a means of mitigating the effects of human resource shortages in medically underserved rural areas, the Columbia University Stroud Center has developed the Program for Outreach to Interprofessional Services and Education in Medically Underserved Areas (POISE). POISE has been developed and implemented in collaboration with the Consortium of New York Geriatric Education Centers, which combines the research and teaching resources of four universities and three medical schools in New York (Toner, Ferguson, & Sokal, 2009). POISE aims to incorporate interprofessional and interdisciplinary education as a means of reducing the effects of the fast-paced growth of the older population and human resource shortages on the health care of older persons in medically underserved areas. The interprofessional component of POISE facilitates healthcare providers' understanding of the roles of a variety of disciplines working within the geriatric healthcare system. Through a combination of interactive teaching modalities, which include role-playing exercises and facilitated group discussions, POISE participants come to understand that many professional roles overlap across disciplines and that it is possible to communicate better to reduce inefficient overlap. Participants also develop an understanding of the shared roles of different disciplines such that healthcare providers can efficiently share some professional roles in the face of human resource shortages.

The interdisciplinary component of POISE reinforces the interprofessional component, but it also contributes uniquely to participants' understanding of the advantages of effective interdisciplinary teamwork. It builds participants' knowledge and skills in team development, team management, team maintenance, and systematic problem-solving techniques. This is achieved primarily through the use of the POISE interdisciplinary team curriculum (Miller & Toner, 1991; Toner, 2002; 1994a, 1994b; Toner, Miller, & Gurland, 1994; Toner & Meyer, in press). The interdisciplinary curriculum emphasizes shared team leadership skills, communication, and systematic problem solving. The curriculum includes: team development exercises (e.g., Defining group members' roles, Leadership Orientations, Establishing Group Norms, Developing a Core Mission Statement); team management exercises (e.g., The Team Contract, Evidence-Based Systematic Problem Solving, Problem Solving Soap Opera Scenarios, Problem Solving Simulations & 'Disaster Prep' Scenarios, and A Method for Developing the Treatment Decision Guide); and team maintenance exercises (i.e. , Team Process Critique, videotape review, and Observations of Groups at Work).

POISE increases the knowledge of healthcare providers in geriatrics and geriatric mental health. POISE may also be making inroads to recruiting and retaining younger healthcare professionals to work with older persons in upstate medically underserved areas. For example, attendance of students from local 4-year and community colleges at POISE programs has increased steadily over the past 4 years. Consequently, community foundations in these medically underserved areas have recently provided scholarship support for professionals-in-training, and collaborative arrangements have been made with local colleges and long-term care facilities.

The purpose of POISE is to develop, implement, evaluate, and sustain interprofessional and interdisciplinary education for geriatric healthcare learners. The POISE curriculum emphasizes improving access to healthcare services, including mental health care for the geriatric population in medically underserved communities. POISE involves educational outreach, which originates from its academic base at Columbia University in New York City, to learners in medically underserved areas throughout New York State. This outreach and integration is facilitated by an internationally renowned faculty of academic psychiatrists, psychologists, social and research scientists, and other health educators linked to the collaborating upstate sites. The faculty includes geriatric specialists from outside New York State, including Canada and the United Kingdom.

POISE has been imbedded in the following programs that operate under the auspices of the Columbia University Stroud Center and the Consortium of New York Geriatric Education Centers in medically underserved areas of upstate New York. The curricula for each of these programs includes both interprofessional and interdisciplinary components. The programs that are primarily unidisciplinary, such as the Statewide Geriatric Psychiatry Residency and Fellowship Programs, include sessions that train the psychiatrist residents and fellows in interprofessional care. This includes a review of the roles of staff on the team from a variety of disciplines and practice assignments when the residents and fellows are leading team meetings. Similarly, the curriculum includes mandatory didactics, experiential exercises, and simulated experiences on interdisciplinary team collaboration.

- **The Statewide Geriatric Psychiatry Residency and Fellowship Programs**: This one- or two-year full-time Columbia University graduate medical education program is accredited by the Accreditation Council of Graduate Medical Education and based at Greater Binghamton Health Center in upstate New York. The program trains fully credentialed psychiatrists in geriatric psychiatry practice in medically underserved areas. The curriculum includes experiential learning through supervised clinical work and didactics and case conferences on a broad range of topics in geriatric psychiatry. The curriculum also includes the interprofessional and interdisciplinary components of POISE. Columbia University faculty travel from their academic base in New York City upstate each week to deliver didactics and provide clinical training to residents and fellows. Similarly, residents and fellows travel from their upstate primary clinical training site to complete week-long monthly rotations at clinical sites serving medically underserved areas in New York City.

- **The Statewide Geriatric Grand Round Series:** A 14-session series of grand rounds and clinical case conferences by the Columbia University Geriatric Psychiatry Fellowship Program faculty is presented annually in Binghamton and Syracuse, which serve predominantly medically underserved regions of New York. The Geriatric Grand Rounds are 2-hour sessions each, which include a wide range of geriatric mental health topics related to psychological, medical/physical (including neurological), social, and environmental issues in the management of geriatric patients. Participants are primarily medical professionals, including psychiatrists, nurses, and other medical doctors, but they also represent a broad range of other disciplines working in the field of aging.

- **The Geriatric Teaching Days and Geriatric Mental Health Teaching Days:** The Geriatric Teaching Days are offered annually at Greater Binghamton Health Center, whose catchment area is primarily medically underserved and rural. The theme for the Geriatric Teaching Days is *Recent Advances in the Care of the Elderly*, and specific topics change annually. The Geriatric Mental Health Teaching Days are 5 teaching days offered over the course of the year in Binghamton, Utica, and Syracuse, in collaboration with partnering hospitals, academic centers, and long-term care facilities. The Geriatric Teaching Days typically involve speakers from a variety of disciplines who address recent advances in their fields related to the current year's topic. In this way, participants are engaged in interprofessional education.

- **The Geriatric Scholar Certificate Program:** This 5-day educational conference held 1 day each week for 5 weeks in the fall (Utica, NY) and the spring (Binghamton, NY) provides professional training in interdisciplinary geriatrics and gerontology. The program is sponsored by the Columbia–New York Geriatric Education Center, in collaboration with the Consortium of New York Geriatric Education Centers and several other academic and clinical geriatric centers, including nursing homes, serving this medically underserved area. The program also receives support from foundations that focus on education of healthcare providers in medically underserved areas, such as the Slocum Dickson Foundation, the Community Foundation of Herkermer and Oneida Counties, and the Community Foundation of the Southern Tier. The Certificate program includes the Geriatric Mental Health Teaching Day and provides continuing education credits for healthcare professionals in the following disciplines: dieticians, nurses, nursing home administrators, physicians, physical therapists, and social workers.

The Geriatric Scholar Certificate Program is a post qualification continuing education program. The curriculum for the 40-hour Geriatric Scholar Certificate Program, which consists of 3 core days and 2 specialty days (i.e., electives) of training in interdisciplinary geriatrics, is endorsed by the national network of Geriatric Education Centers through the Bureau of Health Professions of the Department of Health and Human Services. The curriculum topics provide an overview of the field of geriatric and gerontological practice and includes 3 core days of training with required topics such as: Psychological Development Across the Lifespan, Communication and Sensory Loss in Aging, Geriatric Assessment, Culture and Aging, Bioethics, and Overview of Medicare and Medicaid. The topics for the 2 elective days vary but include one-half day interprofessional education and one full day on the topic of Interdisciplinary Teamwork and Quality of Life Improvement. Table 13-1 provides a day-to-day description of the 5-day agenda for Geriatric Scholar Certificate Program.

The program is cosponsored by a wide range of community, academic, and long-term care partners in the upstate region. The Geriatric Scholar Certificate Program is offered twice each year in a variety of sites in medically underserved areas in upstate New York. There is a faculty exchange between Columbia University and upstate academic and service-oriented centers. The learning objectives of the Geriatric Scholar Certificate Program are listed in Table 13-2 and are designed to meet the national educational guidelines established by the Title VII: Geriatric Education Centers Program, which is funded through the Bureau of Health Professions, Department of Health and Human Services.

- **The Quentin N. Burdick Program for Rural Interdisciplinary Team Training:** This combined on-site and distance learning program utilizes traditional didactics and telehealth and videoconferencing to teach geriatric healthcare teams methods of interdisciplinary team development, team management, and team maintenance. Although the emphasis of this program is interdisciplinary education, content related to interprofessional education is included, particularly as it relates to defining the roles of disciplines on the interdisciplinary team. The curriculum for this program relies heavily on clinical case–based experiential exercises and simulated evidence-based problem solving. The faculty have devoted decades to the development of the curriculum, which has been tailored to healthcare teams in medically underserved areas (Miller & Toner, 1991; Toner, 2002; 1994a, 1994b; Toner et al., 1994)

  - **TeleHealth and Videoconferencing**. The TeleHealth Videoconference Case Consultation Program is the flagship program of the Quentin N. Burdick Program, a federally and private foundation–sponsored effort. The

TABLE 13-1   Geriatric Scholar Certificate Program: Five-Day Agenda

Day 1

Intro. & Overview to Aging in Quality of Life (1)	Physical Changes of Aging (3)
Psychological Development (2) Across the Lifespan	End-of-Life/ Palliative Care (4)

Day 2

Overview of Medicare & Medicaid	Bioethics and Aging
Health Care Ethics and Long-Term Care	Health Issues and Creative Expression of Rural Elders

Day 3

Culture & Aging	Geriatric Rehabilitation

Promoting Wellness & Stress Reduction
  in Geriatric Care
	Communication & Sensory
	  Loss in Aging

Day 4: Geriatric Mental Health Teaching Day

Diagnosis and Course of Dementia (1)	Update on Psychotropic Medications (4)
Treating Geriatric Depression (2)	
Complicated Bereavement and Grief (3)	Alcohol and Prescription Drug Use in Older Adults (5)

Day 5

Choice and Choosing in Quality of Life (1)
Delirium in Elders (2)
Culture Change and Quality of Life in Long-Term Care of Older People (3)
Managing Transitions: Strategies for Assessing the Needs of Older Persons (4)

TeleHealth Videoconference Case Consultation Program includes a series of 10 telehealth videocase conferences annually and connects interdisciplinary healthcare teams from nursing homes and other long-term care facilities in medically underserved areas in upstate New York with Columbia University faculty who provide case consultations originating from studios at the Columbia University Medical Center in New York City. The TeleHealth and Videoconferencing Program involves interdisciplinary faculty from the Columbia University Stroud Center's Statewide Geriatric Psychiatry Residency and Fellowship Program, collaborators at the New York State

TABLE 13-2 Presentation of Educational Objectives

Day 1

Differentiate aging myths from aging realities and identify basic demographic data on aging.

Identify three aspects of psychological development across the life span.

Differentiate the effects of normal vs. abnormal aging on functional competence.

Discuss the physical changes of aging and their impacts on older persons' quality of life.

Discuss quality-of-life issues related to end-of-life and palliative care.

Identify three main approaches to maintaining patient quality of life in palliative care services.

Day 2

Identify unique approaches to better caring for the rural elderly.

Explain the principle of autonomy in ethical decision making.

Understand how Medicaid and Medicare differ and what is covered by both programs.

Recognize the importance of sense of personal identity throughout the aging process.

Day 3

Recognize the functional consequences of communication impairment in older persons, particularly hearing and vision loss.

Outline at least five principles basic to geriatric rehabilitation.

Identify cultural factors impacting assessment of older persons.

Identify three specialized applications of nonpharmacologic pain and stress reduction techniques for the frail elderly.

Day 4: Geriatric Mental Health Teaching Day (GTD)

Identify recent developments in the field of geriatric pharmacology.

Apply nonmedical approaches to managing dementia patients with disturbing behaviors.

Identify medications used to manage these behaviors based on symptoms.

Identify the prevalence of geriatric depressive disorders and the skills needed to assess depressive disorders in older persons.

Recognize the importance of interdisciplinary team meetings and case conferences for improved diagnosis and treatment of mental and physical problems in older persons.

Identify evidence-based approaches to the treatment of complicated bereavement and grief in older persons.

Day 5

Identify methods to transform the admission and assessment process in long-term care of older persons.

Recognize the importance of resident mentoring, and identify methods to implement mentoring.

Explain the critical factors affecting older persons during transitions between home, hospital, and nursing home.

Identify the unique challenges healthcare professionals face in leading the generations.

Psychiatric Institute of the Office of Mental Health, upstate academic collaborators at Utica College and the State University of NY–Upstate Medical Center (Syracuse) and its Clinical Campus at Binghamton, and healthcare practitioners at affiliated clinical sites. Through a grant from the US Department of Agriculture, the New York State Psychiatric Institute at Columbia University Medical Center houses video and teleconferencing equipment with compatible equipment at collaborating satellite sites upstate. This equipment is used to provide face-to-face, real-time dialogue between faculty and consultants at Columbia University Medical Center and upstate, rural clinicians and consumers. In addition to improving mental health care and enhancing interdisciplinary teamwork in upstate rural areas of New York, this service reduces the sense of isolation and frustration experienced by geriatric clinicians and allied healthcare workers in medically underserved rural areas, who often are faced with making difficult clinical decisions regarding complex clinical geriatric patients without the necessary training and skills.

Results

This chapter describes the development and successful implementation of POISE with healthcare professionals serving older persons in medically underserved rural areas in upstate New York. Some evidence, although impressionistic at this point, is provided that POISE increases participants' competency in geriatrics and geriatric mental health knowledge and interprofessional and interdisciplinary practice. This preliminary evidence is provided via participants' ratings that the program objectives for the training were achieved.

The authors note that these data are preliminary and caution that further outcome-based evaluation is necessary to demonstrate these conclusions convincingly. As indicated earlier, this is not primarily a research report of an empirical study. The results of a sample of evaluations demonstrate with preliminary data that the programs were viewed by participants as successful. The results reported in Table 13-3 demonstrate that continuing interprofessional and interdisciplinary education can be implemented successfully in medically underserved rural areas. These programs may help to address health sector shortages and service gaps created by the exodus of healthcare professionals from these areas.

Number of Participants

During the period from spring 2006 to fall 2009, the total number of participants registered in the POISE educational activities in upstate New York was 2667. This number represents repeat attendees; thus, these are not 2667 unique individual participants. Most participants reported that they were currently working with older people.

TABLE 13-3   POISE Participants by Discipline
Upstate New York Programs in MUAs 2006–2009

	Geriatric Psychiatry Fellowship Program at Greater Binghamton Health Center	Statewide Geriatric Grand Rounds Series	Geriatric Teaching Day and Geriatric Mental Health Teaching Day	Geriatric Scholar 5-Day Certificate Program	Burdick Program for Rural Interdisciplinary Team Training: Distance Learning via TeleHealth Clinical Consultations	Total
Allopathic Medicine	11	856	34	46	25	971
Osteopathic Medicine	0	0	4	2	0	6
Medical Student	0	24	8	0	0	32
Nurse Practitioner	0	45	18	23	5	89
Registered Nurse	0	266	308	82	10	666
Licensed P. Nurse	0	14	10	3	1	28
Undergraduate Nursing	0	24	11	12	0	47
Chiropractic	0	0	0	0	0	0
Clergy	0	7	6	6	0	19
Dental Public Health	0	0	0	0	0	0
Health/Nursing Home Admin.	0	53	42	31	10	136
OT/PT/Rec/Speech	0	68	8	11	5	92
Public Health[1]	0	0	1	1	0	2
Preventive Medicine[2]	0	0	1	0	0	1
Clinical Psychology	0	133	5	7	10	155
Psychology Intern	0	20	0	0	0	20
Social Work	0	98	168	37	12	314
Nutritionist	0	17	11	8	2	38
Nurses Aide	0	8	0	12	10	30
Pharmacist	0	14	2	2	3	21
TOTAL	11	1647	633	283	93	2667

[1]Public Health specialists are from any professional discipline and ordinarily receive training at a university-based School of Public Health, which awards public health certificates, and masters and doctoral degrees in Public Health.
[2] Preventive Medicine specialists are medical doctors with specialty training in Preventive Medicine.

Table 13-3 presents a breakdown of the number of participants in all POISE geriatric education programs by healthcare discipline. The disciplines that have the largest number of participants in all POISE programs during this period are the following: medical doctors (n = 971), registered nurses (n = 666), and social workers (n = 314). Although POISE targets certain of its educational programs to medical doctors—primarily because of its roots in geriatric psychiatry—POISE programs in medically underserved areas attract significant numbers of healthcare and nursing home administrators (n = 136) and nurse practitioners (n = 89), who provide primary and specialized health care that may be independent or dependent on physician practice, according to jurisdiction.

Aside from being an educational program, which has been imbedded in the specific programs mentioned above, POISE is also a healthcare rural human resource enhancement and development initiative. The success of this initiative is seen not only in the large number of participants (n = 2667) but in the diversity of its learners. Although primarily a post qualification program, POISE has attracted healthcare workers from all levels, including nurses' aides (n = 30).

Evaluation

POISE has employed standard evaluation methods using pre- and post-education questionnaires, which focus on participants' judgments about the quality of the educational programs. The questionnaires were developed by the Consortium of New York Education Centers and approved for use as an evaluation measure by the federal funding agency, the US Department of Health and Human Services. The validity and reliability of the evaluation questionnaire are currently under study. This systematic, ongoing evaluation insures continuous feedback to the POISE program planners and faculty presenters.

Table 13-4 provides a summary of selected evaluation criteria obtained from participants in the following 2008 and 2009 POISE programs: The Geriatric Scholar Certificate Program (Utica, fall 2008, 2009); the Geriatric Scholar Certificate program (Binghamton, spring 2008, 2009); the Geriatric Teaching Day (Binghamton, spring 2008, 2009); and the Geriatric Mental Health Teaching Day (Utica, fall 2008, 2009). Results were obtained from 369 program participants who completed the evaluation questionnaire. This represents approximately 70% of program participants. The results indicate that the POISE programs are well received by participants. For all evaluation criteria, ratings are made on a 4-point scale ranging from "1–poor" to "4–excellent." The vast majority of participants rated the overall program as "good–excellent" (93% for day 4; 100% for days 3 & 5). The results indicate that participants felt that the objectives for the training had been met.

Table 13-4 represents selected evaluation criteria. Specific comments by participants on the evaluation questionnaire regarding the strengths and weaknesses of the program are not reported here. However, these comments were most useful in helping the authors to revise the curriculum and to mentor speakers who received ratings of "1–poor" or "2–fair."

TABLE 13-4 Evaluation Results

POISE Program Evaluation: Summary Report Geriatric Scholar Certificate Program, Geriatric Teaching Day and Geriatric Mental Health Teaching Day (N = 369)

Evaluation Criterion	Day 1	Day 2	Day 3	Day 4 GTD/GMHTD	Day 5
To what extent was each speaker knowledgeable, organized and effective in presentation?	Speaker 1 1=0%, 2=4%, 3=12%, 4=84% Speaker 2 1=0%, 2=0%, 3=36%, 4=64% Speaker 3 1=0%, 2=4%, 3=24%, 4=72% Speaker 4 1=0%, 2=4%, 3=12%, 4=84%	Speaker 1 1=0%, 2=0%, 3=25%, 4=75% Speaker 2 1=4%, 2=44%, 3=40%, 4=12% Speaker 3 1=0%, 2=20%, 3=47%, 4=33 Speaker 4 1=0%, 2=0%, 3=20%, 4=80%	Speaker 1 1=0%, 2=0%, 3=18%, 4=82% Speaker 2 1=0%, 2=0%, 3=9%, 4=92% Speaker 3 1=4%, 2=4%, 3=35%, 4=61% Speaker 4 1=0%, 2=0%, 3=18%, 4=82%	Speaker 1 1=0%, 2=0%, 3=9%, 4=91% Speaker 2 1=0%, 2=0%, 3=9%, 4=91% Speaker 3 1=0%, 2=0%, 3=9%, 4=91% Speaker 4 1=0%, 2=0%, 3=9%, 4=91%	Speaker 1 1=0%, 2=4%, 3=49%, 4=47% Speaker 2 1=2%, 2=24%, 3=47%, 4=27% Speaker 3 1=0%, 2=2%, 3=30%, 4=67% Speaker 4 1=0%, 2=0%, 3=7%, 4=93%
Overall, to what extent were the teaching methods and aids used appropriately and effectively?	1=0%, 2=4%, 3=25%, 4=71%	1=0%, 2=4%, 3=52%, 4=43%	1=0%, 2=0%, 3=23%, 4=77%	1=0%, 2=0%, 3=9%, 4=91%	1=0%, 2=7%, 3=61%, 4=32%
To what extent have you achieved each objective of this session?	1=0%, 2=0%, 3=24%, 4=76%	1=0%, 2=0%, 3=39%, 4=61%	1=0%, 2=0%, 3=9%, 4=91%	1=0%, 2=0%, 3=9%, 4=91%	1=0%, 2=4%, 3=49%, 4=47%
How was the organization and registration of the overall program?	1=0%, 2=0%, 3=25%, 4=75%	1=0%, 2=0%, 3=29%, 4=21%	1=0%, 2=0%, 3=22%, 4=78%	1=0%, 2=0%, 3=14%, 4=86%	1=0%, 2=2%, 3=25%, 4=73%
Please rate the overall program:	1=0%, 2=4%, 3=52%, 4=43%	1=4%, 2=0%, 3=48%, 4=48%	1=0%, 2=0%, 3=19%, 4=81%	1=0%, 2=0%, 3=14%, 4=86%	1=0%, 2=7%, 3=38%, 4=55%

Note: The rating scale for all criteria ranges from 1 to 4, where 1=poor, 2=fair, 3=good, and 4=excellent.

Lessons Learned for Practice

1. New York State has a higher percentage of older persons than the national average (14% vs. 12% nationally) and suffers from severe human resource shortages, especially in geriatric health care.

2. Severe shortages of gerontologist educators in medically underserved areas of New York have created large gaps in the training of geriatric healthcare workers.

3. The Program for Outreach to Interprofessional Services and Education in Medically Underserved Areas (POISE) has begun to bridge the gaps in the training of geriatric healthcare workers by training 2667 healthcare professionals and allied healthcare providers working in medically underserved areas in upstate New York.

4. Most participants (93% to 100%, depending on specific POISE participant cohorts) rate the POISE educational programs "good–excellent."

5. Pre- and post-test questionnaires about attitudes, perceptions, and motivations for rural practice need to be developed and applied to this population of learners.

There is currently no empirical evidence of the effect of POISE on participants' clinical practice. The authors acknowledge the need to study clinical practice outcomes of POISE that are targeted to a specific region, particularly in medically underserved areas where POISE has been utilized. The authors are exploring with academic colleagues application of geocoding methods, which examine the effects of an intervention (e.g., geriatric health-care education and training) on treatment practices of healthcare trainees in the regions to which they return to clinical practice post-training.

Discussion

The POISE program has made significant inroads to providing continuing geriatric and gerontological education in medically underserved areas of New York State, which have a higher-than-average percentage of older persons and suffer from severe human resource shortages, especially in geriatric health care. POISE has been successful in infusing inter-professional and interdisciplinary, geriatric, and geriatric mental healthcare education, offered with low-cost continuing education credits and contact hours to attract a wide range of disciplines into medically underserved areas of New York State. It remains to be seen, in the face of drastic federal and state cuts during the current recession, how POISE will continue to provide for the educational needs of professionals who work with older persons in medically underserved areas of upstate New York.

References

Baldwin, D., & Tsukuda, R. (1984). Interdisciplinary teams. In C. Cassel & J. Walsh (Eds.), *Geriatric medicine: Medical, psychiatric and pharmacological topics* (Vol. 2, 421–435). New York: Springer-Verlag, Inc.

Barr, H., Koppel, I., Reeves, S., Hammick, M., & Freeth, D. (2005). *Effective interprofessional education: Argument, assumption and evidence.* Oxford (UK): Blackwell Publishing Ltd.

CAIPE (2002). The UK Centre for the Advancement of Interprofessional Education: www .caipe.org.uk.

Curran, V., Sargeant, J., Hollett, A. (2007). Evaluation of an interprofessional continuing professional development initiative in primary health care. *The Journal of Continuing Education in the Health Professions, 27*(4), 241–248.

Krout, J.A., & Maiden, R.J. (2000). *Living in the community: A rural and non- rural comparison. Project 2015: The future of aging in New York.* Albany, NY: New York State Office for Aging.

Maiden, R. (2003). Mental health services for the rural aged: Public policy issues and concerns. *Psychiatry Times, 20*(12), 41–46.

Miller, P., & Toner, J. (1991). The making of a geriatric team. In W. Myers (Ed.), *New techniques in the psychotherapy of older patients.* Washington, DC: American Psychiatric Press.

Roberts, S. (2006, June 13). Flight of young adults is causing alarm upstate. *New York Times,* pp. A1, B4.

Schoevers, R.A., Beekman, A.T., Deeg, D.J., Geerlings, M.I., Jonker, C., & van Tilburg, W. (2000). Risk factors for depression in later life: Results of a prospective community based study (AMSTEL). *Journal of Affective Disorders, 59*(2), 127–137.

Schoevers, R.A., Beekman, A.T., Deeg, D.J., Jonker, C., & van Tilburg, W. (2003). Comorbidity and risk-patterns of depression, generalised anxiety disorder and mixed anxiety-depression in later life: Results from the AMSTEL study. *International Journal of Geriatric Psychiatry, 18,* 994–1001.

Shaw, S. (2008). More than one dollop of cortex: Patients' experiences of interprofessional care at an urban family health centre. *Journal of Interprofessional Care, 22*(3), 229–237.

Toner, J. (1994a). Developing and maintaining links between service disciplines. In J.R.M. Copeland, M.T. Abou-Saleh, & D.G. Blazer (Eds.), *Principles and practice of geriatric psychiatry,* 1021–1026. New York: John Wiley & Sons.

Toner, J. (1994b). Interdisciplinary treatment team training in geriatric psychiatry: A model of university-state-public hospital collaboration. *Gerontology and Geriatrics Education, 14*(3), 25–38.

Toner, J. (2002). Developing and maintaining links between service disciplines (POISE). In J.R.M. Copeland, M.T. Abou-Saleh, & D.G. Blazer, (Eds.). *Principles and practice of geriatric psychiatry* (2nd ed., pp. 795–798). New York: John Wiley & Sons.

Toner, J., Ferguson, D., & Sokal, R. (2009). Continuing interprofessional education in geriatrics and gerontology in medically underserved areas. *Journal of Continuing Education in the Health Professions, 29* (3), 157–162.

Toner, J., & Meyer, E. (in press). The interdisciplinary treatment team as a geriatric mental health resource prior to and during disasters. In J. Toner, T. Mierswa, & J. Howe (Eds.), *Geriatric mental health disaster and emergency preparedness.* New York: Springer Publishing Company.

Toner, J., Miller, P., and Gurland, B. (1994). Conceptual, theoretical and practical approaches to the development of interdisciplinary teams: A transactional model. *Educational Gerontology, 20*(1), 53–69.

US Department of Health and Human Services. (2003). *Rural mental health outreach: Promising practices in rural areas.* Rockville, MD: US Department of Health and Human Services, Substance Abuse and Mental Health Services Administration, Center for Mental Health Services.

York, M. (2007, July 23). Few young doctors step in as upstate population ages. *New York Times,* pp. B1, B4.

Chapter 14

Getting the Home in Nursing Homes

Michael Carter

Several years ago, one of the residents of the nursing home where I practiced expressed her concern to me over the remodeling of the facility. She was upset that too much money was being spent, and she contended that the funds should be allocated to programs for the young whose lives were before them rather than elders like her who were near the end of their lives. "After all," she said, "don't you know that no amount of decorations can change the fact that nursing homes are warehouses for the old awaiting death?" She said that she should know something about that sort of thing in that she was a survivor of Auschwitz.

These poignant words point out one of the critical issues for current nursing homes. The architectural design of nursing homes today is for the ease of the staff or the least costly construction instead of giving full consideration to the fact that these facilities serve as the homes for the residents. Yet few residents would choose to live in a facility that was designed as many of these facilities have been. Long halls, "semiprivate" rooms, bright overhead lighting, institutional furnishings, and loud overhead paging systems all drive home the impression that nursing home residents are living in a hospital-like institution and not a home.

How do people come to leave their own homes and move into a long-term care institution? Institutional living is not often a first choice. But there are times when people are no longer able to perform instrumental activities of living or activities of daily living. This loss means that a move to long-term care may be necessary. The change to a living arrangement in which independence is lost or substantially reduced can be emotionally devastating. The move to a more dependent living arrangement can also portend a potential downward spiral at the end of life.

The type of living arrangement that becomes necessary is determined by the abilities of the person and the nature of outside supporting relationships. Elders can lose their abilities of self-care, and their support system of spouse or other family members may not be able to provide the scope or duration of services required. This usually results in the elder and family making one of the most difficult choices—to move to and live in a long-term care facility. Long-term care facilities vary in the amount and type of direct care that they provide. Assisted living facilities provide limited direct care services, with nursing homes providing the most complex long-term care.

Assisted living facilities emerged in the 1990s as a part of a continuum of care for people who did not require 24-hour care but could no longer live in their own homes independently. There is no national standard as to what is meant by the term *assisted living*, but more than two-thirds of the states require a license for such facilities (Jones, n.d.). These facilities can usually provide assistance with the instrumental activities of daily living, including meal preparation, laundry, shopping, medication management, transportation, and household cleaning. In addition, most assisted living facilities can provide assistance with many of the activities of daily living, including bathing, dressing, grooming, and toileting. The challenges for assisted living become more evident when there are problems with transfer, feeding, continence, and communication. These care needs often require the services of a nursing home.

Nursing homes are designed to provide a higher level of care for people with limitations in their activities of daily living. In addition, these facilities provide nursing assessment and supervision of a number of health-related problems that can easily exceed the capabilities of home care or assisted living facilities. This level of required care is often accompanied by an even greater loss of independence in some of the most basic decisions—when, what, and with whom to eat, use the toilet, bathe, and sleep. These decisions are taken for granted when we live in our own homes.

There have been recent attempts to change the way in which nursing homes make decisions for the residents, allowing much more independence in some of these basic areas. Often, however, architecture becomes an impediment to this change in care delivery, and the many and outdated regulations are problematic.

How did we get to today's nursing home organization and design? What will we need to do to move to a model of care in which maximum independence can be fostered? How can we put the home into nursing homes? Considering the historical developments that led to the modern nursing home in the United States will help lead to some answers to these questions.

The History of the Evolution of Nursing Homes

Nursing homes of today in the United States evolved from the poorhouses of the 1800s and early 1900s (*The Poorhouse Lady*, n.d.). These facilities began as benevolent organizations to provide services for the poor who had no family to care for them and little financial ability to care for themselves. Prior to the poorhouses there were three main approaches to providing care for the poor in the United States. Each of these three approaches was predicated on a local system usually supported by very limited tax dollars. The first system was called outdoor relief. Each county had an overseer of the poor, and this person could provide some very limited funds to support basic needs. The poor would remain in their own homes and just receive relief money. There was usually substantial stigma in using this system. The ideal in America was self-sufficiency, and the very poor without family did not fit this ideal when they required public funds to live.

The second system for "helping" the poor was to auction them off. The pauper was essentially sold to the lowest bidder. This was a form of indentured servitude but was usually time limited. This form of service to the poor was fraught with the potential for abuse and was not widely used in a formal way. There were a number of approaches that were privately operated that were similar, including sharecropping in the South.

The third system of service was for the county to contract with someone or an organization in the community to provide basic food and shelter for the poor. This system evolved into the state-mandated poorhouses in which people lived on the county dole when they were not able to care for themselves. The housing provided was minimal and often crowded. As with the other systems for the poor, the poorhouses did not fit with the notion of self-sufficiency.

During the Depression and under the programs of the New Deal, the idea emerged that the elderly should receive benefits on the basis of need (US Social Security Administration, n.d.). In 1935 President Roosevelt signed the Social Security Act. A section of this act provided matching grants to each state for Old Age Assistance to retired workers. One of the stipulations of the act was that payment could not be made to people living in public institutions. Quickly, private old age homes were developed to replace the publicly operated facilities, including the poorhouses. Private homes were unlicensed and unregulated. This means there were no minimum standards of care. The least expensive methods for construction were those that had several beds in each room.

Following World War II, there were a number of changes in the Social Security Act that changed the face of old age homes. One of the changes was the requirement that all states must begin licensing for nursing homes. Also included was a change that allowed payment of benefits to elderly people who resided in public facilities. By the mid-1950s there was additional legislation that allowed hospitals to build nursing homes as a part of the hospital. This, combined with the earlier Hospital Survey and Construction Act (known as Hill-Burton) that provided federal funds to build hospitals, led to a rapid growth in nursing facilities. The linkage to the hospital meant that these new facilities were built on the same architectural model as the hospital. These new facilities often had very large wards with little privacy, since that was the model of the hospitals during that era. One or a few nurses could observe multiple patients at the same time. Little use was made of the model put forth by Florence Nightingale in her book, *Notes on Hospitals* (1859). Most were austere because few would argue that expensive architecture was appropriate for the poor.

From the 1960s forward, there were many new federal laws that related to the funding of nursing home care or to the ways in which the care should be provided. These new regulations did not relate to the actual design of the living arrangements in the building, and there were many reported cases of fraud, abuse, and abject living situations. Not-for-profit organizations began to be replaced by for-profit systems that quickly understood how to profit from the care of the elderly, even the poor elderly. One of the elements of the emerging systems was to provide care to a maximum number of residents at the lowest costs to meet the minimum new standards. Bedrooms with multiple beds were less expensive to build than private rooms. There was little need to attempt to appease the customer since so many of the residents were receiving public welfare.

In 1986, the Institute of Medicine released its report on improving the quality of care in nursing homes (Committee on Nursing Home Regulation, & Institute of Medicine, 1986). This report led to a variety of new regulations aimed at improving the quality of life for nursing home residents. A number of other policy initiatives were begun in the 1990s with the goal of bringing about substantial change in the way long-term care institutions were designed and operated.

One of the early innovative ideas was the Eden Alternative ("The Eden Alternative philosophy," n.d.) in which there was a reorganization of the key ideas of providing community for elders in living situations, including a change in the habitat. This revisit of living space for elders was designed to return to the elders their autonomy over daily life. This approach attempted to overlay a set of new ideas on existing long-term care facilities. The goal was to flatten hierarchies and to provide the residents with a maximum amount of decision making. There was a good deal of adoption of these ideas but little research showing better resident outcomes (Angelelli, 2004).

The Green House® (NCB Capital Impact, n.d.) was another approach developed with a grant from the Robert Wood Johnson Foundation with the goal of fundamentally changing the way in which long-term care would be delivered. An important part of the Green House was the actual construction design—small numbers of residents (10), private bedrooms and bathrooms, shared living and dining space. However, older building designs were not adapted easily to the goal of transforming the care for nursing home residents. Green House also altered the roles of the care providers. The certified nursing assistant's (CNA) role was expanded to include all aspects of care, including cooking, housekeeping, personal laundry, and personal care. Nurses, physical therapists, occupational therapists, and other professional personnel provided visiting support care. The CNA no longer reported to a nurse but to an administrator. Early on, researchers indicated that the quality of care for Green House residents was generally higher than for comparison nursing homes (Kane, Lum, Cutler, Degenholz, & Yu, 2007).

In 1997 the Pioneer Network (n.d.) was created by a small group of people committed to changing how nursing homes are operated. According to Bowman (2008), the Pioneer Network strongly advocated for moving away from institutional provider-driven models to consumer-driven models. This model has been labeled the *culture change movement*. A great deal of the effort of the Pioneer Network is to work with the Centers for Medicare and Medicaid Services (CMS) to evolve their regulatory system to accommodate this change in care.

The Pioneer Network has focused a good deal of its work on changing architecture to bring about different living environments. For example, current CMS regulation §483.70(d)(1)(ii) requires that each resident is to have 80 square feet of space in his or her bedroom in a shared room. This has become the standard for new nursing home construction, although it was only intended to be the minimum standard. This amount of space will not allow for a chair or computer table should the resident want one. The Pioneer Network has demonstrated that almost no nursing home resident wishes to have a roommate, and most wish to have more of their personal items in their rooms.

Moving to a different model of care is not as simple as it might seem. There are many state and federal regulations that would seem to conspire against putting home in the nursing home beyond the costs of increased private rooms and multiple small buildings (Stone, Bryant, & Barbarotta, 2009). The biggest problems seem to be in life safety codes. These include things like hall width, door structures, kitchen regulations, and a multitude of areas that appear acceptable at first glance but turn out to be a problem. For example, plants are not usually allowed anywhere that they might impede a wheelchair or a bed being moved to assure that nothing restricts egress. These codes do not allow for chairs or other seating to be placed in hallways, even though a resident might need to sit when walking. Various local and state fire codes may not allow for personal items from home to be used in the room.

Fortunately, there are new groups such as the Center of Design for an Aging Society (n.d.) and the Society for the Advancement of Gerontological Environments (n.d.) dedicated to developing new approaches to nursing home environments. These and many other grassroots organizations are pressing for substantial changes in the way that nursing homes are designed and how the care is delivered. All of these efforts seem to be pressing to put the "home" in the nursing home.

Summary

Nursing homes began as an outgrowth of the pauper care system in the United States. Seldom was the quality of the environment a part of the planning for the construction of these facilities. During the late 1940s and early 1950s the construction of new nursing homes seemed to be built on the hospital model, where bunching people together in rather austere bedding arrangements was the most cost-effective. Both of these modes of design had the effect of removing personal independence from the residents.

Over the past 10 to 20 years, several groups have begun to call for a complete change in the culture of nursing homes. This includes a change in the environment, changes in the language, and important changes in the very way that care is organized to allow personal choices to dictate care. All of these changes are focused on maintaining independence for elders as they require assistance from both their architecture and personnel to meet their personal needs in a way that the elder wants these needs met. Little of nursing's focus on care has been a part of these institutions, even though they are called nursing homes. Nursing can take a substantial lead in this new movement.

References

Angelelli, J., (2004). Comparing the characteristics of Eden Alternative early adopters with those who discontinue. *The Gerontologist, 44,* 34.

Bowman, C.S. (2008, April). The environmental side of the culture change movement. Retrieved from Washington, D.C. Centers for Medicare and Medicaid Services website http://www.pioneernetwork.net/Data/Documents/Creating-Home-Bkgrnd-Paper.pdf.

Center of Design for an Aging Society. (n.d.). Making it possible to age with dignity in a supportive environment. Retrieved from http://www.centerofdesign.org/index.html.

Committee on Nursing Home Regulation, and Institute of Medicine. (1986). *Improving the quality of care in nursing homes*. Washington, DC: Academy Press.

The Eden Alternative philosophy. (n.d.). Retrieved from http://www.edenalt.org/our-philosophy.html.

Jones, P.M. (n.d.). Assisted living—A brief history and definition. *Ezine @rticles*. Retrieved from http://ezinearticles.com/?Assisted-Living-A-Brief-History-and-Definition&id=1898892.

Kane, R.A., Lum, T.Y., Cutler, L.J., Degenholz, H.B., & Yu, Tzy-Chyi. (2007). Resident outcomes of small-house nursing homes: A longitudinal evaluation of the initial Green House® program. *Journal of the American Geriatric Society*,55(7), 832–839.

NCB Capital Impact. (n.d.). The Green House® concept. Retrieved from http://www.ncbcapitalimpact.org/default.aspx?id=148.

Nightingale, F. (1859). *Notes on hospitals*. London: John W. Parker and Son.

The Pioneer Network. (n.d.). What is culture change? Retrieved from http://www.pioneernetwork.net/CultureChange/Whatis/.

The Poorhouse Lady. (n.d.). History of 19th century American poorhouses. Retrieved from http://www.poorhousestory.com/history.htm.

Society for the Advancement of Gerontological Environments (n.d.). Welcome to SAGE. Retrieved from http://www.sagefederation.org/.

Stone, R.I., Bryant, N., & Barbarotta, L. (2009, October). *Supporting culture change: Working toward smarter state nursing home regulation* (Commonwealth Fund pub. 1328 Vol. 68). New York, NY: Commonwealth Fund.

U.S. Social Security Administration. (n.d.). Compilation of the Social Security laws. Retrieved from http://www.ssa.gov/OP_Home/ssact/comp-ssa.htm.

Chapter 15

Promoting Healthy Aging with Attention to Social Capital

Carolyn Pierce and Susan Seibold-Simpson

The term *social capital* combines aspects of economics and sociology (Macinko & Starfield, 2001). "Social" refers to living in organized communities and "capital" refers to wealth, property or money (Ehrlich, Flexner, Carruth, & Hawkins, 1980). Generally, authors agree that the concept of social capital includes networks, trust, and norms of reciprocity (a standard within the neighborhood of individuals looking out for and helping each other), or some combination of these terms (Campbell & McLean, 2002; Galea, Karpati, & Kennedy, 2002; Hawe & Shiell, 2000; Kawachi, 2000; Macinko & Starfield, 2001; Putnam, 1995). This chapter reviews what is currently known about social capital as a vehicle to enhance healthy aging of seniors both in the United States and internationally.

Social Capital

It has been suggested that social capital promotes social cooperation (Fukuyama, 2002) and is proposed to facilitate collective action for mutual benefit (Lochner, Kawachi, Brennan, & Buka, 2003). It is also argued that enhancing social capital may alleviate some of the adverse effects of low socioeconomic status, and that strategies to increase social capital should be pursued (Holtgrave & Crosby, 2003). Qualitative research related to the area of social capital supports the concepts clustered as trust, norms of reciprocity, and network membership, and suggests other factors for consideration (Altschuler, Somkin, & Adler, 2004; Ziersch, Baum, MacDougall, & Putland, 2005). For example, respondents in a study by Ziersch et al. (2005) noted that it is important for people in their neighborhood to get along together, including being tolerant, and to have informal interactions for a community to be healthy. In this study, perceived absence of safety (including lack of respect and fear) interfered with trust and reciprocity (Altschuler et al., 2004; Ziersch et al., 2005).

Part of the controversy surrounding the construct of social capital stems from the use of the term "capital" (Navarro, 2004) and the perceived need to separate this construct from existing similar concepts, including social cohesion or social integration (Muntaner,

2004). Controversies have been associated with: (1) the multiple definitions of social capital (Szreter & Woolcock, 2004), (2) the range of different measures of social capital in the research literature (Macinko & Starfield, 2001; Ziersch et al., 2005), (3) the lack of acknowledgement of the impact of politics (Muntaner, 2004), economics, and power relations (Navarro, 2004) on the key aspects of the construct and its proposed benefit to health; (4) whether social capital is accrued at the individual level or group level; and (5) the varying and appropriate level of measurement (e.g., at the neighborhood, block group, or census tract levels, as well as at the state, national, and international levels) (Semaan, Sternberg, Zaidi, & Aral, 2007). As eloquently noted by Kawachi, Kim, Coutts, and Subramanian (2004), "By equating social capital with social networks and support, we would be simply re-labeling terminology, or pouring old wine into new bottles. The concept of social capital surely contributes something additional to the already well-established literature on social networks and support. The novel contribution of social capital, in our view, lies in its collective dimension, i.e., its potential to account for group-level influences on individual health" (p. 683). Despite these controversies, studies incorporating different measures of social capital have proliferated, with authors suggesting the need for additional work to refine the concept and its relationship with health outcomes (Semaan et al., 2007; Szreter & Woolcock, 2004).

Social capital has been closely tied to socioeconomic status and has been demonstrated to co-vary with socioeconomic status. Thus, it is often suggested that when socioeconomic status improves, social capital improves (Drukker, Buka, Kaplan, McKenzie, & van Os, 2005; Drukker, Kaplan, Feron, & van Os, 2003; Franzini, Caughy, Spears, & Esquer, 2005). Social capital has also been demonstrated to mediate the effect of poverty and income inequality on mortality (Gold, Kennedy, Connell, & Kawachi, 2002; Kawachi, Kennedy, Lochner, & Prothrow-Stith, 1997). In a study of 13 low/medium income communities in Texas, social capital (trust and norms of reciprocity) was significantly associated with neighborhood impoverishment and self-reported health (Franzini et al., 2005).

Network Membership

Network membership is a key attribute identified with social capital and may be more easily identifiable than trust or norms of reciprocity. Network membership refers to belonging to groups within a given community and is often measured according to the perceived value provided by this membership. Wood et al. (2008) measured network membership by *if you had a serious personal crisis or problem, how many people living within your suburb could you turn to for comfort and support*. Lindstrom, Hanson, Ostergren, and Berglund (2000) identified subcategories to social networks including: "social anchorage" (to what extent the person belongs to and is anchored within formal and informal groups) and "social participation" (how actively the person takes part in the activities of formal and informal groups in society). These authors also noted that the social networks may provide different types of support, including "instrumental support" (the individual's access to guidance, advice, information, practical services, and material resources from the other persons) and "emotional support" (the opportunity for care, the encouragement of personal value, and feelings of confidence and trust from the other persons).

Integral to the concept of social capital expressed by network membership is the level of network membership and the phenomena of "bonding," "linking," and "bridging." According to Szreter and Woolcock (2004), "bonding" social capital refers to relations between network members who "see themselves as being similar"; "bridging" social capital refers to the relations among network members between people who "know they are not alike in some socio-demographic sense" ; and "linking" social capital refers to the "norms of respect and networks of trusting relationships between people who are interacting across explicit, formal or institutionalized power or authority gradients in society" (p. 655).

Norms of Reciprocity

Norms of reciprocity are often measured by responses to statements such as *most people are helpful* (Kawachi, Kennedy, & Glass, 1999). These norms are frequently represented by actions undertaken by adults in the neighborhood. Wood et al. (2008) listed the following activities for neighborhood reciprocity: *looked after house or garden or collected mail while away; minded, fed or walked their pet; lent them household or garden items or tools; listened to their problems; helped them with odd jobs; provided a lift or transport to shops or school; and cared for, or minded, a child or other family member for them.*

Norms of reciprocity is similar to the concept of *social control* developed by Sampson and Morenoff (1997). Social control relates to neighbors intervening in various ways when people engage in violence or criminal activities.

Trust

Trust refers to the condition of "perceived vulnerability or risk that results from an individual's uncertainty about the motives, intentions, and prospective actions of others they are dependent on and correlates with the individual's beliefs about human nature" (Kramer, 1999, p. 571). Goudge and Gilson (2005) wrote that trust supports cooperation, which enables the achievement of a range of positive outcomes. Judgments are made about the level of risk—for instance, will the trustee act in the best interests of the truster, or in ways that will not be harmful? According to these authors, trust includes knowledge of a combination of social, personal, and political processes. Basically, Ross, Mirowsky, and Pribesh (2001) identified trust as a "belief in the integrity of other people" (p. 569).

The term *trust* is often included in the measurement of trust, as noted by Wood et al. (2008) and colleagues who measured trust by assessing the response to the statements: *Generally, to what extent do you agree that you can trust: most people living in your section of your street or block, most people living in your suburb, and most people generally?*; or Lindstrom and Lindstrom (2006) who asked, *"Do you think most people can be trusted or that you can't be too careful in dealing with people?* Trust has also been measured by asking if individuals know and talk to people in their neighborhood (Ahern & Hendryx, 2005; Boyce, Davies, Gallupe, & Shelley, 2008).

Social Capital and Health

Findings from many studies have demonstrated a relationship between social capital and a variety of health outcomes, including tuberculosis (Holtgrave & Crosby, 2003), sexually transmitted infections (Crosby, Holtgrave, DiClemente, Wingood, & Gayle, 2003; Holtgrave & Crosby, 2003; Semaan et al., 2007), and indeed mortality (Lochner et al., 2003; Skrabski, Kopp, & Kawachi, 2004). Putnam (2004) proposed a variety of mechanisms to explain how social capital improves health, including how social networks affect health-related communication and access to material resources (as in many accounts of health problems in areas of rural poverty), and how social connectedness affects physiological processes. Glass et al. (2004) suggested that their intervention, *Experience Corps*, a volunteer service program designed to improve the lives of urban children and yield health improvements for older persons, improved neighborhood social capital. Farquhar, Michael, and Wiggins (2005) suggested that participation in their community-based participatory prevention research project improved social capital through targeting civic engagement, trust, and social networks.

Nummela, Sulander, Rahkonen, Karisto, and Uutela (2008) found a positive association between high levels of social capital and self-rated health in Finnish elders. In this study, social capital was defined by levels of social participation and trust. Indeed, greater satisfaction with the level of social support was associated with better general cognitive performance, speed, and attention, and a slower decline in episodic memory for elders living in Florida (Hughes, Andel, Small, Borenstein, & Mortimer, 2008). Similarly, de Souza and Grundy (2007) found that Brazilian elders who participated in a community-based program that involved adolescents and elders in memory sharing and reminiscence activities increased the tendency of the elders to rate neighbors as helpful, to consider most people as honest, and to consider their family relationships as good.

Social Capital in Older Persons

The unique circumstances surrounding social capital in older persons was recently showcased in 11 European countries with the Survey of Health, Aging, and Retirement in Europe (SHARE) (Sirven & Debrand, 2008). In this research, social participation was found to contribute to the number of individuals reporting good or very good health. Age was a powerful predictor of decline in health status. While lower income was also found to be related to lower levels of self-rated health (SRH), persons with higher levels of education and more intellectual jobs reported higher levels of SRH. It was also found that retired people and those persons without children in the household were more likely to participate in social activities. The authors concluded that most of the countries would benefit from increased participation in voluntary associations. Two very positive examples of social capital were found in Greece, which has outstanding involvement in religious activities, and in Switzerland, which had the highest levels of SRH. However, the "rate of return" for social involvement was actually highest in Germany, where there was a lower level of involvement in community activities, but this level made a larger contribution to SRH.

Another survey, the British Household Panel Survey (Gray, 2009), involved a longitudinal survey of persons over 60 years of age in Great Britain that focused on the benefits of emotional and practical support from friends and relatives. This population reported a poorer level of support among persons who were childless or had lived alone for a long period of time. In contrast, a rich level of support was found among those who interacted often with others and who saw their neighborhood as a positive social environment. Interestingly, being active in organizations had less of an effect on feelings about social support than informal social relationships. Professional and managerial groups were found to be of more benefit than those attended by working-class elders, even though both were considered to be "well-networked."

A lack of reciprocity, as an indicator of social capital, was associated with poorer self-rated health and depression in both US and German respondents to a national telephone survey (Pollack & von dem Knesebeck, 2004). Civic mistrust in this research was associated with poorer self-rated health in both countries. Levels of participation in community activities were higher in the United States, mainly in church attendance and charity activities. These differences were attributed by the authors to such macro-level features such as history, culture, and economics.

Several studies of elders have shown that economic and marital situations are important indicators of social capital. In a large survey of older persons in the United Kingdom (Arber, 2004), the most materially disadvantaged elders were divorced women. The authors described how gender-powered relationships shaped material well-being and social connectedness in later life. Similarly, Grundy and Sloggett (2003) found that older men and women with no educational qualifications experienced "bad" or "very bad" health. More specifically, bad health was more commonly seen among those who were unmarried. Persons with no social support tended to rate their health as poorer as well. Tenants' ratings of their health was poorer than the ratings of owners-occupiers, while those persons receiving income support reported the most prevalent level of poor health.

Lack of community involvement was described by Berry (2008) as those elders who were "aging, participating less" (p. 533). The author also reported low levels of contact with community activities in spite of a high level of contact with neighbors. However, perceptions about participation were generally positive in spite of lower levels of belonging and optimism and higher levels of distress. The respondents tended to be positively oriented toward community activities even though they were often deprived of the opportunity to attend due to increasing age and financial circumstances (Berry, 2008).

Levels of social capital have also been identified as affecting caregivers of the elderly. Donohue, Dibble, and Schiamberg (2008) suggested that by increasing bridging and bonding social capital available to caretakers, elder mistreatment might be prevented. These effects were noted in both home care and long-term care facilities.

Social Capital and Rural Communities: A Critical Need

Social capital has not been extensively studied in rural areas (Nummela et al., 2008). However, Greiner, Li, Kawachi, Hunt, and Ahluwalia (2004) studied community involvement and found that low-density areas have socially active populations that are working to solve problems through community activities. Kim and Kawachi (2006) found that outside of core urban areas, effects of community trust, informal social interactions, and electoral participation on one's health were more beneficial. This was especially true within non-core urban areas and rural areas, in contrast with their hypothesis of stronger associations for informal social interactions in urban areas.

Additionally, Davis and Bartlett (2008) found that rural elders' preferences for independent living are often thwarted by distance, isolation, housing options, income, access to services, and transportation. Recently, local facilities in this research, such as shops, post offices, banks, gas stations, and public transport, were found to be disappearing. The authors held that loss of local services and the urban-centric views of many healthcare organizations contributed to the marginalization of rural elders by making the negative circumstances of aging in place a challenge.

However, it has recently been shown that the isolation experienced by rural seniors in Australia was somewhat offset by use of the Internet to maintain access to friends and family (Russell, Campbell, & Hughes, 2008). While these findings were encouraging, they also pointed to the fact that most of the Internet users were married, home-owning English-speaking men and women in good health, and thus Internet usage was not universal. The authors pointed to the need for policies to improve access to the Internet resources to generate social capital.

Using Social Capital to Support Healthy Aging

Social capital serves as a useful tool to support communities that are currently transitioning from a standard of care involving "aging in place" to the more forward-thinking concept of "aging in the community" (Eilers, Lucey, & Stein, 2007). Cannuscio, Block, and Kawachi (2003) suggested alternatives to seniors living alone or in gated communities by replacing those locations with planned care environments or "vertically integrated" (i.e., high-rise) housing (p. 398). These communities have been shown to promote reciprocal and intergenerational exchange between elders and the surrounding community. These innovative living formations may consist of assisted-living situations to provide independent, residential living with some personal and health-related assistance within a communal structure.

Similarly, Bronstein, McCallion, and Kramer (2006) described the development of an "aging prepared community" within the Elder Network of the Capital Region in Albany,

New York, area. The goal of this network was to enhance well-being and to sustain elders' independence by connecting available services and working to correct gaps in services. To that end, a consortium was created that includes various health and human services, state and local governments, the local faith community, and a university. One important feature of this network was the Internet-based information and assistance program that was successful in increasing awareness with education and training, while fostering partnerships among all of the constituents to improve care for older persons.

Another important model for elder care is the Eden Alternative, which is a not-for-profit organization promoting deinstitutionalizing of seniors. The Eden Alternative has trained 17,000 associates and includes over 200 registered homes in the United States, Canada, Europe, and Australia (http://www.edenalt.org). The philosophy of the Eden Alternative is to develop elder-centered community habitats where Mother Nature is called upon to provide interaction with plants, animals, and children. Variety and spontaneity in daily life are infused as an alternative to boredom. Traditional bureaucracy is deemphasized, and seniors are involved in the decision-making process. Positive outcomes are evidenced by the continuing promotion of human growth with companionship and meaningful activities and interactions.

Conclusion

This review has shown that promoting social capital within the scope of developing environments that are conducive to healthy aging has unfulfilled potential. Environments that promote networks, reciprocity, and trust provide frameworks not only for delivering health care, but also for meeting the critical need of elders for nurturing relationships within a multigenerational society. "Aging in the community" should be the commitment that we make to elders in both urban and rural settings.

References

Ahern, M.M., & Hendryx, M.S. (2005). Social capital and risk for chronic illnesses. *Chronic Illness*, *1*(3), 183–190.

Altschuler, A., Somkin, C.P., & Adler, N.E. (2004). Local services and amenities, neighborhood social capital, and health. *Social Science & Medicine*, *59*, 1219–1229.

Arber, S. (2004). Gender, marital status, and ageing: Linking material, health, and social resources. *Journal of Aging Studies*, *18*, 91–108.

Berry, H. (2008). Social capital elite, excluded participators, busy working parents and aging, participating less: Types of community participants and their mental health. *Social Psychiatry & Psychiatric Epidemiology*, *43*, 527–537.

Boyce, W.F., Davies, D., Gallupe, O., & Shelley, D. (2008). Adolescent risk taking, neighborhood social capital, and health. *Journal of Adolescent Health*, *43*, 246–252.

Bronstein, L., McCallion, P., & Kramer, E. (2006). Developing an aging prepared community: Collaboration among counties, consumers, professionals and organizations. *Journal of Gerontological Social Work*, *48*, 193–202.

Campbell, C., & McLean, C. (2002). Ethnic identities, social capital and health inequalities: Factors shaping African-Caribbean participation in local community networks in the UK. *Social Science & Medicine, 55,* 643–657.

Cannuscio, C., Block, J., & Kawachi, I. (2003). Social capital and successful aging: The role of senior housing. *Annals of Internal Medicine, 139,* 395–399.

Crosby, R.A., Holtgrave, D.R., DiClemente, R.J., Wingood, G.M., & Gayle, J.A. (2003). Social capital as a predictor of adolescents' sexual risk behavior: A state-level exploratory study. *AIDS & Behavior, 7*(3), 245–252.

Davis, S., & Bartlett, H. (2008). Healthy ageing in rural Australia: Issues and challenges. *Australian Journal in Ageing, 27,* 56–60.

de Souza, E., & Grundy, E. (2007). Intergenerational interaction, social capital, and health: Results from a randomized controlled trial in Brazil. *Social Science & Medicine, 65,* 1397–1409.

Donohue, W.A., Dibble, J.L., & Schiamberg, L.B. (2008). A social capital approach to the prevention of elder mistreatment. *Journal of Elder Abuse & Neglect, 20,* 1–23.

Drukker, M., Buka, S.L., Kaplan, C., McKenzie, K., & van Os, J. (2005). Social capital and young adolescents' perceived health in different sociocultural settings. *Social Science & Medicine, 61,* 185–198.

Drukker, M., Kaplan, C., Feron, F., & van Os, J. (2003). Children's health-related quality of life, neighbourhood socio-economic deprivation and social capital. A contextual analysis. *Social Science & Medicine, 57*(5), 825–841.

Ehrlich, E., Flexner, S.B., Carruth, G., & Hawkins, J.M. (1980). *Oxford American dictionary.* New York: Avon Books.

Eilers, M., Lucey, P., & Stein, S. (2007). Promoting social capital for the elderly. *Nursing Economics, 25,* 304–307.

Farquhar, S.A., Michael, Y.L., & Wiggins, N. (2005). Building on leadership and social capital to create change in 2 urban communities. *American Journal of Public Health, 95*(4), 596–601.

Franzini, L., Caughy, M., Spears, W., & Esquer, M.E.F. (2005). Neighborhood economic conditions, social processes, and self-rated health in low-income neighborhoods in Texas: A multilevel latent variables model. *Social Science & Medicine, 61,* 1135–1150.

Fukuyama, F. (2002). Social capital and development: The coming agenda. *SAIS Review, 22*(1), 23–37.

Galea, S., Karpati, A., & Kennedy, B. (2002). Social capital and violence in the United States, 1974–1993. *Social Science & Medicine, 55,* 1373–1383.

Glass, T.A., Freedman, M., Carlson, M.C., Hill, J., Frick, K.D., Ialongo, N., et al. (2004). Experience Corps: Design of an intergenerational program to boost social capital and promote the health of an aging society. *Journal of Urban Health, 81*(1), 94–105.

Gold, R., Kennedy, B., Connell, F., & Kawachi, I. (2002). Teen births, income inequality, social capital: Developing an understanding of the causal pathway. *Health & Place, 8,* 77–83.

Goudge, J., & Gilson, L. (2005). How can trust be investigated? Drawing lessons from past experience. *Social Science & Medicine, 61,* 1439–1451.

Gray, A. (2009). The social capital of older people. *Aging & Society, 29,* 5–31.

Greiner, K.A., Li, C., Kawachi, I., Hunt, D.C., & Ahluwalia, J.S. (2004). The relationships of social participation and community ratings to health and health behaviors in areas with high and low population density. *Social Science & Medicine, 59,* 2303–2312.

Grundy, E., & Sloggett, A. (2003). Health inequalities in the older population: The role of personal capital, social resources and socio-economic circumstances. *Social Science & Medicine, 56,* 935–947.

Hawe, P., & Shiell, A. (2000). Social capital and health promotion: A review. *Social Science & Medicine, 51,* 871–885.

Holtgrave, D.R., & Crosby, R.A. (2003). Social capital, poverty, and income inequality as predictors of gonorrhoea, syphilis, chlamydia and AIDS case rates in the United States. *Sexually Transmitted Infections, 79*(1), 62–64.

Hughes, T., Andel, R., Small, B., Borenstein, A., & Mortimer, J. (2008). The association between social resources and cognitive change in older adults: Evidence from the Charlotte County healthy aging study. *Journals of Gerontology: Series B: Psychological & Social Sciences., 63B,* 241–46.

Kawachi, I. (2000). Social cohesion and health. In A.R. Tarlov & R.F. St. Peter (Eds.), *The society and population health reader: A state and community perspective* (Vol. II, pp. 57–74). New York: The New Press.

Kawachi, I., Kennedy, B., & Glass, R. (1999). Social capital and self-rated health: A contextual analysis. *American Journal of Public Health, 89*(8), 1187–1193.

Kawachi, I., Kennedy, B., Lochner, K., & Prothrow-Stith, D. (1997). Social capital, income inequality, and mortality. *American Journal of Public Health, 87,* 1491–1498.

Kawachi, I., Kim, D., Coutts, A., & Subramanian, S.V. (2004). Commentary: Reconciling the three accounts of social capital. *International Journal of Epidemiology, 33*(4), 682–690.

Kim, D., & Kawachi, I. (2006). A multilevel analysis of key forms of community- and individual-level social capital as predictors of self-rated health in the United States. *Journal of Urban Health, 83*(5), 813–826.

Kramer, R.M. (1999). Trust and distrust in organizations: Emerging perspectives, enduring questions. *Annual Review of Psychology, 50,* 569–598.

Lindstrom, C., & Lindstrom, M. (2006). "Social capital," GNP per capita, relative income, and health: An ecological study of 23 countries. *International Journal of Health Services, 36*(4), 679–696.

Lindstrom, M., Hanson, B.S., Ostergren, P.O., & Berglund, G. (2000). Socioeconomic differences in smoking cessation: The role of social participation. *Scandinavian Journal of Public Health, 28*(3), 200–208.

Lochner, K.A., Kawachi, I., Brennan, R.T., & Buka, S.L. (2003). Social capital and neighborhood mortality rates in Chicago. *Social Science & Medicine, 56,* 1797–1805.

Macinko, J., & Starfield, B. (2001). The utility of social capital in research on health determinants. *Millbank Quarterly, 79*(3), 387–427.

Muntaner, C. (2004). Commentary: Social capital, social class, and the slow progress of psychosocial epidemiology. *International Journal of Epidemiology, 33,* 674–680.

Navarro, V. (2004). Commentary: Is capital the solution or the problem? *International Journal of Epidemiology, 33,* 672–674.

Nummela, O., Sulander, T., Rahkonen, O., Karisto, A., & Uutela, A. (2008). Social participation, trust, and self-rated health: A study among ageing people in urban, semi-urban, and rural settings. *Health & Place, 14,* 243–253.

Pollack, C., & von dem Knesebeck, O. (2004). Social capital and health among the aged: Comparisons between the United States and Germany. *Health & Place, 10,* 383–391.

Putnam, R.D. (1995). Tuning in, tuning out: The strange disappearance of social capital in America. *Political Science & Politics, December,* 664–683.

Putnam, R.D. (2004). Commentary: 'Healthy by association': Some comments. *International Journal of Epidemiology, 33,* 667–671.

Ross, C.E., Mirowsky, J., & Pribesh, S. (2001). Powerlessness and the amplification of threat: Neighborhood disadvantage, disorder, and mistrust. *American Sociological Review, 66*(4), 568–592.

Russell, C., Campbell, A., & Hughes, I. (2008). Ageing, social capital and the Internet: Findings from an exploratory study of Australian "silver surfers.' *Australian Journal on Ageing, 27,* 78–82.

Sampson, R.J., & Morenoff, J.D. (1997). Ecological perspectives on the neighborhood context of urban poverty: Past and present. In J. Brooks-Gunn & G.J. Duncan (Eds.), *Neighborhood poverty: Policy implications in studying neighborhoods* (Vol. II, pp. 1–22). New York: Russell Sage Foundation.

Semaan, S., Sternberg, M., Zaidi, A., & Aral, S.O. (2007). Social capital and rates of gonorrhea and syphilis in the United States: Spatial regression analyses of state-level associations. *Social Science and Medicine, 64,* 2324–2341.

Sirven, N., & Debrand, T. (2008). Social participation and healthy aging: An international comparison using the SHARE data. *Social Science & Medicine, 67,* 2017–2026.

Skrabski, A., Kopp, M., & Kawachi, I. (2004). Social capital and collective efficacy in Hungary: Cross sectional associations with middle aged female and male mortality rates. *Journal of Epidemiology & Community Health, 58,* 340–345.

Szreter, S., & Woolcock, M. (2004). Health by association? Social capital, social theory, and the political economy of public health. *International Journal of Epidemiology, 33,* 650–667.

Wood, L., Shannon, T., Bulsara, M., Pikora, T., McCormack, G., & Giles-Corti, B. (2008). The anatomy of the safe and social suburb: An exploratory study of the built environment, social capital and residents' perceptions of safety. *Health & Place, 14*(1), 15–31.

Ziersch, A.M., Baum, F.E., MacDougall, C., & Putland, C. (2005). Neighbourhood life and social capital: The implications for health. *Social Science & Medicine, 60,* 71–86.

Chapter 16

Making Community Events Accessible to Older Adults

Geriatric Nurses Collaboration

Beth E. Barba and Anita S. Tesh

It is important that people remain engaged with each other and with the community as they grow older. But for many elders it becomes increasingly difficult to navigate the larger environment well enough to continue their participation in community programs and other events. This chapter recognizes the potential leadership of geriatric nurses as consultants in helping community event planners to make gatherings elder accessible. Experienced geriatric nurses are familiar with the importance of collaborating with other healthcare providers to ensure optimal care for older adults. However, they may be less practiced at working with those outside the health care field. Geriatric nurses have much to offer those who are planning events that may include older adults. Input from a geriatric nurse can ultimately improve the experience for the older adults who participate. Today's older adults want to be socially active and engaged in their communities, and geriatric nurses can help this happen!

Anyone planning for an audience that includes older adults can attest to the challenges of creating events that are safe, meaningful, and, most of all, enjoyable for aging participants. For example, advancement staff at universities need to understand what alumni or older guests face when they enter the setting, from menu selections and audiovisual needs and scheduling to transportation and mobility considerations. Wedding planners, community events planning committees, and other social activities organizers face similar challenges. When positive experiences and goodwill are at stake, it is imperative that event planners understand the issues older adults may face. Geriatric nurses are in an ideal position to advise and educate event planners about the aging process and about strategies that will make events more accessible and appropriate for older participants. Such a collaboration can have broad-reaching effects on the quality of life of community-dwelling older adults.

Geriatric nurses may contribute their expertise through volunteer activities, as part of community-focused employment, or as paid consultants to event planners. For example, a nurse might volunteer to help ensure that a local craft fair is accessible and agreeable to older adults, but serve as a paid consultant to a tour company or other for-profit venture.

When collaborating with event planners, geriatric nurses should keep in mind that event planners may not share the focus on health and safety that is second nature to healthcare providers. It may be necessary to introduce a scheme such as Maslow's Hierarchy of Needs to be used for prioritizing actions (Maslow, 1970) and to lay the foundation for problem solving. It may be helpful to frame the discussion with the following questions:

1. What are the benefits of having older adults participate in this event?
2. What challenges will participating older adults pose for staff, volunteers, and other participants?
3. What challenges will participating in our event pose to older adults?
4. How can we minimize these challenges and prevent problems?
5. How will we know if our modifications/plans are successful?

Many of the challenges in planning and organizing events for older individuals are associated with the physiological changes that occur in aging bodies. These challenges include loss of eyesight and hearing, decreased sharpness of the senses (taste, touch, and smell), slowness or decrease in cognitive processes, weaker bones and muscles, frequent and perhaps urgent sense of urination, need for fluids, and cardiopulmonary conditions, such as peripheral neuropathy and orthostatic hypotension. Reflection on these normal age-related changes within the context of the preceding questions will often lead event planners themselves to identify a variety of changes they could make. Geriatric nurses can foster this discussion by directing the people with whom they are collaborating to consider four main themes: loss of hearing or eyesight, physical impairment, bodily needs and functions, and cognitive-based suggestions.

Loss of Hearing and Eyesight

When we consider aging, it is typical to immediately think of the loss of hearing and eyesight. Hearing impairment is the most common sensory impairment in old age (AGS Panel, 2004). Also, a study produced by Murphy et al. (2002) found that 62.5% of older adults in the United States between the ages of 80 and 97 years had auditory impairment. Out of the population sampled (aged 53 to 97 years), the prevalence of hearing impairment and loss was 24.5%; this percentage increased with age. Clearly, hearing impairment is common in older adults and should be addressed when preparing for an event. Those with hearing impairment may not be able to hear high-pitched sounds and may have difficulty distinguishing sounds when background noise is present.

Visual impairment can occur due to a number of diseases and illnesses that arise with increasing age (glaucoma, cataracts, etc.). The US Centers for Disease Control and Prevention's Morbidity and Mortality weekly report (2006) reported visual impairment statistics for older adults (over 50 years) in five states (Iowa, Louisiana, Ohio, Tennessee, and Texas). In these states the prevalence of visual impairment ranged from 14.3% in Iowa to 20.5% in Ohio (US Centers for Disease Control and Prevention, 2006). With increasing age, older adults may lose peripheral vision, be sensitive to glare, and have decreased ability to judge depth as well as decreased color recognition.

With this information, geriatric nurses may suggest several changes to make in event planning. For example, one should eliminate background noise when possible, lower pitch when speaking to older adults, and choose venues for meetings and gatherings that avoid high-traffic areas, thus decreasing background noise and creating a quieter environment. When making speeches and giving instructions, it is important to get an older audience's attention prior to speaking, to speak more clearly and slowly, and to provide written handouts with instructions. A key suggestion is to determine who has hearing impairments prior to an event, so they can be seated closer to the speaker. To address visual impairment, large-print nametags could be given out to attendees and staff, to avoid their having to squint or use corrective lenses. Large signs might be posted for the location of the event as well as directions to restrooms. Refreshments should be labeled clearly for those with extremely poor eyesight. Transportation could be arranged for those who may not be safe drivers. Finally, for those burdened with hearing and/or eyesight impairments, it is important to be patient during interactions. Discussion of the logistics of the event will allow the geriatric nurse to help the event planner to identify additional creative strategies to customize the event to the older participant.

Physical Impairments

As people age, physical tasks become more difficult due to a variety of aging- and disease-related effects on muscles and bones. Normal neurological changes of aging include decreased reaction time and loss of balance. These changes can lead to more frequent falls, which may result in fractures or broken bones, muscle stiffness, and loss of muscular strength and endurance. In Stevens' (2005) study on the prevalence of falls in older adults, she discovered that more than a third of all older adults in the United States fall each year. This research also indicated that 20% to 30% of those who fall suffer moderate to severe injuries that reduce mobility and independence. Given these alarming statistics, it is essential for the geriatric nurse to educate event planners about the impact of these physical impairments and ways to enhance safety. Understanding the normal changes in reaction time will help event planners to develop realistic schedules or timelines for events.

Obviously, it is also important to provide assistance to older participants who are physically disabled or impaired. For those with faulty balance, assistance should be offered when walking on unstable surfaces. Signs should be posted clearly for directions to the event. Assistance could include wheelchairs as well as human assistance by staff or volunteers. Transportation should also be available to carry older adults as close to the building as possible, in order to limit walking distances. Club cars (i.e., golf carts) can be a good option for this, if the event is located a distance from parking or paved surfaces. Those assisting could go the extra step and escort the attendees directly to their seats and provide nametags. It is helpful to discover who has impairments ahead of time so that requirements for access can be anticipated before the event. It may also be beneficial to designate additional handicapped or reserved parking for older participants.

The geriatric nurse should encourage the event planner to allow wide aisles between tables, so those with assistive walking devices can maneuver around them. Seating should be widely available throughout the setting for those who cannot stand or walk for long periods of time. If possible, chairs should be arranged with space around each, rather than in rows. During events where guests are seated for long periods of time, the geriatric nurse should suggest planning frequent breaks so that older participants' muscles do not stiffen and so people can visit the restroom. As with those with hearing and/or visual problems, it is important to be patient and understand those with physical impairments. The geriatric nurse can facilitate this by helping event planners to think ahead and have proactive plans for dealing with physical limitations.

Adequate preparations for ensuring the safety and comfort of older adults often require more staff or volunteers than for events that only serve younger people. It is typically necessary to allow more time for each step of an event, such as getting seated, changing rooms, or serving from a refreshment line or buffet. Finally, it is essential that the geriatric nurse help the event planner to develop a plan in case of a fall or other injury. It should be designated ahead of time who will assist the injured person, who will call for medical assistance, and who will address the concerns of the other participants/guests. This plan should also ensure that injuries or illness are handled quietly and discreetly, with minimal disruption of the event or embarrassment to the older adult.

Bodily Needs and Functions

In planning events in which older adults are the primary guests, one should be aware of bodily adaptations to aging. Normal changes of aging affect eating, drinking, and elimination. The number of taste buds decreases, as does the amount of saliva produced while eating. The senses of smell and touch are also declining. Fluid intake should be increased to avoid risk of dehydration. The recommended amount of water consumption by older adults is 6 to 8 glasses or 1500 mL of water per day (Khan & Tariq, 2004). Urinary incontinence (UI) is also a growing issue with age. According to research at Emory University, the prevalence of UI in older adults is between 30% and 50% (Johnson & Ouslander, 1999). All of these changes require adaptations by those planning events involving food, beverages, and the location of restrooms.

In particular, the geriatric nurse should emphasize the importance of clear and prominent signs directing guests to the nearest restrooms. With such a high percentage of older adults suffering from UI and urgency, restrooms need to be clearly labeled and close to the venue. This will be particularly crucial for those with physical impairments, who may take longer to get to the restroom. It can be helpful to point out restroom locations early in an event. This can be done as part of an orientation for older adults as they enter the venue. An adequate number of staff or volunteers should be designated to assist those with mobility problems to the restroom, and to identify those who seem "lost" and may be in search of facilities.

The geriatric nurse can help event planners to understand that, given the importance of staying hydrated, refreshments should be continuously available and clearly labeled. Water should always be available for older adults even if other refreshments are not planned. Because of decreased sense of taste, menus should consist of foods with stronger tastes that are easy to eat and digestible. The geriatric nurse should encourage event planners to avoid foods that roll (such as nuts) or food that may be challenging to cut with a knife and fork. A plated meal that is brought out to each person may be a great way to accommodate special food and beverage needs (e.g., diabetics may need sugar-free dessert and unsweetened iced tea). A served meal can also help those with physical impairments, so they do not have to stand for a lengthy period of time in a buffet line. If a buffet line or refreshment table is used instead of a served meal, food should be arranged to minimize reaching and provide easy access. Food and beverage labels may be helpful. In preparing menus, it is important to keep physiological changes in mind to ensure that the event is enjoyable for all participants.

Decline in Cognitive Functioning

Loss of short-term memory is considered a normal change of aging. It is also estimated that 1.0% to 2.5% of older, cognitively healthy adults will become cognitively impaired (not including dementia) each year (Plassman et al., 2008). In 2002, Plassman and her colleagues estimated that there were approximately 5.4 million people 71 years of age or older in the United States who suffered from a decline in cognitive functioning without dementia. Cognitive impairment exists in a range of severity, and most people with mild to moderate impairment remain in the community. Further, an individual's cognitive status may fluctuate over time, even over the course of the day. For example, a person who is alert and oriented in the morning, particularly in a familiar setting, may become disoriented when fatigued, particularly in an unfamiliar setting. It is essential for geriatric nurses to convey to event planners that one cannot judge cognitive function by appearances. A well dressed, pleasant, socially gracious person may not be fully oriented, but may instead be an expert at adaptation and confabulation; likewise, fully oriented persons may become confused over the course of a long event.

With such a high prevalence of cognitive decline, it is necessary for the geriatric nurse to collaborate with event planners to consider this issue when planning events and functions. As with physical impairments, it is helpful to identify participants with cognitive impairment before the event, which will allow staff or volunteers to be readily available and particularly sensitive to their needs. Seating and other arrangements should allow easy access to their designated formal or informal caregivers. It will also be helpful to provide a quiet place where older adults can take a break from the festivities; this is particularly important for those with more moderate cognitive impairment.

Even for attendees with only mild cognitive decline, it may be necessary to alter or adjust presentations or speeches to ensure that older adults receive the information correctly. Geriatric nurses should advise event planners that presentations should be kept simple and to the point for all older adult audiences. Visuals should be in large font, microphones should be clear and crisp, and speakers should speak slowly. Everyone's attention should be fully directed to the speaker before beginning the speech. It is best if the entire presentation is no longer than 15 minutes. Clip art and moveable additions should be kept to a minimum since they can be confusing to follow, even for younger persons. It is also important not to overload attendees with information: keep the slides less crowded with words. Instructions and a copy of the presentation could be provided for those who have trouble keeping up with a presenter.

Geriatric nurses should help event planners build in accommodations for the short-term memory loss and decreased reaction time that accompany normal aging. If an event has multiple steps or stages, it is important to review each next step as it unfolds rather than expect participants to remember a sequence of directions, guidelines, or locations. When giving tours, one should move slowly and increase the amount of time allotted for individuals to look around.

The modifications required for accommodating participants with cognitive decline can seem daunting to event planners. However, the experienced geriatric nurse can help the event planner to understand that older adults with cognitive impairment still need and benefit from social interactions with their families and the community. They may be a part of the legacy of the institution or group and still have much to contribute. The time and effort devoted to including them in events is a wise investment in the organization or groups' culture and future effectiveness.

Putting It All Together: Simulation

Nothing helps us to understand others like walking in their shoes. In addition to discussing the preceding questions and themes, the geriatric nurse should consider doing an "aging simulation" in which the event planners experience their event through the simulated eyes and ears of an older adult. This may be particularly helpful if the event being planned is complex or if the event planners have relatively little experience with older adults. Simulations of the effects of aging can be arranged using standardized materials such as the SECURE Aging Sensitivity Training kit (SECURE, 2009). If standardized materials aren't available, hearing loss can be simulated by placing cotton balls in the ears. Visual changes, such as cataracts, can be simulated by eyeglasses blurred by Vaseline or with central black spots mimicking macular degeneration. Gloves can be used to simulate loss of the sensation of touch, and tape around finger joints can simulate loss of mobility. Add a cane or walker, and have the event planner role play an older adult through a version of the event, such as entering the venue, locating a seat, reading the menus, hearing verbal directions, and eating the planned refreshments. Simulations of this sort are particularly beneficial if a group of event planners engage simultaneously. Their entire perspective on the event may shift dramatically!

Conclusion

In our aging society, most events are likely to include older adults. Collaborating with event planners to ensure that the events are safe and enjoyable for this growing demographic is a fruitful and rewarding new area for geriatric nurses to apply their expertise. Geriatric nurses need to ensure that event planners have a basic understanding of the normal aging process and of changes they can make to help older participants to have an enjoyable and meaningful experience. Once event planners understand the basics of age-related changes (including loss of hearing and eyesight, physical impairment, bodily needs and functions, and changes in cognitive functioning), they will be better able to develop strategies to help create a safer and more welcoming environment for aging participants. These strategies may include decreasing background noise, speaking more clearly and slowly, providing physical assistance, and displaying easy-to-read signs for restrooms and refreshments, among others. Finally, it is important to be patient and understanding when working with older adults. Developing these plans can be challenging, but with the changes made, events will be more appropriate for older attendees. Event planners themselves will be able to identify many of the strategies once geriatric nurses help them to ask the appropriate questions and equip them with the necessary skills to develop meaningful answers. Geriatric nurses can also help the event planners to prioritize their plans based on implications for safety and hierarchy of need. This is an ideal opportunity for geriatric nurses to collaborate with other professionals and community groups to enhance the well-being of older adults in the community. Their leadership in this capacity can assist elders in navigating the sometimes daunting barriers that might otherwise eventually limit or prevent their continued attendance at community events.

References

AGS Panel. (2004). *Geriatrics at your fingertips 2004–2005* (6th ed.). American Geriatrics Society. Malden, MA: Blackwell Publishing.

Johnson, T.M., & Ouslander, J.G. (1999). Urinary incontinence in the older man. *Medical Clinics of North America, 83,* 1247–1266.

Khan, I.J., & Tariq, S.H. (2004). Urinary incontinence: Behavioral modification therapy in older adults. *Geriatric Incontinence, 20,* 499–509.

Maslow, A. (1970). *Motivation and personality* (2nd ed.). New York: Harper & Row.

Murphy, C., Schubert, C., Cruickshanks, K., Klein, B., Klein, R., & Nondahl, D. (2002). Prevalence of olfactory impairments in older adults. *Journal of the American Medical Association, 288,* 2307–2312.

Plassman, B.L., et al. (2008). Prevalence of cognitive impairment without dementia in the United States. *Annals of Internal Medicine, 148,* 427–434.

SECURE. (2009). SECURE aging sensitivity training program. http://www.leememorial.org/shareclub/secure.asp.

Stevens, J. (2005). Falls among older adults—risk factors and prevention strategies. *Journal of Safety Research, 36,* 409–411.

US Centers for Disease Control and Prevention. (2006). *Morbidity and mortality weekly report, 55*(49), 1321-1325.

Chapter 17

Giving Voice to Vulnerable Populations: Rogerian Theory

Sarah H. Gueldner, Geraldine R. Britton, and Susan Terwilliger

The human condition of vulnerability is a concept of vital concern to nurses in that a large portion of nursing practice is spent either helping individuals who find themselves in a vulnerable position or helping them avoid vulnerability. However, nursing has been slow in developing theoretical constructs of vulnerability within a nursing perspective (Spiers, 2000). Traditional definitions of vulnerability are framed within an epidemiological approach to identify persons and groups at risk for harm. Groups most often labeled as vulnerable include the elderly, children, the poor, people with disability or chronic illness, people from minority cultures, and captive populations such as prisoners and refugees (Saunders & Valente, 1992). Labels of vulnerability are customarily applied in relation to socioeconomic, minority, or other stigmatizing status (Demi & Warren, 1995) and reflect a tendency to blame the victim rather than the prevailing social structures. The generally accepted marker for vulnerability has been the inability to function independently in accord with the values of a particular society. Fortunately, there is growing dialogue about vulnerability from the perspective of the person experiencing it, a view that is more congruent with the philosophical stance of nursing (Morse, 1997; Spiers, 2000).

The Rogerian conceptual system (Rogers, 1992), which focuses on the person as integral with and inseparable from his or her environment, holds considerable relevance as an innovative nursing framework to use in addressing the problem of vulnerability. Accordingly, the remainder of this discussion is directed toward application of the theoretical base of Rogerian nursing science to the human condition of vulnerability, particularly as it relates to elderly populations. Because persons who are vulnerable are at greater risk for not being heard, the last part of the chapter describes the Wellbeing Picture Scale (WPS),* a 10-item innovative picture-based tool that offers a menu of paired pictures rather than words, giving people who may not be able to read English text a more user-friendly way of expressing their sense of well-being.

---

*An electronic copy of the Wellbeing Picture Scale and the scoring key may be obtained without cost by contacting Sarah Hall Gueldner at shg13@case.edu.

A Rogerian Perspective of Vulnerability

According to Martha Rogers, energy fields are the fundamental unit of everything, both living and nonliving. The fields are without boundary and dynamic, changing continuously. Two energy fields are identified: the human field and the environmental field. Rogers emphasized that humans and environments do not *have* energy fields; rather, they *are* energy fields. Likewise, she insisted that the human field is unitary and cannot be reduced to a biological field, a physical field, or a psychosocial field. As postulated by Rogers, human and environmental fields flow together in a constant mutual process that is unitary rather than separate. Within this worldview, humans are energy fields that exist in constant mutual process with their immediate and extended environmental energy field, which includes, and cannot be separated from, other living and nonliving fields. She also postulated that both human and environmental energy patterns change continually during this process. The inseparability of the human energy field from its immediate and extended environmental energy field is perhaps the most central feature of the Rogerian conceptual system.

Phillips and Bramlett (1994) asserted that the mutual human–environmental field process can be harmonious or dissonant. Resonant with Rogers' science, these researchers posit vulnerability as an emergent condition that arises when there is dissonance within the mutual human–environmental field process. This view is consistent with Rogerian scholar Barrett's (1990) theory of power, which associates power with individuals' knowing participation in change within their mutual human–environmental process for the betterment of the whole, including themselves. These authors perceive vulnerability as the opposite of powerful, a condition that may occur when an individual is unable or does not choose to participate in an informed and purposeful way in change. Persons in this situation essentially have no voice and may be intentionally or unintentionally left behind in a compromised position. Within this line of thinking, an individual's sense of dissonance or disharmony within the mutual human–environmental field process would be viewed as a manifestation of vulnerability, placing individuals or groups at risk. Barrett developed the text-based tool, Power as Knowing Participation in Change (PKPC), to measure this concept; a subscale of the tool addresses awareness as an essential feature of knowing participation.

Lack of knowing participation may be associated with a number of scenarios. Individuals may be uninformed or misinformed about situations involving their unique human–environmental field process, or they may be unable to participate due to one or more specific circumstances such as illness (e.g., stroke or dementia) or injury (e.g., hip fracture). Common situations that may limit or prevent knowing participation include compromised vision or hearing, aphasia, difficulty with mobility, and confusion or dementia. Other circumstances that may limit knowing participation include any situation that hinders a person from engaging in sufficient communication within the community; examples might include lack of transportation or limited language facility. Insufficient means or the inability to move about freely may diminish presence, making it more difficult, if not impossible, to be "at the table" to achieve representation. Stigmatized individuals or groups such as single mothers, persons who are homeless, and persons perceived as unattractive or different are also at risk for a lack of information or misinformation that may lead to inappropriate participation based on misjudgment. Indeed, information may actually be withheld if participation is not welcome.

Parse's (2003) theory of community becoming, also an extension of Rogers' nursing science, is particularly applicable to the theoretical tenet of vulnerability. She defines community in terms of the relational experience of being "in community" and describes it as a resource, dynamic and continuously changing to represent the good of the individual to achieve the best for all. According to her definition, community is not a location or a group of people who have similar interests; rather, community is the human connectedness with the universe, including connectedness with what she terms "yet-to-be possibles." This view represents a paradigm shift, wherein vulnerability is an emergent characteristic of the community in process that occurs when an individual or group becomes disconnected from the group and therefore from needed resources. Parse describes a nontraditional model of health service for individuals and families who have become disconnected from resources. The process involves envisioning possibilities and inviting others to capture the vision, thus energizing the community to build partnerships to overcome the disconnect.

Within this conceptualization, vulnerability arises as an emergent characteristic when connectedness is compromised by a lack of communication or flawed communication that leads to exclusion from resources. Vulnerability might be seen as an unfortunate estrangement from the process of community. According to this view, persons who are at particular risk for vulnerability are those who for some reason are unable to call enough attention to their needs to garner the support of their community.

Based on Parse's (1997) "human becoming" perspective, her view of nursing practice also differs from traditional nursing practice in that the nurse does not offer standardized professional advice or opinions stemming from the nurse's own value system. Rather, according to Parse, nursing involves a "true presence with and respect for the other" wherein the nurse dwells with the person or family to enhance their perceived "possibles." Parse points out that it is essential to go with vulnerable persons to where they are rather than to attempt to judge, change, or control them. It is in dwelling with the individual in discussion that meanings emerge, and it is in this process of illuminating meaning that possibilities for transcendence are seen.

In Parse's words, "The nurse in true presence with person or family is not a guide or a beacon, but rather an inspiring attentive presence that calls the other to shed light on the meaning of moments of his or her life. It is the person or family in the presence of the nurse that illuminates the meaning and mobilizes the capacity to transcend and move beyond. The person is coauthor of his or her own health…choosing rhythmical patterns of relating while reaching for personal hopes and dreams" (Parse, 1997, p. 40). She continues, "True presence is a special way of *being with* in which the nurse bears witness to the person's or family's own living of value priorities. True presence is an interpersonal art grounded in a strong knowledge base 'reflecting the belief that each person knows *the way* somewhere within self'" (Parse, 1997, p. 40). Certainly, nowhere is it more important to respect the person as he or she is than when working with those who are vulnerable.

Parse describes a humanitarian model of nursing practice based on true presence and profound respect. Use of this model enables people to find actions that increase their ability to knowingly participate in change to improve their position, thus becoming less vulnerable. Parse refers to this process as the search for the possible beyond the now.

However, in even this overall positive system some are likely to find themselves in vulnerable circumstances. Some individuals and groups (such as young children) are placed at risk because they cannot speak for themselves and depend on others to advocate for them. Likewise, sick or frail members of the community may be too weak or impaired to participate knowingly (or sufficiently) in the change process to advance their betterment. They may not be mobile enough, think clearly enough, or be articulate enough to capture community attention and garner the resources they need.

Individuals or families at special risk for vulnerability include those who

- Have energy-draining illnesses or conditions such as stroke, heart attack, cancer, or depression.
- Are not included in the dominant culture.
- Have compromised language facility, putting them at greater risk for being unheard.
- Are out of their familiar turf (i.e., new in the community and do not know the "rules" or avenues for help).
- Are unable to comprehend information (i.e., never learned to read, have diminished vision or hearing, are unconscious or have dementia, or are unable to comprehend English).
- Have illness or injury that limits independence (i.e., broken hips that make it more difficult to stay physically connected with the community).
- Lack the ability to access services needed for everyday life (i.e., means for obtaining food, place to live, health services).
- Are in a position of diminished visibility (e.g., live in a remote area or are homebound, becoming disconnected from community notice).

It is generally recognized that many elders encounter disabling circumstances that place them within these categories of vulnerability.

Viewed from Parse's theory of community becoming, the approach to overcoming vulnerability is a matter of reconnecting the person or group to the community. This sometimes happens naturally through family and friends or through social institutions and/or programs such as churches and civic organizations. But it may take the focused attention and time of individuals, such as nurses, to help the person or family as they gain insight about the possibilities that are available to them.

Giving Voice: An Application of Rogerian Nursing Science

To address the lack of voice that is so intricately associated with the experience of vulnerability, this section describes a simple picture tool, the WPS, developed within the Rogerian conceptual system to amplify the voice of persons who otherwise might not be heard (Gueldner et al., 2005).

The WPS is a 10-item non–language-based pictorial scale that measures general sense of well-being as a reflection of the mutual human–environmental field process. It was originally designed as an easy-to-administer tool for use with the broadest possible range of adult populations, including persons who have limited formal education, do not speak English as their first language, may not be able to see well, or may be too sick or frail to respond to lengthier or more complex measures. Ten pairs of 1-inch drawings depicting a sense of high or low well-being are arranged at opposite ends of a seven-choice, unnumbered, semantic differential scale. The 10 items included are eyes open and closed, shoes sitting still and running, butterfly and turtle, candle lit and not lit, faucet running full and dripping, puzzle pieces together and separated, pencil sharp and dull, sun full and partially cloud covered, balloons inflated and partially deflated, and lion and mouse. Individuals are asked to view each of the 10 picture pairs and mark the point along the scale between the pictures to indicate which they feel most like, for example, a lighted candle or an unlit candle. The brief instructions for the WPS were translated, and the scale has been administered in Taiwanese, Japanese, Korean, Egyptian, and Spanish. Psychometric properties for the tool were established in a sample of 1027 individuals in the United States, Taiwan, and Japan; the sample was 56% Asian, 34% white, and 10% African-American or Hispanic. The overall Cronbach's alpha was found to be 0.8795 across the three countries. Five of the 10 items were completely consistent across countries (puzzle, balloon, sun, eyes, and lion), and all others were consistent across two of the three countries. The scale has since been administered in South Korea, Egypt, and Botswana, Africa.

Conceptual Formulation of Well-Being

Rogers maintained that, "the purpose of nursing is to promote health and well-being for all persons wherever they are" (1992, p. 258). According to Hills (1998), well-being is generally defined as a relative sense of harmony and satisfaction in one's life. Smith (1981) and Todaro-Franceschi (1999) defined health as movement toward self-fulfillment or realization of one's potential, a view that is congruent with Parse's (1997) theory of human becoming. Newman (1994) does not distinguish health from well-being but singularly defines it as a manifestation of expanding consciousness that may occur during, but is not separate from, the experience of illness. This view is supported by the work of Hills (1998), who demonstrated a relationship between well-being and awareness.

Conceptually, the WPS assesses the energy field in regard to four characteristics judged to be associated with well-being: frequency of movement (i.e., intensity) within the energy field, awareness of one's self as energy, action emanating from the energy field, and power as knowing participation in change within the mutual human–environmental energy field process.

Frequency

The term *frequency* denotes the intensity of motion within the energy field(s). It is postulated that higher frequency is associated with a greater sense of well-being and that it is experienced as a sense of vitality.

Awareness

Awareness refers to the sense an individual has of his or her potential for change within the mutual human–environmental field. It signals readiness for moving toward one's potential and is postulated to be positively associated with a sense of well-being. The concept of awareness is congruent with Newman's (1994) theory of health as expanding consciousness and Parse's (1997) theory of human becoming (unfolding). Barrett (1990) included a subscale of awareness in her PKPC tool, and Hills (1998) discussed enlightenment as a manifestation of expanded awareness, higher-level field motion, and well-being. Awareness is postulated to be a positive manifestation of the dynamics of the mutual human–environmental field process.

Action

Action is conceptualized as an emergent of the "continuous mutual human–environmental field process" (Rogers, 1992), reflecting the frequency of the human energy field. Action is viewed as an expression of field energy associated with well-being. Examples of action include activities associated with daily living, such as preparing food, eating, personal grooming, participating in social events, exercising, or doing chores, as well as actively engaging in innovative thinking or the creation of art forms.

Power

As described by Barrett (1990), power is the capacity of an individual to engage knowingly in change. Barrett defined it as the degree to which an individual is able to express energy as power to create desired change within his or her human–environmental energy field process. When power is prominent, it is postulated that one would have a sense of confidence; conversely, it would follow that powerlessness is associated with a sense of vulnerability. Power might also be conceptualized as the capacity of an individual to commute the three aforementioned conditions (energy expressed as frequency, awareness, and action) into an emergent sense of well-being.

WPS Development

The more than 10 years of developmental work and field testing of early versions of the WPS revealed a correlation with several other tools designed to measure aspects of well-being within the Rogerian framework (Gueldner, Bramlett, Johnston, & Guillory, 1996). Johnston (1994), in a sample of nursing home residents and community-dwelling elders, reported a highly significant correlation (r = 0.6647) between the WPS tool and her Human Field Image Metaphor Scale, which uses two- or three-word metaphors to measure general self-image. Gueldner et al. (1996) found an even stronger correlation (r = 0.7841) between the WPS and Barrett's (1990) PKPC tool, which measures an individual's capacity for awareness, choices, freedom to act intentionally, and involvement to bring about harmony in the human–environmental field process.

Davis (1989), in a matched sample of 30 men 19 to 51 years of age who had been hospitalized for traumatic injuries and 30 noninjured men, demonstrated positive significant correlations between the score on the WPS and scores on the PKPC tool (p = 0.002) and Rosenberg's self-esteem scale (p = 0.02). She also found a difference in the between-group mean scores that approached significance (p = 0.059), warranting further consideration in a larger sample.

Hindman (1993), in a sample of 40 nursing home residents and 40 community-dwelling older adults, demonstrated a significant correlation (p = 0.001) between the mean score on the WPS and humor as measured by the Situational Humor Response Questionnaire. She also found that the mean score was higher for the community-dwelling group of older adults (p = 0.001) than for their counterparts who lived in the nursing home and that individuals who perceived their income as adequate scored higher (p = 0.05) than those who perceived their income to be less than adequate. Older participants scored lower (p = 0.05) on the WPS.

Gueldner et al. (2005) administered the WPS and the Geriatric Depression Scale (GDS) to 215 older adults who were attending lunchtime events at six senior centers in a nonurban county in upstate New York. Approximately two-thirds of the sample were female and one-third was male, with a mean age of 75.8 years and a range of 55 to 97 years. A significant negative correlation (r = -.585; p = -.01, two-tailed) was found between the WPS and the GDS scores, providing preliminary evidence that the WPS could serve as a reliable screening device for depression in independently dwelling elders. The mean score for the GDS was 2.58, with a range of 0 to 14; the mean score for the WPS was 52, with a range of 16 to 70. One-fifth (20%) of those who participated in the study scored above the cutoff of 5 (indicating some concern for depression) on the GDS; 10% scored above 8 on the GDS, and three individuals scored an alarming 13–14 on the GDS. These findings support the potential ability of the more user-friendly WPS to screen for depression in community-dwelling elders.

The WPS was used by Liu (2004) to test the effectiveness of a 3-week rehabilitation program in a sample of 30 older persons (mean age 76 years) who had sustained sudden disablement due to hip fracture or orthopedic surgery. She found a significant increase in the mean scores of the WPS (p = .01) from pre- to post-test, and reported a negative correlation (p = -.001) between age and the WPS score. She reported a Cronbach's alpha of .84 for the WPS, which is generally consistent with the Cronbach's alpha of .88 reported in the initial three-country research study.

The WPS was recently administered by nursing students in a one-on-one format, along with the GDS, to a sample of nursing home residents in upstate New York, and preliminary analyses indicated that the residents had little difficulty responding to the picture pairs. Since this was the first time the WPS was tested in a nursing home sample, invitations to participate in the study were limited to those scoring within the top two categories of the Minimum Data Set (a measure of capacity for independent living that is given at the time of nursing home admission). The facility also administers the GDS routinely, so the participants had taken it at least one time previously.

Summary

In summary, the work by Gueldner et al. (1996), Hills (1998), and Johnston (1994) confirmed a high correlation between scores on the WPS and other measures of well-being developed within the Rogerian conceptual system. Additionally, the work of Davis (1989), Hills (1998), Hindman (1993), and Gueldner et al. (2005) have demonstrated a high correlation between the WPS tool and a number of established measures of well-being developed by other disciplines. Preliminary studies by Abbate (1990) and Terwilliger (2007) demonstrated the potential usability of the tool in children. Liu's study (2004) confirmed the effectiveness of the WPS as a pre- and post-evaluation of a rehabilitation program following a disabling orthopedic event. Additionally, preceding studies have shown that elders, even some in nursing homes, were able to respond to the paired picture scale and make their marks themselves or convey their answers to the person administering the scale. Supported by these findings, the WPS is offered as a general measure of well-being mediated through frequency, awareness, action, and power emanating within an individual's mutual human–environmental field process.

Conclusion

Given these findings, the WPS is offered as a general index of well-being for use with international populations who might have difficulty reading English text. The instrument has the potential to give voice to those who are too sick or weak to participate in studies that require lengthy measures of well-being and, perhaps, even to persons with mild to moderate cognitive impairment. A secondary purpose of the tool rests in its potential for use as an easy-to-administer clinical indicator of well-being across a wide sector of community and clinical settings, including assisted living and nursing home facilities. The demonstrated usability of the scale with elders offers a promising option for giving voice to compromised elders, which is the important first step in reducing their vulnerability.

References

Abbate, M.F. (1990). *The relationship of therapeutic horsemanship and human field motion in children with cerebral palsy.* Unpublished master's thesis, Georgia State University, Atlanta.

Barrett, E.A.M. (1990). A measure of power as knowing participation in change. In O.L. Strickland & C.F. Waltz (Eds.), *The measurement of nursing outcomes: Measuring client self-care and coping skills* (Vol. 4). New York: Springer.

Davis, A.E. (1989). *The relationship between the phenomenon of traumatic injury and the patterns of power, human field motion, esteem and risk taking.* Unpublished doctoral dissertation, Georgia State University, Atlanta.

Demi, A.S., & Warren, N.A. (1995). Issues in conducting research with vulnerable families. *Western Journal of Nursing Research, 17,* 188–202.

Gueldner, S.H., Bramlett, M.H., Johnston, L.W., & Guillory, J.A. (1996). Index of Field Energy. *Rogerian Nursing Science News, 8*(4), 6.

Gueldner, S.H., Michel, Y., Bramlett, M.H., Liu, C.F., Johnston, L.W., Endo, E., et al. (2005). The Well-being Picture Scale: A refined version of the Index of Field Energy. *Nursing Science Quarterly, 18*(1), 42–50.

Hills, R. (1998). *Maternal field patterning of awareness, wakefulness, human field motion and well-being in mothers with 6 month old infants: A Rogerian science perspective.* Unpublished doctoral dissertation, Wayne State University, Detroit, Michigan.

Hindman, M. (1993). *Humor and field energy in older adults.* Unpublished doctoral dissertation, Medical College of Georgia, Augusta.

Johnston, L.W. (1994). Psychometric analysis of Johnston's Human Field Image Metaphor Scale. *Visions: Journal of Rogerian Nursing Science, 2,* 7–11.

Liu, C.F. (2004). The relationship between well-being and functional ability in older women recovering from an acute episode of disablement. Unpublished doctoral dissertation, The Pennsylvania State University, State College.

Morse, J.M. (1997). Responding to threats to integrity of self. *Advances in Nursing Science, 19,* 21–36.

Newman, M.A. (1994). *Health as expanding consciousness.* New York: National League for Nursing.

Parse, R.R. (1997). The human becoming theory: The was, is, and will be. *Nursing Science Quarterly, 10*(1), 32–38.

Parse, R.R. (2003). *Community: A human becoming perspective.* Sudbury, MA: Jones and Bartlett.

Phillips, B.B., & Bramlett, M.H. (1994). Integrated awareness: A key to the pattern of mutual process. *Visions, 2,* 7–12.

Rogers, M.E. (1992). Nursing science and the space age. *Nursing Science Quarterly, 5,* 27–34.

Saunders, J.M., & Valente, S.M. (1992). Overview. *Western Journal of Nursing Research, 14,* 700–702.

Smith, J.A. (1981) The idea of health: A philosophical inquiry. *Advances in Nursing Science, 4,* 43–49.

Spiers, J. (2000). New perspectives on vulnerability using emic and etic approaches. *Journal of Advanced Nursing, 31,* 715–721.

Terwilliger, S. (2007). *A study of children enrolled in a school-based physical activity program with attention to overweight and depression.* Unpublished doctoral dissertation, Binghamton University, Binghamton, NY.

Todaro-Franceschi, V. (1999). *The enigma of energy.* New York: Crossroad.

Section V

Practice Imperatives

Chapter 18

Creating a New Philosophy for Elder Care

Eric D. Newman

Blame my parents. When I was 8 years old, they bought me a seemingly innocuous poster for my room: three turtles travelling down a river. The third turtle was paddling furiously, the second turtle was paddling furiously, but the first turtle had climbed out of its shell, had flipped the shell over, was sitting in it, and was using two oars to effortlessly navigate the river. The title of the poster read, "There's always a better way." I never realized it until later in life, when my healthcare position afforded me the opportunity to really "test the waters," but this poster summed up my personal mantra. My hope is that after reading this chapter, I will interest some of you and maybe light a fire under a few of you to challenge the status quo, to redesign healthcare delivery, and to strive to work as a team for the betterment of those we serve—our patients. And nowhere is the need to improve healthcare delivery greater than in the care of our rapidly growing number of elders.

This chapter will be divided into several sections. First, I will briefly summarize the sad state of health care today. Next, I will focus on problem solving—the wrong way and the right way. A few practical healthcare redesign examples, both small and large, will follow. I will then end with a few final thoughts, to keep you interested, amused, and hopefully empowered.

Health Care Today

We are in a crisis. Health care in the United States is costly and of only mediocre quality (Harrington, 2003; Harrington & Newman, 2007; Lofgren, Karpf, Perman, & Higdon, 2006; US Institute of Medicine & Committee on Quality of Health Care in America, 2001). Higher costs lead to a decrease in access to care, and mediocre quality leads to illnesses and complications that could have been avoided. The end result is needless suffering for our patients, and what the Japanese call "muda," or needless waste. Not an enviable position for a country that prides itself on being and delivering the best for its citizens.

The problems with healthcare quality were wonderfully articulated in a landmark pub-lication from the Institute of Medicine over 8 years ago, *"Crossing the Quality Chasm: A New Health System for the 21st Century"* (US Institute of Medicine & Committee on Quality of Health Care in America, 2001). Now class, let's have a show of hands:

How many of you have read the full report (360 pages)?
How many of you have read the executive summary (45 pages)?
How many of you have read the brief report (8 pages)?
How many of you have watched a reality show on television this past week?

If this was a lecture, the audience response would be 0%, 5%, 10%, and 90%. So my first challenge to you is shut the television off and read the Chasm report. It if resonates, read on—we want you to be our caregivers. If it doesn't resonate, please pick another profession.

The Chasm report reflected that the growth in knowledge now is greater than at any point in medical history. In addition, while technology and medical science have moved forward at a rapid pace, the healthcare delivery system has not been able to keep up, lead-ing to unequal and often inferior quality of care. Their conclusion was not unexpected: "The American health care delivery system is in need of fundamental change" (US Insti-tute of Medicine & Committee on Quality of Health Care in America, 2001).

The Chasm report also nicely outlines six categories or domains of care that should be improved, which are easily remembered by the mnemonic **STEEEP**. We need to strive to deliver health care that is **S**afe, **T**imely, **E**ffective, **E**fficient, **E**quitable, and **P**atient-centric. This can be accomplished by redesigning our outdated and ineffective care processes, effectively using information technology, developing patient-centric healthcare teams, coordinating care, and measuring how we are doing. Table 18-1 summarizes some of the many redesign opportunities that can be considered.

TABLE 18-1   Health Care Redesign Opportunities

- Patient access to visits—new and established
- Clinical data gathering, recording, analysis, storing
- Electronic technology support
- Physician–physician communication methods
- Patient communication methods
- Accessing medical knowledge
- Practice provider composition and roles
- Disease state management
- Care process management

In summary, we are caught in a "perfect storm." There are increasing problems with traditional health care, our therapies are more complex and more effective, the expectations for a better outcome are increasing, revenues are at risk and tied to performance, overhead continues to increase, hassles are increasing, and person-power is decreasing relative to demand. The inevitable conclusion: It's not whether to redesign our delivery of care, but what to do and how to do it.

Problem Solving—The Wrong Way

The tribal wisdom of the Dakota Indians, passed on from generation to generation, says that "When you discover that you are riding a dead horse, the best strategy is to dismount." This is a wise and prudent action. However, in health care, we employ more advanced strategies, such as:

- Buying a stronger whip
- Changing riders
- Appointing a committee to study the dead horse
- Arranging visits to see how others ride dead horses
- Lowering the standards so that dead horses can be included
- Promoting the dead horse to a supervisory position
- Hiring outside contractors to ride the dead horse
- Harnessing several dead horses together to increase speed
- Providing additional funding and/or training to increase the dead horse's performance
- Rewriting the expected performance requirements for all horses
- Doing a productivity study to see if lighter riders would improve the dead horse's performance
- Declaring that, as the dead horse does not have to be fed, it is less costly, carries lower overhead and therefore contributes substantially more to the bottom line than do some other horses
- Reclassifying the dead horse as living impaired

The bad news is that most of us have been part of a problem-solving workgroup where such solutions have actually been proposed and implemented. The good news is that there *are* effective ways to implement change and solve problems, and it's perfectly fine to propose and implement a "far out" idea (innovation)—as long as it is tested and monitored in a well-defined fashion.

Problem Solving—The Right Way

Most of us spend our days in "crisis mode"—stamping out the fires of today, with little time left for horizon thinking and planning. Some of us have the pleasure of working in the area of redesign, and a few of us have had the extraordinary opportunity of doing innovative work.

Innovative thinking can be divided into three concepts: taking a different view, challenging the old way, and assuming the impossible. I will illustrate each with an example. Dean Kamen took a different view of transportation. Instead of creating technology to go longer distances faster, he instead focused on going shorter distances more efficiently. His invention, the Segway®, improved transportation efficiency in many different sectors, including large manufacturing plants, the police force, the tourist industry, and those with walking disabilities (Sawatzky, Denison, & Tawashy, 2009).

Challenging the old way often involves flipping the usual pathway 180 degrees. In surgeries such as total joint replacement, the usual paradigm is to educate, then operate, then rehabilitate. By flipping this around and beginning with rehabilitation (termed "prehabilitation"), the outcomes can improve for patients (Jaggers, Simpson, Frost, Quesada, Topp, Swank, & Nyland, 2007).

The final example, assuming the impossible, gets to the center of innovative thinking. When the medical profession and society were faced with the problem of what to do if a heart stops beating, the response was to create a system of transportation that would get these patients to care sooner and train large numbers of lay people to try and keep patients alive until more definitive care could be rendered by trained personnel. But what if you asked a child the same question: "What would you do if the heart stops beating?" The child might reply, "Have the heart start itself." This simple reframing of the problem, assuming the impossible, led directly to the development of the implantable defibrillator and the automatic external defibrillator (AED)—the latter device now incorporated directly into basic life support training and available in many public locations ("Part 4: Adult Basic Life Support," 2005).

Let us move from innovation to the practical skill set of problem solving. As a physician, I always considered myself an excellent problem solver. I was trained to effectively query a patient about salient symptoms, gather objective information through physical examination and a few tests, and with this limited data set formulate a likely differential, ordered according to statistical likelihood. This paradigm serves us well when we deal with an individual patient, but falls apart when we are trying to solve problems in healthcare delivery. If we go right to the solution, without first understanding the problem, we will likely miss opportunities to improve quality and reduce waste, and we are more likely to actually reduce quality and increase costs.

Problem solving, fortunately, is quite easy if you follow a set of linear steps, and do not skip any steps (Harrington & Newman, 2007). An analogy I give to healthcare providers is that problem solving is like doing a procedure; you follow a certain set of steps in order. You would never, for example, operate, and *then* do your sterile preparation. Problem solv-

TABLE 18-2   Problem-Solving Steps

- Define the problem.
- Analyze the problem.
- Develop some solutions.
- Test a solution.
- Measure the results of testing.
- Reassess, retest, and remeasure.

ing is no different. Table 18-2 shows the basic steps involved in solving problems. They work in industry, they work in health care, and sometimes they have even worked in solving family problems (although teenagers are notoriously resistant to change)!

Defining the problem turns out to be a commonly missed but incredibly important first step. When defining a problem, it is important that it sits within your sphere of control, that a cause is not assumed, and that there is no solution in mind. Here is a bad way of framing a problem: "If I only had enough professional staff, our patient backlog would be taken care of." First, this statement assumes causality (that the reason for the backlog is not enough providers). Second, it already provides the solution (hire more providers). A better way to frame the problem is, "We cannot see our patients in a timely fashion." When we frame the problem in this fashion, there are no false assumptions, and more potential solutions are available.

Once defined, the problem then needs to be analyzed. There are many methodologies for doing this, but two common ones are root cause analysis and the fishbone diagram. Root cause analysis is commonly used to discover why a medical error has occurred in a hospital setting, as an example. I find using a fishbone diagram to be more intuitive and easier to grasp. Fishbone diagrams are also called "cause and effect" or Ishikawa diagrams. Kaoru Ishikawa developed the concept over 40 years ago to improve production in the Kawasaki Shipyards in Japan. A fishbone diagram is a picture of the factors that are thought to produce a certain result (the main spine), with big arrows representing contributing factors that could produce this result pointing to the main spine (Harrington & Newman, 2007). Figure 18-1 shows a sample fishbone diagram for lengthy appointments, with the main contributing categories of people, equipment, materials, and process.

Now that we have defined and analyzed our problem, it is time to develop some solutions. This often involves starting with a brainstorming session and finishing with a separate prioritization session. Brainstorming involves getting a larger group of participants to generate a long list of solutions. Someone needs to serve as leader and someone else as scribe. No one is criticized, everyone gets to participate, and lots of solutions and exaggerated ideas are encouraged. A second, smaller group then gets together and prioritizes

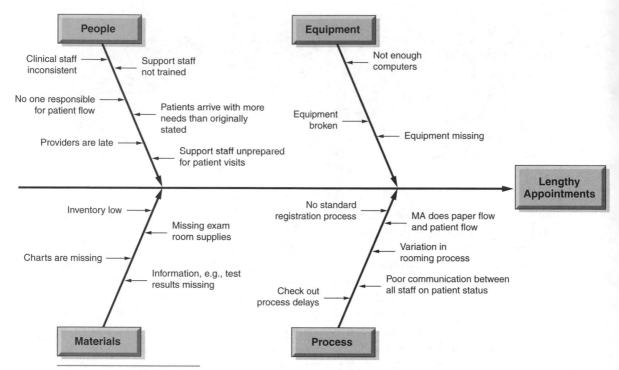

Figure 18-1 Fishbone (cause and effect) of lengthy appointments.

this long list of solutions, focusing on ease of implementation and potential impact as guiding principles.

To recap, we have defined our problem, analyzed our problem, and developed some solutions. Now it is time to test a solution, measure the results, and reassess, remeasure, and retest. This is the core of PDSA methodology—Plan, Do, Study, Act (Berwick, 1998; Harrington & Newman, 2007). PDSA allows for small-scale, rapid-cycle testing of a solution. This is crucial, as it often takes multiple passes (cycles) of testing to improve a particular problem, and many of the cycles will fail. (In truth, there is no failure, just a learning opportunity to change and improve.) The results of the preceding cycle drive the design and testing of the next cycle.

Why is it so important to test on a small scale? Because we are working in a system (Newman, & Harrington, 2007; Nolan, 1998). A system is a set of interdependent variables that work together to achieve a common goal. Systems in health care are often referred to as clinical microsystems. An example might be a healthcare team that includes nurses, secretaries, front desk office staff, and physicians, all circling around the patient. Systems, however, are inherently unruly, and it is difficult to predict the upstream and downstream effects. If a change is introduced into a system of care before small-scale testing, that

TABLE 18-3 PDSA Cycle to Improve "No-Show" Rate

- Plan
  - Decrease new patients who "no-show"
  - More slots will then be available
  - Call all scheduled new patients during the daytime 2 days before their scheduled visit
- Do
  - For 2 weeks
  - Call all scheduled news 2 days before appt
  - Monitor whether patient is reached and how (in person, left message, not reached) and work effort (minutes per appt scheduled)
- Study
  - 80 patients called
  - 50% of patients reached in person
  - No-show rate higher for left message and not reached
  - Cost per appointment calls (minutes / 60 * [salary + benefits]) = $1.00 × 80 patients = $80
  - No-shows averted and filled with alternative patients = 6 × $200/consult = $1200
  - Net additional revenue = $1200 – $80 = $1120 per 2 weeks = $29,120/year
- Act
  - For Cycle 2
    - Call at night to see if yield is better
  - For Cycle 3
    - Capture best time/# to reach to see if reaching a person increases

change could worsen a particular healthcare problem, and even worse, if not properly monitored, it might never be discovered. All of us have probably been affected by some administrative decision that created a ripple effect throughout the workplace—well-meaning in its origin, but a failure in its implementation due to a lack of respect for the unpredictable nature of the system in which the decision was introduced. It wasn't tested before it was rolled out.

As an example of how simple and effective PDSA can be, let's tackle the area of patients who "no-show" for a clinic visit. We would like to decrease our "no show" rate. Table 18-3 shows how the PDSA might look. The end result after 2 weeks is more patients receiving care, and $29,000 additional revenue. Not bad for a simple 2-week test!

In our rheumatology practice, we have applied PDSA methodology to solve very small problems (how to queue up patients after they exit the elevator and try to check in *en masse* at the front desk), medium-sized problems (improving callback for needed testing), and very large problems (improving access to specialty care, how to best manage a population of patients with disease through organized healthcare delivery programs) (Newman, Harrington, Olenginski, Perruquet, & McKinley, 2004; Newman et al., 2006; Olenginski, Newman, Hummel, & Hummer, 2006). Our work on advanced access on the specialty side has resulted in a fascinating journey for us in the field of rheumatology (Newman, Harrington, Olenginski, Perruquet, & McKinley, 2004). We have improved our access to care from over 60 days to just a few days, and the results have been sustainable now for over 8 years. The preceding references will provide more detail for interested readers, but each of these highly successful projects was accomplished using PDSA as the core tool.

Final Thoughts

To be successful at healthcare redesign, there are a few basic necessities. You need a champion. You need buy-in and commitment. You need a team with all players present—doctors, nurses, office assistants, and administrative personnel—all on an even footing, all empowered to effect change, all circling around the needs of the patient. You need incentives, or at the least no disincentives—you don't want to make your team eat the stick while you are beating them with the carrot. You need to develop problem-solving skills; a great place to start is the Institution for Healthcare Improvement (www.IHI.org). You need to have someone on the team capable of entering and tracking data; a simple spreadsheet usually suffices.

A good place to start in redesigning healthcare delivery is to look at the existing rules, regulations, and flows of your clinical microsystem. Chances are excellent that there are both an overabundance of unnecessary steps and significant variation in practice habits. Consider taking a five-senses tour—walk through your own work area as though you were a patient—smell, listen, see, taste, feel. You may smell the nauseating aroma of burnt popcorn, hear a worker shout, *"Are you receiving black lung benefits?"* at the front desk, see magazines from 7 years ago strewn around the waiting area, taste hardened water from the clinic water fountain as you swallow a virtual pill, or feel the coldness and dirtiness of the exam room floor on bare feet. Evaluate your clinic's "vital signs"—access, cycle time, staff satisfaction, patient satisfaction. Simplify workflows, and measure constantly. Aim for a few quick wins, build on your skills, ask questions, and learn as a team from your experiences. There are no failures, just learning opportunities.

Health care is one of the noblest professions. Improving the lives of those we serve—be it one-on-one, or thousands at a time—is one of the most rewarding activities I can imagine. We owe it to our patients and to society to improve the quality and efficiency of our healthcare delivery, and we have the tools and ability to do so. To quote my sister-in-law, a biology teacher in New Hampshire, "if you're not part of the solution, you're part of the precipitate." So I urge you to go forth and conquer. And a good place to begin is to improve access and delivery of all dimensions of health care for our elders, who are among the most vulnerable segments of the population, and are growing rapidly in number.

I would like to dedicate this chapter to my parents, for providing the right genetic wiring and the right environment, and to my good friend and colleague J. Timothy Harrington, MD, for his expertise, mentorship, and willingness to let me tilt at windmills by his side.

—EDN

References

Berwick, D.M. (1998). Developing and testing changes in delivery of care. *Annals of Internal Medicine, 128*(8), 651–656.

Harrington, J.T. (2003). A view of our future: the case for redesigning rheumatology practice. *Arthritis & Rheumatism, 49*(5), 716–719.

Harrington, J.T., & Newman, E.D. (2007). Redesigning the care of rheumatic diseases at the practice and system levels: A two part article. Part 1 – Practice level process improvement (Redesign 101). *Clinical and Experimental Rheumatology, 25*(6 Suppl 47), 55–63.

Jaggers, J.R., Simpson, C.D., Frost, K.L., Quesada, P.M., Topp, R.V., Swank, A.M., & Nyland, J.A. (2007). Prehabilitation before knee arthroplasty increases post-surgical function: A case study. *The Journal of Strength and Conditioning Research, 121*(21), 632–634.

Lofgren, R., Karpf, M., Perman, J., & Higdon, C.M. (2006). The U.S. health care system is in crisis: Implications for academic medical centers and their missions. *Academic Medicine, 81*(8), 713–720.

Newman, E.D., & Harrington, J.T. (2007). Redesigning the care of rheumatic diseases at the practice and system levels. A two part article. Part 2 – System level process improvement (Redesign 201). *Clinical and Experimental Rheumatology, 25*(6 Suppl 47), 64–68.

Newman, E.D., Harrington, T.M., Olenginski, T.P., Perruquet, J.L., & McKinley, K. (2004). "The rheumatologist can see you now": Successful implementation of an advanced access model in a rheumatology practice. *Arthritis & Rheumatism, 51*(2), 253–257.

Newman, E.D., Matzko, C.K., Olenginski, T.P., Perruquet, J.L., Harrington, T.M., Maloney-Saxon, G., et al. (2006). Glucocorticoid-induced osteoporosis program (GIOP): A novel, comprehensive, and highly successful care program with improved outcomes at 1 year. *Osteoporosis International, 17*(9), 1428–1434.

Nolan, T.W. (1998). Understanding medical systems. *Annals of Internal Medicine, 128*(4), 293–298.

Olenginski, T.P., Newman, E.D., Hummel, J.L., & Hummer, M. (2006). Development and evaluation of a vertebral fracture assessment program using instant vertebral assessment (IVA) and its integration with mobile dxa. *Journal of Clinical Densitometry, 9*(1), 72–77.

Part 4: Adult Basic Life Support. (2005). *Circulation, 112*, IV-19–IV-34.

Sawatzky, B., Denison, I., & Tawashy, A. (2009). The Segway for people with disabilities: Meeting clients' mobility goals. *American Journal of Physical Medicine & Rehabilitation, 88*(6), 484–490.

US Institute of Medicine & Committee on Quality of Health Care in America. (2001). *Crossing the quality chasm: A new health system for the 21st century.* Washington, D.C.: National Academy Press.

Chapter 19

Evidence-Based Pain Management

Katherine R. Jones

Managing Persistent (Chronic) Pain in Older Adults

Pain is a commonly occurring problem, and it is particularly prevalent in older adults. Between 25% and 50% of community-dwelling older adults and 45% to 85% of nursing home residents experience persistent pain (American Geriatrics Society [AGS], 2002; Charette & Ferrell, 2007; Horgas & Yoon, 2008). Unfortunately, both malignant and non-malignant pain in the elderly is frequently unrecognized, and when recognized it is often underassessed and undertreated (Charette & Ferrell, 2007; Hadjistavropoulos et al., 2009). Clinicians are often uncertain on how best to achieve optimum management of this common problem (Barber & Gibson, 2009). The evidence supporting pharmacological interventions for managing pain in older persons is inadequate, given the pharmacokinetic and pharmacodynamic changes that occur with aging (Barber & Gibson, 2009). In addition, clinicians are naturally conservative when prescribing pain medication, due to the major known predictors of adverse drug reactions—aging, inappropriate combinations of medications, and polypharmacy (Barber & Gibson, 2009).

Inadequate treatment of pain is associated with functional impairment, falls, slow or delayed rehabilitation and healing, changes in mood, decreased socialization, disturbances in sleep and appetite, and greater healthcare utilization and costs (American Geriatrics Society Panel on Pharmacologic Management of Persistent Pain in Older Persons, 2009). Because of the pervasive influence of pain, there is an overall reduced quality of life for those who are affected (Herr et al., 2006; Zanocchi et al., 2008). Several organizations and associations have developed clinical practice guidelines that have focused on this problem. In addition, multiple systematic reviews have analyzed the research evidence related to specific aspects of persistent pain management. This chapter will review the most recent evidence and recommendations for assessing and managing persistent pain in the older adult.

Sources of Pain

Persistent pain may be the result of musculoskeletal conditions, cancer and cancer treatment, neuropathic conditions, trauma, or limb amputation (AGS Panel, 2009;

Hadjistavropoulos et al., 2009). Obesity may be a contributing factor, since obese elders are twice as likely, and severely obese elders more than four times as likely, to have persistent pain (McCarthy, Bigal, Katz, Deby, & Lipton, 2009). Surgery and other invasive procedures and therapies are also associated with pain, as are various psychological conditions. For example, residents in nursing homes may describe a culmination of existential pain and suffering associated with loss of loved ones, loss of former home, health, and independence, and loss of connectedness (Gudmannsdottier & Halldorsdottir, 2009).

Assessment and Management of Pain

The process of pain management in the older person begins with recognition of pain. A systematic process for identifying pain should be in place. When pain is identified, efforts must be made to identify the source of the pain, as this influences the selection of appropriate interventions (American Geriatrics Society, 2002). There may be more than one source of pain, but it is also possible that no specific source of persistent pain can be identified. A thorough assessment of the pain follows, including location of the pain, level of pain intensity or severity, quality of pain (throbbing, aching), duration and frequency of the pain, what brings it on or makes the pain worse, and what makes the pain better or more tolerable. For example, stair climbing might make the pain worse while heat makes the pain better. The impact of pain on physical and psychosocial functioning should be determined during the assessment. Information about previous experiences with pain, including past approaches to pain management, should also be gathered as part of a comprehensive history and physical examination.

Pain Assessment Tools

The best indicator of pain is the individual's own self-report (AGS, 2002). This is true even if the person has mild or moderate cognitive impairment (AGS Panel, 2009; Hadjistavropoulos et al., 2007). Simple questions and screening tools can be used to determine both the presence and the intensity of the pain. The McGill Pain Questionnaire (MPQ), Brief Pain Inventory (BPI), and Geriatric Pain Measure are validated multidimensional tools for the assessment of pain, but they are difficult to implement in the practice setting (Charette & Ferrell, 2007). Unidimensional tools focus on one domain of pain, usually pain intensity. Pain intensity tools include numeric rating scales, verbal descriptor scales, faces pain scales, and pain thermometers. Reliability and validity for these tools have been fair to good when used in the older population (Charette & Ferrell, 2007). However, the validity and reliability are not as strong when they are used to assess pain intensity in older adults with lower educational levels, deficits in vision and hearing, and moderate to advanced cognitive impairment (Herr & Garand, 2001). The verbal descriptor scale is most sensitive and reliable in older adults with mild to moderate impairment (Taylor, Harris, Epps, & Herr, 2005), and is usually preferred by older adults (Jones et al., 2005), but studies have shown that the Faces Pain Scale for reporting pain intensity may be preferred by African Americans and Hispanics (Taylor & Herr, 2003; Jones et al., 2005).

For those who are nonverbal or with severe cognitive impairment, an observational tool is usually used. The person is observed during rest and movement and is assessed on items such as vocalizations and verbalizations, facial expressions, guarding, and rubbing a body part (Herr et al., 2006). Changes in typical behaviors are also a possible indicator of the presence of pain, such as increased pacing or resistance to care. The American Society for Pain Management Nursing has published five key principles to guide pain assessment in nonverbal populations: obtain self-report if at all possible; investigate for possible pathologies that could produce pain; observe for behaviors that may indicate pain; solicit surrogate reports; and use analgesics to evaluate whether pain management causes a reduction in the behavioral indicators thought to be related to pain (Herr et al., 2006).

There are at least 14 tools for assessing pain in the nonverbal or cognitively impaired adult. Bjora and Herr (2008) reviewed six of these and concluded that there is no single tool with sufficient validity and reliability to warrant recommendation for broad adoption in clinical practice. While and Jocelyn (2009) reviewed four systematic reviews of behavioral pain intensity tools and reported that no consensus could be reached on which tool to use in clinical practice. McAuliffe, Nay, O'Donnell, & Fetherstonhaugh (2009) recommend an individualized approach to pain assessment in the cognitively impaired or nonverbal older adult, which includes (a) knowing the person by caring for them for an extended period of time; (b) providing more education and training to staff about pain and its assessment and management; (c) using the selected tools consistently; (d) conducting baseline assessments to be able to discern changes in behaviors; and (e) having the same person conduct the assessments whenever possible.

Pharmacological Management

Although older adults are at increased risk for adverse drug reactions (Horgas & Yoon, 2008; AGS Panel, 2009), the use of analgesics in managing persistent pain in older persons is widely supported and guided on the basis of clinical experience and consensus among specialists in geriatrics and pain management (Barber & Gibson, 2009). However, careful selection of drugs is required, with consideration of both the physiological status of the older person and the presence of multiple diseases and clinical conditions (Kean, Rainsford & Kean, 2008). The American Geriatrics Society (2009) has identified general principles for pharmacological management that apply to all older persons. These include:

- Start low, go slow (low initial doses followed by upward titration).
- Use least invasive route of administration—usually oral.
- Round-the-clock dosing for persistent pain.
- Rapid-onset, short-acting analgesics for severe, episodic pain or breakthrough pain.
- Premedicate before activities that can be expected to precipitate pain (dressing change, physical therapy).

- Combine pharmacological with nonpharmacological pain management therapies to enhance pain relief.
- Consider that more than one drug may be needed to attain the therapeutic endpoint.

Acetaminophen: Acetaminophen (paracetamol) is recommended as the first-line therapy for mild to moderate pain (AGS Panel, 2009). When used at recommended doses, it is relatively safe with low gastrointestinal and renal toxicity (Barber & Gibson, 2009). However, patients, family members, and clinicians need to be aware of the maximum safe dose of acetaminophen (4 grams per 24 hours, or lower if certain comorbidities are present), and the "hidden" sources of this medication in various combination drugs (Vicodin, Percocet). Liver failure is an absolute contraindication for acetaminophen (AGS Panel, 2009). Relative contraindications include hepatic insufficiency, renal impairment, and chronic alcohol abuse or dependence (AGS Panel, 2009; Barber & Gibson, 2009). Other known risk factors for hepato-toxicity associated with acetaminophen use include poor nutrition and dehydration; potential drug interactions may occur with anticoagulants, drugs affecting gastric emptying, and hepatic enzyme inducers such as hypnotics and anti-epileptics (Barber & Gibson, 2009).

NSAIDs: Non-steroidal anti-inflammatory drugs (NSAIDs) have been used frequently for pain treatment in older persons, especially for those with inflammatory osteo- and rheumatoid arthritic conditions, headache, and low back pain (Barber & Gibson, 2009). NSAIDs include nonselective COX inhibitors and COX-2 selective inhibitors. This class of drugs has undergone the greatest amount of scrutiny in the recent past. Major contraindications to the use of NSAIDs include active GI bleeding and peptic ulcer disease, chronic kidney disease, heart failure, and NSAID-sensitive or aspirin-sensitive asthma (Barber & Gibson, 2009). Relative contraindications include hypertension, H. pylori, history of peptic ulcer disease or GI bleeding, bleeding tendency, hepatic, renal or cardiac impairment, concomitant use of corticosteroids or SSRIs, and older age (AGS Panel, 2009; Barber & Gibson, 2009). Individuals should not take more than one NSAID or COX-2 inhibitor at a time for pain control, and if taking aspirin for cardio-prophylaxis should not use ibuprofen (AGS Panel, 2009). Specific NSAIDs (ketorolac, mefenamic acid, piroxicam, meloxicam, oxaprozin, naproxen) are not recommended for use in older persons due to their elevated risk of toxicity (Barber & Gibson, 2009). Potential drug interactions include antihypertensives, ACE inhibitors, diuretics, high-dose methotrexate, anticoagulants, lithium, oral hypoglycemic agents, and probenecid (Barber & Gibson, 2009). An FDA black-box warning has been issued regarding the dose-dependent GI and renal effects of NSAIDs (Barber & Gibson, 2009). Potential NSAID toxicity may be avoided through co-administration of misoprostol, high dose H2-receptor antagonists, or proton pump inhibitors (Barber & Gibson, 2009; AGS Panel, 2009).

COX-2 selective inhibitor NSAIDs may have fewer significant GI adverse effects, but may still have other NSAID-related toxicities and higher cardiovascular risk. Celecoxib has been used successfully with many elders, while rofecoxib and valdecoxib have been withdrawn from the market because of adverse cardiovascular events (AGS Panel, 2009). The most recent AGS guideline panel (2009) concluded that its previous recommendation suggesting a trial of NSAIDs if acetaminophen is ineffective in relieving pain is often a risky strategy in older adults. Instead, the panel urges individual consideration of the use of NSAIDs, taking into account the individual's comorbidities and other medications, as well as previous positive use of NSAIDs for relieving pain. The panel's formal guideline recommendation is that both nonselective NSAIDs and COX-2 selective inhibitors be considered only rarely, and used with extreme caution, in highly selected individuals (AGS Panel, 2009) (Table 19-1).

Similarly, Barber & Gibson (2009) recommend that acetaminophen be used for mild to moderate pain, and that low-dose corticosteroids be used for inflammatory arthritic conditions. However, Kean, Rainsford, and Kean (2008) believe that traditional NSAIDs remain a good choice in the management of arthritis and musculoskeletal disorders in the elderly, especially if given with a proton pump inhibitor. They assert that the cardiovascular, renal, and hypertensive risks of selective COX-2 inhibitors should be avoided; instead, nonselective NSAIDs in conjunction with a PPI or H2-receptor blocker should be administered, believing this combination provides significant protection from the development of GI symptoms and ulcer complications. Kean et al. (2008) also acknowledge that the use of COX-2 inhibitors may be appropriate in selected cases. Clearly, consensus has not been reached on the use of either type of NSAID for mild and moderate pain in the older population.

Barber & Gibson (2009) issued a series of recommendations regarding NSAID use in the older person. These include considering alternatives; using NSAIDs with a short half-life; using the smallest dose possible for the shortest duration possible; not combining COX-2 inhibitors with nonselective NSAIDs; and avoidance of concomitant use of NSAIDs and aspirin that is intended to provide cardio-protection. Finally, aspirin acts as a nonreversible COX inhibitor, and has no role in the treatment of persistent pain in the elderly (Barber & Gibson, 2009). It is associated with adverse GI effects, and it interacts with corticosteroids, anticoagulants, and alcohol (Barber & Gibson, 2009).

Opioids: Opioids are indicated for severe pain that has not responded to nonopioid drugs (Barber & Gibson, 2009). Opioids are a potentially effective and safe therapy for various types of persistent pain, particularly in light of the evidence that the use of NSAIDs may result in serious GI and CV events (AGS Panel, 2009). However, the potential for adverse effects, drug–drug interactions, and drug–disease interactions is higher in the elderly, given pharmacokinetic and pharmacodynamic changes, higher incidence of comorbid disease, and greater likelihood of polypharmacy (Barber & Gibson, 2009). The physiological changes that occur with aging, combined with increased age-related brain sensitivity to opioids, requires lower initial doses and slower titration until effective analgesia is achieved (Barber & Gibson, 2009; Chou et al., 2009). The use of narcotics thus requires close supervision in the elderly, especially those with cognitive decline (Barber & Gibson, 2009; Keane et al., 2008). Short-acting opioids may be safer for initial therapy because they have a shorter half-life and a lower risk of inadvertent overdose. Interestingly,

TABLE 19-1 Medications Used to Relieve Pain in Older Persons

Drug Category/ Name	Indication	Adverse Effects/ Contraindications/ Precautions
Acetaminophen (Paracetamol)	First-line therapy Mild to moderate pain Lacks anti-inflammatory effects	• Maximum safe dose: 4 grams per 24 hours; less if decreased liver function • Be aware of "hidden sources" in combination drugs • Contraindicated in liver failure; relative contraindication in hepatic insufficiency, renal impairment, chronic alcohol abuse • Has ceiling effect
NSAIDs (Non-steroidal anti-inflammatory drugs)	Mild to moderate inflammatory or non-neuropathic pain; pain not relieved by acetaminophen	• Current recommendation: Use rarely and with caution in older adults, due to toxic effects; consider on individual basis only • Has ceiling effect
Non-selective COX Inhibitors Ibuprofen Choline magnesium Trisalicylate Ketoprofen Nabumetone Naproxen		• Contraindicated in peptic ulcer disease, active GI bleeding, chronic kidney disease, heart failure, NSAID-sensitive asthma; also with alcohol use, steroids, anticoagulants • Relative contraindication in hypertension, H. pylori, history of peptic ulcer disease, or GI bleeding; hepatic, renal, or cardiac impairment • FDA box warning regarding dose-dependent GI and renal effects of NSAIDs; GI bleeding or ulceration, fluid retention and edema

TABLE 19-1 Continued

Drug Category/ Name	Indication	Adverse Effects/ Contraindications/ Precautions
Non-selective COX Inhibitors (cont.)		• If used, co-administer miso-prostol, H_2-receptor antagonists, or proton pump inhibitor
		• Avoid indomethacin; ketorolac
Cox-2 Inhibitors Celecoxib Valdecoxib (taken off market) Rofecoxib (taken off market)		• Fewer GI effects; higher cardiovascular adverse effects
		• Contraindicated in severe hepatic impairment; asthmatics with ASA triad; advanced renal disease; concurrent use of diuretics and ACE inhibitors; anemia
Opioids Hydrocodone Oxycodone Codeine	Moderate to severe pain that has not responded to nonopioids Moderate pain (with or without acetaminophen, ASA)	• Common adverse effects: constipation, nausea, sedation, cognitive changes, pruritis, respiratory depression (if doses too high or titrated up too quickly), urinary retention, dry mouth, dizziness, orthostatic hypotension.
Morphine Hydromorphone Fentanyl ER morphine ER oxycodone Transdermal fentanyl	Severe pain—short-acting and long-acting agents	• Avoid methadone, levorphanol, propoxyphene— long half-lives
		• Avoid meperidine, propoxyphene—toxic metabolites
		• Avoid butorphanol, buprenorphine, pentazocine, nalbuphine—ceiling effect

(continues)

TABLE 19-1 Continued

Drug Category/ Name	Indication	Adverse Effects/ Contraindications/ Precautions
Opioids (cont.)		• Cautious use with respiratory depression, asthma, emphysema, alcohol use; history of drug abuse or dependence; OxyContin must be swallowed whole
		• Be aware of total dose of acetaminophen or ASA being given
Tramadol (Narcotic–like agent)	Relieves moderate to severe pain; now available in sustained release	• Fewer side effects than opioids or NSAIDS
		• Low abuse and diversion potential
		• If renal insufficiency, reduce dose by 50%
		• Side effects: dizziness, drowsiness, constipation, nausea, fatigue, headache
		• Reduces threshold for seizures
Adjuvant drugs: administer with or without other analgesics		
Corticosteroids (prednisone, dexamethasone)	Inflammatory disease, neuro pathic pain	• Use for short-term control of pain
Tricyclic antidepressants (TCAs)(nortriptyline, desipramine)	Neuropathic pain	• Avoid tertiary TCAs (amitriptyline, doxepin, imipramine)
		• FDA warning: extreme caution using desipramine if family history of sudden death, cardiac dysrhythmias
		• Side effects: sedation, dry mouth, constipation, urinary retention

TABLE 19-1   Continued

Drug Category/ Name	Indication	Adverse Effects/ Contraindications/ Precautions
Nontricyclic anti-depressants (SSRIs)—selective serotonin reuptake inhibitors (citalopram, paroxetine, fluoxetine, sertraline)	Neuropathic pain; fibromyalgia	• Efficacy not as good as TCAs; side effects: nausea, headache, insomnia, drowsiness, increased blood pressure. Gradual rather than abrupt discontinuation required
Nontricyclic anti-depressants (SNRIs)—mixed serotonin and nor-epinephrine uptake inhibitors (duloxetine; venlafaxine, desvenlafaxine)	Neuropathic pain; fibromyalgia	• Must be swallowed whole; ceiling effect • Contraindicated: hepatic or renal insufficiency • Gradual rather than abrupt discontinuation required
Anticonvulsants (carbamazepine, gabapentin, pregabalin)	Neuropathic pain; neuralgia, fibromyalgia, post-stroke pain	• Side effects: drowsiness, fatigue, dizziness, slurred speech, headache, nausea, weight gain • FDA warning: suicidal thoughts or actions
Muscle relaxants (baclofen)	Muscle spasms, neuropathic pain	• Requires slow tapering when discontinued
Hormone (calcitonin)	Bone pain, bone metastases	• Side effects—nausea, vomiting, anorexia, unusual taste
Biphosphonate	Bone metastases, bone pain	• Side effects—nausea, esophagitis, hypocalcemia
Topical Agents		
NSAIDs	Inflammatory pain	• Superior safety profile to oral formulations; adverse effects in 10–15%, rash, pruritis
Capsaicin	Diabetic neuropathy, postherpetic neuralgia, arthritic pain	• Need to apply for at least 6 weeks; side effect: local burning
Topical lidocaine (cream or patch)	Neuropathic pain; LBP, osteoarthritis post-herpetic neuralgia	• Contraindicated in liver failure • FDA warning: potentially serious hazards

there is no evidence from randomized clinical trials (RCTs) that shows that any one opioid is superior to another for initial therapy (Chou et al., 2009). Management of breakthrough pain should address the cause of the pain or precipitating factors (if possible), and lessen the impact of the pain when it occurs (Chou et al., 2009). Short-acting or rapid-onset as-needed opioids may be effective (Chou et al., 2009). A recent Cochrane review reported that oral transmucosal fentanyl citrate may be an effective treatment in the management of breakthrough pain (Zeppetella & Ribeiro, 2009).

The most common adverse effects of opioids are constipation, nausea, vomiting, sedation, and cognitive changes (Barber & Gibson, 2009). Most of the adverse effects decrease over time (with the exception of constipation), as the individual develops a tolerance for the drug. Bowel regimens for constipation include increased fluid and fiber intake, stool softeners, and laxatives (Chou et al., 2009). Nausea and vomiting tend to diminish over days or weeks, and may benefit from a number of different anti-emetic therapies, either oral or rectal forms (Chou et al., 2009). Sedation or clouded mentation tends to decrease over time; there is no evidence to recommend specific pharmacological strategies to reduce opioid-related sedation (Chou et al., 2009). Pruritis (itching) and myoclonus (muscle contractions) are also common side effects (Chou et al., 2009). Respiratory depression may occur if the doses are too high initially, are titrated up too quickly, or are combined with other drugs that have this adverse effect (Chou et al., 2009). Although many clinicians and family members fear development of addiction to opioids, older age is significantly associated with low risk for opioid misuse and abuse (AGS Panel, 2009). Underuse of opioids in the older person may be a more serious problem, due to fears of addiction, costs, constipation, and social stigma (AGS Panel, 2009). It is interesting to note that ongoing use of opioids in treating persistent pain in the elderly may involve a lower level of life-threatening risk than that of NSAIDs (Barber & Gibson, 2009).

Tramadol is an effective analgesic for relief of moderate to severe pain. Kean et al. (2008) see a role for minor narcotic-like agents such as Tramadol, either as a primary analgesic or as a supplement to traditional NSAIDs. Tramadol does not suppress respiratory function, has a low incidence of cardiac depression, causes significantly less dizziness and drowsiness than morphine, and presents significantly less risk of drug abuse and addiction (Kean et al., 2008). The pharmacokinetic properties of Tramadol do not differ in older compared to younger adults, so it can be used safely in older patients who may be at increased risk from serious adverse effects of NSAIDs and opioids (Kean et al., 2008). The recent availability of sustained-release or long-acting formulations enable more consistent blood levels of the drug and its active metabolite, and a prolonged dosage interval. Side effects include drowsiness, dizziness, vertigo, fatigue, and headache. Doses should be reduced if renal insufficiency is present. Tramadol lowers the threshold for seizures, so it should not be used in individuals who have seizure disorders or are at risk for seizures (Barber & Gibson, 2009). Pentazocine (neuropsychiatric), pethidine (seizure), dextropropoxyphene (neural and cardiac), meperidine (toxic metabolites) and methadone (long half-life) are not recommended for use in older persons (Barber & Gibson, 2009).

Adjuvants: Adjuvant drugs may be used alone or in combination with nonopioid or opioid analgesics for the management of pain. The AGS panel (2009) guideline states that all patients with neuropathic pain are candidates for adjuvant analgesics. Tricyclic antidepressants (TCAs) provide a moderate level of pain relief for one of three persons with neuropathic pain (Barber & Gibson, 2009; Saarto & Wiffin, 2009) However, tertiary tricyclic antidepressants (amitriptyline, imipramine, doxepin) should be avoided because of their higher risk for adverse effects, especially anticholinergic effects and cognitive impairment (AGS Panel, 2009). The preferred TCA for use in older persons is nortriptylline (Barber & Gibson, 2009). Mixed serotonin and norepinephrine-uptake inhibitors (SNRIs) (duloxetine) are effective for various neuropathic pain conditions and fibromyalgia (AGS Panel, 2009). A second-generation SSRI (selective serotonin-reuptake inhibitor), venlafaxine, was also effective against neuropathic pain (Saarto & Wiffin, 2009). SSRIs are generally better tolerated by patients (Saarto & Wiffin, 2009).

The anticonvulsant drugs carbamazepine, gabapentin and pregabalin have beneficial effects in various neuropathic pain conditions and more benign side effects profiles than the older anticonvulsants (AGS Panel, 2009; Barber & Gibson, 2009; Wiffin, Collins et al., 2009; Wiffin, McQuay, Rees, & Moore, 2009). A recent Cochrane review, however, recommended withholding anticonvulsants until other interventions have been tried (except in the case of trigeminal neuralgia) (Wiffin , McQuay, & Moore, 2009). Pregabalin was found to have the most benefit when used for postherpetic neuralgia and painful diabetic neuropathy, but was not helpful in fibromyalgia (Moore, Straube, Wiffin, Derry, & McQuay, 2009). Carbamazepine had little effect in post-stroke syndrome pain (Wiffin, Collins et al., 2009). The evidence also suggests that gabapentin is not superior to carbamazepine (Wiffin, Collins et al., 2009).

Baclofen, a muscle relaxant, serves as a second-line drug for paroxysmal neuropathic pain, severe spasticity, demyelinating conditions, and other neuromuscular disorders. Possible side effects are dizziness, somnolence, and GI symptoms. Baclofen requires a slow tapering period when it is discontinued (AGS Panel, 2009). Calcitonin is a hormone that may be helpful in bone pain, post osteoporotic vertebral compression fractures and pelvic fractures, and bone metastases of cancer, and is a second-line treatment for some neuropathic conditions (AGS Panel, 2009). Patients should be monitored for nausea, vomiting, anorexia, unusual taste sensation, and altered blood levels of calcium and phosphorus (AGS Panel, 2009). Biphosphonates may be helpful in patients with metastatic cancer and multiple myeloma. A recent Cochrane review concluded that there is evidence to support the effectiveness of biphosphonates in providing some pain relief from bone metastases, and they should be considered where analgesics and/or radiotherapy are inadequate (Wong & Wiffin, 2009). Side effects are nausea, esophagitis, and occasional hypocalcemia (AGS Panel, 2009).

All adjuvant drugs should be started at the lowest therapeutic dose possible and carefully titrated up and monitored for effectiveness and adverse reactions (AGS Panel, 2009). Some agents have a delayed onset of action; for example, gabapentin may take 2 to 3 weeks to demonstrate effectiveness (AGS Panel, 2009), so it should not be discontinued prematurely.

Topical Agents: Topical NSAIDs (diclofenac and salicylate derivatives) may be a safe and effective short-term alternative (AGS Panel, 2009) for some individuals. Two diclofenac topical preparations have received FDA approval for pain management. A recent study (Underwood et al., 2008) compared the use of oral NSAIDs for chronic knee pain in the elderly with the application of topical NSAIDs. Oral NSAIDs produced more adverse (minor) effects than topical NSAIDs. Some subjects with more widespread or severe pain, however, preferred the oral route. Topical lidocaine in the form of a 5% patch may be effective for postherpetic neuralgia, although it is not as good as oral gabapentin or tricyclic antidepressants. It is easy to use, nontoxic, and has few drug interactions (AGS Panel, 2009). Topical lidocaine is most appropriate for localized neuropathic or non-neuropathic pain (AGS Panel, 2009). It is contraindicated in advanced liver failure. Topical capsaicin cream may be applied repeatedly in low-dose form (.075%) or as a single application of a high-dose (8%) patch. It may provide a degree of pain relief to some patients with painful neuropathic conditions (Derry, Lloyd, Moore, & McQuay, 2009), as well as arthritis and herpes zoster. However, 30% of patients cannot tolerate the burning sensation, which may last for several months. Newer formulations are appearing that contain agents to help reduce the burning sensation (AGS Panel, 2009).

Nonpharmacological Interventions for Pain Management

The plan of care for all older individuals should include nonpharmacological strategies for managing the pain. Behavioral treatments may also improve mood, anxiety, functioning, and quality of life, and may decrease the need for analgesic medication (Norelli & Harju, 2008). It is important to explore the individual's attitudes and beliefs, preferences, and experiences with the various nonpharmacological strategies. Some therapies, such as cognitive-behavioral strategies, may not be appropriate for persons with cognitive impairments. Physical strategies such as use of heat and cold are generally safe and effective but must be monitored carefully. Lunde, Nordhus, and Pallesen (2009) conducted a meta-analysis of cognitive and behavioral interventions for chronic pain in older adults (over 60), with a focus on treatment effectiveness. The results indicated that cognitive and behavioral interventions were effective based on self-reported pain, but did not improve depressive symptoms, physical functioning, or medication use. Reid et al. (2008) conducted a review of self-management (SM) strategies (yoga, massage, tai chi, and music) to reduce pain among older adults in community settings. The results suggested that a broad range of SM programs may provide benefits for adults with chronic pain, but that more research is required to establish the efficacy of the programs in diverse age and ethnic groups.

Morone and Greco (2007) conducted a structured review of eight mind-body interventions (biofeedback, progressive muscle relaxation, meditation, guided imagery, hypnosis, tai chi, qi gong, and yoga) for older adults with chronic nonmalignant pain. The authors concluded that the eight interventions were feasible in the older population but often required modifications tailored for older adults. There was not sufficient evidence to conclude that these interventions reduced chronic nonmalignant pain. A recent clinical trial (von Trott, Wiedemann, Reishauer, Willich, & Witt, 2009) compared qi gong or exercise therapy (24 sessions each) to a waiting list control group. There was no difference in average neck pain level, neck pain and disability, or quality of life (SF-36) after 3 and 6 months.

Norelli and Harju (2008) reviewed the evidence for some of the behavioral approaches used to address pain management in older adults. Biofeedback resulted in significant decreases in pain measures for headache; progressive muscle relaxation led to greater pain reduction and improved sleep in older adults experiencing diverse chronic conditions; mindfulness meditation improved pain and mood and reduced stress in other studies. Touch therapies (healing touch, therapeutic touch, Reiki) may also have a modest effect on pain relief (So, Jiang, & Qin, 2009). However, the evidence is inconclusive regarding whether transcutaneous electro-stimulation (TENS) therapy is effective for cancer pain in adults (So, Jiang, & Qin, 2009). Rutjes et al. (2009) also could not confirm that TENS is effective for pain relief for osteoarthritis of the knee.

Conclusion

Persistent pain is a frequently occurring problem in older adults. The general plan of care includes a comprehensive assessment, pharmacological interventions, nonpharmacological interventions, and reassessment for effectiveness and adverse effects. Although NSAIDs have long been a component of the pharmacological management of inflammatory pain in older adults, recent clinical practice guidelines recommend their use in only rare instances. Acetaminophen, and carefully selected opioids and adjuvant drugs, are the preferred alternatives, although there are dissenting opinions expressed in the literature. Nonpharmacological interventions are an important component of the pain plan of care. However, more and larger studies need to be conducted to more firmly establish their individual effectiveness for reducing pain in older adults.

References

American Geriatrics Society. (2002). The management of persistent pain in older persons. *Journal of American Geriatrics Society, 50*, S205–S224.

American Geriatrics Society Panel on Pharmacologic Management of Persistent Pain in Older Persons. (2009). Pharmacologic management of persistent pain in older persons. *Journal of American Geriatrics Society, 57*, 1331–1346.

Barber, J.B., & Gibson, S.J. (2009). Treatment of chronic non-malignant pain in the elderly. Safety considerations. *Drug Safety, 32*, 457–474.

Bjoro, K., & Herr, K. (2008). Assessment of pain in the nonverbal or cognitively impaired older adult. *Clinics in Geriatric Medicine, 24*, 237–262.

Charette, S.L., & Ferrell, B.A. (2007). Rheumatic diseases in the elderly: Assessing chronic pain. *Rheumatic Disease Clinics of North America, 33*, 109–122.

Chou, R., Fanciullo, G.J., Fine, P.G., Adler, J.A., Ballantyne, J.C., Davies, P., et al. (2009). American Academy of Pain Medicine Opioids Guidelines Panel: Clinical guidelines for the use of chronic opioid therapy in chronic noncancer pain, *Journal of Pain, 10*(2), 113–130.

Derry, S., Lloyd, R., Moore, R.A., & McQuay, H.J. (2009).Topical capsaicin for chronic neuropathic pain in adults. *Cochrane Database of Systematic Reviews, 4,* #00075320-06078.

Gudmannsdottier, G.D., & Halldorsdottir, S. (2009). Primacy of existential pain and suffering in residents in chronic pain in nursing homes: A phenomenological study. *Scandinavian Journal of Caring Sciences, 23,* 317–327.

Hadjistavropoulos, T., Herr, K., Turk, D., Fine, P., Dworkin, R., & Helme, R. (2007). An interdisciplinary expert consensus statement on assessment of pain in older adults. *Clinical Journal of Pain, 23,* 1–42.

Hadjistavropoulos, T., Marchildon, G.P., Fine, P.G., Herr, K., Palley, H.A., Kaasalainen, S., & Beland, F. (2009). Transforming long-term care pain management in North America: The policy-clinical interface. *American Academy of Pain Medicine, 10,* 506–520.

Herr, K., Coyne, P., Key, T., Manworren, R., McCaffery, M, Merkel, S., et al. (2006). Pain assessment in the nonverbal patient: Position statement with clinical practice recommendations. *Pain Management Nursing, 7,* 44–52.

Herr, K.A., & Garand, L. (2001). Assessment and measurement of pain in older adults. *Clinical Geriatric Medicine, 17,* 457–478.

Horgas, A.L., & Yoon, S.L. (2008). Pain management. In E. Capezuti, D. Zwicker, M. Mezey, & T. Fulmer (Eds.), *Evidence-based geriatric nursing protocols for best practice* (3rd ed., pp. 199–222). New York: Springer Publishing Company.

Jones, K.R., Fink, R., Hutt, E., Vojir, C., Pepper, G., Scott-Cawiezell, J., & Mellis, B.K. (2005). Measuring pain intensity in nursing home residents. *Journal of Pain & Symptom Management, 30,* 519–527.

Kean, W.F., Rainsford, K.D., & Kean, I.R.L. (2008). Management of chronic musculoskeletal pain in the elderly: Opinions on oral medication use. *Inflammopharmacology, 16,* 53–75.

Lunde, L.H., Nordhus, I.H., & Pallesen, S. (2009). The effectiveness of cognitive and behavioral treatment of chronic pain in the elderly: A quantitative review. *Journal of Clinical Psychology in Medical Settings, 16,* 254–262.

McAuliffe, L., Nay, R., O'Donnell, M., & Fetherstonhaugh, D. (2009). Pain assessment in older people with dementia: Literature review. *Journal of Advanced Nursing, 65,* 2–10.

McCarthy, L.H., Bigal, M.E., Katz, M., Deby, C., & Lipton, R.B. (2009). Chronic pain and obesity in elderly people: Results from the Einstein aging study. *Journal of American Geriatrics Society, 57,* 115–119.

Moore, R.A., Straube, S., Wiffen, P.J., Derry, S., & McQuay, H.J. (2009). Pregabalin for acute and chronic pain in adults, *Cochrane Database of Systematic Reviews, 4,* 00075320-05800.

Morone, N.E., & Greco, C.M. (2007). Mind-body interventions for chronic pain in older adults: A structured review. *Pain Medicine, 8,* 359–375.

Norelli, L.J., & Harju, S.K. (2008). Behavioral approaches to pain management in the elderly. *Clinics in Geriatric Medicine, 24,* 335–344.

Reid, M.C., Papaleontiou, M., Ong, A., Breckman, R., Wethington, E., & Pillemer, K. (2008). Self-management strategies to reduce pain and improve function among older adults in community settings: A review of the evidence. *Pain Medicine, 9,* 409–424.

Rutjes, A.W.S., Nuesch, E., Sterchi, R., Kalichman, L., Hendriks, E., Osiri, M., et al. (2009). Transcutaneous electrostimulation for osteoarthritis of the knee. *Cochrane Database of Systematic Reviews, 4,* 00075320-01745.

Saarto, T., & Wiffin, P.J. (2009). Antidepressants for neuropathic pain. *Cochrane Database of Systematic Reviews, 4*, 00075320-04448.

So, P.S., Jiang, Y., & Qin, Y. (2009). Touch therapies for pain relief in adults. *Cochrane Database of Systematic Reviews, 4*, 00075320-05251.

Taylor, L.J., Harris, J., Epps, C.D., & Herr, K. (2005). Psychometric evaluation of selected pain intensity scales for use with cognitively impaired and cognitively intact older adults. *Rehabilitation Nursing, 30*, 55–61.

Taylor, L.J., & Herr, K. (2003). Pain intensity assessment: A comparison of selected pain intensity scales for use in cognitively intact and cognitively impaired African-American older adults. *Pain Management Nursing, 4*, 87–95.

Underwood, M., Ashby, D., Carnes, D., Castelnuova, E., Harding, G., Hennessy, E., et al. (2008). Topical or oral ibuprofen for chronic knee pain in older people. The TOIB study. *Health Technology Assessment, 12*(22), iii–iv, ix–155.

von Trott, P., Wiedemann, A.M., Reishauer, A., Willich, S.N., & Witt, C.M. (2009). Qigong and exercise therapy for elderly patients with chronic neck pain (QIBANE): A randomized controlled study. *Journal of Pain, 10*, 501–508.

While, C., & Jocelyn, A. (2009). Observational pain assessment scales for people with dementia: A review. *British Journal of Community Nursing, 14*, 438–442.

Wiffin, P.J., Collins, S., McQuay, H.J., Carroll, D., Jadad, A., & Moore, R.A. (2009). Anticonvulsant drugs for acute and chronic pain. *Cochrane Database of Systematic Reviews, 4*, 00075320-01128.

Wiffin, P.J., McQuay, H.J., & Moore, R.A. (2009). Carbamazepine for acute and chronic pain in adults. *Cochrane Database of Systematic Reviews, 4*, 00075320-04450.

Wiffin, P.J., McQuay, H.J., Rees, J., & Moore, R.A. (2009). Gabapentin for acute and chronic pain. *Cochrane Database of Systematic Reviews, 4*, 00075320-04451.

Wong, R.K.S., & Wiffin, P.J. (2009). Biphosphonates for the relief of pain secondary to bone metastases. *Cochrane Database of Systematic Reviews, 4*, 00075320-01585.

Zanocchi, M., Martinelli, E., Luppino, A., Gonella, M., Gariglio, F., Fissore, L., et al. (2008). Chronic pain in a sample of nursing home residents: Prevalence, characteristics, influence on quality of life (QoL). *Archives of Gerontology & Geriatrics, 47*, 121–129.

Zeppetella, G., & Ribeiro, M.D.C. (2009). Opioids for the management of breakthrough (episodic) pain in cancer patients. *Cochrane Database of Systematic Reviews, 4*, 00075320-03307.

Chapter 20

Preventing Functional Decline in Hospitalized Older Adults—An Exemplar for Nursing Education

Laura Sutton, Meredeth Rowe, and Marie P. Boltz

Case Study

Nancy Martin is an 88-year-old widowed woman who is now living in a secure dementia unit at a small long-term care facility. She was admitted to the facility 7 months earlier after her son and daughter-in-law could no longer care for her. Mrs. Martin has moderate Alzheimer's disease, diagnosed about 7 years earlier. She has moderate memory loss and still remembers most of her family by name. She recognizes facility staff, church acquaintances and friends, usually without recalling their names. She is disoriented to date, month, and year and believes she lives in an apartment rather than a long-term care facility. She is able to respond to questions with appropriate answers. Mrs. Martin is incontinent of urine, but not stool; is dependent upon a walker for ambulation; and maintains an excellent appetite. She eats independently when food is given to her but requires assistance with cutting meat and opening certain packaged foods. She needs assistance in dressing and bathing.

Functional decline accelerated dramatically during two hospitalizations prior to admission to the long-term care facility, with marked increase in the need for assistance with daily functional tasks. The need for assistance exceeded what could be provided by relative caregivers and therefore, formal care was required. Prior to the first hospitalization for pneumonia, Mrs. Martin required support for most instrumental activities of daily living (IADL) (Lawton & Brody, 1969), such as making meals, transportation, managing finances, and medication, but was independent in all other basic activities of daily living (ADL). She needed prompting to take her medicine, and sometimes to wash her hair and bathe. Her mood was pleasant, and she was generally cooperative with the daily routine. She lived in independent senior citizen housing with monitoring and assistance from her son. Following the first hospitalization, the family decided she could no longer live by herself. She was less stable when walking, weaker, and experienced significant weight loss. She moved into her son's home. She attended adult day services each weekday while her son and his wife went to work. Her high level of physical functioning made community care possible.

Unfortunately, a second hospitalization due to a fractured hip 3 months later precipitated major changes in her functional status. Even after a significant recuperation period in a rehabilitation center, she never regained the ability to complete ADL (dressing, toileting, bathing) independently nor to walk without a walker. Thus, risk for falling became very acute because she would try to walk without the walker or refuse assistance from others. She developed urinary incontinence and became more aggressive with certain caregivers. These changes were primarily due to loss of physical strength as well as a rapid decrease in cognitive status related to acute delirium with hospitalization. Thus, this level of functional decline made it necessary for her to move to a formal long-term care setting.

Overview of Functional Decline During Hospitalization

The number of older adults is increasing, not only in the United States but throughout the world. Consequently, the number of older adults admitted to hospitals with a variety of acute illnesses and exacerbations of chronic illnesses will also increase, as will the number of those over 65 living in the community (Brummel-Smith & Gunderson, 2007).

Reasons for hospitalization in older adults include exacerbation of an already existing health problem, onset of new acute illness, or an event such as a fall-related injury. One of the complications of hospitalization is decline in functional status. Early studies found that functional decline from admission baseline may occur as early as 1 to 2 days after hospitalization. With or without functional impairment prior to hospitalization (Fortinsky, Covinsky, Palmer, & Landefeld, 1999), as many as 20% to 40% of older adults may experience a significant decline in functional ability resulting from even relatively short hospital stays (Landefeld, Palmer, Kresevic, Fortinsky, & Kowal, 1995). This decline can lead to permanent functional disability, increased risk of rehospitalization, less independence, and even admission into assisted-living, long-term care facilities, or in more severe cases, death (Wakefield & Holman, 2007). Decreased functional status also contributes to increased hospital length of stay and healthcare costs (Counsell et al., 2000). Thus, change of functional status in older adults is important in determining prognosis during hospitalization through postdischarge. It is crucial to develop and implement strategies that prevent decline and maintain functional abilities of older adults to ensure that negative outcomes are prevented and home placement is preserved.

This chapter examines the contributing factors, assessment, and prevention of functional decline in hospitalized older adult using a case study exemplar. It also suggests collaborative educational strategies for undergraduate and graduate nursing students. Together, these strategies can facilitate the provision of excellent care to hospitalized older adults, and specifically, care aimed at the prevention of functional decline during the hospital stay.

Causes of Functional Decline in Older Adults Before and During Hospitalization

From a broader perspective, functional status is determined by physiological, environmental, and social variables such as physical mobility, nutrition, cognitive status, depression, illness, and social interactions or support (Kresevic, 2008; Wakefield & Holman, 2007). These variables affect whether one can care for his/her own bathing, eating, toileting, rest activities, medication management, and other activities that help to determine independence.

There are many reasons why older adults may experience functional decline, either at home or in long-term or acutecare settings. Some of the primary reasons for decline are impaired cognitive status, decreased nutritional status due to decreased appetite and intake, impaired mobility, and inadequate pain control (Arora et al., 2009). Other risk factors may include advanced age, poor vision and hearing, incontinence, skin breakdown, and polypharmacy (Fletcher, 2005; McCusker, Kakuma, & Abrahamowicz, 2002). The variables discussed here are important since nursing interventions can be directed toward their prevention or treatment during the hospital stay.

Delirium or Impaired Cognition

Delirium in older adults may be caused by changes in environment, polypharmacy, dehydration, pain, immobility, sensory loss, hypoxia, and nosocomial infections such as pneumonia and urinary tract infections (Fick & Mion, 2008). It is estimated that delirium superimposed upon dementia may occur in 89% of hospitalized patients (Fick, Agostini, & Inouye, 2002). Delirium may lead to a variety of symptoms, such as increased confusion, lethargy, aggression, and even hallucinations (Boustani & Buttar, 2007). These symptoms may lead nursing staff to restrict the older adults' activities in order to prevent injuries such as falls, or the older adult with delirium may get out of bed unattended and fall.

As a result, delirium superimposed upon dementia or cognitive impairment may compound functional disability (Brummel-Smith & Gunderson, 2007; Salvi et al., 2008). Sands et al. (2003) found that older adults with cognitive deficits such as dementia at hospital admission were less likely than those without cognitive deficits to recover prehospitalization ability to perform ADLs, even 3 months after discharge. They were also more likely to be admitted to long-term facilities after discharge. The findings suggested that cognitive functioning alone was predictive of postdischarge functional status.

Decreased Nutritional Status

Malnutrition or poor nutritional status may also contribute to functional decline of older adults (Salvi et al., 2008). Inadequate food intake may also be associated with depression, dementia, pain, and social interaction, all of which may contribute to decreased functional performance. It can result in decreased muscle mass, decreased strength and power, and a subsequent loss of balance and activity (Haber, 2004). In a descriptive study that examined outcomes of 259 older adults who were either malnourished (18.5%) or at nutritional risk (81.5%) at admission to acute care, researchers found a significant difference in functional ability between those at risk and those classified as malnourished (Feldblum et al., 2007). The study concluded that low food consumption, lower cognitive functioning, and increased depression contributed to malnourishment in older adults.

Impaired Mobility

Older adults are especially vulnerable to functional decline because of age-related changes in cardiovascular and musculoskeletal systems (Graf, 2006; 2008). These changes include decreased musculoskeletal mass, balance, cardiac output, and aerobic capacity. Increased incidence of chronic disease, disability, and pain are also associated with aging.

Activity restrictions during hospitalization due to illness, surgery, and acute pain contribute to even more muscle weakness and deconditioning, decreased bone mass, and orthostatic hypotension. Decreased ambulation, often due to illness, inadequate staffing, or staff's lack of awareness of the need for mobility, plays a major role in the rapid advance of functional decline. For example, in a study of 118 hospitalized older adults 55 and older, researchers observed that hospitalized older adults walked very little in the hall during a 3-hour period (median time 5.5 minutes), even those perceived by nurses as able to walk alone (Callen, Mahoney, Grieves, Wells, & Enloe, 2004).

Inadequate Pain Control

Studies show that older adults have many pain-related acute and chronic conditions that interfere with physical and functional activities (Thomas, Mottram, Peal, Wilkie, & Croft, 2007). In any population, acute or persistent pain limits activity and range of motion; but especially for older adults, persistent or chronic pain is extremely common, affecting as many as 50% of community dwellers and 80% of nursing home residents (American Geriatrics Society Panel on Persistent Pain in Older Persons [AGS], 2002; Potter & Titman, 2007). Chronic conditions such as arthritis, osteoporosis of the spine, joint disorders, and peripheral vascular disease lead to depression, decreased socialization, sleep disturbances, impaired ambulation, and increased medication use. Furthermore, lack of clinician knowledge about pain assessment and management in older adults often leads to ineffective pain management strategies (Blyth et al., 2008). Ineffective pain management further contributes to deconditioning, malnutrition, falls, muscle pain, and even increased mortality and morbidity in the older adult population (Potter & Titman, 2007).

Thus, the constellation of problems contributing to decreased functional status during and after hospitalization is complex. Lack of awareness of risk factors by interdisciplinary healthcare providers and lack of interventions to prevent functional decline also contribute to immediate and long-term negative outcomes.

> Several factors were associated with Mrs. Martin's functional decline. First was the onset of delirium during the first hospitalization, which resulted in increased confusion and frequent attempts to exit the bed over the elevated side rails for toileting needs. The delirium was exacerbated by strategies used to control her agitation, including benzodiazepines and restraints, and a urinary catheter to control her incontinence. Additionally, her hearing aids were rarely offered or worn, adding to confusion and the appearance of not being oriented. She remained in bed for most of the hospital stay, which contributed to rapidly diminished muscle strength and overall deconditioning. In the second hospitalization, she verbalized significant hip pain after surgery for her fracture, but opiate analgesia was withheld and nonopioid analgesics were not administered. Staff feared she would become even more confused if the analgesics were given.
>
> At the time of discharge, increased cognitive impairment and decline in functional status led the hospitalist physician and caseworker to recommend that Mrs. Martin be placed in formal long-term care. She was unable to recover her prehospital level of function, and long-term care placement was made permanent.

Prevention Strategies for Decreased Functional Decline in Hospitalized Older Adults

Strategies to decrease the incidence of delirium and to improve nutrition and mobility are integrated into the care plan for prevention of functional decline. Interdisciplinary collaboration and communication, assessment, interdisciplinary interventions such as ambulating, monitoring medications, toileting schedules, improved education and communication with the older adult and family, limited use of restraints, and removal of urinary catheters and adaptive equipment may improve or even prevent functional decline (Counsell et al., 2000; Kresevic, 2008).

Some study findings even suggest that functional decline in acute illness may be reversed (Sager & Rudberg, 1998; Sager et al., 1996). Community and home-based interventions to improve functional status after discharge may be more effective when patients at high risk are targeted during hospitalization rather than more broadly applied interventions (McCusker, Bellavance, Cardin, Belzile, & Verdon, 2000).

Collaboration and Communication

In today's healthcare settings, an interdisciplinary approach is essential to monitor and intervene for the variety of psychosocial, cognitive, physical, and functional disabilities that occur in older adults (Fernandez, Callahan, Likourezos, & Leipzig, 2008), and communication is key to an effective interdisciplinary approach. Identification of the roles of family, friends, nurses, APNs, physical therapists, occupational therapists, students, and other members of the care team is essential in improving patient function (Covinsky et al., 1998; Kresevic & Holder, 1998). Assessment findings, goals, interventions, and a realistic trajectory of outcomes are discussed with the older adult and family/caregivers for achieving the best functional outcomes.

Education of the older adult and family/caregivers about the importance of activity and independent functioning also helps to improve participation and enhances functional independence (Graf, 2006; Kresevic, 2008). Older adults and their families need to understand the importance of proper exercise, socialization, mentally challenging activities, pain management, adherence to medications, potential side effects, and adequate nutrition (Kresevic, 2008).

Assessment

Multidisciplinary and multidimensional assessment, with age-appropriate interventions, may be the most important determinants for improving functional status and preventing functional decline in older adults regardless of setting (Counsell et al., 2000; Sennour, Counsell, Jones, & Weiner, 2009). Continual assessment of functional status for changes and modifications to the plan of care reveal the older adult's ability to be independent or to need help from family and others. Although functional decline may occur prior to and during hospitalization, functional assessment provides a systematic way to identify strengths and weaknesses of the older adult and to develop strategies for improved functional outcomes across acute care and community settings (Covinsky et al., 2003; Kleinpell, 2007; Wakefield & Holman, 2007).

Therefore, a change in functional status prior to and during hospitalization is an important indicator in older adults and may accompany acute or chronic illness or disability (Ham, Sloane, Warshaw, Bernard, & Flaherty, 2007). Functional assessment should be included in routine admission and daily assessments, as should history, physical, and diagnostic assessments (Kane & Thomas, 2000). It is also important to determine pre-admission functional status in order to have a baseline with which to compare changes related to hospitalization and to develop strategies to improve functional status before discharge. It is critical for determining goals of treatment, which, at minimum, should aim to restore baseline functional status before discharge (Wakefield & Holman, 2007).

Routine assessment should thus include an evaluation of the risk for functional decline upon admission to the hospital (Kresevic, 2008) and a comprehensive assessment of the patient's ability to perform ADLs and IADLs. It includes capacity to ambulate independently or with assistance, consideration of sensory and cognitive skills required for ambulation (Campbell, Seymour, & Primrose, 2004; Freedman, Martin, & Schoeni, 2002), and what resources are needed to ambulate. Comprehensive assessment may also include associated risk factors, such as nutritional and fluid status; diminished cognitive status; activity and physical therapy orders; effects of pain and pain-related medications; effects of other medications on mobility/IADLs/ADLs; social interactions and cognition; and the impact of the physical environment on enhancing or hindering independent function. An excellent resource for functional status assessment may be accessed at http://www.ConsultGeriRN.org (Hartford Institute for Geriatric Nursing, 2008). Table 20-1 provides a list of some well-established tools used for functional assessment.

TABLE 20-1　Common Tools to Measure Functional Status

Measurement Tool	Author	Functions Measured
Barthel Index of Activities of Daily Living (Barthel IADLs)	(Mahoney & Barthel, 1965)	ADLs of physical functioning: bathing, grooming, continence, stair-climbing, and ability to propel a wheelchair
Confusion Assessment Method (CAM)	(Inouye et al., 1990)	Delirium: acute onset and fluctuating course, inattention, disorganized thinking, and altered level of consciousness
Cornell Scale	(Alexopoulos, Abrams, Young, & Shamoian, 1988)	Depression in probable dementia and non-dementia patients. Uses agitation/psychosis, disruption in rhythms, and negative symptoms such as weight loss and loss of interest
Geriatric Depression Scale (GDS)	(Sheikh & Yesavage, 1986)	Depression in mentally ill, mild or moderate cognitive impairment
Get-Up-and-Go test	(Mathias, Nayak, & Isaacs, 1986)	Balance during sitting and standing; gait steadiness

(continues)

TABLE 20-1   (Continued)

Measurement Tool	Author	Functions Measured
Hospital Admission Risk Profile (HARP)	(Sager et al., 1996)	Uses age, cognitive function, and IADL function prior to admission to determine risk for developing functional decline when hospitalized
Katz Activity of Daily Living Scale (Katz ADL)	(Katz, Down, Cash, & Grotz, 1970)	ADLs: bathing, dressing, eating, toileting, hygiene, transferring
Lawton Instrumental Activities of Daily Living (IADL)	(Lawton & Brody, 1969)	Ability to use telephone, shopping, food preparation, laundry, mode of transportation, responsibility for own medications, housekeeping, ability to handle finances
Mini-Cognitive Assessment (Mini-Cog)	(Borson, Scanlan, Brush, Vitaliano, & Dokmak, 2000)	Routine screening for cognitive impairment
Mini-Mental State Examination (MMSE)	(Folstein, Folstein, & McHugh, 1975)	Orientation, attention, memory, concentration, language, constructional ability
Mini-Nutritional Assessment (MNA)	(Guigoz, Lauque, & Vellas, 2002)	Presence of risk factors for malnutrition in older adults

Questions to Consider: Assessment

1. What is the role of the adult or geriatric advanced practice nurse in the assessment of Mrs. Martin's functional status? What other healthcare providers would be included in her care?

2. What assessment variables are included in the undergraduate student's nursing care plan?

3. What preadmission variables made Mrs. Martin at increased risk for functional decline during hospitalization?

4. Which assessment tools are helpful in determining Mrs. Martin's functional status? Why?

5. What diagnostic tests should be ordered at hospital admission and post discharge?

Decrease Incidence of Delirium

Interacting with the environment through sensory stimulation and activity may improve cognitive function (Fick & Mion, 2008). Hearing aids and eyeglasses are important for orientation, along with monitoring older adult patients' responses to constant noise, light, and multiple healthcare providers asking questions. Monitoring the number and effects of multiple medications, including sedatives, hyponotics, and opioids, is also imperative. These may increase agitation or induce hallucination and disorientation. Currently, the typical response to agitation is often increased pharmacological intervention and/or physical restraints, which decrease mobility and have the potential to create even more disorientation (Cotter, 2005; Fick & Mion, 2008).

Improve Mobility

Interventions that promote mobility, increase endurance, and minimize bed rest should be a standard of care for hospitalized older adults (Fick & Mion, 2008; Kleinpell, 2007). Physical activity should be alternated with rest periods. Graf (2006) suggests an interdisciplinary collaborative activity plan that improves patient activity levels. Early referral to physical and possibly occupational therapy, and frequent ambulation (with or without assistive aids, depending on assessment) helps to minimize muscle deconditioning.

Following discharge, outpatient rehabilitation in the home requires client and family education and commitment to an exercise routine in order to continue muscle strengthening. This is especially difficult when the client has cognitive deficits. Education that includes not only the exercises, but also the reason for continued exercise is essential because Medicare, private insurance, or Medicaid reimbursement is time-limited (Murer, 2006). Prior to any activity, assessment for pain and interventions such as medications to reduce pain will enhance activity (Covinsky et al., 1998).

Improve Nutritional Status

Activity associated with mealtime may encourage patients to eat more than when in bed or when alone (Graf, 2006). Sitting in a chair or going to a dining room not only gets older adults out of bed to eat, but also increases mobility, prevents associated complications from immobility such as skin breakdown, and increases the older adult's socialization and food intake.

Aggressive nutritional support not only improves nutritional status but also may increase functional status (Wells & Dumbrell, 2006). Nutritionists or dieticians are an important part of the interdisciplinary team. Modifying meals to smaller amounts at more frequent intervals may make it easier for older adults to ingest and digest foods. Foods with higher levels of spices or strong tastes may not be tolerated well. However, mild spices may enhance flavor and food intake when salt is restricted. Good oral and dental care is also imperative for sufficient food intake for optimum nutrition.

In addition to nutritional supplements, Ham and colleagues (Ham et al., 2007) suggest use of the Modified Food Pyramid for Mature Adults (70 or older) (Tufts University, 2002). This strategy recommends eight, 8-ounce glasses of water, additional vitamin supplements (calcium, vitamin D, and vitamin B_{12}), increased complex carbohydrate and decreased refined carbohydrates, decreased amounts of proteins with saturated and partially hydrogenated fats, and increased monounsaturated and polyunsaturated omega-3 fats. Examples of these foods include fish, beans, nuts, and vegetable oils, with less red meat, butter, and refined carbohydrates such as sweets.

Questions to Consider: Prevention Strategies

1. What communication strategies between staff and family could be used to improve continuity of care?

2. What strategies might the geriatric nurse practitioner and APN graduate and undergraduate nursing students suggest to prevent delirium, falls, and functional decline?

3. What might the geriatric nurse practitioner order to prevent deconditioning?

4. Consider which medications might increase delirium during hospitalization. What alternatives might be ordered to decrease this risk?

Collaborative Educational Nursing Strategies

Several educational strategies may enhance the functional status of older adults in acute care and in the community. They are based on a collaborative model in which undergraduate and graduate advanced practice (APN) nursing students collaborate in the classroom, in seminars, and in clinical settings to assess the functional status of older adults and to plan and implement interventions that prevent or reduce functional decline.

Case Studies

At the beginning of their respective didactic courses, faculty provide both undergraduate and graduate APN nursing students with the same exemplar case study. Course content is coordinated between graduate and undergraduate courses so topics are similar each week. Course objectives, however, are based on students' educational level. Each week, faculty provides the students with additional information about the older adult and his/her family and environment. Students then discuss the assessment data and plan of care. For example, in the case study used in this chapter, Mrs. Martin fell and broke her hip. The students discuss prevention strategies for falls. The undergraduate student focuses on environmental issues, the need for toileting, and Mrs. Martin's ability to ambulate safely by herself. The graduate student focuses on medication orders and side effects, diagnostic tests for fractures and treatment.

Seminars

Students and undergraduate/graduate faculty may meet weekly or biweekly to discuss the case study presented in class. The purpose of the seminar is to explore options for effective assessment and plan of care for the older adult in the case study. This discussion between graduate and undergraduate nursing students provides insight into the levels of nursing practice and the different roles of nursing. The graduate class includes adult and geriatric nurse practitioner students and adult and geriatric clinical nurse specialists. In addition, clinical leader graduate students may be included to provide a unit-based generalist perspective regarding the implementation of care.

Clinical Interdisciplinary Rounds

Each week both undergraduate and graduate students participate together in interdisciplinary rounds focusing on older adults. Together, they discuss the nursing practice plan of care from levels of practice and its contribution to the interdisciplinary plan of care. This could be done in weekly post conference seminars or at the time of the rounds.

Case Study Exemplar—Clinical Practice and Education Implementation

The following baseline vulnerabilities predisposed Mrs. Martin to functional decline during hospitalization: advanced age, dementia, baseline functional impairment, pain, and sensory (hearing) impairment. Additionally, acute illness (pneumonia) associated with delirium contributed to her functional loss. The following iatrogenic care practices exacerbated impairment: bed rest, lack of exercise and a toileting plan, the use of benzodiazepines, inaccessible hearing aids, inadequate pain assessment and management, use of physical restraints, not engaging the family in care planning and provision, and use of a Foley catheter.

The cornerstone of care aimed at preventing functional decline is diligent and continuing comprehensive assessment of functional status. The geriatric nurse practitioner (GNP) worked with the primary nurse and nursing students to assess the baseline cognitive and physical function of the patient. First, they asked the family if Mrs. Martin had "severe memory problems" and/or was diagnosed as having dementia or Alzheimer's disease (AD). Mrs. Martin's son responded that she had been diagnosed 7 years earlier with AD; but he also asserted that despite her dementia, Mrs. Martin was typically able to communicate her basic needs and follow simple requests. He described changes in mental status ("more confused") and occasional "sleepiness" alternating with periods of being "hyper" that began in the last 12 hours. The APN student conducted the Mini-Cog screening (Borson, Scanlan, Brush, Vitaliano, & Dokmak, 2000), which demonstrated cognitive impairment. Mrs. Martin was able to recall only one of three words and failed the clock drawing test. The nurse then used the Confusion Assessment Method (CAM) (Inouye et al., 1990) to confirm the presence of delirium.

The patient's functional status was assessed with the Barthel Instrumental Activities of Daily Living tool (Barthel IADL) (Mahoney & Barthel, 1965) and the Katz Index (Katz, Down, Cash, & Grotz, 1970). The nurse also interviewed the family, inquiring about baseline functional status (status two weeks prior to admission) and the patient's current functional status. Together, the primary nurse and the APN student noted that IADL was significantly impaired (dependent in all aspects). ADL status had declined dramatically over the past 48 hours, in which Mrs. Martin had developed new onset of urinary incontinence, demonstrated difficulty getting dressed and bathed, and required one-person assistance for unsteady gait. Mrs. Martin did demonstrate good range of motion, good motor strength, and ability to follow one-step commands with physical cueing.

During the interdisciplinary rounds, the primary nurse, the GNP, the APN, and undergraduate students discussed assessment findings. The goals for Mrs. Martin's care were to address her need for safety and prevent the complications of delirium, including functional decline, falls, nutritional problems, infection, and skin breakdown. The GNP and APN graduate student collaborated with the hospitalist to evaluate the following studies to determine the etiology of delirium: urinalysis, complete blood count (CBC) with differential count, B12 and folate levels, thyroid function test, full chemistry panel including serum albumin and prealbumin (PAB), and a chest X-ray. The chemistry panel revealed elevated blood urea nitrogen (BUN) and the chest X-ray indicated pneumonia. Other diagnostics were negative. An intravenous infusion was begun for hydration as well as administration of IV antibiotics. Oxygen administered via nasal cannula addressed the low O2 saturation. The GNP determined that the Cornell Scale (Alexopoulos, Abrams, Young, & Shamoian, 1988) was negative for depression.

Together, the primary nurse collaborated with the GNP to develop the initial plan and discussed it with the undergraduate students in seminar. The plan was reviewed with the interdisciplinary team during rounds:

- *Prevention of functional decline:* The interdisciplinary plan of care consisted of physical/occupational therapy consult, walking the patient to the toilet before and after meals (not leaving unattended in the bathroom), logging incontinence episodes to create an individualized toileting program, assisting Mrs. Martin out of bed three times a day to include meals, and ambulation per the physical therapist recommendation. Meals were to be provided when she was up in the chair. During breakfast, the nursing assistant planned to remain with her, cueing her to eat and drink. The nurse secured a volunteer to sit with the patient when she was up in the chair at lunchtime. Her son and daughter-in-law planned to visit at dinner time and help her to eat.

- *Fall/fall-related injury prevention:* Safety interventions included a room close to the nurse's station, safety checks conducted every 15 minutes, a sensor alarm on the bed, and an adjustable-height bed in the lowest position. These interventions to prevent functional decline and to address urinary incontinence were considered integral components of the fall prevention program. Mrs. Martin also received nonskid socks to wear when she was out of bed.

- *Prevention of nutritional compromise:* The plan of care included monitoring intake (food and fluid) and securing a nutritionist consult.

- *Prevention of skin breakdown:* A pressure-relieving mattress, daily skin assessments, and the plan for nutrition (previously described) were instituted.

- *Correct delirium:* In addition to the medical workup to prevent delirium, Mrs. Martin was provided the following preventive/corrective interventions: hearing aid and assess preference for hearing amplifier; monitor for nonverbal expressions of pain; and implementation of plan to prevent functional decline and prevent falls/fall-related injury and nutritional problems. Additionally, physical and chemical restraints were to be avoided. A very low dose of Haldol was prescribed for the first 24 hours. The IV site was camouflaged with cling wrap and covered with Mrs. Martin's sweater. The family was encouraged to bring in familiar objects from home, including her blanket and photos, and to inform staff about how to best address Mrs. Martin and how to provide sources of comfort for her, including spiritual music.

- *Family education:* Written instructions were reviewed and included manifestations of delirium, symptoms to report, and Mrs. Martin's plan of care.

The nutritionist assessed Mrs. Martin using the Mini-Nutritional Assessment tool (MNA) (Guigoz, Lauque, & Vellas, 2002); Mrs. Martin's nutritional laboratory values, her basal metabolic index (BMI), and other parameters were within normal range. She recommended a soft diet for Mrs. Martin, and a snack was provided (according to her son, her preference was a ½ cheese sandwich or vanilla yogurt) when she ate less than 50% of her meal. Within 24 hours of admission to the floor, Mrs. Martin's IV was discontinued. The physical therapist recommended ambulation in the hall 100 feet, three times a day, starting on Day 2, progressing to 200 feet, three times a day on Day 3. This recommendation was implemented. The incontinence log was reviewed and her toileting plan was adjusted to include toileting at 7:00 A.M. if awake, before and after meals, and at bedtime.

Mrs. Martin was discharged home on Day 4. At the day of discharge she was experiencing occasional incontinence, was able to ambulate 200 feet with minimal assistance, and was able to respond to two-step verbal commands and three-step commands with cueing. A referral was made to a skilled nursing facility to monitor her pulmonary status, cognitive status, and functional status. Additionally, physical therapy and a home health aide were prescribed as well as a medical social worker to explore adult day care options and return to home.

Summary

Obviously, some older adults, especially those with cognitive deficits, are at greater risk for the negative effects of hospitalization. With the interventions and educational strategies discussed in this chapter, the most vulnerable may be able to avoid or minimize the devastating functional decline that is now associated with the hospitalization of older adults. An individualized interdisciplinary-based plan of care such as the one described in this exemplar should be designed and implemented for every older adult and his/her family upon admission to acute care settings. The outcome of this plan can result in improved quality of life for older adults and their families.

References

Alexopoulos, G., Abrams, R., Young, R., & Shamoian, C. (1988). Cornell scale for depression in dementia. *Biological Psychiatry, 23*(3), 271–284.

American Geriatrics Society Panel on Persistent Pain in Older Persons. (2002). The management of persistent pain in older persons. *Journal of the American Geriatrics Society, 50*, S205–S224.

Arora, V., Plein, C., Chen, S., Siddique, J., Sachs, G., & Meltzer, D. (2009). Relationship between quality of care and functional decline in hospitalized vulnerable elders. *Medical Care, 47*(8), 895–901.

Blyth, F., Rochat, S., Cumming, R., Creasey, H., Handelsman, D., Le Couteur, D., et al. (2008). Pain, frailty and comorbidity in older men: The CHAMP study. *Pain, 140*(1), 224–230.

Borson, S., Scanlan, J., Brush, M., Vitaliano, P., & Dokmak, A. (2000). The mini-cog: A cognitive 'vital signs' measure for dementia screening in multi-lingual elderly. *International Journal of Geriatric Psychiatry, 15*(11), 1021–1027.

Boustani, M., & Buttar, A. (2007). Delirium. In R. Ham, P.D. Sloane, G. A. Warshaw, M.A. Bernard, & E. Flaherty (Eds.), *Primary care geriatrics: A case-based approach* (5th ed., pp. 210–218). New York, NY: Mosby-Elsevier.

Brummel-Smith, K., & Gunderson, A. (2007). Caring for older patients and an aging population. In R. Ham, P.D. Sloane, G.A. Warshaw, M.A. Bernard, & E. Flaherty (Eds.), *Primary care geriatrics: A case-based approach* (5th ed., pp. 3–13). New York, NY: Mosby-Elsevier.

Callen, B., Mahoney, J., Grieves, C., Wells, T., & Enloe, M. (2004). Frequency of hallway ambulation by hospitalized older adults on medical units of an academic hospital. *Geriatric Nursing, 25*(4), 212–217.

Campbell, S., Seymour, D., & Primrose, W. (2004). ACMEPLUS Project. A systematic literature review of factors affecting outcome in older medical patients admitted to hospital. *Age and Ageing, 33*(2), 110–115

Cotter, V. (2005). Restraint free care in older adults with dementia. *Keio Journal of Medicine, 54*(2), 80–84.

Counsell, S., Holder, C., Liebenauer, L., Palmer, R., Fortinsky, R., Kresevic, D., et al. (2000). Effects of a multicomponent intervention on functional outcomes and process of care in hospitalized older patients: A randomized controlled trial of acute care for elders (ACE) in a community hospital. *Journal of the American Geriatric Society, 48*(12), 1572–1581.

Covinsky, K., Palmer, R., Fortinsky, R., Counsell, S., Stewart, A., Kresevic, D., et al. (2003). Loss of independence in activities of daily living in older adults hospitalized with medical illnesses: Increased vulnerability with age. *Journal of the American Geriatric Society, 51*(4), 451–458.

Covinsky, K., Palmer, R., Kresevic, D., Kahana, E., Counsell, S., Fortinsky, R., et al. (1998). Improving functional outcomes in older patients: Lessons from an acute care for elders unit. *Joint Commission Journal on Quality Improvement, 24(2)*, 63–76.

Feldblum, I., German, L., Castel, H., Harman-Boehm, I., Bilenko, N., Eisinger, M., et al. (2007). Characteristics of undernourished older medical patients and the identification of predictors for undernutrition status. *Nutrition Journal, 6*, 37.

Fernandez, H., Callahan, K., Likourezos, A., & Leipzig, R. (2008). House staff member awareness of older inpatients' risks for hazards of hospitalization. *Archives of Internal Medicine, 168*(4), 390–396.

Fick, D., Agostini, J., & Inouye, S. (2002). Delirium superimposed on dementia: A systematic review. *Journal of the American Geriatric Society, 50*(10), 1723–32.

Fick, D., & Mion, L. (2008). How to try this: Delirium superimposed on dementia. *American Journal of Nursing, 108*(1), 52–60.

Fletcher, K. (2005). Immobility: Geriatric self-learning module. *MEDSURG Nursing, 14*(1), 35–37.

Folstein, M., Folstein, S., & McHugh, P. (1975). "Mini-Mental State": A practical method for grading the cognitive state of patients for the clinician. *Journal of Psychiatric Research, 12*, 189–198.

Fortinsky, R., Covinsky, K., Palmer, R., & Landefeld, C. (1999). Effects of functional status changes before and during hospitalization on nursing home admission of older adults. *Journals of Gerontology Series A: Biological Sciences and Medical Sciences, 54*(10), M521–526.

Freedman, V., Martin, L., & Schoeni, R. (2002). Recent trends in disability and functioning among older adults in the United States: A systematic review. *Journal of the American Medical Association, 288*(24), 3137–3146.

Graf, C. (2006). Functional decline in hospitalized older adults. *American Journal of Nursing, 106*(1), 58–67.

Graf, C. (2008). The hospital admission risk profile: The HARP helps to determine a patient's risk of functional decline. *American Journal of Nursing, 108*(8), 62–71.

Guigoz, Y., Lauque, S., & Vellas, B. (2002). Identifying the elderly at risk for malnutrition: The mini nutritional assessment. *Clinics in Geriatric Medicine, 18*, 737–757.

Haber, D. (2004). *Health promotion and aging* (3rd ed.). New York: Springer Publishing Co.

Ham, R., Sloane, P., Warshaw, G., Bernard, M., & Flaherty, E. (2007). *Primary care geriatrics: A case-based approach* (5th ed.). Philadelphia, PA: Mosby Elsevier.

Hartford Institute for Geriatric Nursing. (2008). *ConsultGeriRN.org*. Retrieved from http://consultgerirn.org.

Inouye, S., van Dyck, C., Alessi, C., Balkin, S., Siegal, A., & Horwitz, R. (1990). Clarifying confusion: The confusion assessment method. A new method for detection of delirium. *Annals of Internal Medicine, 113*(12), 941–948.

Kane, D., & Thomas, B. (2000). Nursing and the "F" word. *Nursing Forum, 35*(2), 17–24.

Katz, S., Down, T.D., Cash, H.R., & Grotz, R.C. (1970). Progress in the development of the index of ADL. *Gerontologist, 10*(1), 20–30.

Kleinpell, R. (2007). Supporting independence in hospitalized elders in acute care. *Critical Care Nursing Clinics of North America Focusing on Acute Care of the Hospitalized Elderly, 19*(3), 247–252.

Kresevic, D., & Holder, C. (1998). Interdisciplinary care. *Clinics in Geriatric Medicine, 14*(4), 787–798.

Kresevic, D.M. (2008). Assessment of function. In D.Z.E. Capezuiti, M. Mezey, & T. Fulmer (Eds.), *Evidence-based geriatric nursing: Protocols for best practice.* New York: Springer Publishing Co.

Landefeld, C., Palmer, R., Kresevic, D., Fortinsky, R., & Kowal, J. (1995). A randomized trial of care in the hospital medical unit especially designed to improve the functional outcomes of acutely ill older patients. *New England Journal of Medicine, 332*, 1338–1334.

Lawton, M.P., & Brody, E.M. (1969). Assessment of older people: Self-maintaining and instrumental activities of daily living. *Gerontologist, 9*(3), 179–186.

Mahoney, F.L., & Barthel, D.W. (1965). Functional evaluation: The Barthel index. *Maryland State Medical Journal, 14*, 61–65.

Mathias, S., Nayak, U., & Isaacs, B. (1986). Balance in elderly patients: The "get-up and go" test. *Archives of Physical Medicine and Rehabilitation, 67*(6), 387–389.

McCusker, J., Bellavance, F., Cardin, S., Belzile, E., & Verdon, J. (2000). Prediction of hospital utilization among elderly patients during the 6 months after an emergency department visit. *Annals of Emergency Medicine, 36*(5), 438–445.

McCusker, J., Kakuma, R., & Abrahamowicz, M. (2002). Predictors of functional decline in hospitalized elderly patients: A systematic review. *Journals of Gerontology Series A: Biological Sciences and Medical Sciences, 57*(9), M569–577.

Murer, C. (2006). Caps are back: Are you provider based? Medicare sets new financial limitations on therapy reimbursements. *Rehabilitation Management, 19*(5), 46–47.

Potter, J., & Titman, H. (2007). Persistent pain. In R. Ham, P.D. Sloane, G.A. Warshaw, M.A. Bernard, & E. Flaherty (Eds.), *Primary care geriatrics: A case-based approach* (5th ed., pp. 350–359). New York, NY: Mosby-Elsevier.

Sager, M., & Rudberg, M. (1998). Functional decline associated with hospitalization for acute illness. *Clinics in Geriatric Medicine, 14*(4), 669–679.

Sager, M., Rudberg, M., Jalaluddin, M., Franke, T., Inouye, S., Landefeld, C., et al. (1996). Hospital admission risk profile (HARP): Identifying older patients at risk for functional decline following acute medical illness and hospitalization. *Journal of the American Geriatrics Society, 44*(3), 251–257.

Salvi, F., Giorgi, R., Grilli, A., Morichi, V., Espinosa, E., Spazzafumo, L., et al. (2008). Mini nutritional assessment (short form) and functional decline in older patients admitted to an acute medical ward. *Aging Clinical and Experimental Research, 20*(4), 322–328.

Sands, L., Yaffe, K., Covinsky, K., Chren, M., Counsell, S., Palmer, R., et al. (2003). Cognitive screening predicts magnitude of functional recovery from admission to 3 months after discharge in hospitalized elders. *Journals of Gerontology Series A: Biological Sciences and Medical Sciences, 58*(1), 37–45.

Sennour, Y., Counsell, S., Jones, J., & Weiner, M. (2009). Development and implementation of a proactive geriatrics consultation model in collaboration with hospitalists. *Journal of the American Geriatrics Society, 57*(11), 2139–2145.

Sheikh, J. L., & Yesavage, J. A. (1986). Geriatric depression scale (GDS): Recent evidence and development of a shorter version. *Clinical Gerontologist, 5*, 165.

Thomas, E., Mottram, S., Peat, G., Wilkie, R., & Croft, P. (2007). The effect of age on the onset of pain interference in a general population of older adults: Prospective findings from the North Staffordshire Osteoarthritis Project (NorStOP). *Pain, 129*(1–2), 21–27.

Tufts University. (2002). *TUFTS food guide pyramid for older adults*. Retrieved from http://nutrition.tufts.edu/docs/guidelines.pdf.

Wakefield, B.J., & Holman, J.E. (2007). Functional trajectories associated with hospitalization in older adults. *Western Journal of Nursing Research, 29*(2), 161–177. doi: 10.1177/0193945906293809

Wells, J., & Dumbrell, A. (2006). Nutrition and aging: Assessment and treatment of compromised nutritional status in frail elderly patients. *Journal of Clinical Interviews and Aging, 1*(1), 67–79.

Chapter 21

Caring for the Elderly in the Emergency Department

Candy Blevins and Martha H. Bramlett

Introduction

There are sweeping changes occurring in America's population. Advances in health care, disease prevention and diagnosis, and the everyday environment have produced incredible results. Unique in American history, more people are reaching and surpassing the age of 65 than ever before. According to the US Census Bureau (2008), 12.3% of the American population is now age 65 and over. By the year 2030, the senior population is expected to grow from its present 33.8 to 70 million people (United States [U.S.] Census Bureau, 2003). The fastest-growing cohort, those over age 85, will increase from 4 million to 19 million adults by 2050.

In turn, this newest trend in population statistics is presenting new challenges in emergency healthcare delivery. As the growth of the senior population continues to rise, the elderly will become proportionately greater consumers of emergency health care. Dramatic economic changes, status of insurance coverage, current functional status of the patient, and injury and acuity of illness all contribute to the elderly patient's decision to seek care at an emergency department (ED). The rapid rise in the number of ED visits by the elderly requires us to know more about the changes that occur in the older adult and to identify those changes that will influence the successful health outcome of the elderly ED patient. The elderly present with unique medical and sociological needs that may be embedded within preexisting health complexities. As a result, they typically use more resources during their stay in the emergency department. Senior patients are more likely to arrive by ambulance and have higher acuity levels. They average 30 more minutes per visit and are more likely to be admitted to the hospital, to require admission to an ICU, and to require more staff time (Aminzadeh & Dalziel, 2002; Richardson, 2003; Ross et al., 2003). Compared to younger patients, however, studies have found the elderly are less likely to seek care from an ED inappropriately (Aminzadeh & Dalziel, 2002; Richardson, 2003). Geriatric patients present to EDs with signs and symptoms of depression, dementia, incontinence, problems with mobility, multiple health complexities, and multiple home medications (Amimzadeh & Dalziel, 2002; Ross et al., 2003).

Barriers to Care

There are currently barriers to quality care of seniors in the emergency department. Recent surveys among physicians and other healthcare workers report that healthcare workers feel less comfortable treating seniors. Specifically, they feel that the elderly are more difficult to evaluate and more time-consuming to diagnose and treat (Sanders, 1996). Other studies report that healthcare workers think the elderly are unable to learn or understand their circumstances, are unable to participate in decision-making, and are unable to interact with their environment (Collison, 1992; Jackson, 1989). These attitudes directly affect the quality of care seniors receive during an ED stay.

Bias, including ageism, is common in American culture. Growing old is viewed as an unfortunate state often accompanied by failing cognitive and physical viability. Healthcare workers are not immune to this type of thinking. Many view the elderly as depressing, senile, untreatable, or rigid (Reyes-Ortiz, 1997). Physicians and others may become frustrated or angry when confronted by an elderly patient's physical or cognitive limitations (Nelson, 2005). The ED is often visited by patients from nursing homes who are ill with significant medical issues, and who present with acute changes in their health status. This type of visit can contribute to an unbalanced or negative view of the older adult. Negative reinforcement can perpetuate the myth of aging, leading to a focus on disease management instead of prevention.

Seniors have issues that are specific to their age and development. Yet healthcare workers are offered little education to address the needs of this population. In one survey, 69% of ED physicians reported a lack of continuing education on geriatric emergency medicine. Indeed, 53% of residency-trained emergency physicians report deficient education on the emergency care needs of seniors during their residency (Sanders, 1996). Nurses are affected by the lack of geriatric education as well. Unfortunately, comprehensive geriatric nursing education has not been included in basic nursing education or in nursing continuing education programs to the degree needed (Hartford Institute for Geriatric Nursing, 2000). A survey conducted by the Hartford Institute for Geriatric Nursing (2000) revealed that ED nurses believed they had inadequate knowledge of older adult norms, yielding inaccurate assessments of the elderly. There is a clear need for geriatric-trained workers to provide education to colleagues, serve as a resource for the staff, and help meet the emergency care needs of this population.

Other barriers affect emergency care of the elderly. Compensation programs for assessing and treating the elderly can take longer and may reimburse poorly. The elderly may not be aware of community resources that can help them with activities of daily living. Underutilization of these resources may limit the success of the health care plan. Communication is a vital aspect of all human interaction, but the elderly may suffer from impairments that hinder effective communication. Thus ED healthcare workers must develop communication techniques specific to older patients, their families, and caretakers.

Impact on the Healthcare System

The significant impact of the elderly on EDs is undeniable. In studies conducted from 1993 to 2003, the visit rate by elderly patients increased by 26% (Pitts, Hiska, Yu, & Burt, 2006). Visits by persons 65 and over are expected to double from 6.4 million to 11.7 million visits by 2015. The elderly accounted for 263 million ambulatory care visits in 2006 (Centers for Disease Control and Prevention[CDC], 2006). Persons age 75 and older had the second-highest per capita rate of visits to the ED at a ratio of 60.2 per 100, or 10.2 million. Among patients over 65 years of age, 24.6% were triaged as immediate or emergent. Additionally, 6 million seniors arrive at the ED by ambulance (Pitts et al., 2006). In a study conducted by MacLean (2000), 60% of ED managers reported a rise in the number of visits by the elderly.

As a result of the surge in the numbers of seniors seeking health care in the ED, patient outcomes have been negatively affected. EDs find themselves facing reduced patient satisfaction scores. Elderly patients complain of unmet needs and inadequate discharge education, and they often feel ignored by the healthcare staff (Jones, Young, LaFleur, & Brown, 1999).

Health outcomes are negatively affected as well. Senior patients are more likely to suffer adverse health outcomes following discharge from the ED. The elderly have soaring admission rates (30–50% compared to 10–20% of the younger population). They are likely to have repeat ED visits at rates of 24% at 3 months and 44% at 6 months (Salvi et al., 2007). Seniors are more likely to suffer functional decline (10–45% at 3 months), and institutionalization and death (10% at 3 months). Poor utilization of community resources, inadequate discharge planning, and poor assessment technique and documentation contribute to the problems faced by older adults in the emergency department.

Healthcare providers agree that current delivery systems and the episodic model of medical care does not adequately meet the needs of the elderly. The goal of the emergency department is to provide timely medical care and interventions to patients with acute illness or injury. The system breaks down, however, when an older patient with complex medical issues, impaired cognitive and/or physical functioning, and poor social support arrives seeking emergency health care.

Theoretical Framework

As more seniors seek ED services now and into the future, it will be clear that current modes of treatment are simply inadequate to meet their needs. However, the needed changes should not occur at random. Newly designed models of geriatric emergency health care should include interventions targeted to the needs of the elderly. Due to the unique nature of this vulnerable population, specialized skills and knowledge are needed to manage their health effectively. Revised systems of care should consider the growth and development of the older adult and generate understanding of the elder adult's dynamic state of health.

When designing healthcare interventions, it is most helpful to have practical guidelines from which to structure new models of caring. A theoretical framework is crucial to the change process. Theory is a set of facts, propositions, or principles used to explain and predict phenomena. Nursing models, for instance, use assessment, planning, and implementation to design interventions specific to the needs of a population. Thus, the application of theory or a nursing model gives us both a meaningful framework and a way to measure the effectiveness of the interventions.

The Roper-Logan-Tierney Model of Nursing describes aging as a life process based upon 12 essential activities of living, or ALs. These functions include: maintaining a safe environment, communication, breathing, nutrition/hydration, elimination, washing/dressing, thermoregulation, mobility, working/playing, sexuality, sleeping, and death/dying (Roper, Logan, & Tierney, 2000). Roper, Logan, and Tierney's model proposes that throughout a human lifetime, one moves along a bidirectional continuum of dependence and independence (Roper et al., 2000). The more one can maintain ALs without help, the more independence is achieved, and the more help needed to meet ALs, the more dependent one becomes. It is expected that infants and children will be dependent on others for assistance with activities of living. During the maturation process, one eventually attains independence through mastery of all activities of living. It is the goal of the maturing human being to achieve independence and self-maintenance.

In the senior adult, many factors can influence the ability to maintain self-care. Psychological factors (emotion, cognition, spiritual beliefs, and understanding), biological factors (overall health, current medical issues, and injury), sociocultural factors (impact of society and culture, expectations, values, and social class), environmental factors (impact of environment on individuals and individuals on environment) and politicoeconomic factors (impact of politics, government, and economy) can profoundly affect ALs, and ultimately the elder's position on the dependence-independence continuum (Roper et al., 2000).

The Roper-Logan-Tierney Model enables providers to predict the likelihood of success of planned health outcomes among the elderly. The greater the ability to perform self-care (independence) the older adult has, the more likely he/she will be able to stay in compliance with the treatment plan. The inability to perform one or more of the 12 essential life functions independently makes it less likely the older adult will be able to maintain treatment plan compliance.

This model can benefit emergency geriatric health care in many ways. The theoretical framework, based on activities of living, can provide for holistic and comprehensive assessment. From the comprehensive assessment, targeted interventions can be designed to improve the quality of emergency health care for seniors, and the outcomes can be measured.

Roper, Logan, and Tierney's (2000) essential activities of living reflect the growth and development of the older adult. Their model promotes a holistic approach to the older adult and allows providers to gain a clearer picture of the needs and issues faced by the elderly patient. Using the activities of living as a basis of assessment will enable healthcare workers to gauge changes in health status using measurable terms and less subjectivity. Since the model examines other facets of living such as psychological, environmental, and sociocultural influences, these can all be considered in the assessment and subsequent development of a therapeutic healthcare plan. The application of a theoretical framework enables healthcare workers to more accurately assess and document health issues for more effective referral to community resources, social services, and other multidisciplinary resources.

Recommendations

The secret to resolving any challenge is to first examine the nature of the challenge. The same process can be applied to improving geriatric emergency care. Assessment is the single most important aspect of an ED visit. Inadequate education about the elderly directly affects assessment, diagnosis, treatment, and discharge planning (Luk, Or, & Woo, 2000). Health outcomes are likely to be negatively affected. In a study conducted by Miller, Lewis, Nork, and Morley (1996), 77% of discharged elderly patients reported at least one unmet need. Forty percent needed clarification of discharge instructions (Jones et al., 1999). Assessment of the elderly must encompass the entirety of the person in order to detect crucial health issues that may be hidden within comorbidities, polypharmacy, atypical symptomologies, ineffective communication, and physical and cognitive dysfunctions (Salvi et al., 2007).

The purpose of the assessment process is to determine diagnosis, screen for treatable disease or injury, and create a mutually acceptable therapeutic plan of care accompanied by complete documentation (Luk et al., 2000). In many circumstances, appropriateness of referral to other resources and placement in long-term care facilities can be initiated in the ED. Many geriatric assessment forms have been created to assess various aspects of the elderly patient; these can be located in the literature. What is vital to any geriatric assessment is that the assessment must incorporate a holistic approach in order to obtain accurate information.

Arthur Sanders (1996) developed 11 principles of geriatric emergency care that should be considered when assessing an older adult. The principles reflect the life functions that

Roper, Logan, and Tierney describe, and therefore make these principles valuable in creating new interventions that will generate quality geriatric emergency care. A detailed description of these principles follows.

Principle 1. Complexities of Presentation. The first principle to consider is one previously discussed. An elderly patient's presentation is most often complex. Symptoms may be difficult to discern. Often, the older adult will describe multiple symptoms that inundate the medical provider with possibilities, or conversely, will not be able to describe any symptoms other than "something isn't right."

Principle 2. Atypical Symptoms. The elderly patient may present with symptoms that are atypical for the given illness or disease. This can cause misdiagnosis, premature discharge, and increased mortality rates (Sanders, 1996). Healthcare providers must always be cognizant of this second principle of geriatric emergency care.

Principle 3. Comorbidities. The third principle to be aware of is the presence of comorbidities. The elderly patient's symptoms may be related to their preexisting disease, or the comorbidities may have a profound impact on the new health concern.

Principle 4. Polypharmacy. Polypharmacy is a common and potentially life-threatening occurrence. The average elderly adult takes five prescription drugs and two over-the-counter drugs daily in the United States (Sanders, 1996). Logically, the more drugs a person takes, the greater the risk of interaction or other adverse side effects. Adverse drug reactions account for 5% of all admissions by the elderly (Sanders, 1996). Weakness, decreased functional status, and change in cognitive function are common ED complaints of the elderly and may result from polypharmacy.

Principle 5. Cognitive Status. Principle 5 reiterates the importance of recognizing cognitive impairment among the elderly. Sanders (1996) states that 30% to 40% of all elderly ED patients will have some cognitive dysfunction. Recognition of cognitive impairment is vital for determining the extent of medical testing and discharge status.

Principle 6. Physiological Efficiency. It is important to understand that the aging process affects the efficiency of human physiological processes. As a result, Principal 6 reminds providers that some diagnostic tests have age specificity.

Principle 7. Functional Reserve. As previously stated, the aging process induces change in the physiological processes of the body. As a result of these changes, providers must be aware that the elderly are likely to have decreased functional reserve. While performing normal activities of living, the elderly may function well. When stressed by illness or injury, their functional reserve may be depleted quickly.

Principle 8. Social Support System. The elderly may have inadequate social supports. Often they must rely on caregivers to help them with activities of living. Principle 8 holds that this domain is instrumental in discharge planning. It also reminds us that those who will help the elderly after discharge will need appropriate discharge education.

Principle 9. Baseline Health Status. It is important for healthcare providers to have knowledge of the older patient's baseline health status. This information can be used to discern functional decline and to assist in diagnosis and treatment.

Principle 10. Psychological Assessment. Principle 10 upholds the importance of psychological assessment. Emotional problems can influence somatic complaints. Psychological problems may disguise underlying health issues or may even be a result of a physiological issue.

Principle 11. Assessment for Abuse and Other Relevant Issues. Lastly, Principle 11 is perhaps the most crucial in terms of a complete geriatric assessment. Observing elders in the ED provides an opportunity to discover relevant issues that may affect the overall well-being of the older adult. Issues such as substance abuse, elder abuse, and depression may not be readily evident, but they are nonetheless critical.

Sanders' principles of geriatric emergency care intertwine with Roper, Logan, and Tierney's Model of Nursing. Indeed, the two form a net that supports and comforts the elderly patient through thoughtful assessment, holistic caring, and application of specialized knowledge. Ultimately, the result can be an improved state of emergency health care for the elderly.

Comprehensive geriatric assessment is an opportunity not only to resolve the current health concern, but also to improve the overall quality of life for the elderly patient (Sanders, 1996). The information obtained from the thorough assessment will help to identify the needs of the patient and to promote referral to multidisciplinary resources. Additionally, discharge planning can be accomplished that will support patient compliance with the therapeutic healthcare plan.

Specialized knowledge and skills are vital to providing quality emergency health care to the older adult. Medical and nursing programs must begin to recognize the importance of these skill sets in providing health care in the future. Current research suggests there are serious inadequacies in basic nursing and medical education programs, as well as in continuing education, for healthcare workers involved in caring for the elderly (Sanders, 1996; Hartford Institute for Geriatric Nursing, 2000). It follows that changes to current models of geriatric emergency healthcare delivery must include changes to current curriculum and instruction.

Very few emergency departments now use geriatric specialists such as geriatric consult teams or geriatric nurse practitioners in their departments. Expanded roles such as these offer the elderly the expertise of a specialist, and offer the facility the benefit of a role model, educator, and change agent (Salvi et al., 2007). New models of geriatric emergency health care include Geriatric Emergency Departments or Observation Units dedicated to evaluating seniors exclusively. But not all facilities or EDs are capable of supporting these interventions. Therefore it is important to recognize the value of continuing education for staff and utilization of a multidisciplinary approach.

Knowledge and skill in providing quality geriatric emergency healthcare are crucial. To help providers to gain this knowledge and skill, short, user-friendly assessment forms would be invaluable. These forms would serve several purposes: provide a framework for a comprehensive geriatric assessment; create a method of accurate, complete documentation; enhance identification of social needs; and incorporate a means of identifying appropriate referrals to community resources.

Results of Interventions

Research into the effects of specialized geriatric emergency care is promising. Patients receiving an assessment from a geriatric nurse specialist were less likely to have gone to a nursing home 30 days after their ED visit than those receiving the usual care, at a difference of 0.7% compared to 3% (Mion et al., 2003). Additionally, 56% had been referred to a community resource versus 1% of the usual care patients. Those who were assessed by a geriatric nurse specialist had fewer hospital admission days (0.6) than the usual care group (1.6) and fewer nursing home admissions at 30 days (2% versus 7%) and 120 days (3% versus 10%) as reported by Mion et al., (2003). These statistics illustrate the potential positive effect of specialized emergency care for the elderly on health outcomes. Indeed, positive health outcomes result in improved well-being and quality of life, and a reduction in overall health care costs. Further research into the effectiveness of specialized geriatric emergency health care delivery is still needed.

Conclusion

Current research indicates that the elderly are not satisfied with their ED visits. Lower satisfaction scores, unmet needs, and inattentive staff are common complaints among senior patients and families. Additionally, the elderly maybe discharged from the ED without appropriate referrals to community resources. Many are discharged without consideration of their ability to perform self-care activities.

As the population of seniors in America continues to rise over the next few decades, the emergency healthcare system will need to adapt and embrace the difficult challenges of caring for the elderly in the ED. Emergency health care will be sought in departments where elderly patients present with complex medical needs that require greater time and resources, more in-depth diagnostic studies, and additional staff. The unique challenges faced by EDs include lack of geriatric care education in basic health care programs and continuing education, disinterest among new-to-practice professionals in caring for the elderly, lack of staff support—such as geriatric nurse specialists, whose responsibility is to ensure optimal emergency nursing care for seniors—ageism, and conflicting cultural norms regarding aging. As the number of elderly increases, it seems certain that these practice issues will continue to challenge EDs now and well into the future.

The older patient's odds of achieving successful health outcomes are based upon the ability to perform activities of daily living. The Roper-Logan-Tierney Model of Nursing (Roper et al., 2000) explains and predicts this phenomenon through a dependent-independent continuum. The continuum describes 12 essential life functions. Inability to perform one or more of these functions hampers older adults' ability to manage a plan of care successfully. Sanders' (1996) eleven (11) principles of geriatric emergency care reviews the essential components of geriatric assessment. These principles align with Roper,

Logan and Tierney's Model of Nursing, thus providing a solid foundation on which to rebuild the current models of emergency health care delivery for the elderly. Traditional methods of providing emergency health care for the elderly no longer meet the complex needs of seniors. Change is both needed and imminent.

References

Aminzadeh, F., & Dalziel, W. (2002). Older adults in the emergency department: A systematic review of patterns of use, adverse outcomes, and effectiveness of interventions. *Annals of Emergency Medicine, 39*(3), 238–247. Retrieved from doi:10.1067/mem.2002,121523

Caplan, G.A., Gideon, A., Williams, A.J., Daly, B., & Abraham, K. (2004). A randomized, controlled trial of comprehensive geriatric assessment and multidisciplinary intervention after discharge of elderly from the emergency department—the DEED II study. *Journal of the American Geriatrics Society, 52*(9), 1417–1423.

Centers for Disease Control and Prevention. (2006). *Ambulatory care utilization estimates for 2006.* Retrieved from www.cdc.gov

Collison, D. (1992). Nurses' attitudes to the elderly are crucial. *New Zealand Nursing Journal, 85*(4), 2–8.

Hartford Institute for Geriatric Nursing. (2000). *Fast facts: Emphasis needed on geriatric nursing.* Retrieved from http://www.hartfordign.org

Jackson, M. (1989). Geriatric versus general medical wards: Comparison of patient's behaviours following discharge from an acute care hospital. *Journal of Advanced Nursing, 14*(1), 906–914.

Jones, J., Young, M., LaFleur, R., & Brown, M. (1999). Effectiveness of an organized follow-up system for the elderly released from the emergency department. *Academic Emergency Medicine, 4*(12), 1147–1152.

Luk, J., Or, K., & Woo, J. (2000). Using the comprehensive geriatric assessment technique to assess elderly patients. *Hong Kong Medical Journal, 6*(1), 93–97. Retrieved from http://www.hkmj.org/index.html.

MacLean, S. (2001). *2001 ENA benchmark guide: Emergency departments.* Des Plaines, IL: Emergency Nurses Association.

Miller, D., Lewis, L., Nork, M., & Morley, J. (1996). Controlled trial of geriatric case finding and liaison service in an emergency department: Trends for decreasing emergency department visits. *Journal of the American Geriatrics Society, 44* , 513–520.

Mion, L., Palmer, R., Meldon, S., Bass, D., Singer, M., Payne, S., Lewicki, L., Drew, B., Connor, J., Campbell, J., & Emerman, C. (2003). Case finding and referral model for emergency department elders: A randomized clinical trial. Annals of emergency Medicine, 44(1), 57–68.

Nelson, T. (2005). Ageism: Prejudice against our feared future self. *Journal of Social Issues, 61*(2), 207–221. DOI 10;1111/J.1540-4560.2005.00402.x.

Pitts, S., Hiska, R., Yu, J., & Burt, C. (2006). *National hospital ambulatory medical care survey: 2006 emergency department summary* (National Health Stats Report No. 7). Retrieved from Centers for Disease Control and Prevention website: http://www.cdc.gov/nchs/

Reyes-Ortiz, C. (1997). Physicians must confront ageism. *Academic Medicine, 72*(10), 831.

Richardson, B. (2003). Overview of geriatric emergencies. *The Mount Sinai Journal of Medicine, 70*(2), 75–84.

Roper, N., Logan, W., & Tierney, A. (2000). *The Roper-Logan-Tierney model of nursing: Based on activities of living.* Philadelphia, PA: Churchill Livingstone.

Ross, M., Compton, S., Richardson, D., Jones, R., Nittis, W., & Wilson, A. (2003). The use and effectiveness of an emergency department observation unit for elderly patients. *The Annals of Emergency Medicine, 41*(5), 668–677.

Salvi, E., Morichi, V., Grilli, A., Giorgi, R., De Thommaso, G., & Dessi-Fulgheri, P. (2007). The elderly in the emergency department: A critical review of problems and solutions. *Internal and Emergency Medicine, 2*(4), 292–301.

Sanders, A. (1996). *Emergency care of the elderly.* Society for Academic Emergency Medicine. Retrievd from http://www.saem,org/saemdnn/Education/Education Resources/EmergencyCare oftheElderPerson/tabid/305/Default.aspx.

United States Census Bureau. (2003). *Projections of the total resident population by 5-year age groups, and sex with special age categories: Middle series, 1999 to 2000* (NP-T3-A). Retrieved from www.census.gov/population/projections/nation/summary/np-t3-a.pdf

United States Census Bureau. (2008). State and County Quick Facts. Modified April 22, 2010. Retrieved from http://quickfacts.census.gov/qfd/states/00000.htm.USAQuickFacts.

Chapter 22

Cognitive Rehabilitation in People with Dementia

Nikki L. Hill and Ann M. Kolanowski

Introduction

Dementia is common in older adults, affecting approximately 10% of people over age 65 and up to 50% of those over age 85 (American Academy of Neurology, 2001). It is caused by a variety of underlying pathologies, the most common of which is Alzheimer's disease (AD), and all of which lead to progressive decline in memory and other cognitive functions (Zarit & Zarit, 2007). Disturbances in language, visuospatial skills, intellectual abilities, and memory are persistent and continually worsen over time, leading to significant impairments in functional abilities (American Psychiatric Association, 1994; Cummings & Mega, 2003). Family caregivers also face challenges and negative outcomes, including high emotional stress (Alzheimer's Association & National Alliance for Caregiving, 2004) and depression (Yaffe et al., 2002). Additionally, cost to the healthcare system is significant, tripling the cost of care for Americans age 65 and over (Alzheimer's Association, 2009). However, early diagnosis and appropriate treatment that includes interventions for family members may result in significant cost savings (Weimer & Sager, 2009).

There is interest in the development of nonpharmacological interventions to prevent or compensate for brain damage associated with degenerative neurological disorders such as Alzheimer's disease. Cognition-based interventions for people with dementia (PWD) have shown promise in their potential to slow disease progression and improve quality of life (De Vreese, 2001; Woods, Thorgrimsen, Spector, Royan, & Orrell, 2006; Yu et al., 2009). Cognitive rehabilitation is one cognition-based method that embraces a person-centered, holistic approach to intervention. The person with dementia, along with family members, works collaboratively with professional staff in order to identify goals, modify intervention components throughout dementia progression, and improve everyday, personally relevant problems or functional limitations (Clare, 2005; Woods & Clare, 2008). In this chapter we will:

1. Provide an overview of cognitive rehabilitation, including its definition and distinction from other cognition-based interventions.

2. Discuss the theoretical basis supporting the use of cognitive rehabilitation in people with dementia.

3. Introduce the clinical application of cognitive rehabilitation, including specific techniques used and approaches to implementation.

4. Review the research efficacy of cognitive rehabilitation in healthy older adults, individuals with mild cognitive impairment, and those with dementia.

5. Identify implications for practice and research related to interventions for PWD.

Differentiating Cognitive Rehabilitation from Other Cognition-Based Approaches

Cognition-based approaches as interventions for PWD include cognitive stimulation, cognitive training, and cognitive rehabilitation, although the boundaries of each of these therapies is often unclear, resulting in their frequent interchangeable use in the literature (Clare, Woods, Moniz-Cook, Orrell, & Spector, 2003; Woods, Spector, Prendergast, & Orrell, 2005). In order to facilitate an understanding of what distinguishes cognitive rehabilitation from other approaches, we will define the concept and explore the differences between the three concepts.

Definition of Cognitive Rehabilitation

Cognitive rehabilitation is a cognition-focused psychological approach for people with dementia involving "a collaboration between client, family member (where appropriate) and professionals aimed at devising and carrying out an individually-planned intervention that addresses negotiated, personally meaningful goals which are directly relevant to specific aspects of cognitive functioning as these impact on everyday life" (Clare, 2005, p. 334). It is, therefore, a personally tailored intervention rather than one specific protocol. Although limiting disability and enhancing capability are inherent components (Cappa, 2008; Londos et al., 2008; Moniz-Cook, 2008), the focus is on improving the everyday functioning of the person with dementia rather than altering any particular area of cognitive function in isolation (Wilson, 2008). Additional important themes of cognitive rehabilitation include collaboration between the person with dementia, family caregivers, and professional staff to determine goals (Kurz, Pohl, Ramsenthaler, & Sorg, 2009; Mimura & Mimura, 2007) as well as use of a practical approach to selecting intervention components in which individual needs are considered (Clare, Woods, Moniz-Cook, Orrell, & Spector, 2003; Mateer, 2005).

Alternative Cognition-Based Interventions

Cognitive stimulation is the most generalized approach to cognition-focused interventions. Based on the evidence that continued engagement in mentally stimulating activities may provide cognitive benefits, including a decreased risk of developing dementia (Wilson et al., 2002) as well as improved cognition after a dementia diagnosis (Spector, Woods, & Orrell, 2008), cognitive stimulation aims to improve overall cognitive and social functioning through group activities/discussions based on reality orientation principles (Clare, 2003). Research supports the benefits of cognitive stimulation programs on cognition and quality of life in people with Alzheimer's disease that are comparable to benefits of pharmacological therapies (Spector et al., 2008). Combining cognitive stimulation therapy with an acetylcholinesterase inhibitor may provide even greater cognitive benefits (Matsuda, 2007). Cognitive stimulation is typically nonspecific regarding both the domain of cognition that is targeted and the individually desired outcomes. The goal is to improve general cognitive function using generalized approaches. Older adults are often encouraged by both healthcare providers and media messages to remain mentally active in order to potentially slow cognitive decline, which reflects current research on the effectiveness of cognitive stimulation.

  Cognitive training refers to a more specific and structured intervention in which standardized tasks are developed that target a particular cognitive function, such as memory, attention, or problem-solving (Clare, Woods et al., 2003) and may be tailored to individual functional level (Woods & Clare, 2008). The client practices these tasks repeatedly over time, typically at progressive levels of difficulty, either individually or in a group setting. Cognitive training programs have been shown to improve memory, attention, reasoning, and processing speed in older adults without cognitive impairment (Ball et al., 2002; Smith et al., 2009), as well as improving memory, learning, executive functioning, activities of daily living, and decision-making in people with early-stage Alzheimer's disease (Sitzer, Twamley, & Jeste, 2006). Therefore, the evidence supports the effectiveness of cognitive training as well. However, interventions seem to be more effective when they focus on cognitive deficits that are specifically related to the dementia process and each individual's current functional ability (Yu et al., 2009), highlighting the additional benefits of personally tailored interventions.

Contrasting Cognition-Based Approaches

In summary, cognitive stimulation is a nonspecific cognition-focused approach that does not target any individual aspect of cognition. Cognitive training is more specialized; the intervention is delivered as a training program and aims to improve specific areas of cognition. Cognitive training may be tailored to ability level for the person with dementia, although this is not a prescribed intervention component. Both cognitive stimulation and cognitive training share the mutual goal of improving cognitive ability at a broad level, whether that is overall cognition or one aspect of it. In comparison, cognitive rehabilitation encompasses a more holistic and personalized approach to managing the cognitive limitations of people with dementia. The focus of cognitive rehabilitation is less concerned with maintaining or improving cognition overall, but is rather an individualized approach that meets everyday goals of the person with dementia.

Use of Cognitive Rehabilitation in People with Dementia

Historically, cognitive rehabilitation has been an intervention used for those with acute brain injury such as cerebrovascular accident rather than progressive, degenerative conditions such as Alzheimer's disease. However, maximizing function and well-being as well as minimizing excess disability are rehabilitative goals that have been similarly justified in people with dementia (Clare & Woods, 2001). Although the implementation of rehabilitation for survivors of brain injury began as early as World War I (Wilson, 2008), the first instances of cognitive rehabilitation use for people with dementia don't appear in the scientific literature until the 1980s and not to a great extent until the early 2000s. In recent years, our understanding of the process of brain aging and related pathology has developed significantly. Previously, damage to the brain due to aging was considered unavoidable, and the occurrence of neuronal loss, regardless of cause, was deemed permanent. Our belief was that neuronal regeneration does not occur and the brain does little to compensate in the face of injury. However, more recent research has shown that the brain is in fact quite adaptable to damage through both protective effects (Stern, 2006) and compensation (Duffau, 2006). The ability of the brain to adapt to degenerative processes supports the potential of rehabilitative efforts to halt or slow the disease process in people with dementia. Interventions that enhance protective effects (cognitive reserve) and stimulate compensatory effects (brain plasticity) may offer significant benefits.

Cognitive Reserve

Although the pathophysiological process of Alzheimer's disease has been understood for some time, clinical experience often demonstrates a wide variation in disease presentation and progression given the same level of underlying pathology. Observation of these differences by clinicians and scientists led them to question: Why do some people with similar neurodegenerative changes exhibit a wide variation of disease manifestation? Research supports the idea of cognitive reserve as an explanation for these observations.

The concept of cognitive reserve reflects the hypothetical ability of the brain, at varying individual capacities, to withstand a certain level of injury or disease before the manifestation of clinical dementia (Whalley, Deary, Appleton, & Starr, 2004). Some individuals exhibit a robust response of this protective mechanism, resulting in increased maintenance of cognitive ability, while the same amount of brain damage causes severe disability in others. Similarly, some people may exhibit extensive dementia symptoms but on autopsy are not found to have profound pathology. Hence, cognitive function is not solely dependent upon amount of brain insult as a result of dementia, but is instead mitigated by a variety of factors such as intelligence, level of education, occupation, and leisure activities (Stern, 2003; Whalley et al., 2004). Higher levels of intelligence, educational achievement, and occupational success lead to higher cognitive reserve due to more efficient processing. Cognitively stimulating leisure activities such as reading, writing, crossword puzzles, or group discussions increase cognitive reserve, although the relative effectiveness of each activity is unclear (Hall et al., 2009). Understanding and using the protective effects of leisure activities later in life may prolong the onset of cognitive impairment in dementia by enhancing cognitive reserve (Hall et al., 2009; Stern, 2006). Behavioral modifications, such as intellectual and physical activity interventions, for example, have the potential to strengthen these mechanisms (Mattson, Chan, & Duan, 2002). Therefore, development of interventions that increase cognitive reserve may provide protective benefits to PWD.

Brain Plasticity

In addition to the inherent neuroprotective effects of genetic and lifestyle factors, the aging brain also remains quite dynamic in its ability to compensate for neurodegenerative effects. Brain plasticity refers to the ability of the brain to reorganize itself such as during the learning process or after sustaining nervous system damage (Duffau, 2006). In order to optimize brain function, this process of remodeling continues throughout the entire life span.

A certain level of cognitive decline does occur during the aging process, most notably in relation to memory tasks requiring high levels of attention and effort as opposed to involuntary tasks (Buckner, 2004). However, there also exists a "plastic" potential to improve cognitive performance given the proper conditions (Jones et al., 2006). This brain plasticity demonstrates a link to cognitive reserve, as compensatory mechanisms appear to be better utilized by those with more highly preserved cognitive capacity (Pariente et al., 2005). Both environmental enrichment (Jankowsky et al., 2005) and increased activity levels (Calero-García, Navarro-González, & Muñoz-Manzano, 2007) have been associated with neuronal stimulation leading to improved cognitive function. A high level of activity over the entire life span is associated with a higher cognitive function in old age, but it is the maintenance of that activity throughout the aging process itself that contributes to brain plasticity later in life (Calero-García et al., 2007). This plasticity appears to be maintained, to some extent, throughout early-stage Alzheimer's disease (Fernández-Ballesteros & Fernández, 2005).

The mechanisms of brain plasticity are likely multiple, including neuronal regeneration, development of new neural connections, and compensatory use of alternative brain regions to bypass damaged areas (Bach-y-Rita, 2003; Limke & Rao, 2002). Neural stem cells remain present in the brain and may be able to replace damaged neurons and supporting cells, possibly throughout the aging process, in response to environmental demands (Mattson et al., 2002). Brain reorganization may result in unique neural communication methods in which distant brain sites are activated without synaptic transmission, resulting in the compensatory use of unaffected regions (Bach-y-Rita, 2003). This communication may occur by release of neurotransmitters that travel beyond the synapse in order to reach remote receptors. The implication for Alzheimer's disease is that intact brain areas may be able to take over the functions of damaged brain areas if trained appropriately, such as through rehabilitation efforts.

Functional Imaging

The development of new imaging techniques such as functional magnetic resonance imaging (fMRI) has allowed us to see precisely which areas of the brain are activated by memory and learning tasks, and to compare these activities in people with dementia to those in older adults without dementia. These studies have provided strong evidence that those with Alzheimer's disease can compensate for neuronal loss through altered activation of brain areas during cognitive tasks (Rocca & Filippi, 2006). Although research supports the process of compensatory use of brain areas, it is mixed regarding whether new areas are recruited or existing areas are used to a greater degree. Individuals with Alzheimer's disease have been shown to use brain regions unique to healthy older adults when performing a memory task, and the use of these areas was associated with better performance (Grady et al., 2003). The stimulation of several areas is important for rehabilitation efforts since it may suggest a global adaptation to the disease process rather than a task-specific one. However, when a different form of memory task was used in a similar study, people with Alzheimer's disease were found to recruit the same brain regions as healthy older adults but to a larger extent, rather than using new brain regions (Gould et al., 2006). The activation patterns of those with Alzheimer's disease completing a memory task were the same as those of healthy older adults performing a more difficult version of the same task.

These differences in findings highlight the complexity of the underlying mechanisms at play in brain plasticity. Different types of demands on the brain of a person with Alzheimer's disease may result in a variety of compensatory mechanisms. Additionally, although increased activation occurs during cognitive tasks in people with dementia, several brain regions such as the hippocampus experience a decrease in activation as the disease progresses (Masdeu, Zubieta, & Arbizu, 2005). Therefore, an optimal time window may exist for implementation of effective rehabilitative interventions.

Summary of Theoretical Support

In summary, the theoretical basis for cognitive rehabilitation has support in the research literature. Due to advances in technology we will continue to broaden our understanding of how the brains of people with Alzheimer's disease can combat its degenerative effects, and to what extent. The concept of cognitive reserve offers an explanation for the variety of clinical manifestations of dementia in individuals with similar brain pathology, and the continued discovery of the components that enhance this reserve will enable the development of effective interventions. Brain plasticity is an important component as well, since research supports the existence of a dynamic process of reorganization in the brains of those with dementia when confronted with a cognitive demand such as a memory task. The presence of this plasticity supports the use of rehabilitation as a potentially beneficial component to the treatment of neurological diseases (Duffau, 2006).

Clinical Application of Cognitive Rehabilitation

Rehabilitation refers to a process occurring within the disabled person, rather than something imposed externally, during which the individual gains and uses the knowledge and skills necessary for optimal physical, psychological, and social functioning (McLellan, 1991). As a rehabilitation program, cognitive rehabilitation encompasses a variety of techniques that may be employed to improve function through collaborative effort, in this case cognitive function such as attention or memory. Interventions depend upon individual client goals, involve families and caregivers in the process, and embrace a pragmatic approach to caring for those with cognitive deficits (Clare, 2008; Wilson, 2008).

Techniques employed within a cognitive rehabilitation program either attempt to utilize intact cognitive abilities to the greatest extent possible or use compensatory aids and strategies to reduce the demand on memory (Clare, 2003). Components may include, but are not limited to, techniques such as spaced retrieval, mnemonics, errorless learning, and external memory aids. Although the methods used vary, the individualization of the intervention to address the difficulties most relevant to the person with dementia is the hallmark of cognitive rehabilitation. Interventions may include several of these components, or they may use other techniques that are thought to be beneficial in addressing the individual's goals. For example, cognitive rehabilitation programs for older adults with mild cognitive impairment or dementia have included addressing empowerment issues (Nomura et al., 2009) as well as self-assertiveness training and stress management (Kurz et al., 2009). A review of the most common techniques used with PWD within a cognitive rehabilitation framework is presented, along with a discussion of applying the principles of rehabilitation to a cognitive intervention and including caregivers as targets of the intervention.

Common Techniques

Spaced Retrieval
Spaced retrieval is a technique whereby information is learned and then repetitively recalled over increasing periods of time (Hawley, 2008). For example, if someone has trouble recalling a loved one's name, they gradually attempt to learn and recall the information over a longer and longer time frame. First, they would be taught the name. Next, they would attempt to recall it after 5 seconds, after 10 seconds, and so on. If successful, the

time between recall attempts is lengthened, gradually expanding to long retention intervals during which the subject is distracted from the task at hand through conversation or other methods in order to increase the difficulty level.

Errorless Learning

Errorless learning is not one specific technique, but rather a principle used during the learning process in order to prevent errors and promote the acquisition of correct information on every trial, rather than using a trial-and-error approach that encourages guessing (Clare & Jones, 2008). This is accomplished by breaking the task into small steps, providing necessary guidance prior to task performance, encouraging the participant to avoid guessing, correcting errors immediately, and/or using cues (Sohlberg, 2005). Cues may be provided with either decreasing or increasing assistance (Clare, 2008). For example, when attempting to learn a face-name association, an individual may be shown a photograph and first asked to remember the name when shown the full name minus one letter, then when given the name minus two letters, and so on. (decreasing assistance or vanishing/fading cues). Alternatively, a portion of the name could be given initially, and then a letter added every few seconds if the participant is not able to remember, until he or she successfully completes the task (increasing assistance). Errorless learning may be most beneficial for people with more extensive cognitive impairment (Clare & Jones, 2008; Metzler-Baddeley & Snowden, 2005), and learning conditions that require more effort, rather than less, may be more beneficial in early-stage dementia (Dunn & Clare, 2007).

Mnemonics

Mnemonics, or mnemonic devices, are a variety of strategies used to help clients remember a piece of information. For example, associating an individual's face with another person by the same name that you are able to remember, or pairing a piece of information with a mental visual cue. Similar techniques may be used along with spaced retrieval and other methods to provide additional memory support. Additionally, external memory aids such as a memory notebook to remember daily activities or an alarm as a reminder to take a medication may be used as a primary cognitive rehabilitation strategy or more likely as one component of a program (Robert, Gelinas, & Mazer, 2009; Schmitter-Edgecombe, 2008).

Application of a Rehabilitative Framework

In order to achieve goals that improve everyday problems, the person with dementia and his or her support network must be involved in identifying both priorities and objectives of the intervention. The collaborative process identifies the most relevant difficulties for the client and his or her family members based on the impact of cognitive change in their daily life, and strategies are developed that consider the client's functional abilities, social context, and emotional responses (Woods & Clare, 2008). The cognitive rehabilitation process is not static, but rather evolves with both the degenerative aspect of dementia and the client's needs over time.

Considering the degenerative nature of the dementia process, it should be determined whether a significant improvement in cognitive function over time is a realistic goal for these individuals (Ávila, Carvalho, Bottino, & Miotto, 2007). Although the plasticity of the brain may allow for a certain level of compensation under optimal conditions, the activation of these mechanisms is not completely understood. Regenerative or compensatory mechanisms of brain function may be limited during the course of progressive brain damage caused by the underlying pathology of advanced Alzheimer's disease or other forms of dementia. Maintenance of functional ability when possible and improvement in perceived quality of life may be more realistic objectives (Boccardi & Frisoni, 2006; Ford, 1996), but still extremely important goals for individuals living with dementia and their loved ones. Particularly in individuals with an advanced stage of dementia, improvement of social interaction, mood, and overall well-being may be the most appropriate goals (Boccardi & Frisoni, 2006). Ethical issues should be considered as well; orientation to reality may be painful for a person with dementia, and coping mechanisms may be impaired as a result of the disease process. All of these considerations highlight the importance of collaborative goal identification and the personalization of cognitive rehabilitation based on each individual's current functional status and needs.

Caregivers as Intervention Recipients

Relatives and caregivers of PWD are often included in cognitive rehabilitation interventions, and they may be corecipients of the intervention, such as improving their coping skills (Onor et al., 2007). The collaborative nature of these interventions provides a prime opportunity for tailoring a program to meet both the needs of the person with dementia and his or her family caregiver, which would ideally improve the overall experience of what is commonly referred to as the *caregiving dyad*. Intervention components for family caregivers may involve counseling programs and group sessions as an adjunct to cognitive rehabilitation for the person with dementia. Such programs can educate the caregivers about the disease process and accompanying behaviors, identify social and support resources, and improve coping skills (Nomura et al., 2009; Onor et al., 2007).

Evidence of the Effectiveness of Cognitive Rehabilitation

In order to explore the full body of evidence as it relates to the care of older adults, efficacy research regarding its use in healthy elders, those with mild cognitive impairment, and PWD will be reviewed in this section.

Efficacy in Healthy Older Adults

The potential effectiveness of cognitive rehabilitation to improve or maintain memory performance in older adults experiencing normal, age-related cognitive changes may delay dementia onset or even prevent its occurrence. However, research in this area is somewhat limited at present. A systematic review of all randomized controlled trials of cognitive interventions for healthy older adults found no evidence of delayed or slowed progression to AD, but the limitations of existing research were identified as a problem in the scientific literature (Papp, Walsh, & Snyder, 2009). It has been demonstrated that cognitive rehabilitation, when implemented with older adults with normal cognitive decline, may result in improved memory performance, goal management, and psychosocial status, which includes overall well-being, happiness, coping strategies, and quality of life (Winocur, Craik et al., 2007; Winocur, Palmer et al., 2007). Although research on the use of cognitive rehabilitation specifically as a cognition-based intervention is limited at this point, it does show enough promise to justify future research into its use in prevention or slowing of mild cognitive impairment or dementia.

Efficacy in Mild Cognitive Impairment

Cognitive rehabilitation interventions for older adults with mild cognitive impairment (MCI) have demonstrated improvement in a variety of outcomes. A review of therapies used in MCI treatment identified several approaches that may be of benefit, including mnemonics, spaced retrieval, vanishing cues, and errorless learning (Peters & Winocur, 2006), all of which can be used within a rehabilitation program. When an established cognitive rehabilitation intervention originally used in traumatic brain injury was implemented in people with MCI, subjects demonstrated improvement in cognition, occupational performance, and quality of life (Londos et al., 2008). In another study, individuals with MCI were compared to those with early-stage AD (Kurz et al., 2009). The MCI group exhibited significantly improved mood, activities of daily living, and episodic memory, while the gains in the AD group were nonsignificant (Kurz et al., 2009). Similar benefits in people with MCI, including improvements in everyday memory and use of memory strategies, have also been demonstrated (Kinsella et al., 2009). In addition to demonstrated improvements on rehabilitative goals, one case study of cognitive rehabilitation use in MCI found changes in brain activation on fMRI consistent with decreases in sensory activation and increases in memory-related activation after the intervention (Clare et al., 2009). Considering the possibility that MCI may be an early stage of AD (Petersen et al., 2006), positive outcomes within this population are important to consider along the continuum of dementia care.

Efficacy in People with Dementia

A 2001 comprehensive review of the literature found that memory rehabilitation for people with Alzheimer's disease has the potential to be both clinically effective and useful to the person with dementia (De Vreese, 2001). Subsequently, a 2003 systematic review (updated in 2006) that evaluated the effectiveness of cognitive rehabilitation interventions for people with early-stage Alzheimer's disease or vascular dementia found no randomized controlled trials (RCTs) of individualized cognitive rehabilitation (Clare, Woods et al., 2003). However, the authors' review of the available evidence found possible benefits in learning, development of compensatory strategies, enhanced functional skills, and goal attainment for PWD.

Not All Cognitive Rehabilitation Is Alike

Due to the confusion in the use of the terms *cognitive training, cognitive stimulation*, and *cognitive rehabilitation*, research that is labeled cognitive rehabilitation in the literature may in fact not meet criteria to be correctly designated as such (Galante, Venturini, & Fiaccadori, 2007; Rozzini, 2007). This is seen most notably in the lack of personally tailored interventions or goals that are most relevant to the person with dementia. It is important to consider the actual aspects of the intervention implemented when reviewing research findings. When rehabilitation programs have been tailored to address the individualized goals of people with dementia (such as remembering the names of people in their social group, alleviating repetitive questioning of family caregivers, or improving occupational performance in household tasks), significant improvements in those areas have been found in several case studies (Clare et al., 2000; Clare, Wilson, Carter, & Hodges, 2003; Clare, Wilson, Carter, Hodges, & Adams, 2001). These gains may be maintained to higher-than-baseline levels after discontinuation of the interventions for as long as 2 years (Clare et al., 2001). Spaced retrieval and errorless learning, when used together and tailored to the identified needs of the person with dementia, were successful in helping subjects to relearn previously forgotten instrumental activities of daily living, hence potentially increasing autonomy (Thivierge, Simard, Jean, & Grandmaison, 2008). Incorporation of a memory notebook and alarm in order to minimize daily memory difficulties decreased the instances of memory failures and improved engagement in everyday activities for people with dementia; these measures also decreased depressive symptoms, anxiety, and stress in their caregivers (Bottino, 2005; Schmitter-Edgecombe, 2008). Rehabilitation programs conducted on an individual basis may be more effective at improving activities of daily living (Ávila et al., 2007), while those conducted on a group basis may be better suited to reducing anxiety, depression, and behavioral symptoms (Ávila et al., 2007; Onor et al., 2007).

Awareness as a Contributing Factor

Another potential contributor to the effectiveness of cognitive rehabilitation is the awareness of cognitive impairments in PWD. Personal awareness of cognitive deficits may be important to the success of the intervention, and alternatively, lack of awareness may limit cognitive rehabilitation effectiveness or eliminate consideration of the intervention for the individual at that time (Akhtar, Moulin, & Bowie, 2006; Clare, Wilson, Carter, Roth, & Hodges, 2004; Hardy, Oyebode, & Clare, 2006). Considering the importance of collaboration throughout the rehabilitation process, individuals who are unaware of their cognitive impairments or deny their existence are limited in their ability to participate in the intervention. Alternative cognition-based interventions or a modification of the typical cognitive rehabilitation approach may be more appropriate in these cases.

Combination with Pharmacological Therapy

Comprehensive dementia treatment is often a combination of both pharmacological and nonpharmacological approaches. Cognitive rehabilitation is an intervention that may be easily applied alone or in conjunction with pharmacological therapy. When acetyl-cholinesterase inhibitors (AChE-I) were used concurrently with cognitive rehabilitation, improvement in targeted areas was the same as that attained in those who received cognitive rehabilitation alone (Clare, Wilson, Carter, Roth, & Hodges, 2002). For Alzheimer's disease patients on stable doses of AChE-I, it has been found that a cognitive rehabilitation program produced improvements in face-name association, orientation, processing speed, and specific functional abilities (Loewenstein & Acevedo, 2006). These gains were maintained over time, even after the discontinuation of the cognitive rehabilitation intervention. Additionally, when AChE-I treatment alone was compared to AChE-I treatment plus cognitive rehabilitation, both cognitive and neuropsychological test scores improved significantly in addition to a nonsignificant reduction of psychiatric symptoms as reported by caregivers (Bottino, 2005). Therefore, rehabilitation may be an important supplement to pharmacological therapy that offers additional benefits beyond what is provided by medication alone. Indeed, improvements in targeted areas as identified by the person with dementia may provide significant, noticeable benefits that are directly related to daily activities.

Nursing Implications

Cognitive rehabilitation has been studied almost entirely within the field of psychology. Nursing has largely failed to embrace its potential as a nursing intervention, but limited research has considered the contribution of nurses within a cognitive rehabilitation program. Community nurses have demonstrated some use of memory strategies (Cross, Broomfield, Davies, & Evans, 2008), and the use of interdisciplinary teams that include nurses has been recommended for cognitive rehabilitation programs (Garrison, Ringholz, & Lindeman, 2000; Moniz-Cook, 2008; Raggi, 2007). Nurses are strategically poised to help develop, implement, and evaluate these programs, and hence, potentially to improve outcomes for PWD. It is therefore crucial that nurses become more involved in the implementation of cognitive rehabilitation for persons with dementia.

Applying the Nursing Process

The nursing process (assessment, diagnosis, planning, implementation, evaluation) is highly applicable to cognitive rehabilitation; it is both person-centered and goal-oriented, both of which are key components of the intervention. Functional assessment, including ability to perform ADLs, is a frequent baseline measure, used both to determine target areas and to evaluate progress (Bottino, 2005; Moniz-Cook, 2008; Talassi, Guerreschi, Feriani, Bianchetti, & Trabucchim, 2007; Thivierge et al., 2008). Assessment of cognitive status, such as the Mini-Mental Status Exam (Folstein, Folstein, & McHugh, 1975), also contributes to intervention planning and evaluation (Ávila et al., 2007; Dunn & Clare, 2007; Nomura et al., 2009; Souchay, 2008). Nurses commonly conduct these assessments, particularly in regard to PWD, and can use this data to begin tailoring a cognitive rehabilitation intervention. Additional cognitive rehabilitation criteria that are common in nursing assessments are risk for falls (Garrison et al., 2000), depression screening (Onor et al., 2007; Woods, 1996), and measurements of caregiver burden (Bucks et al., 2002; Farina et al., 2006).

Any number of nursing diagnoses may be appropriate, including chronic confusion, impaired memory, or self-care deficit, as well as caregiver role strain or compromised coping when including family members in the intervention (NANDA, 2008). Due to the personalized nature of the intervention (targeting personally relevant everyday problems), nursing diagnoses will be highly variable depending upon each person's needs. Planning and implementation of interventions may be conducted by nurses, or it may be a collaborative process with other members of the healthcare team, including psychologists and social services. Increasing participation and engagement in life activities, rather than reducing impairment itself, is a worthwhile goal (Wade, 2005), especially in those with more advanced dementia. The usefulness of the intervention for rehabilitation nurses or nurses working in memory clinics is a particularly important consideration. Evaluation of program effectiveness is ongoing and is vital to modifying the intervention as cognitive abilities progressively decline.

Use in Nursing Practice

Cognitive rehabilitation can be an important tool for all nurses who work with older adults, particularly those with early-stage dementia. Most likely settings for implementation include outpatient psychiatric programs, memory clinics, or even long-term care facilities. Programs generally include education about memory processes and dementia, formal practice of cognitive exercises targeted to individual goals, instruction for implementing techniques in daily life, and support for caregivers. Although formal practice over a set period of time, such as biweekly sessions for several months, is an important component, the intervention requires continual practice by the client and caregiver at home as well. Clients should be provided with more than a training program; instead, they should be given a variety of memory strategies that will serve them in a variety of contexts. Implementation of a cognitive rehabilitation program in nursing practice is guided by an intervention protocol described by Moniz-Cook (2008) that was used in memory clinics.

Assessment

In the current framework for applying cognitive rehabilitation (Moniz-Cook, 2008), the intervention is considered psychological treatment; a trained psychologist conducts the session while a nurse assists as an interviewer. However, the suggested tool for qualitative assessment of the client and caregiver is similarly applicable to professional nurses. The Hull memory clinical protocol includes assessment of several domains: cognitive function, behavioral changes, and memory concerns; personality, self-role identity, and coping style; mood; and carer characteristics (Agar, Moniz-Cook, Elston, Orbell, & Wang, 1997; Moniz-Cook, 2008; Teri et al., 1992). Although this protocol includes assessment based on tests not within nursing practice, each of these domains can be similarly assessed with instruments used within nursing. Although a thorough discussion of available tools is beyond the scope of this chapter, the Hartford Institute for Geriatric Nursing offers extensive resources in their Try This series, including assessment instruments and demonstrations of their use (Hartford Institute for Geriatric Nursing, 2009).

Education

Education of clients and caregivers should begin with describing the dementia process and how memory is affected. A dementia diagnosis is, understandably, quite terrifying. Providing a safe place where questions can be answered and disease progression discussed is essential to the foundation of the collaborative care process. Programs may be group-based and follow a prescribed outline of educational material, or they may be individual, based on each client's needs. Some individuals may embrace the opportunity to meet with a group and share a common experience, while others may prefer to maintain their privacy. These distinctions are based on clinical judgment as well as facility resources and agenda.

Before beginning any protocol of cognition-focused strategies or techniques, education about their content and use must also be provided. Due to the collaborative component of cognitive rehabilitation, clients will not simply be recipients of the intervention, but rather active participants in a team process. This process itself should also be well described to clients and caregivers in order to facilitate participation and success.

Goal-Setting

Participants will be asked to work with the nurse to identify personal goals that are applicable to their everyday lives. Overcoming practical difficulties of cognitive impairment, increasing participation in social activities, promoting adaptive behavior, supporting the coping abilities of both the person with dementia and his or her caregivers, reversing excess disability, alleviating depression or anxiety, and supporting personal identity are all potential goals of treatment that can be addressed through personally tailored nursing interventions. It is important, however, to be specific when goal-planning. There should be no expectation that achievement of a goal would, as a result, positively influence cognition overall or lead to generalized improvement in other functional areas. Goals may relate to remembering names of friends in a social group, managing a calendar of daily activities, or alleviating repetitive questioning of a caregiver. Desired outcomes should also be attainable; a reduction in memory failures, for example, may be more appropriate than their elimination.

Specific Strategies and Techniques
Development of cognitive rehabilitation program strategies may draw on a variety of methods, some of which have been discussed in this chapter, such as errorless learning or mnemonics. This rehabilitative approach is a pragmatic one; in other words, it employs what is needed for each person. The caregiving dyad implements these techniques or strategies together, although with guidance from the nurse. Options, based on identified goals, may include the use of verbal and visual cues in conversation and daily tasks, improving retained memory skills through the use of techniques such as spaced retrieval, or using memory aids such as notebooks, calendars, and alarms (Moniz-Cook, 2008; Schmitter-Edgecombe, 2008). The nurse may also suggest additional resources such as support groups in order to meet the identified needs of the client and caregiver. Although some intervention components are applicable to nursing practice directly, others may be collaborative efforts among members of the healthcare team or may require a referral for services. The following is recommended for consideration within a holistic approach to cognitive rehabilitation (Moniz-Cook, 2008):

- Problem-solving and practical coping needs
- Sustained social and emotional support services for clients and caregivers, either in groups or individually
- Counseling or cognitive therapy for mood disorders and emotional distress (clients and caregivers)
- Arrangements for discussion with others experiencing cognitive impairment
- Evaluation and enhancement of vulnerable family systems

Future Research

Although the emerging use of cognitive rehabilitation for people with dementia appears promising, further research is necessary in order to develop the intervention as well as to test its effectiveness. In addition to the need for randomized controlled trials (Clare, Woods et al., 2003), longitudinal data regarding its effectiveness over time and ability to halt or slow the progression of underlying pathology is essential (Kurz et al., 2009). Such research could potentially support its use as an intervention that preserves functional ability, delays dementia onset, and therefore decreases healthcare costs. There is a noticeable void in the evidence regarding its potential use in long-term care facilities. Both the feasibility and effectiveness of cognitive rehabilitation programs in institutional environments is particularly important since many people with dementia will eventually require placement in these facilities. Its usefulness for people with more advanced dementia has also been largely unexplored. Additional areas of future development in research and practice that have been identified are coordination of dementia management networks to facilitate use of the intervention (Moniz-Cook, 2008), the effectiveness of specific techniques when used individually (Clare, 2003), and the development of standardized programs with multidisciplinary teams (Onor et al., 2007).

In summary, cognitive rehabilitation is an intervention that has, as yet, not been thoroughly researched and lacks an extensive empirical basis. However, evidence from non- and quasi-experimental studies is intriguing and provides support for further scientific inquiry in this area. Overall, findings are cautiously positive (Clare, Woods et al., 2003). At its core, cognitive rehabilitation is the translation of person-centered care into rehabilitation practice for people with dementia. Nurses, although traditionally utilized as support staff within cognitive rehabilitation programs, possess the knowledge and skills to effectively implement the intervention, and should therefore consider its use in their own practice.

References

Agar, S., Moniz-Cook, E.D., Elston, C., Orbell, S., & Wang, M. (1997). Measuring the outcome of psychosocial interventions for family caregivers of dementia sufferers: A factor analytical model. *Aging and Mental Health, 1,* 166–175.

Akhtar, S., Moulin, C.J.A., & Bowie, P.C.W. (2006). Are people with mild cognitive impairment aware of the benefits of errorless learning? *Neuropsychological Rehabilitation, 16*(3), 329–346.

Alzheimer's Association. (2009). *2009 Alzheimer's disease facts and figures.* Retrieved from http://www.alz.org/national/documents/report_alzfactsfigures2009.pdf

Alzheimer's Association, & National Alliance for Caregiving. (2004). *Families care: Alzheimer's caregiving in the United States 2004.* Retrieved from http://www.alz.org/national/documents/report_familiescare.pdf

American Academy of Neurology. (2001). *Detection, diagnosis and management of dementia.* Retrieved from http://www.aan.com/professionals/practice/pdfs/dementia_guideline.pdf

American Psychiatric Association. (1994). *Diagnostic and statistical manual of mental disorders* (4th ed.). Washington, D. C.: American Psychiatric Association.

Ávila, R., Carvalho, I. A.M., Bottino, C.M.C., & Miotto, E.C. (2007). Neuropsychological rehabilitation in mild and moderate Alzheimer's disease patients. *Behavioural Neurology, 18*(4), 225–233.

Bach-y-Rita, P. (2003). Theoretical basis for brain plasticity after a TBI. *Brain Injury, 17*(8), 643–651.

Ball, K., Berch, D.B., Helmers, K.F., Jobe, J.B., Leveck, M.D., Marsiske, M., et al. (2002). Effects of cognitive training interventions with older adults: a randomized controlled trial. *JAMA, 288*(18), 2271–2281.

Boccardi, M., & Frisoni, G. B. (2006). Cognitive rehabilitation for severe dementia: Critical observations for better use of existing knowledge. *Mechanisms of Ageing and Development, 127*(2), 166–172.

Bottino, C. M. C. (2005). Cognitive rehabilitation combined with drug treatment in Alzheimer's disease patients: A pilot study. *Clinical Rehabilitation, 19*(8), 861–869.

Buckner, R. (2004). Memory and executive function in aging and AD: Multiple factors that cause decline and reserve factors that compensate. *Neuron, 44*(1), 195–208.

Bucks, R.S., Byrne, L., Haworth, J., Wilcock, G., Hyde, J., Emmerson, C., & Spaull, D. (2002). Interventions in Alzheimer's disease. *International Journal of Geriatric Psychiatry, 17*(5), 492–493.

Calero-García, M. D., Navarro-González, E. & Muñoz-Manzano, L. (2007). Influence of level of activity on cognitive performance and cognitive plasticity in elderly persons. *Archives of Gerontology and Geriatrics, 45*(3), 307–318.

Cappa, S. (2008). Rehabilitation of cognitive disorders. In S. Cappa, J. Abutalebi, J.F. Demonet, P. Fletcher, & P. Garrard (Eds.), *Cognitive neurology: A clinical textbook* (pp. 499–505). New York: Oxford University Press.

Clare, L. (2003). Cognitive training and cognitive rehabilitation for people with early-stage dementia. *Reviews in Clinical Gerontology, 13*(1), 75–83.

Clare, L. (2005). Cognitive rehabilitation in early-stage dementia: Evidence, practice and future directions. In P.W. Halligan & D.T. Wade (Eds.), *Effectiveness of Rehabilitation for Cognitive Deficits* Oxford: Oxford University Press, 327–336.

Clare, L. (Ed.). (2008). *Neuropsychological rehabilitation and people with dementia.* New York: Psychology Press.

Clare, L., & Jones, R. S. P. (2008). Errorless learning in the rehabilitation of memory impairment: A critical review. *Neuropsychology Review, 18*(1), 1–23.

Clare, L., van Paasschen, J., Evans, S.J., Parkinson, C., Woods, R.T., & Linden, D.E. (2009). Goal-oriented cognitive rehabilitation for an individual with mild cognitive impairment: Behavioural and neuroimaging outcomes. *Neurocase, 15*(4), 318–331.

Clare, L., Wilson, B., Carter, G., Breen, K., Gosses, A., & Hodges, J.R. (2000). Intervening with everyday memory problems in dementia of Alzheimer type: An errorless learning approach. *Journal of Clinical Experimental Neuropsychology, 22*(1), 132–146.

Clare, L., Wilson, B., Carter, G., & Hodges, J.R. (2003). Cognitive rehabilitation as a component of early intervention in Alzheimer's disease: A single case study. *Aging & Mental Health, 7*(1), 15–21.

Clare, L., Wilson, B., Carter, G., Hodges, J.R., & Adams, M. (2001). Long-term maintenance of treatment gains following a cognitive rehabilitation intervention in early dementia of Alzheimer type: A single case study. *Neuropsychological Rehabilitation, 11*(3–4), 477–494.

Clare, L., Wilson, B.A., Carter, G., Roth, I., & Hodges, J.R. (2002). Relearning face-name associations in early Alzheimer's disease. *Neuropsychology, 16*(4), 538–547.

Clare, L., Wilson, B., Carter, G., Roth, I., & Hodges, J.R. (2004). Awareness in early-stage Alzheimer's disease: Relationship to outcome of cognitive rehabilitation. *Journal of Clinical Experimental Neuropsychology, 26*(2), 215–226.

Clare, L., & Woods, B. (2001). Editorial: A role for cognitive rehabilitation in dementia care. *Neuropsychological Rehabilitation, 11*(3/4), 193–196.

Clare, L., Woods, R.T., Moniz-Cook, E.D., Orrell, M., & Spector, A. (2003). Cognitive rehabilitation and cognitive training for early-stage Alzheimer's disease and vascular dementia. *Cochrane Database of Systematic Reviews, 4*, CD003260.

Cross, S., Broomfield, N.M., Davies, R., & Evans, J.J. (2008). Awareness, knowledge and application of memory rehabilitation among community psychiatric nurses working with dementia. *Dementia, 7*(3), 383–395.

Cummings, J.L., & Mega, M.S. (2003). *Neuropsychiatry and behavioral neuroscience.* New York: Oxford University Press.

De Vreese, L. (2001). Memory rehabilitation in Alzheimer's disease: A review of progress. *International Journal of Geriatric Psychiatry, 16*(8), 794–809.

Duffau, H. (2006). Brain plasticity: From pathophysiological mechanisms to therapeutic applications. *Journal of Clinical Neuroscience, 13*(9), 885–897.

Dunn, J., & Clare, L. (2007). Learning face-name associations in early-stage dementia: Comparing the effects of errorless learning and effortful processing. *Neuropsychological Rehabilitation, 17*(6), 735–754.

Farina, E., Mantovani, F., Fioravanti, R., Pignatti, R., Chiavari, L., Imbornone, E., et al. (2006). Evaluating two group programmes of cognitive training in mild-to-moderate AD: Is there any difference between a 'global' stimulation and a 'cognitive-specific' one? *Aging & Mental Health*, *10*(3), 211–218.

Fernández-Ballesteros, R., & Fernández, B. (2005). Learning potential: A new method for assessing cognitive impairment. *International Psychogeriatrics, 17*(1), 119–128.

Folstein, M.F., Folstein, S.E., & McHugh, P.R. (1975). "Mini-mental state": A practical method for grading the cognitive state of patients for the clinician. *Journal of Psychiatric Research, 12*, 189–198.

Ford, S. (1996). Cognitive rehabilitation of patients with dementia: A review of the effectiveness of learning mnemonics. *International Journal of Rehabilitation & Health, 2*(4), 277–283.

Galante, E., Venturini, G., & Fiaccadori, C. (2007). Computer-based cognitive intervention for dementia: Preliminary results of a randomized clinical trial. *Giornale italiano di medicina del lavoro ed ergonomia, 29*(3 Suppl B), B26–B32.

Garrison, S.J., Ringholz, G.M., & Lindeman, J. (2000). Rehabilitation issues in patients with vascular dementia: Case studies with commentary. *Topics in Stroke Rehabilitation, 7*(3), 20–28.

Gould, R.L., Arroyo, B., Brown, R.G., Owen, A.M., Bullmore, E.T., & Howard, R.J. (2006). Brain mechanisms of successful compensation during learning in Alzheimer disease. *Neurology, 67*(6), 1011–1017.

Grady, C., McIntosh, A., Beig, S., Keightley, M., Burian, H., & Black, S. (2003). Evidence from functional neuroimaging of a compensatory prefrontal network in Alzheimer's disease. *The Journal of Neuroscience, 23*(3), 986–993.

Hall, C.B., Lipton, R.B., Sliwinski, M., Katz, M.J., Derby, C.A., & Verghese, J. (2009). Cognitive activities delay onset of memory decline in persons who develop dementia. *Neurology, 73*(5), 356–361.

Hardy, R., Oyebode, J., & Clare, L. (2006). Measuring awareness in people with mild to moderate Alzheimer's disease: Development of the memory awareness rating scale—adjusted. *Neuropsychological Rehabilitation, 16*(2), 178–193.

Hartford Institute for Geriatric Nursing (2009). *Assessment tools: Try this and how to try this resources.* Retrieved from http://consultgerirn.org/resources

Hawley, K. (2008). Memory interventions and quality of life for older adults with dementia. *Activities, Adaptation & Aging, 32*(2), 89–102.

Jankowsky, J.L., Melnikova, T., Fadale, D.J., Xu, G.M., Slunt, H.H., Gonzales, V., et al. (2005). Environmental enrichment mitigates cognitive deficits in a mouse model of Alzheimer's disease. *The Journal of Neuroscience, 25*(21), 5217–5224.

Jones, S., Nyberg, L., Sandblom, J., Neely, A.S., Ingvar, M., Petersson, K.M., et al. (2006). Cognitive and neural plasticity in aging: General and task-specific limitations. *Neuroscience and Biobehavioral Reviews, 30*, 864–871.

Kinsella, G.J., Mullaly, E., Rand, E., Ong, B., Burton, C., Price, S., et al. (2009). Early intervention for mild cognitive impairment: A randomised controlled trial. *Journal of Neurology, Neurosurgery and Psychiatry, 80*(7), 730–736.

Kurz, A., Pohl, C., Ramsenthaler, M., & Sorg, C. (2009). Cognitive rehabilitation in patients with mild cognitive impairment. *International Journal of Geriatric Psychiatry, 24*(2), 163–168.

Limke, T.L., & Rao, M. (2002). Neural stem cells in aging and disease. *Journal of Cellular and Molecular Medicine, 6*(4), 475–496.

Loewenstein, D., & Acevedo, A. (2006). Training of cognitive and functionally relevant skills in mild Alzheimer's disease: An integrated approach. In D.K. Attix & K.A. Bohmer (Eds.), *Geriatric neuropsychology assessment and intervention* (pp. 261–274). New York: Guilford Publications.

Londos, E., Boschian, K., Linden, A., Persson, C., Minthon, L., & Lexell, J. (2008). Effects of a goal-oriented rehabilitation program in mild cognitive impairment: A pilot study. *American Journal of Alzheimer's Disease & Other Dementias, 23*(2), 177–183.

Masdeu, J.C., Zubieta, J.L., & Arbizu, J. (2005). Neuroimaging as a marker of the onset and progression of Alzheimer's disease. *Journal of Neurological Science, 236*(1–2), 55–64.

Mateer, C.A. (2005). Fundamentals of cognitive rehabilitation. In P.W. Halligan & D.T. Wade (Eds.), *The effectiveness of rehabilitation for cognitive deficits.* New York: Oxford University Press.

Matsuda, O. (2007). Cognitive stimulation therapy for Alzheimer's disease: The effect of cognitive stimulation therapy on the progression of mild Alzheimer's disease in patients treated with donepezil. *International Psychogeriatrics, 19*(2), 241–252.

Mattson, M., Chan, S., & Duan, W. (2002). Modification of brain aging and neurodegenerative disorders by genes, diet, and behavior. *Physiological Reviews, 82*(3), 637–672.

McLellan, D.L. (1991). Functional recovery and the principles of disability medicine. In M. Swash & J. Oxbury (Eds.), *Clinical neurology.* London, UK: Churchill Livingstone.

Metzler-Baddeley, C., & Snowden, J.S. (2005). Brief report: Errorless versus errorful learning as a memory rehabilitation approach in Alzheimer's disease. *Journal of Clinical and Experimental Neuropsychology, 27*(8), 1070–1079.

Mimura, M., & Mimura, S.-i. (2007). Cognitive rehabilitation and cognitive training for mild dementia. *Psychogeriatrics, 7*(3), 137–143.

Moniz-Cook, E. (2008). Assessment and psychosocial intervention for older people with suspected dementia: A memory clinic perspective. In K. Laidlaw & B. Knight (Eds.), *Handbook of emotional disorders in later life: Assessment and treatment* (pp. 421–451). New York: Oxford University Press.

NANDA (2008). *NANDA nursing diagnoses: Definitions and classification, 2007–2008.* Philadelphia: North American Nursing Diagnosis Association.

Nomura, M., Makimoto, K., Kato, M., Shiba, T., Matsuura, C., Shigenobu, K., et al. (2009). Empowering older people with early dementia and family caregivers: A participatory action research study. *International Journal of Nursing Studies, 46*(4), 431.

Onor, M.L., Trevisiol, M., Negro, C., Signorini, A., Saina, M., & Aguglia, E. (2007). Impact of a multimodal rehabilitative intervention on demented patients and their caregivers. *American Journal of Alzheimer's Disease and Other Dementias, 22*(4), 261–272.

Papp, K.V., Walsh, S.J., & Snyder, P.J. (2009). Immediate and delayed effects of cognitive interventions in healthy elderly: A review of current literature and future directions. *Alzheimer's & Dementia, 5*(1), 50–60.

Pariente, J., Cole, S., Henson, R., Clare, L., Kennedy, A., Rossor, M., et al. (2005). Alzheimer's patients engage an alternative network during a memory task. *Annals of Neurology, 58*(6), 870–879.

Peters, K., & Winocur, G. (2006). Combined therapies in mild cognitive impairment. In H.A. Tuokko & D.F. Hultsch (Eds.), *Mild cognitive impairment: International perspectives* (pp. 265–287). New York: Taylor & Francis, Inc.

Petersen, R.C., Parisi, J.E., Dickson, D.W., Johnson, K.A., Knopman, D.S., Boeve, B.F., et al. (2006). Neuropathologic features of amnestic mild cognitive impairment. *Archives of Neurology, 63*(5), 665–672.

Raggi, A. (2007). The effects of a comprehensive rehabilitation program of Alzheimer's disease in a hospital setting. *Behavioural Neurology, 18*(1), 1–6.

Robert, A., Gelinas, I., & Mazer, B. (2009). Occupational therapists' use of cognitive interventions for clients with Alzheimer's disease. *Occupational Therapy International, 17*(1), 10-19.

Rocca, M.A., & Filippi, M. (2006). Functional MRI to study brain plasticity in clinical neurology. *Neurological Sciences, 27* (Suppl 1), S24–26.

Rozzini, L. (2007). Efficacy of cognitive rehabilitation in patients with mild cognitive impairment treated with cholinesterase inhibitors. *International Journal of Geriatric Psychiatry, 22*(4), 356–360.

Schmitter-Edgecombe, M. (2008). Multidyad memory notebook intervention for very mild dementia: A pilot study. *American Journal of Alzheimer's Disease and Other Dementias*, *23*(5), 477–487.

Sitzer, D.I., Twamley, E.W., & Jeste, D.V. (2006). Cognitive training in Alzheimer's disease: A meta-analysis of the literature. *Acta Psychiatrica Scandinavica*, *114*(2), 75–90.

Smith, G.E., Housen, P., Yaffe, K., Ruff, R., Kennison, R.F., Mahncke, H.W., et al. ((2009). A cognitive training program based on principles of brain plasticity: Results from the improvement in memory with plasticity-based adaptive cognitive training (IMPACT) study. *J. Am Geriatr Soc, 57*(4), 594–603.

Sohlberg, M. (2005). Instructional techniques in cognitive rehabilitation: A preliminary report. *Seminars in Speech and Language*, *26*(4), 268–279.

Souchay, C. (2008). Rehearsal strategy use in Alzheimer's disease. *Cognitive Neuropsychology*, *25*(6), 783–797.

Spector, A., Woods, B., & Orrell, M. (2008). Cognitive stimulation for the treatment of Alzheimer's disease. *Expert Review of Neurotherapeutics*, *8*(5), 751–757.

Stern, Y. (2003). The concept of cognitive reserve: A catalyst for research. *Journal of Clinical and Experimental Neuropsychology*, *25*(5), 589–593.

Stern, Y. (2006). Cognitive reserve and Alzheimer disease. *Alzheimer Disease and Associated Disorders*, *20*(2), 112–117.

Talassi, E., Guerreschi, M., Feriani, V., Bianchetti, A., & Trabucchim, M. (2007). Effectiveness of a cognitive rehabilitation program in mild dementia (MD) and mild cognitive impairment (MCI): A case control study. *Archives of Gerontology and Geriatrics*, *44*(1), 391–399.

Teri, L., Truax, P., Logdson, R., Uomoto, J., Zarit, S.H., & Vitaliano, P.P. (1992). Assessment of behavioral problems in dementia: The revised memory and behavioral problems checklist. *Psychology and Aging, 7*, 622–631.

Thivierge, S., Simard, M., Jean, L., & Grandmaison, E. (2008). Errorless learning and spaced retrieval techniques to relearn instrumental activities of daily living in mild Alzheimer's disease: A case report study. *Neuropsychiatric Disease and Treatment*, *4*(5), 987–999.

Wade, D.T. (2005). Applying the WHO ICF framework to the rehabilitation of patients with cognitive deficits. In P. W. Halligan & D. T. Wade (Eds.), *Effectiveness of rehabilitation for cognitive deficits*. Oxford: Oxford University Press.

Weimer, D., & Sager, M. (2009). Early identification and treatment of Alzheimer's disease: Social and fiscal outcomes. *Alzheimer's & Dementia, 5*(3), 215–226.

Whalley, L., Deary, I., Appleton, C., & Starr, J. (2004). Cognitive reserve and the neurobiology of cognitive aging. *Ageing Research Reviews*, *3*(4), 369–382.

Wilson, B. (2008). Neuropsychological rehabilitation. *Annual Review of Clinical Psychology*, *4*(1), 141–162.

Wilson, R., Mendes De Leon, C.F., Barnes, L., Schneider, J., Bienias, J., Evans, D., et al. (2002). Participation in cognitively stimulating activities and risk of incident Alzheimer disease. *The Journal of the American Medical Association, 287*(6), 742–748.

Winocur, G., Craik, F.I.M., Levine, B., Robertson, I., Binns, M., Alexander, M., et al. (2007). Cognitive rehabilitation in the elderly: Overview and future directions. *Journal of the International Neuropsychological Society*, *13*(1), 166–171.

Winocur, G., Palmer, H., Dawson, D., Binns, M., Bridges, K., & Stuss, D. (2007). Cognitive rehabilitation in the elderly: An evaluation of psychosocial factors. *Journal of the International Neuropsychological Society*, *13*(1), 153–165.

Woods, B. (1996). Cognitive approaches to the management of dementia. In R. G. Morris (Ed.), *The cognitive neuropsychology of Alzheimer-type dementia* (pp. 310–326). New York: Oxford University Press.

Woods, B., & Clare, L. (2008). Psychological interventions with people with dementia. In B. Woods & L. Clare (Eds.), *Handbook of the clinical psychology of ageing* (pp. 523–548). West Sussex, England: John Wiley & Sons, Ltd.

Woods, B., Spector, A., Prendergast, L., & Orrell, M. (2005). Cognitive stimulation to improve cognitive functioning in people with dementia. *Cochrane Database of Systematic Reviews, 4,* CD003260.

Woods, B., Thorgrimsen, L., Spector, A., Royan, L., & Orrell, M. (2006). Improved quality of life and cognitive stimulation therapy in dementia. *Aging & Mental Health, 10*(3), 219–226.

Yaffe, K., Fox, P., Newcomer, R., Sands, L., Lindquist, K., & Dane, K. (2002). Patient and caregiver characteristics and nursing home placement in patients with dementia. *Journal of the American Medical Association, 287,* 2090–2097.

Yu, F., Rose, K.M., Burgener, S.C., Cunningham, C., Buettner, L.L., Beattie, E., et al. (2009). Cognitive training for early-stage Alzheimer's disease and dementia. *Journal of Gerontological Nursing, 35*(3), 23–29.

Zarit, S.H., & Zarit, J.M. (Eds.). (2007). *Mental disorders in older adults: Fundamentals of assessment and treatment* (2nd ed.). New York: The Guilford Press.

Chapter 23

The Power of Connection

Nancy Richeson

A colleague Mike Brady and I taught a college course for older adults with early-stage dementia, titled *Health Promotion for the Mind, Body, and Spirit.* The class was offered through the University of Southern Maine's Osher Lifelong Learning Institute. The 12-week class was developed by Buettner & Fitzsimmons to provide people with mild memory loss a dignified and normalized adult education experience. The course provided engaging learning opportunities that focused on promoting healthy aging, even in this at-risk group. Life does not have to end when one is diagnosed with dementia; people can still learn, grow, connect, and contribute to society in meaningful ways.

I have learned this and much more from having the privilege of teaching this course. From the first day of class when the 14 students registered and were screened for cognitive status, depression, and self-efficacy, I knew I was about to touch something within the participants and within myself. That something was an opening of the hearts for both the students and the teachers, letting the other(s) in and helping each other remember that the purpose of life is to achieve a passionate and meaningful life. For me the class has brought me home, reminding me why I have chosen to teach.

Each week as the students walked into class I was flooded with stories, stories of their week, their life, their disease. Stories that addressed the shame and stigma of living with dementia. Stories that articulated fears and sadness about losing their memories, stories of joy and happiness of a life well lived. The shared stories transformed their experiences, helping them to feel their pain, confront their feelings, and cope with their lives. I witnessed how being in connection with others in an empathetic and compassionate way empowers individuals to grow, despite living with a progressive disease. Bearing witness for each other linked the participants to the shared humanity in the classroom. At times this was difficult for the participants and for me. One man commented in a letter he wrote to me, "It is depressing to see how the disease has progressed in others and to know where I am headed." Another participant, a former counselor, struggled with the stigma attached to the disease and was fearful of exposure, having people find out he was attending a class for people with memory loss. A retired professor wrote me a short essay highlighting his awareness of time, stating, "I am almost 25 years over the age of 65, born six days after Jack Kennedy (29 May, 1917) on 4 June 1917." His essay further reflected on his cognitive status; noticing his decline he writes, "I am having difficulty tying my bow tie if I think about it instead of thoughtlessly following a habit."

However, the majority of the participants, despite the pain of recognizing their losses, felt the need for a learning community. As one man, a retired minister, reminded us weekly, "We are in this together, we are not alone." One woman, a retired nurse, stated, "I still want to learn and be with people, even though I have dementia." Yet another woman, in a profound statement pointed out, "We are more alike than different." Yes, we are more alike than different. We all need meaningful connection that provides information and promotes growth throughout our lives. As Virginia Satir (1976, as cited in Intrator & Scribner, 2003) noted in her poem *Making Contact*, the greatest gift to receive and to give is to be seen, heard, and touched [*sic*], when this is done contact has been made (p. 123).

As a teacher with over 15 years of experience, I am grateful for the opportunity to teach this class and engage in a learning community with older adults with memory loss. Recently, I felt I have taken the learning process for granted, and I was looking for inspiration, a way to keep a vibrant heart; this class has encouraged me to continue my life's work. The gift of teaching has been rekindled by the opportunity to teach a group of older adults with memory loss, for I have witnessed courage, compassion, and hope—and for that I am grateful.

Reference

Intrator, S.M., & Scribner, M. (Eds.). (2003). *Teaching with fire.* Brainbridge Island, WA: Jossey-Bass.

Chapter 24

Linking Dental Care with General Health Care

An Opportunity for Nurse Leadership

Frederick J. Lacey and Lynne B. Lacey

Aging and Its Redefinition of Oral Health

For the first time in recorded history, more people in developed countries are over the age of sixty-five. This consequence of fertility decline and increased life expectancy can be attributed to advances in medicine, nutrition, and community health, along with awareness of and participation in individual wellness (United Nations Publications, 2004). In the United States, it is projected that twenty % of the population will be over the age of 65 by 2030. Notable increases in the population growth of oldest-old individuals (those 80 and older) are expected also, with the numbers of frail elderly Americans over the age of 80 comprising 7.3% of the world population. Increasingly the elderly population will become more diverse, reflecting changing demographics. In 2006, 30% of the US population identified itself as a specific ethnic group; black, Hispanic, Native American, or Asian (United States Department of Health and Human Services, 2009). As world populations age, the oral health profile of emergent frail elderly individuals, particularly Americans, is improving. Key factors in these changes include: (1) fluoridation, both municipal and in consumer product form; (2) advances in the quality of dental materials, technology, and procedures; (3) increases in the use of dental services; and (4) improved oral hygiene, leading to the retention of some or all of the natural teeth as people move into advanced age. While this phenomenon provides functional benefits, such as improved nutrition and increased masticatory efficiency, it also presents challenges, as the number of restored tooth surfaces rises and risk factors for root caries, periodontal disease, and oral cancers increase due to systemic and physical age-related changes. The need for preventive and restorative strategies that address the partial or reduced dentitions of the oldest old cannot be underestimated from the viewpoint of diet, nutrition, speech, resistance to systemic disease, pain, social isolation, and positive self-image (Anusavice, 2002; Vargas, Kramarow, & Yellowitz, 2001).

Older Americans will also experience changes in the oral mucosa and supporting structures of the oral cavity, which may be the result of medications, dysphagia (swallowing dysfunction), alveolar bone loss, or multiple disease sequelae (Gooch, Malvitz, Griffin, & Maas, 2005). The cumulative effects of physical, cognitive, and functional limitations may force elders into an institutional or homebound situation with increased need for assistance with (oral) activities of daily living (ADL) such as tooth brushing and eating (Stein & Henry, 2009). Younger, healthier seniors will be able to function independently, living in the community with sufficient support and resources to maintain their physical and oral health. Others will live with chronic health conditions and insufficient resources, making it difficult to obtain dental care in any setting other than an emergency one (Bailey, Gueldner, Ledikwe, & Smiciklas-Wright, 2005). Additionally, oral health care for elders will be increasingly experienced in a competitive system divided by public and private interests. Off-site delivery of dental treatment and private reimbursement create social and economic barriers to care. The emerging complexity of oral care and its relationship to overall health also requires a change in the attitudes and knowledge of elders about the necessity of preventive dental care in the absence of pain. Many of the most common oral diseases, while difficult to treat in the frail elderly and oldest old populations, may be preventable with intervention.

Meeting the Need

Meeting the oral health care needs of elders residing in long–term care (LTC) facilities and homebound situations has a number of dimensions to take into account. Caregivers who wish to implement preventive and treatment options must consider the physical or cognitive limitations of elders. These limitations may make it difficult if not impossible for elders to obtain services in private dental offices. Data from the US Department of Health and Human Services 2008 Chartbook determined that 22% of individuals over the age of 74 had reduced visual acuity even with glasses or contact lenses, and 16% had difficulty hearing or were deaf. Oral pain, diminished psychomotor capacity, and physical impairment were other impediments that kept elders out of the dental office (Clark, 2005; United States Department of Health & Human Services, 2009). Informed consent, transportation, economic, and guardianship issues often become so overwhelming that elders or their families choose to forego dental treatment, complicating future treatment. At issue also is the absence of adequate training of nondental caregivers in oral health information, inappropriate use of or no available oral health supplies, lack of care planning, minimal supervision of caregivers, and oral health intervention documentation discrepancies (Coleman & Watson, 2005).

Nurse Leadership in Oral Health

Nurses who manage and monitor the oral healthcare interventions of vulnerable elders are in a unique position to provide the leadership needed to form oral health partnerships with dental professionals. Through interprofessional education, healthcare professionals can work collaboratively to share knowledge and skills that advance oral and general health outcomes and promote oral health as a valued part of healthy aging (Coleman, 2004a, 2005; Gooch, Malvitz, Griffin, & Maas, 2005; Fellona & DeVore, 1999). Improvements in the quality of oral health interventions require an understanding of:

- Risk factors that contribute to poor oral health.

- The use of oral health assessment tools that clearly define the preventive and treatment needs of vulnerable elders.

- Optimal oral health interventions based on individual oral health assessment, practices based on sound scientific evidence, access to oral hygiene therapeutics and equipment, and educative and supportive customization of interventions.

In addition, educating beyond the caregiver's beliefs, knowledge, and attitudes related to oral health will ensure that people in their care are treated with respect and dignity as human beings, even in the presence of compromised oral health (Jablonski, Munro, Grap, Schubert, Ligon & Spigelmyer, 2008)

Literature Review

Fitzpatrick's (2000) literature review of health practices in the United Kingdom pointed to the variability and inadequacy of oral care in LTC settings.

Gaps in the oral health knowledge base of nurses and other caregivers, the lack of oral hygiene supplies with which to provide care, and heavy workloads placed oral care in low priority. A study of oral care provided by certified nursing assistants (CNAs) in several upstate New York nursing homes determined that adherence to basic oral care standards was low, contrasting markedly with caregivers' self-reported standards of practice (Coleman & Watson, 2005). The Boczko, McKeon and Sturkie (2009) study of American LTC facilities found that the problem of inadequate or nonexistent delivery of oral care persists, with nurses' knowledge of dental caries, periodontal disease, oral cancer, medication, and systemic disease effects on the oral cavity incomplete. Confusion about the efficacy of oral hygiene products and equipment available to elders to perform self-care, or to caregivers who provide oral care for elders under their care, was also evident. These studies and others indicate that while standards for oral care in LTC facilities exist, implementation is uncertain and caregiver training is inadequate (Coleman, 2004b); Hardy, Darby, Leinbach, & Welliver, 2004; Munro & Grap, 2004; Munro, Grap, Jablonski, & Boyle, 2006; Stein & Henry, 2009; Terpenning, 2005; Jablonski, et al, 2008). The oral care of homebound individuals, as well as standards for home health care (HHC) agencies and hospice, has not been well studied. In the United States, agencies receiving federal or state funding must provide caregiver training in personal hygiene and grooming that includes oral hygiene. However, these situations do not require an oral health assessment as part of the nursing assessment. Likewise, federal guidelines offer little information about oral hygiene care

- Use of fluoridated toothpaste that has been accepted by the American Dental Association Council on Dental Therapeutics.

- The effective removal of bacterial plaque using a soft manual or mechanical toothbrush, dental floss, or other interdental cleaning aids such as stimudents or interdental brushes. Oral irrigation may be used to loosen and remove food particles but is not a substitute for plaque removal.

- The use of fluoridated water for drinking and cooking. If municipally fluoridated water is unavailable, bottled water with fluoride should be used.

- Adoption of a healthy diet by reducing fermentable carbohydrate intake, especially between meals.

- Regularly scheduled professional preventive oral health care which includes:
  - Health history and medication review.
  - Updated dental and periodontal charting.
  - Oral cancer screening.
  - Professional oral prophylaxis.
  - Radiographs as prescribed by a dentist.
  - Comprehensive oral examination performed by a licensed dentist.
  - Individualized oral hygiene instruction.
  - Recare and treatment recommendations.

Adapted from: Glassman, et al. (2003). Practical protocols for the prevention of dental disease in community settings for people with special needs: the protocols, p. 161

Figure 24-1 Fundamental oral health care practices traditionally and widely accepted by dental health practitioners

standards or caregiver training competencies (Electronic Code of Federal Regulations, 2008). Medical respiratory, surgical trauma, and neurological intensive care units provide oral care; however, frequency and intervention standards vary widely (Munro & Grap, 2004).

Various protocols have been developed for use in providing oral health interventions to vulnerable populations. Interventions must be considered in terms of those that require a professional diagnosis, prescription, or application and those that do not. To date, there is insufficient evidence to determine a single best approach to oral care to those most vulnerable, since oral health assessment in LTC and HHC is not documented by dental professionals. Fundamental oral health practices that dental professionals are in agreement with were developed in 2003 for populations with special needs. These oral health practices could form the foundation from which specific interventions for vulnerable populations are developed. See Figure 24-1 (Glassman et al., 2003).

The Oral Health Assessment

The oral health assessment is a screening tool used to provide the baseline data needed to advocate and plan for oral health promotion strategies. Appropriate oral assessment criteria are used to identify risk factors for oral disease, individual oral health needs, an individual care plan, equipment needed to meet the care plan objectives, and the need to refer for treatment.

In the United States, federally mandated oral health assessments for elders entering LTC have shifted the responsibility for collection and assessment of baseline oral health information to nurses exclusively. In response, nurse administrators and educators have employed several types of oral health assessment tools within diverse clinical settings to determine which ones best improve the nurses' knowledge, skills, attitudes, and behaviors related to daily oral care. An assortment of tools to assess oral health are available at Best Practices in Nursing Care to Older Adults, a series provided by the Hartford Institute for Geriatric Nursing's Hartford Institute Web site, www.hartfordign.org, or its ConsultGeriRN website, www.ConsultGeriRN.org.

The Minimum Data Set 2.0 (MDS 2.0) developed and monitored by the federal government is the system in common usage for facilities receiving Medicare or Medicaid funding. An oral exam conducted by a licensed dentist or dental hygienist is not required for this initial resident assessment questionnaire. An article by Guay (2005) outlined suggested changes to the MDS 2.0 made by the American Dental Association (ADA) and Special Care Dentistry (SCD). These changes include an oral health quality indicator, which updates the dental content of the MDS to contain language more reflective of the oral health status of elders. The indicator would also provide the information needed to inform the process of assessment and subsequent care planning when used by LTC facility staff. Recommendations also included electronic linkage of the medical SNOMED (Systemized Nomenclature of Medicine) diagnostic coding system to the MDS 2.0 since it has the ADA-developed SNODENT (Systemized Nomenclature of Dentistry) comprehensive, dental diagnostic system embedded into its hierarchy. Codification of oral health status into the patient record would provide access to past medical and dental histories, medication profiles, and drug interactions.

Off-site diagnosis and delivery of dental services presents complications in responding adequately to institutional electronic record keeping. Medical management of oral care requires that data be reliably retrieved and aggregated as well as transmitted electronically and securely. Not all off-site dental offices are electronically capable. Many LTC facilities include weekly or monthly on-site dental visits in their provided services; however, it was found that only 10% of the LTC facilities have equipment available to provide treatment. Care delivered off-site is paid through private pay or third-party insurance. Medicare coverage is not available for off-site care unless the dental treatment is tied directly to alleviation of a medical condition (Pyle, Massie & Nelson, 1998; Pyle, Jasinevicius, Sawyer, & Madsen, 2005). Use of the MDS 2.0 as a short oral health assessment has appeal for ease

Resident's Name_____   Date_____

Examiners Name_____   Score_____

CATEGORY	MEASUREMENT	0	1	2
LYMPH NODES	Observe and feel nodes	No enlargement	Enlarged, not tender	Enlarged and tender
LIPS	Observe, feel tissue, ask resident, family or staff (Esp. primary caregiver)	Smooth, pink moist	Dry, chapped or red at corners*	White or red patch bleeding or ulcer for 2 weeks
TONGUE	Observe, feel tissue, ask resident, family or staff (Esp. primary caregiver)	Normal roughness, pink and moist	Coated, smooth, patchy, severely fissured or some redness	Red, smooth; white or red patch; ulcer for 2 weeks*
TISSUE INSIDE CHEEK, FLOOR, AND ROOF OF MOUTH	Observe, feel tissue, ask resident, family or staff (Esp. primary caregiver)	Pink and moist	Dry, shiny, rough, red or swollen*	White or red patch; bleeding hardness; ulcer for 2 weeks*
GUMS BETWEEN TEETH AND/OR UNDER ARTIFICIAL TEETH	Gently press gums with tip of tongue blade	Pink, small indentations; firm, smooth and pink under artificial teeth	Redness at border Around 1–6 teeth; one red area or sore spot under artificial teeth	Swollen or bleeding gums, redness at border around 7 or more teeth, loose teeth; generalized redness or sores around artificial teeth*
SALIVA (EFFECT ON TISSUE)	Touch tongue blade to center of tongue and floor of mouth	Tissues moist, saliva free flowing and watery	Tissues dry and sticky	Tissues parched and red, no saliva*
CONDITION OF NATURAL TEETH	Observe and count number of decay or broken teeth	No decayed or broken teeth or roots	1–3 decayed or broken teeth/roots*	4 or more decayed or broken teeth/roots; fewer than 4 teeth in either jaw*
CONDITION OF ARTIFICIAL TEETH	Observe and ask resident, family or staff (Esp. primary caregiver)	Unbroken teeth, worn most of the time	1 broken/missing tooth, or worn for eating or cosmetics only	More than one broken or missing tooth, or either denture missing or never worn
PAIRS OF TEETH IN CHEWING POSITION (Natural or Artificial)	Observe and count pairs of teeth in chewing position	12 or more pairs of teeth in chewing position	8–11 pairs of teeth in chewing position	0–7 pairs of teeth in chewing position

Figure 24-2 The Kayser Jones Brief Oral Health Status Examination (BOHSE)

CATEGORY	MEASUREMENT	0	1	2
ORAL CLEANLINESS	Observe appearance of teeth or dentures	Clean, no food particles/tartar in the mouth or on artificial teeth	Food particles/tartar in one or two places in the mouth or on artificial teeth	Food particles/tartar in most places in the mouth or on artificial teeth

Upper dentures labeled: Yes _____ No _____ None_____ Lower dentures labeled: Yes _____ No _____ None _____

Is your mouth comfortable? Yes _____ No _____ if no, explain:

Additional comments:

_____

Figure 24-2 (continued)

Source: Kayser-Jones, J., Bird, W.F., Paul, S.M., Long, L., & Schell, E.S. (1995). An instrument to assess the oral health status of nursing home residents. *The Gerontologist, 35*(6), 814–824. Figure 2, p. 823.
Copyright © The Gerontological Society of America. Reproduced by permission of the publisher.

of clinical usage and electronic integration; however, the reliability of its measurements is questionable due to the limited and vague number of categories reported on and the obsolete nature of the category descriptors. A recent pilot study addressed underreporting of oral health problems by nurses using the MDS 2.0 in skilled nursing facilities. Education sessions targeted to completion of the MDS 2.0 found that while there was no significant change in oral health knowledge, as measured by a pre- and posttest, nurses improved their thoroughness and congruency in completing the MDS 2.0 (Munoz, Touger-Decker, Byham-Gray, & Maillet, 2009).

The Kayser-Jones Brief Oral Health Status Examination (BOHSE) (Figure 24-2) has been tested and used in LTC, HHC, and various community settings since 1995. It has 79% to 83% test-retest reliability, and its dental content validity has been secured by five field experts (Kayser-Jones, Bird, Paul, Long & Schell, 1995). Screening measurements are taken in 10 head and neck categories, with oral health status graded from 0 to 2 in each category. High scoring reflects a higher number of problems identified. The screener is guided through each category using observation, palpation, and questioning skills. The BOHSE provides an easy-to-use and appropriate reference for screeners who do not have in-depth dental training. It includes where and what to ask about, look for, and palpate. Each category is then scored, based on visual oral descriptors. Nurses learning to evaluate oral health with the help of BOHSE will develop a usable knowledge base through repeated, simple matching and identification. With practice, nurses may expand their basic oral health assessment skills for use in referral or customization of care plans for elders.

Electronic interface and linkage of BOHSE into the SNOMED diagnostic coding system has not been studied since this assessment tool does not have the federally mandated universal usage that MDS 2.0 has. The Hartford Institute for Geriatric Nursing of New York University College of Nursing reviewed and recommended BOHSE for use in nursing education in its 2007 best nursing practices educational series (Chia-Hui Chen, 2007).

A third instrument used to evaluate the oral health of elders is the Oral Health Assessment Tool (OHAT) developed by Jane Chalmers for use in Australian Residential Care Centers (Chalmers, King, Spencer, Wright, & Carter, 2005). Similar to the BOHSE, it guides nurses through eight head and neck categories using observation, palpation, and questioning skills with grading from 0 to 2. The OHAT reliability and validity have been tested with the cognitively impaired. In Canada, its use as a training tool has improved nurse accuracy in completing the required Canadian MDS 2.0 for residential and long-term care. The OHAT also has a companion oral healthcare planning tool that is used extensively in Canada (van der Horst & Scott, 2009).

While the burden of oral assessment, oral care, and referral for treatment has fallen primarily upon nurses, the dental profession must take responsibility for broadening its understanding of the institutional structures in which nurses perform their work. Oral assessment and caregiver training should not be developed and implemented in a nursing/medical vacuum; it must include consultative and informational cooperation from dental professionals. Attentiveness to oral disease control and preventive measures based on legitimate scientific evidence and principles of collaboration within multidisciplinary engagement will ensure a complete and thorough approach to the oral health needs of elder patients in the future (Gueldner et al., 2007; Durso, 2005).

Risk Factors Contributing to Poor Oral Health

Dental Caries

Dental caries (decay) is the most commonly shared disease in populations of all ages throughout the world. It may affect the root (cementum) or the coronal (enamel) part of the tooth. Caries are evident when there is extension beyond the surface of enamel or cementum into the underlying dentin. It is visually discernible by a white to deep brown discoloration, or is penetrable by a dental hand instrument called an explorer. It may also be identified on a digital image or radiograph as an area of darker opacity than the surrounding landmarks and tissues. The developmental mechanism is similar in both children and adults with demineralization of enamel or cementum occurring through changes in salivary pH due to metabolization of fermentable carbohydrates by *Mutans streptococci* bacteria contained in plaque that forms on and adheres to tooth surfaces. Acid is produced as a by-product of bacterial metabolization of carbohydrates. Frequency of food intake and the physical characteristics of food (soft or hard) coupled with the timing of consumption determine demineralization. If there is not enough time for the salivary pH to return to neutral levels between acid productions or if there is a decrease in salivary production that reduces the buffering capacities needed to remineralize tooth surfaces, caries development occurs. Once demineralization occurs, lactobacilli found in saliva colonize in and around the carious lesion, and rapid decay progression occurs (Saunders & Meyerowitz, 2005; Anusavice, 2002). Analysis of data found in several surveys, including the National Health and Nutrition Survey (NHANES III), indicates that the rate of coronal caries for those over the age of 65 is similar to the general adult population, while the prevalence of root caries increases with age. Fluoride in municipal drinking water and oral hygiene products help to remineralize coronal tooth surfaces due to continued enamel uptake throughout a person's lifetime. In exposed root dentin, fluoride uptake begins to diminish after the age of 65, though recent studies using fluoride varnishes on exposed dentin surfaces have shown promise in providing short-term protection against decay (American Dental Association Council on Scientific Affairs, 2006a). Elders living in LTC facilities have a higher rate of coronal and root caries than those living in the community (Department of Health and Human Services, 2009). Gingival (i.e.,gum) recession due to normal aging and periodontal disease is a major risk factor for increases in root caries. The most relevant predictor of future dental caries is a recent history of decay. In elders, identification of active and inactive lesions after performing a caries risk assessment is necessary to develop appropriate treatment and oral hygiene regimens. As the number of restored teeth increases in aging populations, the challenge is to prevent primary and secondary decay, especially on exposed root surfaces (Anusavice, 2002; Zero, Fontanna, & Lennon, 2001). Large spaces between teeth may harbor materia alba and plaque on exposed dentin surfaces. Medications causing dry mouth side effects, consumption of sticky, soft foods, radiation therapy for head or neck cancers, and diminished ability to perform oral hygiene skills also contribute to root caries development (National Institutes of Health, 2001; Zero et al., 2001). Planning and monitoring mechanical oral hygiene interventions using a high fluoride content dentifrice can help seniors to reduce decay-producing bacteria as well as improve gingival health. Auxiliary preventive measures such as interproximal oral irrigation or evening mouth rinsing with 0.05% neutral sodium fluoride should also be added to the daily routine (American Dental Association Council on Scientific Affairs, 2006b; Anusavice, 2002).

Periodontal Disease

Distinguishing normal gingival tissue from diseased tissue is most important for determining the risk for the development of root caries, opportunistic oral infections, and associated systemic infections. Periodontal disease is an inflammatory disorder that affects the supporting structures of the teeth. Generally found in adults over the age of 30, it presents increased risks for systemic infection in elders, particularly the oldest-old (United States Department of Health & Human Services, 2009). Early onset or gingivitis may be observed visually by a change in the color of the gingiva from pink to red, with puffiness, bleeding, and sensitivity to brushing or touch. If gingivitis is not corrected with oral hygiene interventions it may progress to moderate or severe periodontal disease (periodontitis). Periodontitis is characterized by a progressive loss of attachment of the periodontal ligament to the gingiva and tooth, and loss of surrounding alveolar bone. It is episodic, with periods of quiescence followed by rapid destruction of the periodontal ligament and bone. The role of gram-negative bacteria found in subgingival, oral surface plaque has been well documented. Gram-negative bacteria colonize subgingival plaque and produce toxins and enzymes that injure tissue, eliciting an immune response. The inflammatory and chronic nature of this disease establishes a systemic bacteremic burden. Destabilization of atherosclerotic plaques contributes to a prothrombic state, heightening the risk of heart attack and stroke (Rethman, 2009).

Control of periodontal disease is particularly important in the management of diabetes mellitus. There is a large evidence base suggesting that poor glycemic control is associated with elevated levels of gingival crevicular fluid. Subsequent gingival inflammation can adversely affect the metabolic control of diabetes (Taylor & Borgnakke, 2008; Mealey, 2006). Grossi et al. (1997) first reported that a reduction of periodontal inflammation was associated with decreases in glycolated levels of hemoglobin. Inflammation may be the common link between periodontal disease and diabetes. Mealey (2006) suggests, however, that more randomized, controlled studies need to be conducted to expand the evidence base.

The increase in severity of periodontal disease due to estrogen deficiency has been associated with osteoporosis and decreased mandibular trabecular bone density. This may result in accelerated tooth loss for postmenopausal women and may negatively impact the survival rates of dental implants in this population (Reinhardt et al., 1999; Mulligan & Sobel, 2005).

This complicated oral disease cannot be diagnosed by visual inspection alone. Instrumentation measurements of the loss of attachment of the periodontal ligament, pocket depth measurements, bleeding upon probing, and radiographic or digital image evaluation of alveolar bone reduction and quality are necessary for diagnosis and for determining the progress of the disease over time. Mechanical oral hygiene interventions and auxiliary preventive measures such as chlorhexidine oral rinses and antibiotics help to reduce gram-negative bacteria and improve gingival health. The use of localized antibiotics inserted directly into periodontal pockets has been helpful in disease control also (Genco, 1996).

Oral and Pharyngeal Cancers

Oral and pharyngeal cancers are closely associated with growing older. The median age of individuals at the time of diagnosis is 64, with over 90% diagnosed as squamous cell carcinoma (SCC) (United States Department of Health and Human Services, 2009). The World Cancer Report predicts an alarming increase in new cancer cases to 15 million yearly by 2020, up from 10 million in 2000. Early detection of premalignant and malignant changes to the most common oral sites, the tongue (30%), lips (17%), and floor of the mouth (14%), and identification of high-risk behaviors can be effective in reducing cancer incidence when combined with patient education efforts (Silverman, 2001). Color, texture induration, and unilateral appearance of the oral tissues provide the visual clues that must be taken into consideration during the oral examination for cancer. Squamous cell carcinoma may present as a persistent mass, nodule, or indurated ulcer with color consisting of red or red and white hues. It has been clearly tied to the precancerous lesion erythroplakia, which has three usual visual presentations—a red, macular lesion, red with a white overlay that cannot be wiped off, or a red lesion speckled with white. Common sites are the lateral borders of the tongue, ventral aspect of the tongue, soft palate, and the floor of the mouth. More than 90% of the lesions identified as erythroplakia exhibit a microscopic diagnosis of carcinoma in situ, SCC, or cell dysplasia (Bsoul, Huber, & Terezhalmy, 2005).

Other associative lesions include leukoplakia, which is the clinical term for any white, oral lesion that cannot be readily diagnosed; such a lesion should be noted in the chart and watched to see if there are changes. Leukoplakia may be found in several areas of the mouth, including the ventral and lateral aspects of the tongue, the buccal (cheek) mucosa and mandibular, and the alveolar ridge area where the tooth sockets are located. It may or may not be premalignant. Identification of leukoplakia should be referred to a dental professional for diagnostic consideration. Verrucous leukoplakia presents visually as a corrugated and fissured white lesion appearing most often on the oral ridges where the tooth sockets are located, the buccal mucosa, or the gingiva. Its rate of malignant transformation is 65% to 100%, and it is seen mostly in women at an average age of 70 years (McIntyre & Oliver, 1999). The tobacco-associated lesions—nicotine stomatitis (red/white) and snuff keratosis (corrugated white)—found most frequently on the buccal mucosa and the gingival, are closely associated with tobacco placement and smoke inhalation irritation (Neville & Day, 2002). These two lesions should not be confused with oral submucous fibrosis seen almost exclusively in South Asian adults who chew betel quid. Characterized by a white, lacelike network extending over the tissue behind the last molar on the mandible area, buccal mucosa, soft palate, uvula, tongue, lips, and other oral structures, this type of fibrosis may also be found in the pharynx and esophagus. While leukoplakic in appearance, significant to the diagnosis is the presence of palpable fibrous bands of tissue. The deposition of fibrous tissue may lead to a size reduction in the opening of the esophagus, dysphagia, masticatory difficulty, speech impediment, sore throat, and decreased tongue function. Betel quid also leaves dark, heavy, sticky deposits on the coronal and root surfaces of teeth, making visual caries identification difficult (Cunha-Gomes, Kavarana, Choudhari, et al., 2003; Jeng, Chang, & Hahn, 2001). Oral lichen planus (OLP) presents as a lacelike network of white raised areas on the buccal mucosa or lateral areas of the tongue. It may extend to the uvula and into the esophagus and is often accompanied by epidermal lichen planus. Patient complaints may consist of burning mouth, metallic taste, dry mouth, and sensitivity to brushing or flossing. This controversial lesion is thought to be a chronic, autoimmune inflammatory condition with an associative risk of SCC; however, not all researchers are in agreement with this conclusion. Some studies indicate that the erosive type of OLP precedes malignancy. Until more definitive information is available, biopsy should be included in any determination of OLP to monitor the lesion's potential for malignant transformation (Bsoul et al., 2005; Hietanen, Paasonen, Kuhlfelt, et al., 1999). Actinic cheilitis is a variation of oral leukoplakia found most often on the lower lip. Visually, it appears as raised white or gray plaques between parallel folds. Predominantly found in men over the age of 40, it is a result of long-term exposure to ultraviolet light and is considered a precursor of SCC of the skin.

Bisphosphonate-Associated Osteonecrosis (BON) of the Jaw

Bisphosphonates, such as Zometa and Aredia used for the intravenous treatment of breast, lung, and other cancers, Paget's disease, hypercalcemia, reduction of bone pain, and skeletal complications from multiple myelomas, are associated with necrosis of the jaw. Invasive dental procedures should be avoided while these drugs are in use. BON is also associated with the use of oral bisphosphonates, such as Fosamax, Actonel, and Boniva, for the treatment of osteoporosis; however it is unclear if an underlying condition is what determines risk for BON (Mulligan & Sobel, 2005). Clinical presentation includes painful soft tissue swelling, loosening of teeth, drainage, and exposed bone. It may occur at the site of a previous tooth extraction or spontaneously. The risk for developing BON is much higher in cancer patients treated intravenously than in osteoporosis patients treated orally. The ADA Council on Scientific Affairs recommends conservative surgical procedures, antibiotic therapy, appropriate use of oral disinfectants, and physician consultation. Chemotherapy patients should have a dental examination prior to therapy, with subsequent examinations to manage oral hygiene (American Dental Association Council on Scientific Affairs; 2006a).

Oral Ulcerations

Any break in the oral epithelium may cause an ulceration that becomes painful or sore when exposed to citrus, salty, or spicy foods. Visually, these lesions appear as a single gray or yellow sphere with an inflammatory red halo surrounding the ulcerated site. Acute in nature, they are painful and heal spontaneously within 3 weeks. Local factors such as trauma due to ill-fitting appliances, sharp teeth or restorations, or self-inflicted, iatrogenic, or nonaccidental injury may cause ulcerations, as may burns from chemicals, cold, heat, radiation, or electricity. Most times, careful questioning of the patient will pinpoint the cause. Chronic trauma will present with a keratotic margin and is of special concern for elders wearing dental appliances or chewing hard foods in areas with missing teeth (Scully & Felix, 2005). Recurrent apthous stomatitis (apthous ulcer) is a common condition affecting approximately 20% of the population. It begins in childhood or adolescence and recurs throughout life. Visually, it presents as clusters of small, round, circumscribed gray or yellow areas surrounded by individual inflammatory haloes. The condition is thought to be present in individuals with a genetic predisposition to it. There is no association with specific bacteria or viruses. Stress, trauma, vitamin B and iron deficiency, use of oral hygiene products containing lauryl sulphate, and immune deficiency are some of the suspected predisposing factors. The most common form found in elderly women is the herpetiform type. It can involve any site on the oral mucosa and begins as small pin-point clusters that progress into a large, ragged, painful ulceration. In some individuals, these lesions occur so often that they become a chronic nuisance requiring constant management with symptom relief. Maintenance of good oral hygiene and the use of chlorhexidine or triclosan mouth rinses can minimize discomfort. Oral antibiotics and corticosteroid agents in pellet, topical, mouthwash, and spray form may also be used under dentist supervision (Neville & Day, 2002; Scully & Felix, 2005).

Oral Infections

Mucosal infections that cause mouth ulcers generally have their etiology in viruses with Coxsackie's, herpes viruses, and enteric cytopathic human orphan (ECHO), the most common. Herpes simplex virus (HSV) lesions are found intraorally throughout the mouth and oropharynx and externally on the lips (herpes labialis/cold sore). Intraorally they present as an irregular, painful, coalesced, red lesion that may be accompanied by lymph node enlargement and fever. Approximately 15% of the population has recurrent herpes infections, most commonly on the lips. Reactivating factors associated with elders include upper respiratory infection, fever, immunosuppression, trauma, and sunlight. Early labial symptoms may include tingling, burning, or itching that rapidly progresses to a pustular lesion within 48 hours. Spontaneous healing takes place within 7 to 10 days, and lip comfort may be managed with a 1% topical pencyclovir application. In immunocompromised individuals, HSV is seen on the dorsal region of the tongue and has a white, dendritic (branching) appearance. Systemic antivirals such as acyclovir or valacyclovir may be used. It is also beneficial to hydrate, provide a bland and soft diet, reduce fever, and control pain (Neville & Day, 2002; Scully & Felix, 2005).

Oral candidiasis is caused by an overgrowth of *Candida albicans* due to changes in the normal balance of protective oral flora. It presents as a red or white flat lesion that may adhere to hard or soft oral mucosa and to removable appliances. Medications, including antibiotics, corticosteroids, and chemotherapeutics may change oral homeostasis, allowing fungi to overgrow. Immune and endocrine deficiencies, xerostomia, cancer radiotherapy, systemic disease, and chronic oral irritation are contributors to the infection. Denture stomatitis with concomitant candidiasis is a condition frequently seen when dentures are ill-fitting, broken, or insufficiently cleaned. Candidal angular cheilosis, found in the tissue folds where the lips come together, is seen with inadequate oral hygiene due to overclosure of the mouth in individuals who do not wear their dentures. A simple reline, adjustment, repair, or replacement of dentures helps to restore the oral tissues to contour and may alleviate this painful problem (Neville & Day, 2002; Scully & Felix, 2005). Control of oral candidiasis is difficult, especially with immunocompromised or chronically ill patients. Topical or systemic antifungal medications can be used to treat the infection, which can be life threatening if allowed to spread to the esophagus or lungs (Munro & Grap, 2004).

Xerostomia is a frequent elder complaint that describes a subjective perception of oral dryness. It may be a serious indication of several underlying systemic conditions, such as dehydration, diabetes, thyroid disorders, and connective tissue diseases or adverse, medication-induced side effects (Atkinson, Grisius, & Massey, 2005). Xerostomia, commonly called dry mouth, is characterized by reduced salivary flow (hyposalivation), which may or may not be accompanied by changes in salivary composition. It is often associated with growing older due to reduced reserves in the salivary glands; however there is no causative evidence to support qualitative or quantitative alterations in salivary gland function due to aging. Medication usage is thought to be the most common reason for reductions in salivary flow. Anticholinergic action, which can affect fluid balance, and sympathomimetic action, which produces viscous saliva with reduced volume, are cited as two side effects (Atkinson et al., 2005). In the US noninstitutionalized population, approximately 50% of people over age 65 take at least one prescription medication, with women over age 65 using the highest number of medications (Kaufman, Kelly, Rosenberg, Anderson, & Mitchell, 2002). The importance of including a medication history with the oral health assessment cannot be overstated. Dryness complaints increase with age due to the synergistic effects of taking multiple medications. Anticholinergic medications include antihistamines, antihypertensives, antidepressants, antipsychotics, antispasmodics, antiemetics, and anti-parkinsonian drugs. Sympathomimetic drugs include decongestants, bronchodilators, appetite suppressants, and amphetamines. As new drugs are introduced, the number of drugs associated with xerostomia grows. New classes include proton pump inhibitors, analgesics, narcotics for pain management, anti-infective agents, some antineoplastic agents, and reverse transcriptase inhibitors for HIV infection (Spolarich, 2009). Polymedicine, or the use of five or more drugs simultaneously, must also be considered, especially in individuals who take four or fewer prescribed medications and self-medicate to control mild pain or allergies with OTC drugs (Williams & Kim, 2005; Kaufman et al., 2002). Diseases of the salivary glands may also cause dryness. Sjögren's syndrome may present as a primary disease unrelated to any autoimmune disease, or a secondary, inflammatory autoimmune disorder. Each includes symptoms of severe oral dryness, burning or itching of the mouth, and difficulty in eating, speaking, or swallowing. There is a permanent reduction in the quantity and quality of saliva produced; however, salivary gland biopsies of Sjögren's patients reveal that 50% of glandular cells remain intact, so there may be a benefit from properly prescribed sialogogues, such as pilocarpine or cevimeline to stimulate salivary gland flow. Xerostomia and dehydration in type 1 diabetes can result from elevated fasting blood glucose levels, medication use, or elevated glycosylated hemoglobin levels. Xerostomia is also associated with autoimmune thyroiditis, chronic graft-versus-host disease, rheumatoid arthritis, and amyloidosis (Fox & Stern, 2002).

Intensive care unit patients may have medical equipment in place that keeps the mouth open continuously, contributing to xerostomia and subsequent plaque accumulation. Stress, anxiety, and fluid imbalances in critical illness also contribute to xerostomia. In studying ventilator-associated pneumonia (VAP) in the intensive care unit, researchers compared nurse-administered tooth brushing using a defined protocol to the use of a foam or glycerin swab with no protocol. They found that tooth brushing decreased the overgrowth of dental plaque containing *Staphylococcus aureus* and pseudomonas, the most common bacterial colonizers of endotracheal tubing. They cautioned, however, that mechanical removal in the absence of microbicidal intervention might increase translocation of organisms to the trachea or bloodstream (Munro & Grap, 2004; Terpenning, 2005; Munro et al., 2006). The use of pediatric-sized toothbrushes (to work around intubation) with a chlorhexidine mouth-rinsing product is recommended if a suction toothbrush is not available. Many suction toothbrushes dispense a 1.5% hydrogen peroxide agent for microbicidal action. Wennström & Lindhe's (1979) study of hydrogen peroxide rinsing suggested its efficacy in reducing plaque levels; however, recent studies dispute this information. Hydrogen peroxide products containing povidone-iodine work synergistically to reduce plaque levels, while hydrogen peroxide, 1.5% has no clinically significant effect on plaque reduction (Maruniak et al., 1992; Hoenderdos et al., 2009). Since usual methods of rinsing and expectoration are diminished, chlorhexidine products in conjunction with mechanical plaque removal and measures to alleviate oral dryness will assist in prevention of VAP and the level of comfort a person experiences while in critical care (Munro & Grap, 2004)

Chemotherapeutic drugs can damage salivary and oral tissues. Changes in flow rates, salivary composition, and systemic immunosuppression advance the progression of periodontal disease, dental caries, and opportunistic infections. Amofostine, a free radical scavenger drug, may be used to lower the incidence of moderate to severe xerostomia in patients experiencing radiation therapy, which includes a significant proportion of the parotid gland; however, this area should be protected as much as possible during therapy (Spolarich, 2009).

Managing Xerostomia

There are several basic strategies used for the management of xerostomia. Environmental, nutritional, and topical management take precedence for short-term relief and oral disease prevention. Small sips of fluoridated water (not bottled), humidification, and avoidance of caffeine, alcohol, and sugary and sticky foods will reduce the subjective sensation of dryness. Chewing sugar-free gum or sucking on sugarless candies and citric acid–containing products such as sugar-free vitamin C tablets, lemon drops, or lozenges can achieve mechanical stimulation of saliva. Patients may also increase salivary flow using a sonic toothbrush with an alcohol-free dry mouth product, such as biotene® oral balance toothpaste or mouthwash (Atkinson et al., 2005; Papas et al., 2007). Commercially available saliva substitutes and lubricants, such as mucopolysaccharide lubricants, biotene® lubricant, or Salivart® aerosol, are available over the counter or as prescribed by a dentist. Patient preferences and comfort will determine what substitutes are used, as will oral myofunctional habits such as tongue thrusting or lip pursing. These may take the form of mouth rinses, lubricating sprays or gels, and chewing gum. The use of clinically applied neutral sodium fluoride varnishes to root surfaces or fluoride gels are indispensable adjunctive therapies in the prevention of dental caries. Rinsing daily, preferably in the evening, with a 0.05% neutral sodium fluoride mouthwash such as ACT® fluoride rinse, ACT® Restoring™ Anticavity mouthwash, or Fluorigard® Anticavity rinse will decrease the incidence of decay. For rampant decay, prescription formula PreviDent® 5000 or 5000+ containing 1.1% neutral sodium fluoride in toothpaste form or rinse may be prescribed by a dentist (Spolarich, 2009; Atkinson et al., 2005; Glassman et al., 2003). A growing body of evidence suggests that chewing gum and lozenges containing xylitol inhibit the growth of strep mutans bacteria, thereby decreasing the incidence of decay (Glassman et al., 2003; Kitchens, 2005). One study indicated that established cases of xerostomia can benefit from humidification of inspired air through commercially available airflow generators of humidified air (Hay & Morton, 2006). Paying attention to diet and nutrition will avoid oral injury and provide comfort. Food choices should be limited to lukewarm foods that are soft, moist, and easy to chew or thinned with liquids such as broth, milk, yogurt, or gravy. Foods that are crunchy, sharp, spicy, or acidic may cut or scrape the oral mucosa and should be avoided. Chewing slowly and sipping liquids between small bites will increase the enjoyment of eating.

Dentures

The average life of a complete denture is almost 18 years. More than half (57%) of denture wearers seldom or never present for routine dental exams and struggle orally with an unstable denture. This instability contributes to plaque accumulation on the palate, on the oral ridges under the denture, and on the denture itself. Plaque accumulation causes malodor, which can be distressing for elders and caregivers (Melton, 2000). Full and partial denture wearers, particularly those with xerostomia or recent weight loss, must be examined by a dentist for fit and comfort. The American Dental Association recommends evaluations at 18-month intervals for edentulous persons (American Dental Association, n.d.) Oral hygiene care is relatively easy and should be completed by the individual if possible. Reminders and coaching to clean and remove dentures in the evening may be needed. Dentures should be brushed to remove plaque. Overnight soaking with a disinfectant product such as Polident® is essential to reduce bacterial and fungal counts on the denture and in the mouth. Soaking also reduces denture odors that may occur due to the porosity of the denture construction material. The disinfectant solution should be renewed daily. Traditional soaking rinses using vinegar and water, while inexpensive, are not recommended because there is no reduction in bacterial count, repeated use may damage denture acrylic, and the taste may be disagreeable. The mucobuccal folds of the cheeks and lips should be checked for plaque and food accumulation, which if present, can be wiped out gently with a glycerin swab or soft washcloth soaked in alcohol free mouth wash. A soft bristled manual toothbrush should be used with caution to clean edentulous mouths since movement or resistance may cause damage to the oral mucosa.

Freshening dentures throughout the day with a disinfecting denture soak of 3–4 minutes or commercially available denture wipes will reduce bacteria and odor. If the mouth is dry, saliva substitutes and lubricants should be encouraged to soothe the oral mucosa (American Dental Association, n.d.) There is little information in the literature that speaks to oral care for the edentulous person experiencing xerostomia. More studies and clinical trials need to be conducted (Turner, Jahangiri, & Ship, 2008)

Dementia

Dementia presents a difficult challenge to healthcare providers, since elders experiencing dementia are often admitted to LTC with a variety of burdensome oral health complications, pain, functional weakness, and varying levels of cognitive impairment. There may not have been dental care for extended periods of time prior to admission, and as dementia progresses, resistance behaviors to oral hygiene interventions become more frequent. These behaviors are not uncommon since the elder may have lost interest in or the capacity needed to perform personal care, therapeutic products may have a strange taste or consistency in the mouth, or there may be an unspoken sense of grief, embarrassment, or rage at the loss of control. Resistance behaviors include screaming, head turning, mouth closing, pushing away, or biting. Viewing these behaviors as symptoms of unmet needs such as pain, insecurity, fear, or medication side effects can guide the caregiver in developing a person-centered relationship with the individual. Institutional practices should take into account the caregiver as central to assisting the elder in working through the behavior. Unvarying caregiver assignments contribute to comfort care because staff has an opportunity to develop a relationship with the person and is likely to notice physical or cognitive changes that require modifications to care. Caregivers may offer choices that allow the person to guide the given care, regardless of disability, ensuring that the process is respectful of the person's privacy, reassuring, inclusive, and safe (Garrett, Baillie, & Garrett, 1989; White, Newton-Curtis, & Lyons, 2008; Stein & Henry, 2009). Caregiver education in the management of difficult behaviors, oral health care in-service education, and changes in caregiver-to-patient ratio assignments must be considered by institutions when implementing person-centered care. More studies are needed to determine how to modify caregiver attitudes and fears so that delivery of basic oral care is consistent with oral care guidelines and standards developed within the LTC and HHC industry (Jablonski et al., 2008; Coleman & Watson, 2005; Coleman, 2004b; Chalmers & Pearson, 2005).

Resources

Most LTC and HHC organizations have developed in-house resources for in-service, family, or caregiver training. Nurses, when making decisions about appropriate training information, must take care to assure that optimal, person-centered oral health interventions are based on individual oral health assessment, sound scientific evidence, and access to appropriate therapeutic aids and equipment. The University of Iowa, through its Geriatric

Education Center, has developed an excellent oral health training resource for persons who have dementia that can be used as a caregiver in-service take-away or as a family resource. The plaque reduction protocol focuses on promoting maximum function and independence, comfort, and autonomy. The contents of this publication can easily transfer to delivery of oral health care for any elder, in any institutional, long-term, or home health care situation. It leads its reader through disease issues and explanations and describes strategies for oral hygiene set-up, environmental considerations, and the supplies needed. There is discussion concerning person-centered communication techniques, including bridging, distraction, chaining, hand-over hand, rescuing, and sequential tasking. It describes a protocol for the mechanical removal of plaque (tooth brushing) and makes a recommendation for prescription microbicidal intervention for gingival bleeding. Its photographic essay is a visual guide to oral hygiene access techniques and approaches to care delivered in upright and prone positions (Chalmers & Spector, 2009).

Another first-rate publication is a self-study module published online by the Southern Association of Institutional Dentists (n.d.) for dental professionals (*Preventive Dentistry for Persons with Severe Disabilities*). This resource provides information on how to follow a care plan based on the oral health assessment. Written for institutional use, it includes toothbrush selection and modification for grip and fine motor control, toothbrushing techniques for adequate plaque removal, flossing techniques, sequential tasking, antimicrobial agents prescribed, use of mouth props, therapeutic restraints, positioning, and communication techniques. Its multidisciplinary approach includes tips for the use of oral hygiene products and ordering information, appropriate team member consultations for specific problems, design and evaluation of an oral hygiene program, and components of a caregiver training program. There is also a source list of institutions willing to share organizational preventive information for program development.

A literature review by Chalmers and Pearson (2005) found that more research is needed to develop and validate oral health assessment tools and staff education programs. They suggest trial preventive oral hygiene care strategies and products, and trial dementia-focused behavior management and communication strategies.

Retaining Independence

Elders can retain independence through sustained oral health educational efforts. A small clinical trial comparing two types of oral health education programs aimed at elders provided strong evidence that oral health promotion can work. Multiple sessions encompassing hands-on education within a small group was compared with verbal instruction and use of a self-training manual. These types of interventions require a more concentrated institutional effort, but the results of this study showed that these efforts are beneficial. Structured interventions of either type with booster sessions and use of oral health equipment individualized to specific risk factors reinforced learning and decreased elders' plaque scores simply by raising the profile of oral hygiene. The type of education presented was not significant (Ribeiro et al., 2009).

Pyle, Massie, and Nelson (1998) identified the benefits of instituting a 6-week oral health education initiative for nursing assistants with quantifiable decreases in plaque indices for elders. While most studies measure caregiver attitudes toward the provision of oral care for elders, there have been no studies measuring the impact of an oral health education program for caregivers on caregiver plaque indices. Researchers support the development of interdisciplinary caregiver education programs targeted toward improving the oral health of elders (Boczko et al., 2008; Chalmers & Ettinger, 2008; Coleman, 2005; Durso, 2005; Glassman et al., 2003; Gooch et al., 2005; Munoz et al., 2009; Pyle et al., 1998).

Future Directions

Federal regulations have placed responsibility for oral health care needs and treatment on LTC facilities, and most specifically on nurses. Studies show, however, that oral health care receives lowest priority on the ever-growing list of duties that caregivers must maintain for elders. Given the limited oral health content in nursing school curricula, the general population's negative attitudes toward oral care, and limited monitoring of care interventions by dental professionals, the nurse is continually challenged to find ways to remove these weighty barriers to care (Fitzpatrick, 2000; Coleman, 2005). At the same time, dental and dental hygiene curricula lack the didactic and clinical experience to treat the functionally dependent and frail elderly (Yoder, 2006).

In practice, dental hygienists routinely appoint patients two to three times a year for at least 15 minutes. A recent study indicated that hygienists had a strong desire to increase their knowledge base about the management of medical conditions related to diabetes. Hygienists also expressed a preference for regular professional continuing education, and the opportunity to interact with other health professionals (Boyd, 2008). Modeled on the precedents set by the nursing profession, and the experiments conducted at the Forsyth Dental Center in the 1970s, a curriculum for the Advanced Dental Hygiene Practitioner (ADHP) is in development to address the unmet oral health needs of underserved populations (Lobene & Kerr, 1979; American Dental Hygienists Association, 2009; Minnesota Passes Legislation, 2009). Among dental hygienists surveyed, there is more support for the ADHP educational pathway than interest in pursuing it; nevertheless, hygienists are in agreement that ADHP's working in alternative oral care settings such as mobile dental health clinics, hospitals, or LTC facilities would benefit elders too frail or ill to travel for off-site care (Lambert, George, Curran, Lee, & Shugars, 2009). The American Dental Association, citing lack of a specific curriculum for ADHP's initiative, has offered its solution to meeting the oral health needs of underserved populations by proposing a new member of the dental health team, the Community Dental Health Coordinator (CDHC). Working independently, yet in partnership with dentists, the CDHC will advocate for provision of a consistent oral health component within a multidisciplinary network of health and social care providers (American Dental Association, 2008). As the use of dental services continues to increase for those who have access, future elders will present with complicated oral rehabilitation that has the potential for both technical and biological complications. Dental implant therapy is one example of treatment that can significantly improve the lives of elders; however, ongoing maintenance and recare visits are important to the success and retention of both fixed and removable prostheses (Stanford, 2007).

The ADHP or the CDHC, as an oral health liaison to the HHC or LTC services network, could more effectively navigate the complex healthcare system. Collection of oral health assessment data, care planning and monitoring, caregiver and family in-service education, oral health outcomes measurement, and dental advocacy through referral and policy recommendations could ensure appropriate and timely attention to oral health care needs. This new member of the dental health team could also address the need many elders have for a dental home if requirements include the utilization of a collaborative work agreement with a licensed dentist. Elders with a dental home, whether it is off- or on-site, are more likely to receive appropriate preventive and routine care, reducing the risk of preventable oral disease and associative infections (Gueldner et al., 2007).

Pioneering partnerships are developing between nursing, dental, and dental hygiene schools and postdoctoral dental residencies to begin a dialogue with dental practitioners about person-centered practice through multidisciplinary collaboration. The nursing-dental alliance at New York University (NYU) pairs nursing and dental hygiene students for evidence-based practice skill sharing that addresses the needs of vulnerable populations. Faculties are collaborating in research and faculty development courses (Westphal, Fumari, & Haber, 2009). The Association of American Medical Colleges (AAMC) and the American Dental Education Association (ADEA) have also formed an academic partnership to share teaching resources across universities. MedEdPORTAL will now include dental education resources, expanding collaboration between medicine and dentistry by providing access to scholarly, high-quality, peer reviewed material (American Dental Education Association, 2009).

Nurse leaders have long recognized that oral health literacy is essential to improved general health outcomes, and they have provided the guidance needed to link the oral health knowledge base to medicine and other healthcare professions. Oral assessment should not become incorporated into the accepted scope of medical practice, nor should it be practiced in dental isolation. Nurses recognize the merit of each individual practice area's education and expertise and respect the clear boundaries that define the roles and responsibilities for diagnosis and treatment. Nursing research and clinical practice have identified deficiencies in the oral health status of LTC and HHC elders. Nurses will continue to provide leadership in this area as the professions move toward the development of an integrated national model for LTC and HHC oral health delivery that is interdisciplinary, grounded in science, guided by research evidence, delivered with best practices, and committed to professional ethics.

References

American Dental Association. (n.d.). *Oral health topics. Dentures: Frequently asked questions.* Retrieved from http://www.ADA.org

American Dental Association. (2008, March 13). ADA offers statement on SF 2895. *ADA News Today.* Retrieved from http://www.ada.org/prof/resources/pubs/adanews/index.asp

American Dental Association Council on Scientific Affairs (Ed.). (2006a). Dental management of patients receiving oral bisphosphonate therapy: Expert panel recommendations. *Journal of the American Dental Association, 137*, 1143–1150. Retrieved from http://jada.ada.org

American Dental Association Council on Scientific Affairs (Ed.). (2006b). Professionally applied topical fluoride: Evidence-based clinical recommendations. *Journal of the American Dental Association, 137*(8), 1151–1159. Retrieved from http://jada.ada.org/cgi/content/full/137/8/1151

American Dental Education Association. (2009, July 17). *New dental resources now on MedEdPORTAL.* Retrieved August 22, 2009, from http://www.adea.org/mededportal/Pages/NewDentalResources.aspx

American Dental Hygienists Association. (2009). *ADHA—Advanced dental hygiene practitioner fact sheet.* Retrieved from http://www.adha.org/media/facts/adhp.htm

Anusavice, K.J. (2002). Dental caries: risk assessment and treatment solutions for an elderly population. *Compendium of Continuing Education in Dentistry, 23*(10), supplement, 12–20.

Atkinson, J.C., Grisius, M., & Massey, W. (2005). Salivary hypofunction and xerostomia: Diagnosis and treatment. *Dental Clinics of North America, 49*, 309–326.

Bailey, R., Gueldner, S., Ledikwe, J., & Smiciklas-Wright, H. (2005). The oral health of older adults: An interdisciplinary mandate. *Journal of Gerontological Nursing, 31*(7), 11–17.

Boczko, F., McKeon, S., & Sturkie, D. (2009). Long-term care and oral health knowledge. *Journal of the American Medical Directors Association, 10*(3), 204–206.

Boyd, L. (2008). Commentary on "survey of diabetes knowledge and practices of dental hygienists." *Access, Sept–Oct*, 40–43.

Bsoul, S.A., Huber, M.A., & Terezhalmy, G.T. (2005). Squamous cell carcinoma of the oral tissues: A comprehensive review for oral healthcare providers. *Journal of Contemporary Dental Practice, 6*(4), 1–16.

Centers for Disease Control and Prevention, and The Merck Company Foundation. (2007). *The state of aging and health in america 2007.* Whitehouse Station, NJ: The Merck Company Foundation.

Chalmers, J., & Pearson, A. (2005). Oral hygiene care for residents with dementia: A literature review. *Journal of Advanced Nursing, 52*(4), 410–419.

Chalmers, J., King, P., Spencer, A., Wright, F., & Carter, K. (2005). The oral health assessment tool—validity and reliability. *Australian Dental Journal, 50*(3), 191–199.

Chalmers, J.M., & Ettinger, R.L. (2008). Public health issues in geriatric dentistry in the United States. *Dental Clinics of North America, 52*(2), 423–446.

Chalmers, J, & Spector, E. (2009). *Oral hygiene care for nursing home residents with dementia* [Brochure]. Iowa City, Iowa: The University of Iowa: Iowa Geriatric Center.

Chia-Hui Chen, C. (2007). The Kayser-Jones Brief Oral Health Status Examination (BOHSE). *Try This: Best Practices in Nursing Care to Older Adults*, (18). The Hartford Institute for Geriatric Nursing, New York University, College of Nursing. Retrieved September, 2009, from www.hartfordign.org

Christensen, G.J. (2005). Special oral hygiene and preventive care for special needs. *Journal of the American Dental Association, 163*(8), 1141–1143.

Clark, G.T. (2005). Orofacial pain and sensory disorders in the elderly. *Dental Clinics of North America, 49*(2), 343–362.

Coleman, P. (2005). Opportunities for nursing-dental collaboration: Addressing oral health needs among the elderly. *Nursing Outlook, 53*(1), 33–39.

Coleman, P., & Watson, N.M. (2005). Oral care provided by certified nursing assistants in nursing homes. *Journal of the American Geriatric Society, 54*, 138–143.

Coleman, P.R. (2004a). Pneumonia in the long-term care setting: Etiology, management, and prevention. *Journal of Gerontological Nursing, 30*(4), 14–23.

Coleman, P.R. (2004b). Promoting oral health in elder care—challenges and opportunities. *Journal of Gerontological Nursing, 30*(4), 3.

Cunha-Gomes, D. Kavarana, N.M., Choudhari, C., Rajendraprasad, J.S., Bhathena, H.M. Desai, P.B., Vyas, J.J., Gangwal, S. (2003) Total oral reconstruction for cancers associated with advanced oral submucous fibrosis. *Annals of Plastic Surgery*, 51(3), 283–289.

Durso, S.C. (2005). Interaction with other health team members in caring for elderly patients. *Dental Clinics of North America*, 49(2), 377–388.

Electronic Code of Federal Regulations. (2008, Winter). Title 42, Chapter IV, Part 418.94; Part 484.36. Retrieved September, 2009, from http://ecfr.gpoaccess.gov

Fellona, M.O., & DeVore, L.R. (1999). Oral health services in primary care nursing centers: Opportunities for dental hygiene and nursing collaboration. *Journal of Dental Hygiene*, 73(2), 69–86.

Fitzpatrick, J. (2000). Oral health care needs of dependent older people: Responsibilities of nurses and care staff. *Journal of Advanced Nursing*, 32(6), 1325–1332.

Fox, R.I., & Stern, M. (2002). Sjögren's syndrome: Mechanisms of pathogenesis involve interaction of immune and neurosecretory systems. *Scandinavian Journal of Rheumatology Supplement*, 116, 3–13.

Garrett, T.M., Baille, H.W., & Garrett, R.M. (1989). *Health care ethics principles and problems*. Englewood Cliffs, N.J: Prentice Hall.

Genco, R.J. (1996). Current view of risk factors for periodontal diseases. *American Journal of Periodontology*, 67(10), 1041–1049.

Glassman, P., Anderson, M., Jacobsen, P., Schonfeld, S., Weintraub, J., White, A., et al. (2003). Practical protocols for the prevention of dental disease in community settings for people with special needs: The protocols. *Special Care in Dentistry*, 23(5), 160–164.

Gooch, B.F., Malvitz, D.M., Griffin, S.O., & Maas, W.R. (2005). Promoting the oral health of older adults through the chronic disease model: CDC's perspective on what we still need to know. *Journal of Dental Education*, 69(9), 1059–1063.

Grossi, S.G., Skrepcinski, F.B., DeCaro, T., Zambon, J.J., Cummins, D., & Genco, R.J. (1997). Treatment of periodontal disease in diabetics reduces glycated hemoglobin. *Journal of Periodontology*, 68(8), 713–719.

Guay, A.H. (2005). The oral health status of nursing home residents: What do we need to know? *Journal of Dental Education*, 69(9), 1015–1017.

Gueldner, S.H., Pierce, C., Beatty, P., Lacey, F.J., Lacey, L.B., Lesperance, L., et al. (2007). A community action mandate for oral health in rural populations. In L.L. Morgan & P.S. Fahs (Eds.), *Conversations in the disciplines sustaining rural populations* (pp. 31–51). New York: Global Academic Publishing.

Gusberti, F., Sampathkumar, P., Siegrist, B.E., & Lang, N.P. (1988). Microbiological and clinical effects of chlorhexidine digluconate and hydrogen peroxide mouth rinses on developing plaque and gingivitis. *Journal of Clinical Periodontology*, 15(1), 60–67. doi: 10.1111/j.1600-051X.1988 .tb01556.x

Hardy, D.L., Darby, M.L., Leinbach, R.M., & Welliver, M.R. (2004). Self-report of oral health services provided by nurses' aides in nursing homes. *Journal of Dental Hygiene*, 69, 75–82.

Hay, K., & Morton, R.P. (2006). Optimal nocturnal humidification for xerostomia. *Head & Neck*, 28(9), 792–796. doi:10.1002/hed

Hietanen, J., Paasonen, M.R., Kuhlefelt, M., & Malmstrom, M. (1999). A retrospective study of oral lichen planus patients with concurrent or subsequent development of malignancy. *Oral Oncology*, 35(3), 278–282.

Hietanen, J., Paasonen, M.R., Kuhlefelt, M., & Malmstrom, M. (1999). A retrospective study of oral lichen planus patients with concurrent or subsequent development of malignancy. *Oral Oncology*, 35(3), 278–282.

Hobdell, M., Petersen, P.E., Clarkson, J., & Johnson, N. (2003). Global goals for oral health 2020. *International Dental Journal, 53*(5), 285–287.

Hoenderdos, N.L., Rosa, N.M., Slot, D.E., Timmerman, M.F., Van der Velden, U., & Van der Weijden, G.A. (2009). The influence of a hydrogen peroxide and glycerol containing mouth rinse on plaque accumulation: A 3-day non-brushing model. *International Journal of Dental Hygiene, 7*(4), 294–298. doi: 10.1111/j.1601-5037.2009.00367.x

Jablonski, R.A., Munro, C.L., Grap, M.J., Schubert, C.M., Ligon, M., & Spigelmyer, P. (2008). Mouth care in nursing homes: Knowledge, beliefs and practices of nursing assistants. *Geriatric Nursing, 30*(2), 99–107. doi: 10.1016/j.gerinurse.2008.06.010

Jeng, J.H., Chang, M.C., & Hahn, L.J. (2001). Role of areca nut in betel quid associated chemical carcinogenesis: current awareness and future perspectives. *Oral Oncology, 37*(6), 477–492.

Kaufman, D.W., Kelly, J.P., Rosenberg, L., Anderson, T.E., & Mitchell, A.A. (2002). Recent patterns of medication use in the ambulatory adult population of the United States: The Slone survey. *Journal of the American Medical Association, 287.3*, 337–344.

Kayser-Jones, J., Bird, W.F., Paul, S.M., Long, L., & Schell, E.S. (1995). An instrument to assess the oral health status of nursing home residents. *The Gerontologist, 35*(6), 814–824.

Kitchens, D.H. (2005). Xylitol in the prevention of oral diseases. *Special Care in Dentistry, 23*(3), 140–144.

Lambert, D., George, M., Curran, A., Lee, J., & Shugars, D. (2009). Practicing dental hygienists' attitudes toward the proposed advanced dental hygiene practitioner: A pilot study. *Journal of Dental Hygiene, 83*(3), 117–125. Retrieved from http://www.adha.org/pub

Lobene, R.R., & Kerr, A. (1979). *The Forsyth experiment: An alternative system for dental care.* Cambridge, MA: Harvard University Press.

Maruniak, J., Clark, W.B., Walker, C.B., Magnusson, I., Marks, R.G., Taylor, M., et al. (1992). The effect of 3 mouthrinses on plaque and gingivitis development. *Journal of Clinical Periodontology, 19*(1), 19–23. doi: 10.1111/j.1600-051X.1992.tb01143.x

McIntyre, G.T., & Oliver, R.J., (1999). Update on precancerous lesions. *Dental Update, 26*(9), 382–386.

Mealey, B.L. (2006). Periodontal disease and diabetes: A two-way street. *Journal of the American Dental Association, 137*(S2), 26S–31S.

Melton, A.B. (2000). Current trends in removable prosthodontics. *Journal of the American Dental Association, 131*(1), 52S–56S.

Metheny, N.A., Boltz, M., & Greenberg, S.A. (2008). Preventing aspiration in older adults with dysphagia. *American Journal of Nursing, 108*(2), 45–46.

Minnesota passes legislation allowing mid-level oral health provider. (2009, May 19). Retrieved from http//www.medicalnewstoday.com

Mulligan, R., & Sobel, S. (2005). Osteoporosis: Diagnostic testing, interpretation, and correlations with oral health—implications for dentistry. *Dental Clinics of North America, 49*, 463–484.

Munoz, N., Touger-Decker, R., Byham-Gray, L., & Maillet, J. (2009). Effect of an oral health assessment education program on nurses' knowledge and patient care practices in skilled nursing facilities. *Special Care in Dentistry 29*(4), 179–185. doi: 10.1111/j.1754-4505.2009.00084.x

Munro, C.L., & Grap, M. (2004). Oral health and care in the intensive care unit: State of the science. *American Journal of Critical Care, 13*, 24–34.

Munro, C.L., Grap, M., Jablonski, R., & Boyle, A. (2006). Oral health measurement in nursing research: State of the science. *Biological Research for Nursing, 8*(1), 35–42.

National Center for Health Statistics. (2009). *Health, United States 2008 with chartbook* (pp. 65, 284–89, 364–65). Washington, DC: US Government Printing Office.

National Institute of Dental and Craniofacial Research. (2009). *Oral health in America: A report of the surgeon general.* Bethesda, MD: National Institutes of Health.

National Institutes of Health. (2001). NIH consensus development conference on diagnosis and management of dental caries throughout life. *Journal of Dental Education, 65*, 935–1179.

Neville, B.W., & Day, T.A. (2002). Oral cancer and precancerous lesions. *CA Cancer Journal Clinics, 52*(4), 195–215.

Papas, A.S., Singh, M., Harrington, D., Ortblad, K., De Jager, M., & Nunn, M. (2007). Reduction in caries rate among patients with xerostomia using a power toothbrush. *Special Care in Dentistry, 27*(2), 46–51.

Pyle, M.A., Jasinevicius, R.T., Sawyer, D.R., & Madsen, J. (2005). Nursing home executive directors' perception of oral care in long-term care facilities. *Special Care in Dentistry, 25*(2), 111–117.

Pyle, M.A., Massie, M., & Nelson, S. (1998). A pilot study on improving oral care in long-term care settings. *Gerontological Nursing, 24*, 112–117.

Reinhardt, R.A., Payne, J.B., Maze, C.A., Patil, K.D., Gallagher, S.J., & Mattson, J.S. (1999). Influence of estrogen and osteopenia/osteoporosis in clinical periodontitis on postmenopausal women. *Journal of Periodontology, 70*(8), 823–828.

Rethman, M.P. (2009, March 31). Chronic periodontitis associated with increased incidence of coronary heart disease: A critical summary. [Review of "Periodontal disease and coronary heart disease incidence: A systematic review and meta-analysis" by L.L. Humphrey, R. Fu, D.I. Buckley, & M. Helfand. *Journal of General Internal Medicine*, 2008:23(12).] Retrieved August 5, 2009, from ADA, Center for Evidence-Based Dentistry.www.ebd.ada.org.

Ribeiro, D.G., Pavarina, A.C., Giampaolo, E.T., Machado, A.L., Jorge, J.H., & Garcia, P.P. (2009). Effect of oral hygiene education and motivation on removable partial denture wearers. *Gerodontology, 26*(2), 150–156.

Roberts, J. (2000). Developing an oral assessment and intervention tool for older people: 3. *British Journal of Nursing, 9*(19), 2073–2078.

Saunders, R.H. & Meyerowitz, C., (2005) Dental caries in older adults. *Dental Clinics of North America, 49*, 293–308.

Scully, C. & Felix, D.H., (2005) Oral medicine—update for the dental practitioner. Apthous and other common ulcers. *British Dental Journal*, 199(5), 259–264.

Silverman, S., (2001) Demographics and occurrence of oral and pharyngeal cancer: the outcomes, the trends, the challenge. *Journal of the American Dental Association, 132S*, 7S–11S.

Southern Association of Institutional Dentists. (n.d.). *Preventive dentistry for persons with severe disabilities*. Retrieved from http://www.saiddent.org.

Spolarich, A.E. (2009). Medication use and xerostomia: Treating drug induced dry mouth. *Dimensions of Oral Hygiene 3*(7), 22–24.

Stanford, C.M. (2007). Dental implants: A role in geriatric dentistry for the general practice? *Journal of the American Dental Association, 138*(9), 34S–40S.

Stein, P., & Henry, R.G. (2009). Poor oral hygiene in long-term care: A continuing education program for nurses. *American Journal of Nursing, 109*(6), 44–50.

Taylor, G.W., & Borgnakke, W.S. (2008). Periodontal disease: Associations with diabetes, glycemic control and complications. *Oral Disease, 14*(3), 191–203.

Terpenning, M. (2005). Geriatric oral health and pneumonia risk. *Clinical Infectious Diseases, 40*(12), 1807–1810.

Turner, M., Jahangiri, L., & Ship, J.A. (2008). Hyposalivation, xerostomia and the complete denture: A systematic review. *Journal of the American Dental Association, 139*(2), 146–150.

United Nations Publications. (2004). Sex and age distribution of the world population. *World Population Prospects: The 2004 Revision*, Vol. II (Highlights), 10, 53–63. Retrieved August 13, 2009, from http://www.un.org/.../population/publications/WPP2004/WPP2004_Volume 3.htm

United States Department of Health and Human Services. (2009, May 21). *Perceived oral health status among adults with teeth in the United States, 1988–94*. Retrieved from www.cdc.gov/nchs/nhanes/Databriefs. htm

Van der Horst, M., & Scott, D. (2009). *Oral health for frail older adults: Oral health assessment tool and care plan* [Power Point Program]. Retrieved from www.rgpc.ca

Vargas, C.M., Kramarow, E.A., & Yellowitz, J.A. (2001). The oral health of older Americans. *Aging Trends, 3*, 1–8.

Verma, S., & Mahalinga, B. (2004). Acceptability of powered toothbrushes for elderly individuals. *Journal Public Health Dentistry, 64*(2), 115–17.

Wennstrom, J., & Lindhe, J. (1979). Effect of hydrogen peroxide on developing plaque and gingivitis in man. *Journal of Clinical Periodontology, 6*(2), 115–130. doi: 10.1111/j.1600-051X.1979.tb02190.x

Westphal, C.M., Fumari, W., & Haber, J. (2009, July). *College of Dentistry/College of Nursing partnership*. Retrieved from http://www.adha.org/publications/specialfeature3.htm

White, D.L., Newton-Curtis, L., & Lyons, K.S. (2008). Development and initial testing of a measure of person-directed care. *The Gerontologist. 48*(1), 114–123. Retrieved from http://gerontologist .gerontologyjournals.org/cgi/reprint/48/suppl_1/114

Williams, B.R., & Kim, J. (2005). Medication use and prescribing considerations for elderly patients. *Dental Clinics of North America, 49*, 411–427.

Yoder, K. (2006, February). A framework for service-learning in dental education. *Journal of Dental Education*, 115–123.

Zero, D., Fontanna, M., & Lennon, A.M. (2001). Clinical applications and outcomes of using indicators of risk in caries management. *Journal of Dental Education, 65*, 1126–1132.

Chapter 25

The Effect of Anticipatory Socialization on Morale in Newly Institutionalized LTC Residents

Samantha Sterns, Susan Allen, and Eva Kahana

The Study

Purpose

Admission to long-term care (LTC) facilities is common for older adults, and adjustment to institutional living has often proven to be difficult. This research examined the impact of anticipatory socialization and institutional stressors on morale of long-term care residents.

Design and Method

Self-reports of 134 LTC residents' morale were obtained at two time points: Time 1, when they first moved into institutions, and Time 2, after 8 months of residence. Morale was measured through the loneliness–dissatisfaction subscale of the Lawton Morale Scale (Lawton, 1975), which for this study is considered to be a general measure of resident well-being. We examined the impact of residents' demographic characteristics, health, and several aspects of anticipatory socialization (Merton & Kitt, 1950) on morale at both Time 1 and Time 2. We also examined the impact of institutional stressors, specifically those related to congregate living (Kleemeier, 1961) and institutional control (Goffman, 1961) on morale at Time 2 (after residents had been living at the facility for 8 months).

Results

Lack of anticipatory socialization was a significant predictor of lower morale at the time of the initial move, but not at Time 2. Rather, residents' health and their perceptions of institutional stressors had the greatest impact on their later well-being.

Implications

This research highlights that positive adaptation into an LTC facility is possible. Educating residents on what to expect prior to the move appears to help them adapt early on, while months later, reducing institutional stressors improves adaptation. Fortunately, a major focus of the culture change movement is to minimize these stressors, hopefully resulting in more residents who adapt well and who have a good morale when living in LTC facilities.

Background and Theory

Transitioning to living in a long-term care facility can be a difficult and lengthy process. Previous research on this topic has shown that residents do not experience an immediate adjustment when moving into long-term care; rather, this adjustment occurs over time. In particular, researchers have identified clear stages that nursing home residents experience in this adjustment process (Brooke, 1989; Lee, Woo, & Mackenzie, 2002; Wilson, 1997). Brooke (1989) found that residents who were disorganized at admission were able to reorganize their lives and built friendships over a 6-month period, and eventually stabilized into their new roles. Similarly, Lee and colleagues identified a four-step process of adjusting: orienting, normalizing, rationalizing, and finally stabilizing. These studies support the concept that there is a distinct process of adjusting to life in an institution, and that eventually many residents are able to adapt. Arguably, if a person was better prepared for a move and in fact made the choice to move into an LTC facility (i.e., more anticipatory socialization), s/he may have an easier time adapting to the new environment.

"Anticipatory socialization" is a process or set of experiences in which individuals come to correctly anticipate the values, norms, and behaviors that will be encountered in a new social setting (Merton, 1957; Merton & Kitt, 1950). Persons could be said to be lacking anticipatory socialization if they experience an abrupt or unwelcome move into an LTC setting. While Merton and Kitt wrote about this process for newcomers on a job, concepts relating to anticipatory socialization have been applied to the process of moving into nursing homes, among other settings. For instance, in a study of nursing home residents, Schwartz (1999) found that an abrupt move into a nursing home was traumatic for older adults, that residents often have limited choice over the decision to move into a long-term care facility, and that many enter against their will. In a study on foster care and nursing home residents, Reinardy and Kane (1999) found that many residents were manipulated into moving, or that the move was inevitable or unwelcome. Additionally, transitions into a nursing home are typically involuntary, with physicians and social workers often the most influential in the decision to move (York & Caslyn, 1977). Given this prior research, we concluded that higher levels of anticipatory socialization could lead to a better morale for residents in long-term care facilities.

Institutional stressors may also affect resident morale. Long-term care provider settings, such as nursing homes, assisted living facilities (ALF), and others, are structured to meet the physical and cognitive needs of typically large groups of elderly individuals with multiple and diverse impairments. In an effort to increase efficiency, institutional providers have established set times and regimens for waking, bathing, dressing, and other daily activities. A move from the community into an LTC setting can be difficult, as residents' daily schedules are no longer self-regulated, but now must be reorganized to fit within this structured setting.

Many of the difficulties experienced in institutions are theorized in the classic text *Asylums* by Goffman (1961). Goffman characterized the "total institution" as an environment where residents live in a congregate setting, with a group of people who live under the same set of rules and who are expected to routinely participate in a number of daily activities together. Goffman also noted that people who live under such conditions typically lose their individualism and live with little autonomy. With many same-age peers doing the same things together daily, institutional life leads to conflict between personal needs and institutional demands. "Institutional control" thus limits residents' choices over daily schedules, food options, and generally what residents can do and when they can do it. While Goffman's research was conducted in mental institutions, his "total institution" theory has been applied to other institutional settings, such as nursing homes (Clark & Bowling, 1990; Shield, 1988). In a study that applies total institution theory, Clark and Bowling (1990) found that the theoretical premise held true in a long-stay hospital ward, but not for smaller nursing homes for the elderly. This study points to the possibility that not all nursing homes can be classified as total institutions, and that certain setups (such as smaller dwellings) may be more accommodating to residents' needs. Other researchers have examined problems that stem from institutional living, but not all used Goffman's theory as a research framework (Gubrium, 1975; Lieberman & Tobin, 1983; Vladeck, 1980). For instance, Gubrium (1975) found that nursing homes limited resident choices by instituting rigid mealtimes and structuring when residents received aid services based on the institution's schedule, and concluded that institutional living limited residents' choices and autonomy. However, in spite of widespread attention to problems faced by LTC residents, there has been relatively little empirical research applying fundamental social theories in the study design, such as the classic work of Goffman (1961) in his studies of the total institution.

The congregate nature of institutional living also poses challenges to new residents (Kleemeier, 1961). Older adults who were living in the community prior to LTC entry may have been living in their own homes, either alone or with family members or friends. In LTC settings, residents often share rooms and eat meals with other older adults who are likely to be strangers to them; thus it is understandable that new residents may encounter difficulties adjusting to the congregate features of nursing homes. In our research, we refer to these difficulties as "congregate stressors." Specifically, we refer to problems with other residents intruding on others' personal privacy and on the inability to be by oneself, as well as difficult interactions between and among staff and residents.

This study sought to bring out sociological insights through the examination of the experiences of institutional living in a sample of 135 residents newly entering one of 14 long-term care facilities. We examined the impact of anticipatory socialization for residents' well-being (Merton & Kitt, 1950). Additionally, we looked at issues of institutional control (Goffman, 1961) and problems associated with congregate living (Kleemeier, 1961). Specifically, we tested whether residents' perceptions of institutional living (i.e., institutional control and congregate living) influenced resident morale.

Rationale and Hypothesis

Based on Merton and Kitt's (1950) concept of anticipatory socialization and aspects of Goffman's (1961) theory of the total institution, our two hypotheses relate to the influence of extra-institutional and intra-institutional factors on residents' quality of life. We hypothesized (I) that the presence of anticipatory socialization would increase both early and later morale, and (II) that the combined impact of congregate and institutional control-based stressors would significantly lower later (i.e., Time 2) morale.

Methods

Sample

The study population consisted of 135 residents over the age of 52, who entered one of 14 LTC facilities located in two large Midwestern cities (Kahana, Kahana, & Young, 1987). Both proprietary and nonprofit charitable or religious institutions were included in the study. Facilities were located in two metropolitan areas and were primarily urban locations with some suburban and rural representation. Half of the institutions had combined nursing home licensure with home for the aged or board and care home licensure. Eleven facilities were sponsored by religious entities (5 Jewish, 4 Protestant, 2 Catholic institutions), but religious sponsorship did not require that residents practice or adhere to that faith. There was an average capacity of 203 beds, and none of the facilities had fewer than 100 beds. Eligibility criteria required that participants be newly admitted (from a community setting) to self-care or intermediate care divisions of these institutions, that they be ambulatory, and that they be able and willing to participate in the interview.

Measures

The outcome measures included morale at Time 1, when residents first entered the facilities; and again at Time 2, after 8 months of living in a facility. At both time points, psychological well-being was measured with the "loneliness–dissatisfaction" portion of Lawton's Morale Scale (1975). This measure for morale was comprised of six items. Two items were framed as questions: "How much do you feel lonely?" and "How satisfied are you with your life today?" with distinct answer choices. For the remaining four items residents were asked to confirm or deny the following statements: "I see enough of my friends and relatives"; "I sometimes feel that life isn't worth living"; "I have a lot to be sad about"; and "Life is hard for me much of the time." Morale scores ranged from 6 (lowest) to 12 (highest). Reliability analysis on the six items from each time wave showed fairly high congruence across items (Time 1 alpha = .75; Time 2 alpha = .75).

Anticipatory socialization was measured at Time 1 by three variables developed to capture multiple dimensions of this construct. They included the following: consideration of alternatives to the move; reluctance to move; and clarity of what to expect after the move. These variables did not load onto a factor and were shown empirically to be separate concepts through an external correlates test. The item "reluctance to move" ranged from 1, "eager to move," to 3, "reluctant to move." The second item was dichotomous, indicating whether or not residents considered alternatives to move. The third and final construct used in the analyses asked about the clarity of the move: "All in all, your picture of what your life will be like in the residence is: 'very clear,' 1, 'clear,' 2, or 'unclear about what to expect,' 3."

Two dichotomous variables were developed to capture residents' responses related to institutional living: institutional control and congregate living. These variables were created based on residents' open-ended responses, measured a few weeks after the first interview. Specifically, respondents were asked: "How much difficulty have you had related to . . . ?": 1. the physical environment, 2. activities, 3. staff, 4. food, 5. other residents, and 6. family. Examples of difficulties categorized under "congregate living" were: "I don't like a large group of people"; "chronic complainer picking on me"; and "other residents come in and out of room." Examples of institutional control are: "7:30 a.m. breakfast, having to get dressed"; "they want you to stay at the same table all the time"; and "I have nothing to do."

Demographic characteristics, including gender, age, race, and immigrant status, were determined by interview questions. Residents' cognitive impairment as reflected by memory deficits was assessed at the time just prior to their moving to the LTC facilities by using the well-known Mental Status Questionnaire (MSQ) (Kahn, Goldfarb, Pollack, & Peck, 1960). This questionnaire provides a brief, objective, and quantitative measurement of cognitive functioning of older adults, appropriate for patient samples (1960). Questions assess respondents' orientation, including knowing the day's date, the current president's name, and the name of the most immediate previous president (10 items). Scores ranged from 0 to 10, with a score of 10 representing no errors (alpha = .73).

Three health measures were included in the analysis. The first question asked respondents about their health compared with others their age, with five answer categories ranging from "very poor" to "excellent." The second question asked respondents how their health was now compared to two years prior, with five answer categories that ranged from "much worse" to "much better." For both single item indicators, a higher value represented better health. A third index of health was "activities of daily living" (ADL), as based on factor analyses and prior literature. The three items comprising ADL include: "Can you still do heavy work around the house?" "Can you still walk half a mile without help?" and "Can you walk up and down the stairs to the second floor without help?" with answer categories of "yes" and "no." The resulting ADL index ranged from 3 (most independent) to 6 (most dependent).

Analysis

To test the preceding hypotheses, we ran two ordinary least-squares regression models; the first on initial morale, when residents first moved into the facilities, and the second on later morale at 8 months post-institutionalization. Key anticipatory socialization predictors were regressed on both initial morale and later morale (to test hypothesis I). At Time 2, we added a third model that included whether residents experienced one or two stressors (congregate and institutional) to determine the relative impact of multiple stressors on morale (to test hypothesis II). Covariates at both waves included demographic characteristics (gender, age, born in the United States or foreign born, married, or widowed) and health characteristics (health compared with others one's age, health compared with two years prior, ADL, and MSQ).

Results

The sample was primarily female (77.8%) and in their late seventies (mean = 78.7). Most were widowed (64.4%), with only 18.5% still married. The sample was racially homogeneous, with over 95% of the sample Caucasian. Regarding immigrant status, 38.5% of residents were born outside the United States (Table 25-1).

The majority of respondents said they were in good health (Table 25-1). Over half of the sample (64.4%) reported their health as "good" or "excellent" compared with others their age, while less than 10% (8.1%) felt that their health was "poor" or "very poor" in comparison with others their age. Additionally, over 50% of the sample indicated that they had very little difficulty with their ADLs, while only about one-fourth of respondents recorded a score of 6, indicating extremely high difficulty with their ADLs (Table 25-1). Furthermore, over half of the sample said that they had no cognitive impairment, while 23.2% had mild cognitive impairment (<3 incorrect responses). There was a fairly substantial portion of the population who felt that their health was "worse" or "much worse" than two years prior (32.6%), with a smaller group (17.0%) who felt that their health was "better" or "much better" in comparison.

Respondents showed relatively high levels of anticipatory socialization (Table 25-2). The majority of respondents either made the decision to move into the facility jointly with others (49.3%) or on their own (43.0%), while only ten (7.7%) had the decision to move made completely by others. For the most part, respondents felt "very clear" or "clear" about what to expect (75.5%), and were "eager" or "somewhat willing to move" (80.7%) to

TABLE 25-1   Sample Characteristics

Study Measures	Distribution % (N)
Gender	
2–Female	77.8 (105)
1–Male	22.2 (30)
Race	
2–Black	2.2 (3)
1–White	97.8 (132)
Age (Mean = 78.7; SD = 7.5)	
52–65	3.7 (5)
65–74	28.2 (38)
75–84	45.2 (61)
85–94	23.0 (31)
Immigrant Status	
1–Born in the USA	61.5 (83)
2–Born outside the USA	38.5 (52)
Marital Status	
Married	18.5 (25)
Widowed	64.4 (87)
Divorced or separated	8.2 (11)
Never married, single	8.9 (12)
Health compared with others your age	
5–Excellent	24.4 (33)
4–Good	40.0 (54)
3–Fair	27.4 (37)
2–Poor	5.9 (8)
1–Very poor	2.2 (3)
Health now compared with two years ago	
5–Much better	5.9 (8)
4–Better	11.1 (15)
3–Same	50.4 (68)
2–Worse	26.7 (36)
1–Much worse	5.9 (8)

(*continues*)

TABLE 25-1 (Continued)

Study Measures	Distribution % (N)	
Instrumental activities of daily living (IADL) problems (Mean = 4.6; SD = 1.0)		
3—Least difficulties	15.6	(21)
4	37.0	(50)
5	23.0	(31)
6—Most difficulties	24.4	(33)
Cognitive functioning (MSQ) (Mean = 8.9; SD = 1.7)		
1–5—Most cognitively impaired	5.2	(7)
6–7	17.0	(23)
8–9	20.0	(27)
10—No cognitive impairment	57.8	(78)

TABLE 25-2 Key Study Variables

Anticipatory Socialization	% (N)
The decision to move was made by	
Yourself only	43.0 (58)
Jointly with others	49.3 (67)
Others only	7.7 (10)
Have you ever visited the residence?	
Yes	81.6 (110)
No	18.4 (25)
Did you consider alternatives to moving to this residence?	
Yes	37.0 (50)
No	63.0 (85)
All in all, your picture of what your life will be like in the residence will be:	
1–Very clear	34.8 (47)
2–Clear	40.7 (55)
3–Unclear what to expect	24.4 (33)

(continues)

TABLE 25-2   (Continued)

Anticipatory Socialization	% (N)
Are you:	
1–Eager to move	38.5 (52)
2–Somewhat willing to move	42.2 (57)
3–Reluctant to move	19.3 (26)

Institutional Living	% (N)
Congregate living	
0–no living	76.3 (103)
1–stressor	23.7 (32)
Institutional control	
0–no stressor	79.3 (107)
1–stressor	20.7 (28)
Number of institutionally related stressors (congregate and autonomy)	
0	63.0 (85)
1	29.6 (40)
2	7.4 (10)

Outcomes	% (N)
Morale scale (Time 1) (Mean = 10.1; SD = 1.7)	
6–7 –Low morale	12.6 (17)
8–9	20.0 (27)
10	14.8 (20)
11	24.4 (33)
12 –High morale	28.1 (38)
Morale scale (Time 2) (Mean = 10.4; SD = 1.8)	
6–7 –Low morale	14.1 (19)
8–9	9.6 (13)
10	16.3 (22)
11	23.7 (32)
12 –High morale	36.3 (49)

the LTC facility. About two-thirds of the sample (63%) did not consider alternatives to moving to their LTC residence.

Relatively few residents (fewer than one-fourth) reported institutional stressors after about a month in the facilities (Table 25-2); 23.7% of the respondents experienced problems related to congregate living, and 20.7% had a problem with institutional control. Only 7.4% experienced problems related to both congregate living and institutional control.

Morale was fairly high for the majority of residents (Table 25-2). At Time 1, 52.5% had a high level of morale (scoring 11–12), while only 12.6% scored extremely low (scoring 6–7). At Time 2, 60% had a high morale (7.5% higher than at Time 1), while only 14.1% scored extremely low (1.5% lower than at Time 1).

Ordinary Least–Squares Results

Regression results reveal different patterns of association on morale at Time 1 and morale at Time 2. Anticipatory socialization variables were significantly associated with initial morale at Time 1, but not later morale, at Time 2 (Table 25-3; Table 25-4). Variables associated with lower morale at Time 1 included a greater reluctance to move to LTC and more uncertainty about what to expect before the move ($b = -.56$, $b = -.52$) (Table 25-3). Demographic patterns also impacted morale differently upon entering LTC facilities versus after 8 months of residence. In multivariate analysis, immigrant status was the only demographic variable significantly associated with lower morale at Time 1 ($b = -.68$) (Table 25-3). By comparison, older age, immigrant status, and poorer health compared with others one's age were significantly associated with morale at Time 2 ($b = -.07$, $b = -.85$, and $b = -.53$, respectively) (Table 25-4, Model 2).

The reporting of both institutional living stressors was significantly associated with lower morale at Time 2 ($b = -1.24$). Reporting one stressor compared to no stressor was not significantly associated with morale at Time 2 ($b = -.28$) (Table 25-4, Model 2).

Discussion

Residents with high levels of anticipatory socialization experienced better morale when first moving into an LTC facility, suggesting they were more able to initially adapt to institutional life than those who lacked this prior socialization. Eight months later, factors that translated to a better morale were better health and experiencing fewer institutional living stressors. Conversely, residents who reported their environments to be problematic were more likely to experience a lower morale. The findings suggest that reducing the negative aspects of congregate living and institutionalization makes resident adaptation easier and may decrease residents' dissatisfaction with life in LTC facilities.

For the majority of residents in this study, the move into LTC was a move they were willing to make. Specifically, our study showed higher levels of resident involvement and choice than has been observed in many studies. We found that 43% of the residents studied here made the decision to move on their own, which is contrary to the findings of a

TABLE 25-3   Regression Analyses of Morale at Time 1 (N = 135)

	b	SE b	Beta
Personal Characteristics			
Gender (1 = female)	.22	.35	.05
Age	−.02	.02	−.07
Immigrant	−.68	.29	−.21*
Married	.64	.49	.15
Widowed	.37	.39	.12
Health compared with others your age	−.27	.18	−.14
Health compared with 2 years ago	−.15	.17	−.08
ADL T1	−.01	.16	−.01
MSQ total T1	−.03	.09	−.04
Anticipatory Socialization			
Consideration of alternatives	.23	.30	.10
Reluctance to move	−.56	.21	−.18*
Uncertain what to expect before move	−.52	.19	−.21*

R = .52

R^2 = .27

Adjusted R^2 = .20

F = 3.70, $p < .001$

Intercept: 14.46

*Significance at the $p < .05$ level

qualitative study of 52 older adults entering nursing homes conducted by Nakashima and colleagues (2004), where only 24% of the sample had made the decision to move themselves. Furthermore, while prior research reports that many residents are manipulated into moving (Reinardy & Kane, 1999), and that a transition into a nursing home is typically involuntary (York & Caslyn, 1977), the majority of residents in our study voluntarily entered nursing homes and had input into the decision to move there. Differences between our data and other studies may be due to the fact that the residents we studied were more physically healthy and had higher levels of cognitive functioning than those in other studies. Future research should expand upon the work on anticipatory socialization by determining the role that physical frailty and cognitive impairment may have on limiting anticipatory socialization.

TABLE 25-4 Regression Analyses of Morale at Time 2 (N = 135)

	Adjusted R^2 = .29			Adjusted R^2 = .31		
	Model 1 $F = 5.52, p < .001$			Model 2 $F = 5.20, p < .001$		
	b SE b Beta Intercept: 19.00			b SE b Beta Intercept: 18.75		
	b	SE b	Beta	b	SE b	Beta
Personal Characteristics						
Gender (1 = female)	.25	.34	.06	.19	.34	.04
Age	−.07	.02	−.30**	−.07	.02	−.27**
Immigrant	−.97	.28	−.26**	−.85	.28	−.23**
Married	.47	.48	.10	.35	.48	.07
Widowed	.57	.38	.15	.62	.38	.17
Health compared with others your age	−.54	.17	−.29***	−.53	.17	−.28**
Health compared with 2 years ago	−.22	.16	−.11	−.18	.16	−.09
ADL T1	.08	.16	.05	.13	.15	.03
MSQ total T1	−.04	.08	−.04	−.05	.08	−.04
Anticipatory Socialization						
Consideration of alternatives	.30	.29	.08	.13	.30	.03
Reluctance to move	−.30	.20	−.12	−.23	.20	−.09
Uncertain what to expect before move	−.29	.19	−.12	−.26	.19	−.11
Institutional living						
None vs. 2 stressors				−1.24	.57	−.18*
None vs. 1 stressor				−.28	.30	−.07
		R = .59			R = .61	
		R^2 = .35			R^2 = .38	

* Significance at the $p < .05$ level, ** $p < .01$, *** $p < .001$

In this study, anticipatory socialization significantly impacted initial well-being, but not later well-being. Other studies have reported findings similar to ours. For instance, in a qualitative study of nursing home residents and direct care staff, Shield (1988) found that residents who were unaware that the move to the nursing home was permanent experienced a more difficult adjustment. Furthermore, while residents initially had a difficult time giving up their autonomous lifestyle in the community, over time they adjusted to the nursing home by recognizing and accepting the safeguards and security as necessary elements of the institution. It is postulated that they also learned to lessen the effects of congregate living by choosing friends and activities that they enjoyed. The findings of this study support our findings that the effects of anticipatory socialization may diminish over time. However, contrary to our findings, one study (Davidson & O'Conner, 1990) found that perceived control over relocation decisions positively impacted health during the first month of residency, but negatively impacted health and morale between the second and fourth months. It is possible that the differences in the findings between this study and ours may be attributable to differences in the institutions studied, or perhaps to the time frames of the interviews; for instance, our second contact was 8 months following study entry, allowing greater time for adjustment than the 4-month period reported in the Davidson and O'Connor study.

Similar to previously discussed research (Goffman, 1961; Gubrium, 1975; Lieberman & Tobin, 1983; Vladeck, 1980, 2003), our research suggests that multiple problems faced in institutional settings lead to lower morale. Specifically, we found that about a fifth of the residents in our study experienced problems related to institutional control, and one-fourth expressed problems related to living in a congregate setting. Common problems reported include those described by Goffman, expressed as complaints related to control over schedules, limitations on what residents could and could not do, and problems related to food choices and food quality. One resident's comments illustrate the heart of Goffman's theory, "This place is a jail. I can't do what I want to when I want to."

It is significant that the majority of respondents (63%) reported no problems. This finding indicates that these residents did not choose to report a problem, or that they experienced no problems, suggesting that the institutional structure was only a problem for a relatively small number of the residents, while the rest were willing and able to adapt fairly easily and quickly to this new environment. A perhaps more probable explanation is that as these questions were asked early on in the move, problems were only reported by respondents who experienced immediate negative reactions to institutional living, and early recognition of a poor person–environment fit had a significant impact on morale for these residents.

We found that factors unrelated to the institution or to anticipatory socialization also significantly impacted later morale. Patient factors including worse physical health, being older, and being an immigrant played a significant role in predicting lower morale at Time 2. It also seems possible that having immigrated from another country may have made the adjustment to institutionalization more difficult due to language barriers and to food preferences. Additionally, it is possible that immigrants may have encountered cultural barriers in interactions with staff and other residents. Finally, different ethnic cultures have different norms. For example, in many cultures children are obligated to take care of their parents, perhaps making living in an LTC facility more problematic for residents who emigrate from other countries. Unfortunately, many LTC facilities do not focus on meeting the needs of different cultural populations (Cohen & Diaz Moore, 1999). In response to the need for culturally appropriate care, Day and Cohen (2000) have developed a series of recommendations in redesigning care environments to be culturally appropriate for dementia patients as well as for cognitively intact patients. However, while there is some research on preferences and expectations of specific cultural groups (Alves, 2005; Heikkila, 2004), more empirical research is needed on how being an immigrant influences adaptation to life in a traditional LTC facility, and on what institutional initiatives can be/have been successful in improving cultural sensitivity.

When considering the factors impacting initial and later morale, we can conclude that different variables impact adjustment throughout the process of living in an institution. We found that anticipatory socialization played a larger role earlier on, while 8 months later it did not. Instead, other factors now played a larger role in morale, including one's age, health, and stressors relating to the institution. Our research therefore identified two distinct stages in a move to an LTC facility: Stage 1, where uncertainty and prior reluctance to moving can overwhelm a resident; and Stage 2, where new concerns about problems in the institution and health become central. In the first stage, the residents who were better prepared and knowledgeable about the move were more successful than others. In the second stage, residents who reported fewer institutionally related problems or health concerns were more successful (i.e., less lonely and dissatisfied) in accepting their more institutionalized way of life. Examining nursing home adaptation using this framework of stages is consistent with prior research that reports differences in adaptation over time (Brooke, 1989; Lee, Woo, & Mackenzie, 2002; Wilson, 1997). This study found that residents at admission were disorganized and had to orient to their new environment, but that over time they were able to normalize, stabilize, and accept their new lives. Similarly, our findings suggest that when residents initially moved into a nursing home, they were still somewhat disengaged from the facility, focusing instead on problems predating their move. Residents later focused on problems related to the institution, rather than factors that occurred prior to their move, suggesting they were more attuned to their current home.

A substantial body of research, including this work, points to potentially positive outcomes and experiences of living in LTC, with many residents having a good adjustment and overall positive psychological well-being. For instance, Street and colleagues (2007) found that in assisted living facilities, higher food quality and resident perception of adequate privacy are associated with better resident well-being. In another study on nursing home residents, Stafford (2003) reported that residents find life in nursing homes meaningful, adapt and find new relationships with people inside the home, and stay involved in activities and developing new roles. In our study, we found that more than half of the residents had a high morale, and have therefore adapted reasonably well to life in an LTC facility. This adaptation may have been due to respondents' resilience, or it may alternatively represent residents "giving in" and thus conforming to the institution's ways.

There are limitations to our study. First, while we had a relatively high level of ethnic variation (i.e., a large immigrant population), one limitation is the low proportions of minorities in the sample. Secondly, the relatively small sample size limited the power, resulting in relatively large standard errors. With a larger sample size we could perhaps have detected more subtle effects. Compared with research in this same area, however, our study did represent a relatively large sample. But regardless of sample size, the findings of this study still inform us about salient issues that can guide policy development related to long-term care.

This study had a number of strengths. While previous studies mainly used an inductive approach, first collecting data and then forming theories to explain it, this research applied hypotheses based on previously developed theories and concepts to objective data. Furthermore, the present study had an advantage over previous research as the data were obtained from in-person interviews with residents of LTC facilities. Moreover, our data is based on a large multiwave quantitative and qualitative data set of several LTC facilities, examining problems facing residents in both the early and the later adaptation phases. The findings are relevant to residents entering assisted living facilities and shed light on how residents adapt to their new environment.

Implications/Conclusions

Findings from this research have important implications for policy and practice, including the need for more resident involvement in decisions regarding LTC placement and altering the nursing home environment to be less institutional. One key implication is the value of involving older adults in the decision to move to LTC. There is literature suggesting patient involvement in making decisions is beneficial in many areas of health care delivery, including in LTC facilities. For instance, in one study, policies in residential care facilities that allow more choice and control were associated with better resident well-being, less use of daily living assistance, and greater integration in the community, among other positive outcomes (Timko & Moos, 2006). Unfortunately, patients are not always involved in their care decisions, especially when an acute care crisis warrants a move. Therefore, it is particularly important to involve persons with physical impairments and/or cognitive impairment in the actual decision process before crises occur. For those elders who are more reluctant to move, it may be useful to have them visit the facilities with their families and have input into *which* facility they would be willing to move to in the event of a health crisis. By educating elders on what they can expect once they move into LTC facilities, it can help them to mentally prepare earlier, making the adjustment process easier and leading to a better transition.

Also, long-term care facilities can potentially lessen the adverse effects of institutional living. Many nursing homes are attempting this transformation, through methods collectively termed "culture change." Some of the key constructs of culture change (Harris, Poulson, & Vlangas, 2006) include: (1) environments designed to be a home rather than an institution, (2) close relationships between staff, family, resident, and community, (3) care and activities directed by residents, (4) staff empowerment, and (5) collaboration and decentralized management. One "culture change" model is the Eden Alternative, a program that strives to achieve a warm, friendly environment that is enjoyable to live in on a day-to-day basis by encouraging meaningful relationships among nursing home residents (Thomas, 1996). This type of program helps improve the institutional environment to some degree, but some research has found that underlying problems with the traditional nursing home structure impair the complete success of the Eden Alternative program (Thomas, 2003). Another model of cultural change is the Green House (Brown, 2007; Rabig, Thomas, Kane, Cutler, & McAlilly, 2006), which advocates small homes created for 10 or fewer residents. Thus, a more family-like setting provides each resident with a private bedroom and bathroom, and with smaller group areas in which to eat and gather. This design offers a setting where there is privacy, and where residents have autonomy and support, in a place that feels more like a home (Brown, 2007). In addition to the above, many US nursing homes have reorganized care to encompass the needs of their specific residents (i.e., to make care resident-centered), demonstrating that the concept of culture change is not a one-solution model. Solutions for nursing homes tend to be specific to both the organization and the needs of its residents and staff. By implementing a spirit of change, it encourages each facility to find solutions to problems that are by their nature, specific. Overall, there appears to be a great potential for the culture change movement to improve the quality of life for both residents and staff, and thus to potentially increase overall morale.

References

Alves, S.M. (2005). Accommodating culturally meaningful activities in outdoor settings for older adults. *Journal of Housing for the Elderly, 19*(3/4), 109–140.

Brooke, V. (1989). Nursing home life: How elders adjust. *Geriatric Nursing, 10*, 66–68.

Brown, M.H. (2007, January). *"Green Houses" provide a small group setting alternative to nursing homes—and a positive effect on residents' quality of life.* Retrieved March 1, 2007, from http://www.rwjf.org/reports/grr/057114.htm?gsa=1

Clark, P., & Bowling, A. (1990). Quality of everyday life in long stay institutions for the elderly. An observational study of long stay hospital and nursing home. *Social Science Medicine, 30*(11), 1201–1210.

Cohen, U., & Diaz Moore, K. (1999). Integrating cultural heritage into assisted living environments. In B. Schwartz & R. Brent (Eds.), *Aging, autonomy, and architecture: Advances in assisted living* (pp. 90–109). Baltimore, MD: John Hopkins University Press.

Davidson, H.A., & O'Conner, B.P. (1990). Perceived control and acceptance of the decision to enter a nursing home as predictors of adjustment. *International Journal of Aging and Human Development, 31*(4), 307–318.

Day, K., & Cohen, U. (2000). The role of culture in designing environments for people with dementia: A study of Russian Jewish immigrants. *Environment and Behavior, 32*, 361.

Goffman, E. (1961). *Asylums: Essays on the social situation of mental patients and other inmates.* Chicago, IL: Aldine Publishing Co.

Gubrium, J. F. (1975). *Living and dying at Murray Manor.* New York: St. Martin's.

Harris, Y., Poulson, R., & Vlangas, G. (2006). Measuring Culture Change Literature Review. CFMC–Medicare Quality Improvement Organization for Colorado. Publication number, PM–411–114 CO

Heikkila, K. (2004). *The role of ethnicity in care of elderly Finnish immigrants*. Sweden: Baran tryck Sollentuna.

Kahana, E., Kahana, B., & Young, R. (1987). Strategies of coping and post institutional outcomes. *Research on Aging, 9*(2), 182–199.

Kahn, R.L., Goldfarb, A.I., Pollack, M., & Peck, A. (1960). Brief objective measures for the determination of mental status in the aged. *American Journal of Psychiatry, 117*, 326–328.

Kleemeier, R.W. (1961). *Aging and leisure: A research perspective into the meaningful use of time*. New York: Oxford University Press.

Lawton, M.P. (1975). The Philadelphia geriatric center morale scale: A revision. *Journal of Gerontology, 30*, 85–89.

Lee, D.T.F., Woo J., & Mackenzie, A.E. (2002). Cultural context of adjusting to nursing home life. *Chinese Elders' Perspectives, 42*(5), 667–675.

Lieberman, M., & Tobin, S. (1983). *The experience of old age: Stress, coping and survival*. New York: Basic Books.

Merton, R.K. (1957). *Social theory and social structure*. New York: Free Press.

Merton, R.K., & Kitt, A. (1950). *Contributions to the theory of reference group behavior*. Glencoe, Illinois: Free Press.

Nakashima, M., Chapin, R.K., Macmillian, K., & Zimmerman, M. (2004). Decision making in long-term care: Approaches used by older adults and implications for social work practice. *Journal of Gerontological Social Work, 43*(4), 79–102.

Rabig, J., Thomas, W., Kane, R.A., Cutler, L.J., & McAlilly, S. (2006). Radical redesign of nursing homes: Applying the green house concept in Tupelo, Mississippi. *Gerontologist, 46*(4), 533–539.

Reinardy, J., & Kane, R.A. (1999). Choosing an adult foster home or a nursing home: Resident's perceptions about decision making and control. *Social Work, 44*(6), 571–585.

Schwartz, M.C. (1999). From home to nursing home: The last transition—the reality and the challenge. *Journal of Geriatric Psychiatry, 32*(2), 241–247.

Shield, R.R. (1988). *Uneasy endings: Daily life in an American nursing home*. Ithaca, NY: Cornell University Press.

Stafford, P.B. (Ed.) (2003). *Gray areas: Ethnographic encounters with nursing home culture*. Santa Fe, NM: School of American Research Press.

Street, D., Burge, S., Quadagno, J., & Barrett, A. (2007). The salience of social relationships for resident well-being in assisted living. *The Journals of Gerontology Series B: Psychological Sciences and Social Sciences, 63*, S129–S134.

Thomas, W. (1996). *Life worth living: How someone you love can still enjoy life in a nursing home—the Eden Alternative in action*. Acton, MA: VanderWyk & Burnham.

Thomas, W. (2003). Evolution of Eden. In A.S. Weiner & J.L. Ronch (Eds.), *Culture change in long-term care* (pp. 141–158). New York: Hawthorn Press, Inc.

Timko, C., & Moos, R.H. (2006). Choice, control, and adaptation among elderly residents of sheltered care settings. *Journal of Applied Social Psychology, 16*(8), 636–655.

Vladeck, B.C. (1980). *Unloving care: The nursing home tragedy*. New York: Basic Books.

Vladeck, B.C. (2003). Unloving care revisited: The persistence of culture. *Journal of Social Work in Long-Term Care, 2*(1/2), 1–9.

Wilson, S.A. (1997). The transition to nursing home life: A comparison of planned and unplanned admissions. *Journal of Advanced Nursing, 26*, 864–871.

York, J., & Caslyn, R. (1977). Family involvement in nursing homes. *The Gerontologist, 17*(6), 500–505.

Chapter 26

Poetry for Caregivers of Older Adults: Easing the Burden

Lori Kidd

She was feeling very sorry for herself that morning as she pulled into the parking lot of the rehab facility. She was a single middle-aged woman caring for her mother. Her only brother and his family lived out of state, so the burden of care fell on her. Some days it didn't feel like a burden to help care for your best friend, but other days, she felt so very alone. When a voice called out her name, she turned around to see her girlfriend in the parking lot beside her. Such a welcome surprise! But when her friend wrapped her arms around her in a hug of greeting, she burst into tears. . . .

The purpose of this chapter is to discuss stresses associated with being a caregiver for an older adult, and to briefly examine nursing interventions and strategies that can help reduce those stresses. A particular focus will be the unique burden associated with being a family caregiver for older adults with dementia. Recent research describing a pilot of a poetry writing intervention to help dementia family caregivers will be presented in some detail, along with a discussion of how expressive therapies may help caregivers.

Caregivers for Older Adults—Who Are They?

Caregiving can be a lonely job. Yet for one in five people over the age of 18 in the United States, it is a daily reality (National Alliance for Caregiving/American Association of Retired Persons [NAC/AARP], 2004). And days can turn into years. The average duration of care provided by caregivers is more than 4 years (National Alliance for Caregiving, and American Association of Retired Persons, 2004). With estimates that the elderly population will double between 2000 and 2030, even more persons will become caregivers for older adults in the future (Federal Interagency Forum on Aging-Related Statistics, 2000).

Formal caregivers are compensated for their efforts. They are professionals, skilled and trained in their duties. They choose to engage in activities that assist others, and embark upon careers of service that they find rewarding. Informal caregivers, however, often find their duties suddenly thrust upon them, perhaps by choice, perhaps because there is no one else available. They are not financially compensated for their efforts. Greater than 60% are female (NAC/AARP, 2004). The role of older adult caregiver is assigned to spouses, children, extended family members, sometimes even friends. Caregiving inevitably involves burden because of its physical, psychological, and financial demands; however, there is great variation in whether that burden is heavy or light, shared or unshared, borne with joy or sadness. One caregiver talks about her role:

> I'm not really a caregiver; it made me realize that I enjoy it because I love him . . . and it's so hard because he's not who I loved, and he's a totally different person and he's like a stranger, and so I love who he was, so I guess I still love him (crying) . . . I do love him, and these are my reasons for doing what I'm doing.

Another caregiver speaks of having what it takes:

> . . . you have to have a passion for what you do (caregiving is a tough job), and I think that you have to truly have a love for people, and I hope it shows that . . .

Several research studies have documented positive effects of caregiving on family members with dementia, including gratification, feeling uplifted, and gaining satisfaction and mastery of challenges (Kinney & Stephens, 1989; Lawton, Kleban, Moss, Rovine, & Glickman, 1989; Motenko, 1989). In their study of formal and informal family caregivers for those with mild dementia, Andren and Elmstahl (2005) found the coexistence of moderate burden and great satisfaction. They concluded that caregivers can experience satisfaction despite feeling simultaneously burdened. It is a professional and ethical mandate for nurses to promote wellness in their clients and family members. Thus, when the caregiving experience results in positive emotions, these emotions should be reinforced to strengthen the caregivers themselves and the caregiving bond.

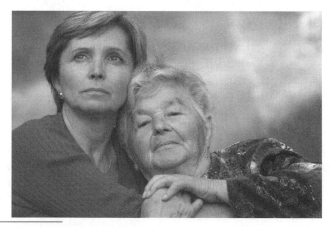

Figure 26-1   © absolut/ShutterStock, Inc.

The burden of caregiving, however, is frequently associated with more negative outcomes. The majority of empirical evidence cites adverse consequences related to the ongoing strain of the caregiver role. When that role unexpectedly appears and becomes a long-term journey punctuated by requirements for assistance, hospitalization, institutionalization, and multiple losses, caregiving may indeed become a "career" (Aneshensel, Pearlin, Mullan, Zarit, & Whitlatch, 1995). Adjusting to being a caregiver is challenging . . .

> I've got to accept the way he is, and not be so critical and I've got to realize that I can't ask him to do things for me anymore . . . like one of the ladies at church says, "We always thought that they would be around to take care of us, and here we are taking care of them," and I said "Yeah, right."

. . . and the journey is filled with loss.

> I'm having a hard time visiting her, because it's hard to see her there and you know she used to have flower gardens and worked in the yard, and she used to go to this nursing home and sing with the church group and visit people there, and you know she was always baking and cooking . . . and now . . . she plays with the dolls at the nursing home, but other than that she doesn't really do anything, and each time you see her, you see her health going down a little bit more.

While shouldering the burden of caregiving, the caregiver asks,

> . . . regardless of what I did, did I do enough? Years of tending. It's like jello melting and slipping through your fingers. No matter how much care I provided or tried to do . . .

Caregiver Stress and Burden

Financial costs of caregiving are high. The 2000 US Census estimated that 4.5 million people were diagnosed with Alzheimer's disease (Hebert, Scherr, Bienias, Bennett, & Evans, 2003). US businesses experience losses of over $61 billion each year due to work absences of their employees caring for loved ones with Alzheimer's disease. In addition, the annual cost of care for each individual diagnosed with Alzheimer's disease is estimated to range between $18,000 for mild Alzheimer's to over $36,000 for severe illness (Nichols et al., 2008). In 2004, caregivers helping to provide for an elder adult not a spouse averaged spending of over $200/month (NAC/AARP, 2004). Caregivers must try to balance the demands of caregiving with multiple demands of work, home, and other social obligations.

Heavy economic costs of caregiving pale, however, in comparison to physical and psychological costs imposed on caregivers. Physical costs of caring for a family member with dementia are great. The course of a neurobiological dementing illness is unpredictable, frequently long, and full of ambiguity (Baumgarten et al., 1992). Strain may occur to the point of increasing the risk of poor health (Wright, Clipp, & George, 1993; Schulz, O'Brien, Bookwala, & Fleissner, 1995), compromising immune system functioning

(Shaw et al., 1997), and increasing the risk of mortality (Schulz & Beach, 1999). In a meta-analysis (summary of multiple research studies), Schulz, Vistainer, and Williamson (1990) found that caregivers were more likely to experience psychiatric and physical morbidity than the general population. Many caregivers are older themselves and must work hard to maintain their own health to care for another. A middle-aged spouse caregiver wonders:

> [W]ill I still be in shape and physically and mentally together enough when this phase of my life changes and I am not the direct caregiver anymore to have the vigor to do anything? That really scares me. I don't want to wear out.

Caregiving produces more emotional than physical strain. One-third of caregivers (35%) surveyed rated their stress level as 4 of 5 on a 5-point scale. Those experiencing the greatest emotional stress were: female (40% vs. 26% male respondents); white or Hispanic (36% vs. 30% African American and 23% Asian American); and in fair or poor health (35% of those providing the most intense care). Almost one-third of caregivers (29%) reported a need for more help or information in managing emotional and physical stress. Those caring for someone with dementia reported even higher stress levels than other types of caregivers (42% vs. 32%) (NAC/AARP, 2004). In the words of a child caregiver:

> I was angry at the beginning. I've been angry for a long time and guilty, too, because I didn't want to be around her . . . there's a lot of guilt . . . I still am in denial . . . I just want her to straighten up and be like she's supposed to be.

Although heaviness of caregiving burden and intensity of care most predict physical and emotional health-related problems (Talley & Crews, 2007), caregiving at any level or degree can produce adverse psychological consequences for the caregiver. Adverse psychological outcomes such as depression and anxiety are more likely to develop in women than men, and are associated with greater responsibility for care tasks, more hours spent

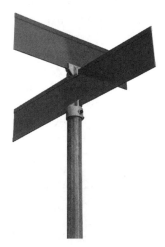

Figure 26-2 © R. Gino Santa Maria/Shutterstock, Inc.

on caregiving, and greater physical and mental decline of the care recipient (Yee & Schulz, 2000).

Dementia caregivers suffer even more negative consequences. Caring for a person with dementia has been associated with decreased psychological well-being of the caregiver (Bell, Araki, & Neumann, 2001; George & Gwyther, 1986; Zarit, Reever, & Bach-Peterson, 1980). Caregivers are at greater risk for depressive symptoms whether residing with or separately from the demented care recipient (Gibson, Butkus, Jenkins, Mathur, & Liu, 1997). Self-report on research studies with those caring for elders with dementia have consistently shown greater depression and anxiety than peers matched for age and gender (Schulz, 2000). Perceived stress can predict depression in caregivers (Etters, Goodall, & Harrison, 2008).

Help for the Helper

Nursing educators must spread the word that caregivers need attention and help. The nursing profession must mobilize an arsenal of interventions to help protect and defend all caregivers—and particularly, dementia caregivers—from negative consequences of caregiving. One way of assisting dementia caregivers is to directly affect behavior of the care recipient. Interventions such as day care help to improve behavioral and psychological symptoms in the demented individual; in turn, stress for the caregiver is reduced (Mossello et al., 2008). Another way to help reduce depressive symptoms in caregivers is to help provide meaning to care. If caregivers can feel satisfaction in their role or believe that caregiving helps them to grow in some way, their depression may be lessened and they may have increased self-esteem (Noonan & Tennstedt, 1997).

In the Stress Process Model, individuals cope with stress in several ways. One way is to modify or change the situation. A second way is to alter the meaning of the problem. Finally, one may manage the stress or learn better ways to accommodate to it (Pearlin & Schooler, 1978). In the Stress and Coping Model, problem-focused and emotion-focused strategies of coping are proposed (Lazarus & Folkman, 1984). Problem-focused strategies directly confront the problem or redefine it, while emotion-focused strategies help to reduce the caregiver's perception of burden and alleviate psychological distress. One caregiver speaks about her experience of poetry writing as an emotion-focused strategy:

> [I]t takes you away in your mind . . . relaxing . . . you can get out your feelings and move on . . . you kind of let go of it . . . just let it disintegrate a little bit. It's on paper now and it's passed, it's over. . . .

Psychosocial interventions such as education, support groups, and family and individual counseling may address caregiver stress at several levels. Education may help to provide strategies for dealing with problem behaviors. Through informal support groups, caregivers may redefine their approaches and perspectives about their role and their loved ones as others share their own learning, successes, and failures. Counseling may help caregivers accept their situations and temper their reactions to stress, so as not to be overwhelmed. In general, research supports psychosocial interventions as a means of reducing psychological distress in caregivers for persons with dementia (Brodaty, Green, & Koschera, 2003; Manepalli, Desai, & Sharma, 2009; Mohide, Pringle, Streiner, Gilbert, & Muir, 1990; Ostwald, Hepburn, Caron, Burns, & Mantell, 1999; Roberts et al., 1999; Zarit, Anthony, & Boutselis, 1987). Schulz et al. (2002) suggested that no single method would effectively reduce stress and burden for caregivers, noting that a variety of methods may be required.

One more innovative method of stress and burden reduction is the use of expressive therapies. Expressive therapies make use of creative arts such as music, dance, drama, art, and writing to encourage release and integration of emotion. The process of creation itself is emphasized and is more important than the final product.

Expressive Writing

Expressive writing can have great power. Used by ordinary people to record life events or capture stressful moments, "poets and novelists have . . . drawn on traumatic life experiences for inspiration . . . and have used writing as a means of transformation and healing." (Connolly Baker & Mazza, 2004, p. 141). Writing can force people to pause and reflect, to gain greater clarity, self-understanding, and closure (Connolly Baker & Mazza, 2004).

Much evidence-based research about the effectiveness of writing on health has been published. Linking emotions to writing seems to bestow greater benefit. Theories about why this happens include catharsis or release of emotion, increased insight, and active inhibition (King, 2002; Pennebaker, 1989). Pennebaker (1989) proposed that emotional expression, verbal or written, required confronting stressful thoughts and feelings, then restructuring thoughts about them. Thus, individuals can safely discharge pent-up emotion that may be weakening their immune systems and making them ill. Although many of Pennebaker's studies were conducted with college students, others have found expressive writing a useful tool. For example, expressive writing has been used as a psychosocial intervention to promote resilience in older adults and caregivers (Caldwell, 2005); to help elders cope with loss in later life (Caplan, Haslett, & Burleson, 2005); and to reduce stress or improve health in family caregivers (Mackenzie, Wiprzycka, Hasher, & Goldstein, 2007).

Why Poetry?

Poetry has been used as a method of healing therapy for many years. Poetry is "an expressive therapy not limited by space, time, organization, rhyme, form, placement on paper, or even word structure" (Springer, 2006, p. 69). The symbols and images of poetry reflect the thoughts, moods, and beliefs of the writer.

In those suffering from trauma, the value of poetry lies in its ability to unite the emotional, sensory right brain unable to assimilate overwhelmingly painful experiences with the verbal, cognitive left brain (Springer, 2006). The language of poems can alter brain wave patterns and provide a "bridge" between the halves of the brain (Springer, 2006, p. 71). Some of poetry's other uses include: growth during times of loss, coping with fears, creating meaning from life and its experiences; discovering self and improving self-esteem; understanding and relating to experiences shared by others; and nurturing creativity (Springer, 2006). Poetry writing can be cathartic. It can help the poet gain insight and feel pride and increased self-confidence. It may be pleasurable and fun (Bolton, 1999). Poetry writing—and reworking of poem content—also may help caregivers gain a sense of control (Bolton, 1999); this could be especially valuable to dementia caregivers who often function in unpredictable and out-of-control situations.

A Poetry-Writing Intervention for Dementia Family Caregivers

A pilot study tested the effectiveness of a poetry-writing intervention on outcomes of self-transcendence, resilience, depressive symptoms, and subjective caregiver burden in a sample of 20 caregivers for older adults with dementia. The researcher believed that poetry writing might be an intervention that would encourage persons to choose positive attitudes such as self-transcendence—the ability to rise above difficult life situations—and resilience—bouncing back from stressful life events. Poetry writing would be trialed to see if it decreased depressive symptoms, such as feelings of sadness, fatigue, and unhappiness, and caregiver burden, or the sense that life was being impacted in negative ways by the caregiving role.

The study was guided by a synthesis of Reed's theory of self-transcendence and the individual personality development theories of Adler and Frankl. Reed (1993) stated that nurses can directly intervene to influence inner resources such as self-transcendence in individuals. The theories of Frankl (1969) and Adler (1956) helped support the identification of nursing interventions that would promote the ability to transcend and create meaning from experiences. Poetry writing was seen as a specific nursing intervention that would help family caregivers to transcend stresses, affirm meaning, and achieve positive outcomes by encouraging caregiver expression of emotion. It could also offer distraction or redirection from unpleasant caring tasks, and enhance positive feelings about the care recipient.

A semistructured interview format was used to collect data. Four instruments were administered: the Self-Transcendence Scale, the Resilience Scale, the Center for Epidemiologic Studies–Depression (CES-D) and the Zarit Burden Interview (short form). Participants in both groups were also interviewed about their poetry-writing experiences. Demographic data were collected and used to describe both groups. Analysis was descriptive and involved the examination of trends in the data relative to outcome variables. In addition, analysis of poem theme content with "member checks" of randomly chosen participants was conducted. The feasibility of the research protocol and of conducting a larger clinical trial was also assessed.

In this 12-week longitudinal study, the researcher expected to see positive changes in instrument scores (increased self-transcendence and resilience and decreased depressive symptoms and caregiver burden) after the groups wrote poems at either interview Time 1 or interview Time 2 and at the end of the study (interview Time 3). She especially expected the interviews about the poetry-writing experience to yield rich qualitative data.

After the first interview, Group A caregivers were asked to write at least three poems over the next 4 weeks. Poems could be about any topic the caregiver chose. Group B caregivers were asked to wait and not write poems. At the second interview, all caregivers again completed the study instruments and the researcher asked Group A caregivers what it was like for them to write poetry. Another month passed, during which Group B caregivers were asked to write at least three poems. Group A caregivers were told they could write more poems or not if they chose. At the third interview, all participants completed the study instruments again, and the researcher asked Group B participants about their experience of writing poetry.

The demographic makeup of the caregivers in the study was 85% female, with an average age of just over 60 years. Nineteen of 20 participants were white, with one African American caregiver. Group A was slightly younger than Group B, while more males were in Group B (3 of 10). This may have affected outcomes of the study by group, as female caregivers tend to experience more depression and burden than male caregivers (Rose-Rego, Strauss & Smyth, 1998; Gallachio, Siddiqi, Langenberg, & Baumgarten, 2002; Campbell et al., 2008). Older adults also tend to have greater self-transcendence (Young & Reed, 1995; Stinson & Kirk, 2006). Results for these groups in this study supported previous research findings, in that women had lower scores on self-transcendence and resilience and higher scores on depressive symptoms and caregiver burden, while older participants had higher scores on self-transcendence and resilience and lower scores on depressive symptoms and caregiver burden.

At the end of the study, changes on instrument scores were barely perceptible or changed in an unanticipated direction. Analysis of group means suggested that, after writing poetry, most participants were slightly less self-transcendent, less resilient, more depressed, and felt greater caregiver burden. Yet individual scores and interview data demonstrated evidence to contradict these negative trends. Not only did individuals within each group have substantial changes in their scores in a positive direction, but 18 of the 20 participants stated that they would probably continue to write poetry or incorporate poetry writing into future journaling. One encouraging finding was that over half (60%) of Group A participants chose on their own to write poems during the month they were not specifically requested to by the researcher.

Caregiver Poetry

Poems of caregivers reflected study outcomes of self-transcendence, resilience, depressive symptoms, and caregiver burden. Self-transcendence was the theme most commonly identified by readers. Following is an example from a spouse caregiver referring to her awareness of a higher power (God):

> . . . each day when I wake, I know that you care,
> I talk to you and have no doubts that you're there
> . . . Your sovereignty and love is what keeps me afloat,
> Without you I'd feel more pain, like being lost in a boat.
> . . . You've been my guide through all of my years,
> You've held me and loved me through laughter and tears.

An adult child caregiver wrote about how she transcended life challenges in her poem "Creator":

> To love and not to hate
> To give and not to receive
> To live life in its fullness
> To have gratitude for all things
> To humbly go in submission relying totally on your will
> To understand that letting go of myself
> Gives you complete control

A spouse caregiver who spoke in interview about deliberately trying to elevate her mood through her poetry showed resilience when she wrote:

> Bright sun, warm days
> Hearts swell sending glad rays
> Hope and cheer
> Courage without care
> Knowing deep inside
> Love resides there.

Burden sometimes resulted from caregivers' struggles to manage concrete symptoms of dementia:

> I don't know what you remember
> I'm afraid to say Dad, remember this?
> . . . It hurts when I know you did but you say you don't recall.
> . . . I hate difficult conversation.

An adult child caregiver who scored high initially on depressive symptoms and caregiver burden instruments wrote a poem filled with self-pity and anger:

It's hard Sometimes
　Not to whine
　　Not to think how hard I've got it
　　　No partner
　　　No help
　　　　No one to love me . . .
. . . I just want to whine
　To cry
　　To shout to the Stars
　　　I am SOMEONE
　　　　God damn it!

The caregiver who wrote the preceding poem was one of the success stories of the poetry-writing study. She found poetry writing to be such an excellent release that she missed it and felt tension build up on days she didn't write. Although she noted that nothing helped that much on days she was tired, she believed that writing poetry was most helpful for her in maintaining balance. In addition, her scores on depressive symptoms and caregiver burden dropped dramatically after she began writing poetry.

Reflecting the complexities of the caregiving role and human beings themselves, sometimes depressive symptoms, caregiver burden, and self-transcendence coexisted simultaneously:

Alone—so alone
As I sob in despair
Wait-no-not alone
God is always with me
Holding me.
No longer alone.

A spouse caregiver whose mate was experiencing greater cognitive decline scored high on measures of depressive symptoms and burden, yet her poem reflected her intent to "soldier on":

Run away, far away from here
Nothing will move, stuck like glue
Float, float away from here
Free, Free and happy always to
Stay right here.

Caregiver Interviews

In the interviews about the experience of poetry writing, caregivers talked about a number of benefits. The majority of caregivers felt a sense of pride and accomplishment in being able to do the task of writing poems, as many had not written poetry in a number of years;

perhaps last as a school assignment. Some caregivers spoke of experiencing a release of emotion or catharsis:

"[I]t allowed me to express what I was feeling. . . ."

"I liked the release that it gave me for my emotions . . . I think poetry organizes thoughts and feelings together. . . ."

Others gained greater acceptance of their loved ones and their illnesses and felt more empathy for the person for whom they were caring.

"[W]riting the poems put more, brought more of a personal feeling to it that 'well yeah, this is an Alzheimer's patient, but don't forget that it's your dad, because so often I find that I do do that . . . this is somebody that I love and it really has helped me to be more aware of remembering that side of it."

"It made me more sympathetic, you know. I just saw how fragile my mom is. It made me almost feel sorry, you know, because I can't imagine what it is like sitting around some place 24–7 and just looking around and sometimes not knowing where you're at."

Still others became more self-aware as they reflected on their caregiver role:

"[It] consolidated my feelings and capsulated them. Helped me to label my own feelings . . . because I've been able to clarify what I've been going through, I can accept it a little bit more."

Several caregivers seemed to express in laymen's terms the value of separating the emotional right brain from the verbal left brain:

"[R]educing emotion to words I think gives you a different perspective . . . something tangible to attach to the intangible emotion. . . ."

" . . . (poems) . . . like a snapshot . . . It's a brief, encapsulated, simple form of just encapsulating some feelings . . . it kind of freezes in time and memory. . . ."

Some caregivers found poetry writing a welcome distraction and noted that it had the potential to change their thoughts or mood:

"It gave me a purpose and something that I knew I had to be thinking about."

"It kept my mind occupied . . . it made me wake up and listen more to certain things, be more focused and attentive . . . it kept me more upbeat. . . . I wasn't thinking the bad thoughts all the time."

One caregiver spoke of writing poems with a deliberate intention to elevate her mood. Others found the task fun, creative, and a positive challenge:

"[I]t was positive stress."

"[I]t's like music . . . it's like singing instead of talking. . . . It's more art than just writing in a journal and then complaining . . . it's a creation."

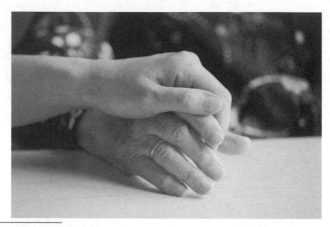

Figure 26-3   © Tyler Olson/ShutterStock, Inc.

One adult child caregiver who began the study with high scores for depressive symptoms and caregiver burden considered employing poetry writing as a strategy to help forge a greater bond between herself and her mother:

> My mother used to write poetry and she can't write anymore, but she can talk, so I'm wondering if we could do something together on tape and maybe that would help us both. . . .

Conclusion

Caring for an older adult can become an arduous "career" that can tax an individual to his or her utmost limits. It is critical that those caring for an older adult or even those who know or work with someone caring for an older adult be aware of the myriad challenges. In this chapter, evidence-based research demonstrating the negative outcomes of the caregiver role was briefly described, as were some of the psychosocial interventions found to be effective in reducing stress and burden. The particular challenges of the role of dementia caregiver were highlighted. Finally, an overview of methods and results of a recently completed research study piloting a poetry-writing intervention for dementia caregivers was presented.

It would be far too simplistic to suggest that the complexities of caring for a demented adult can be resolved with any one solution; however, strategies that reduce negative outcomes and promote positive outcomes hold promise. As one caregiver noted after she reflected on her experience of being in the poetry-writing study, "(being in the study) helped me see that I'm up to the challenge (of caregiving)." For the sake of older adults and those who love and care for them, let's help ease burdens. Then all caregivers can be equal to the challenge.

References

Adler, A. (1956). *The individual psychology of Alfred Adler: A systematic presentation in selections from his writings*. New York: Basic Books.

Andren, S., & Elmstahl, S. (2005). Family caregivers' subjective experiences of satisfaction in dementia care: Aspects of burden, subjective health and sense of coherence. *Scandinavian Journal of Caring Science, 19*, 157–168.

Aneshensel, C.S., Pearlin, L.I., Mullan, J.T., Zarit, S.H., & Whitlatch, C.J. (1995). *Profiles in caregiving: The unexpected carer*. San Diego: Academic Press.

Baumgarten, M., Battista, R.N., Infante-Rivard, C., Hanley, J., Becker, R., & Gauthier, S. (1992). The psychological and physical health of family members caring for an elderly person with dementia. *Journal of Clinical Epidemiology, 45*, 61–70.

Bell, C., Araki, S., & Neumann, P. (2001). The association between caregiver burden and caregiver health-related quality of life in Alzheimer disease. *Alzheimer Disease and Associated Disorders, 15*, 129–136.

Bolton, G. (1999). "Every poem breaks a silence that had to be overcome": The therapeutic power of poetry writing. *Feminist Review, 42*, 118–133.

Brodaty, H., Green, A., & Koschera, A. (2003). Meta-analysis of psychosocial interventions for caregivers of people with dementia. *Journal of the American Gerontological Society, 51*, 657–664.

Caldwell, R. (2005). At the confluence of memory and meaning—Life review with older adults and families: Using narrative therapy and the expressive arts to re-member and re-author stories of resilience. *Family Journal, 13*(2), 172–175.

Campbell, P., Wright, J., Oyebode, J., Job, D., Crome, P., Bentham, P., et al. (2008). Determinants of burden in those who care for someone with dementia. *International Journal of Geriatric Psychiatry, 23*(10), 1078–1085.

Caplan, S.E., Haslett, B.J., & Burleson, B.R. (2005). Telling it like it is: The adaptive function of narratives in coping with loss in later life. *Health Communication, 17*(3), 233–251.

Connolly Baker, K., & Mazza, N. (2004). The healing power of writing: Applying the expressive/creative component of poetry therapy. *Journal of Poetry Therapy, 17*(3), 141–154.

Etters, L., Goodall, D., & Harrison, B.E. (2008). Caregiver burden among dementia patient caregivers: A review of the literature. *Journal of the American Academy of Nurse Practitioners, 20*, 423–428.

Federal Interagency Forum on Aging-Related Statistics. (2000). *Older Americans 2000: Key indicators of well-being*. Washington, DC: Author.

Frankl, V.E. (1969). *The will to meaning: Foundations and applications of logotherapy*. New York: The World Publishing Company.

Gallachio, L., Siddiqi, N., Langenberg, P., & Baumgarten, M. (2002). Gender differences in burden and depression among informal caregivers of demented elders in the community. *International Journal of Geriatric Psychiatry, 17*, 154–163.

George, L.K., & Gwyther, L.P. (1986). Caregiver well-being: A multidimensional examination of family caregivers of demented adults. *Gerontological Society of America, 26*, 253–259.

Gibson, D., Butkus, E., Jenkins, A., Mathur, S., & Liu, Z. (1997). *The respite care needs of Australians: Respite review supporting paper 1*. Canberra: Australian Institute of Health and Welfare.

Hebert, L.E., Scherr, P.A., Bienias, J.L., Bennett, D.A., & Evans, D.A. (2003). Alzheimer disease in the US population: Prevalence estimates using the 2000 Census. *Archives of Neurology, 60*, 1119–1122.

King, L.A. (2002). Gain without pain: Expressive writing and self-regulation. In S.J. Lepore & J.M. Smyth (Eds.), *The writing cure: How expressive writing promotes health and emotional well-being* (pp. 119–134). Washington, DC: American Psychological Association.

Kinney, J.M., & Stephens, M.A. (1989). Hassles and uplifts of giving care to a family member with dementia. *Psychology of Aging, 4*, 402–408.

Lawton, M.P., Kleban, M.H., Moss, M., Rovine, M., & Glickman, A. (1989). Measuring caregiver appraisal. *Journals of Gerontology: Psychological Sciences, 44*, P61–P71.

Lazarus, R.S., & Folkman, S. (1984). *Stress, appraisal, and coping.* New York: Springer.

Mackenzie, C.S., Wiprzycka, U.J., Hasher, L., & Goldstein, D. (2007). Does expressive writing reduce stress and improve health for family caregivers of older adults? *The Gerontologist, 47*(3), 296–306.

Manepalli, J., Desai, A., & Sharma, P. (2009). Psychosocial-environmental treatments for Alzheimer's disease. *Primary Psychiatry, 16*(6), 39–47.

Mohide, E.A., Pringle, D.M., Streiner, D.L., Gilbert, J.R., & Muir, G. (1990). A randomized trial of family caregiver support in the home management of dementia. *Journal of the American Geriatrics Society, 38* (4), 446–454.

Mossello, E., Caleri, V., Razzi, E., DiBari, M., Cantini, C., Tonon, E., et al. (2008). Day care for older dementia patients: Favorable effects on behavioral and psychological symptoms and caregiver stress. *International Journal of Geriatric Psychiatry, 23*, 1066–1072.

Motenko, A.K. (1989). The frustrations, gratifications, and well-being of dementia caregivers. *Gerontologist, 29*, 166–172.

National Alliance for Caregiving, and American Association of Retired Persons (2004). *Caregiving in the US.* Washington, DC: National Alliance for Caregiving.

Nichols, L.O., Chang, C., Lummus, A., Burns, R., Martindale-Adam, J., Graney, M.J., et al. (2008). The cost-effectiveness of a behavior intervention with caregivers of patients with Alzheimer's disease. *Journal of the American Geriatrics Society, 56*, 413–420.

Noonan, A.E., & Tennstedt, S.L. (1997). Meaning in caregiving and its contribution to caregiver well-being. *The Gerontologist, 37*, 785–794.

Ostwald, S.K., Hepburn, K.W., Caron, W., Burns, T., & Mantell, R. (1999). Reducing caregiver burden: A randomized psychoeducational intervention for caregivers of persons with dementia. *The Gerontologist, 39*, 299–309.

Pearlin, L.J., & Schooler, C. (1978). The structure of coping. *Journal of Health and Social Behavior, 19*, 2–21.

Pennebaker, J.W. (1989). Confession, inhibition, and disease. In L. Berkowitz (Ed.), *Advances in experimental social psychology, Vol. 22* (pp. 211–244).

Reed, P.G. (1993). The theory of self-transcendence. In M.J. Smith & P. Liehr (Eds.), *Middle range theories for nursing* (pp. 145–166). New York: Springer.

Roberts, J., Browne, G., Milne, C., Spooner, I., Gafni, A., Drummond-Young, M., et al. (1999). Problem-solving counseling for caregivers of the cognitively impaired: Effective for whom? *Nursing Research, 48*, 162–172.

Rose-Rego, S.K., Strauss, M.E., & Smyth, K.A. (1998). Differences in the perceived well-being of wives and husbands caring for persons with Alzheimer's disease. *The Gerontologist, 38*, 224–230.

Schulz, R. (Ed.). (2000). *Handbook on dementia caregiving: Evidence-based interventions for family caregivers.* New York: Springer.

Schulz, R., & Beach, S.R. (1999). Caregiving as a risk factor for mortality: The caregiver health effects study. *Journal of the American Medical Association, 282*, 2215–2219.

Schulz, R., O'Brien, A., Bookwala, J., & Fleissner, K. (1995). Psychiatric and physical morbidity effects of dementia caregiving: Prevalence, correlates, and causes. *The Gerontologist, 35*, 771–791.

Schulz, R., O'Brien, A., Czaja, S., Ory, M., Norris, R., Martire, L.M., et al. (2002). Dementia caregiver intervention research: In search of clinical significance. *Gerontologist, 42*(5), 589–602.

Schulz, R., Vistainer, P., & Williamson, G.M. (1990). Psychiatric and physical morbidity effects of caregiving. *Journals of Gerontology: Psychological Sciences, 45*, 181–191.

Shaw, W.S., Paterson, T.L., Semple, S.J., Ho, S., Irwin, M.R., Hauger, R.L., et al. (1997). Longitudinal analysis of multiple indicators of health decline among spousal caregivers. *Annals of Behavioral Medicine, 19*(2), 101–109.

Springer, W. (2006). Poetry in therapy: A way to heal for trauma survivors and clients in recovery from addiction. *Journal of Poetry Therapy, 19*(2), 69–81.

Stinson, C.K., & Kirk, E. (2006). Structured reminiscence: An intervention to decrease depression and increase self-transcendence in older women. *Journal of Clinical Nursing, 15*(2), 208–218.

Talley, R.C., & Crews, J.E. (2007). Framing the public health of caregiving. *American Journal of Public Health, 97*(2), 224–228.

Wright, L., Clipp, E., & George, L. (1993). Health consequences of caregiver stress. *Medical Exercise and Nutritional Health, 2*, 181–195.

Yee, J.L., & Schulz, R. (2000). Gender differences in psychiatric morbidity among family caregivers: A review and analysis. *The Gerontologist, 40*(2), 147–164.

Young, C.A., & Reed, P.G. (1995). Elders' perceptions of the role of the group psychotherapy in fostering self-transcendence. *Archives of Psychiatric Nursing, 9*(6), 338–347.

Zarit, S.H., Anthony, C.R., & Boutselis, M. (1987). Interventions with care givers of dementia patients: Comparison of two approaches. *Psychology of Aging, 2*, 225–232.

Zarit, S.H., Reever, K.E., & Bach-Peterson, J. (1980). Relatives of the impaired elderly: Correlates of feelings of burden. *The Gerontologist, 20*(6), 649–655.

Chapter 27

Home Is Where the Heart Is

Evelyn G. Duffy

Home is where the heart is, and it is increasingly becoming the site of the provision of health care. After decades of decline, home health care and house calls have become the fastest growing areas of health care. While health care can be provided in the home to any age patient, one study found that over 90% of house calls by physicians are made to elderly patients (Meyer & Gibbons, 1997). Florence Nightingale was clairvoyant when she made the statement in 1867, *"My view, you know, is that the ultimate destination is the nursing of the sick in their own home. I look to the abolition of all hospitals . . . but no use to talk about the year 2000"* (Lundy, Utterback, Lance, & Bloxsom, 2009, p. 971). She couldn't possibly have known about the changes in Medicare reimbursement that would transform care that is provided in the home. The decision in the 1980s to increase the coverage of home health care resulted in a huge increase in home health agencies (Lundy et al., 2009). Consequently millions of homebound older adults were able to receive care from a variety of health professionals who would otherwise have been inaccessible. These changes in Medicare reimbursement were happening at the same time that the technological revolution made it possible to provide sophisticated monitoring equipment in the home, as well as access to portable diagnostic equipment. Now we are beyond the year 2000 and almost any service that is available in the hospital setting can also be provided in the home, just as Florence had foreseen.

House calls by physicians had drastically declined after World War II. There were probably as many reasons that this decline occurred as there were physicians who stopped making house calls. Perhaps the attitude existed that the quality of care provided in the home was inferior to that provided in a clinic setting, where the new technology that appeared after the war was available to better diagnose and treat. Even after technology became more readily available in the 1980s and home health agencies were increasing the home care they provided, physicians who made house calls were still few in number. One challenge to the physicians who would be willing to make house calls was the poor reimbursement by Medicare. Home health nursing services were reimbursed at a higher level than house call visits, and physicians couldn't afford to provide the service. The impact of improved reimbursement that resulted from the passage of the Balanced Budget Act of 1997 saw a 43% increase in house calls by physicians from 1998 to 2004 (Moore, 1998; Landers et al., 2005). The Balanced Budget Act also liberalized Medicare coverage of physician assistants and nurse practitioners, and now they have become major contributors to house calls by providers (Moore, 1998; Landers et al., 2005). Nurse practitioners are especially well prepared for house calls with their professional emphasis on patient teaching, caregiver support, comfort and function (Landers, 2006).

Benefits of Care in the Home

The goal of home health care as stated in the official Medicare booklet about home health benefits is to "help you get better, regain your independence, and become as self-sufficient as possible. If you have long-term health problems, the goal of home health care is to maintain your highest level of ability or health, and help you learn to live with your illness or disability" (Centers for Medicare & Medicaid Services, 2007, p. 2). Regardless of whether an older adult has an acute episode of illness or is burdened with chronic health issues, the goal of home health care is to help him or her to function at the highest level possible. Functional independence is a key goal of gerontological health care. Providing care in the home offers opportunities to advance that goal that are unavailable in office settings. The ability to see a patient function in the home environment allows the providers to see the patient as a person rather than as a disease. This perspective may result in a different approach to decision making, with a higher regard for the effect the decision has on individuals and their families.

The decline in the percentage of older adults residing in nursing homes is another advantage of the accessibility to house calls and home health care. While there are other factors that contribute to this phenomenon, the decline in nursing home residence from 1985 to 2004 (24% among older adults age 65–74 and a 37% in decline in those age 75 and over) coincides well with the rise in home health care and house calls (Federal Interagency Forum on Aging-Related Statistics, 2008). If an older adult is functionally dependent because of either a physical or an emotional illness, remaining at home is not without its costs to individuals and their families. However, remaining at home is the desire of most, and for most represents a level of independence not equated to living in a nursing home.

Home Health Care

Home health care agencies offer services from multiple disciplines, as well as personal care and light housekeeping by aides. In order for the service to be covered by Medicare, the patient must have a skilled nursing or therapy need, and be homebound (Landers, 2006). The Centers for Medicare and Medicaid Services state that "homebound means that leaving home takes considerable and taxing effort. A person may leave home for medical treatment or short, infrequent absences for non-medical reasons, such as a trip to attend religious services. You can still get home health care if you attend adult day care" (Centers for Medicare & Medicaid Services, 2007, p. 3). When there is a skilled need, other services such as home health aides, nutritional counseling and social work will also be covered, but they cannot be the primary reason for home health care (Levine, Boal, & Boling, 2003). Only a physician can establish and approve the plan of care, and the physician is responsible for recertifying the patient for home health services every 60 days. Physicians do not need to be making home visits themselves in order to oversee the care, and they are reimbursed for their certification and recertification of care (Landers, 2006; Levine et al., 2003).

Medicare is not the only payor for home health care services. Medicaid provides health care coverage for those with low income (Lundy et al., 2009). If a patient has Medicare and Medicaid, Medicare would be the first source of coverage. Coverage under Medicaid may have fewer constraints than the requirements for reimbursement by Medicare. For example, neither homebound status nor skilled services are required. The home health care does have to be certified and recertified by a physician, as is required by Medicare. Benefits offered by private insurance, including long-term care insurance, may also include home health coverage.

House Calls

Unlike home health care that requires the patient to be homebound, house calls do not have the same constraint. From the American Academy of Home Care Physicians Web site the following is noted, "Medicare explicitly stated in 2001 that physician home visits to patients are covered even if the patient is not homebound. Justification for a home visit must be documented, but the patient being homebound is only one of many reasons a home visit may be appropriate. Patient convenience and patient request are not the type of justifications Medicare is looking for, however" (Ratner, 2002). The number of house calls made annually is increasing, but they still represent a very small percentage of all outpatient care. While it is estimated that there are over one million older adults who are permanently homebound, and many others are homebound temporarily due to illness or injury, in 2004 it was reported that 2,060,029 house calls were billed, which represented less than 1% of all outpatient services (Landers et al., 2005; Levine et al., 2003). Providers who make house calls must depend more on their clinical skills than on technology, because it is possible to have blood drawn and X-rays taken in the home, but it is not as easy as sending the patient down the hall to the phlebotomist or the radiology department in a hospital or office. In his Fourth Annual Nicholas J. Pisacano Lecture, Dr. Ian Whinney challenged his physician audience to return to their roots. He described the home visit as more than a utilitarian act, "It says, I care enough about you to leave my office and come to see you on your ground" (McWhinney, 1997, p. 433). Physicians, nurse practitioners, and physician assistants are not the only providers of medical care in the home. Podiatrists, dentists, and most recently pharmacists are also venturing into the home care arena.

Functional Health and Older Adults

Care in the home offers a unique opportunity to partner with older adults to help them achieve the highest level of health. The World Health Organization (WHO) definition of health as stated in the 1948 *Preamble to the Constitution of the World Health Organization* is "Health is a state of complete physical, mental and social well-being and not merely the absence of disease or infirmity" (World Health Organization, 2003). For older adults, health is measured in the ability to function as independently as possible. The partnership requires the expertise of multiple disciplines to address the three aspects noted in the WHO definition: physical, mental, and social well-being. Not only does the home environment support providers' ability to make a holistic assessment, the disciplines involved can make a joint visit and practice true interdisciplinary collaboration. This collaboration is so crucial that it is required for Medicare certification of a home health agency (Lundy et al., 2009).

Functional health is the result of multiple factors. A classic paper published in 1995 outlined the elements of a practical functional assessment (Fleming, 1995). The paper makes the point that assessment of functional health is more than just an evaluation of activities of daily living; rather, the assessment involves evaluation of basic self-care activities as well as the instrumental activities necessary for function in the community. Mobility is a key to function and requires an assessment of gait, balance, and joint motion and strength. Mental health, which includes cognitive ability, affective status, and substance use, has a major impact on functional activities and safety. Sensory function, hearing, and vision are also key aspects of functional health. Adequate nutrition provides the energy that is essential to perform the activities of daily living and to maintain good health and promote healing. To maintain an elder's physical, mental, and social well-being, providers must assess and address deficits in all of these areas. The complex nature of optimum functioning is another reason that interdisciplinary collaboration is necessary.

Unwin and Jerant (1999) suggest a mnemonic to help guide the care of patients in the home. INHOMESSS stands for immobility, nutrition, home, other people, medication, examination, safety, spirituality, and services. The mnemonic was initially introduced in 1991 as INHOME safety; spirituality and services were added later to provide a more holistic picture of the patient. Immobility, which includes activities of daily living, and nutrition are areas also addressed in the Fleming paper. Home environment includes the dwelling as well as the neighborhood where the patient resides. The category of "other people" is an assessment of social support and caregivers. The house call visit offers opportunities to comprehensively evaluate medication use, to complete a thorough physical examination, and to address issues of safety and spirituality. Areas that may take a back seat in office settings present themselves readily in the home, where personal items such as religious symbols may offer an avenue for discussion of their meaning to the patient and the family.

While it is possible to evaluate these elements in the office setting, in the home the provider can see firsthand the challenges to the patient's function, such as an unsafe neighborhood, a dwelling that is in ill repair, poor lighting, lack of handrails, cupboards that require excessive reaching, or doorways that cannot accommodate the width of assistive devices. In the office setting, patients can only be asked to describe how they perform day-to-day activities; in the home the provider can have the patient demonstrate those activities. There is no need to have them tell you how they get in and out of the bathtub; you can go into the bathroom with them and have them SHOW you how they do it. Shelves and refrigerators can be inspected, and the management of medications can be observed and supervised. Whether it is the nurse, physician, or one of the therapists providing the care, the success of care provided in the home can be measured by the effect it has on function.

The Home Visit

Whatever the profession of the person making the home visit, there are many practical issues to be considered. From the time that providers step into the car or other form of transport, they have to be aware of their own need for safety. The importance of timing visits to minimize the possibility of being out after dark in unfamiliar areas, as well as organizing the schedule to decrease the transit time, requires careful planning. Just as the providers need to assess the safety of the neighborhood for the sake of the patient, they need to keep that factor in mind for their own safety. Similarly, just as the dwelling may compromise the patient's health, wooden stairs up to the door of the home that are rotted and broken can challenge the health and safety of the provider. Vicious unleashed animals are another challenge to safety. Once inside the home, responding tactfully when bugs or rodents invade your property is a technique not usually required in institutional settings. The microscopic bugs are also a concern, and good hygiene to prevent transmission of disease should be a part of any practice; however, this may be more challenging in the home.

In the office and institutional setting the providers are the authority, setting the rules and controlling the encounter. Just the opposite is true in the home, where the patient is the authority and can set limits on the encounter. The provider is a guest and needs to act accordingly. While inspection of cupboards and refrigerators can offer important information about the patient's health, the provider must have permission in order to perform that inspection. Blaring radios, or television programs, children or animals running around, and phone calls that the patient answers all offer challenges to the provider, who has a goal to complete the care but is not in the position to control this environment. Another type of distraction may be created by the patient who wants to delay the departure of the provider for as long as possible. Time constraints are present in home health and health call practices just as they are in any setting, but limiting the time of the visit when the provider is in the patient's home can be even more challenging (Lundy et al., 2009).

Professionals who choose to provide care in the home need to be comfortable in an independent role. With the technology that is now available, the isolation that was experienced in the past is decreased, but placing a call on a cell phone or connecting with a laptop is not the same as having another professional step into the room, discuss the assessment, and assist with decision making (Lundy et al., 2009). Maintaining proper boundaries in a setting where the professional is visiting can be a challenge, especially when the patient/provider relationship has been long term. A relationship of trust must be established, but the caring professional can find it a challenge not to blur the roles of provider and friend.

Case Examples

The Well Elder Living Alone

Mrs. G has been widowed for 15 years; she has no children. Her closest relative lives 500 miles away. She owns her own home in an older neighborhood of a large metropolitan city. She has lived in the neighborhood for 40 years. When she and her husband purchased the home the neighborhood was full of young families, and the men all worked at the steel plant. Now the plant is closed and there are few residents on the block whom Mrs. G recognizes. In the past 2 years many owners abandoned their homes, and they are boarded up. Mrs. G would like to move to a senior apartment, but she would never be able to sell her home, so she installed a security system and obtained a life line that she wears all the time. Mrs. G does not drive, and her arthritis makes it impossible for her to use public transportation. A friend from church takes her to the hairdresser once a week and then they go grocery shopping.

On one of her shopping trips the neighbor suggested that they try out the blood pressure machine in the pharmacy. Mrs. G had a very high reading, so her friend encouraged her to see a doctor. Mrs. G "didn't like doctoring and hadn't been seen by one for many years." Her friend knew of a House Calls practice at the nearby medical center, and Mrs. G agreed to see a doctor if the doctor would come to her. While Mrs. G does not meet the Medicare definition of homebound, her resistance to health care and her immediate health need, along with her willingness to have a provider come to her, would satisfy the requirements of medical necessity for a house calls visit.

The house call was thorough and included the comprehensive assessment of function. Mrs. G was independent in her basic activities of daily living and was only dependent in instrumental activities for transportation. The assessment did uncover some depressive symptoms and some unresolved grief both for the loss of her husband and for the loss of her safe and comfortable neighborhood. Physically Mrs. G was a well elder, but in addition to the arthritis, she was diagnosed with hypertension and elevated cholesterol. She was started on two medications. Because the providers made a house call, they could see the challenges to Mrs. G's safety. However, it was also possible to see how well she was managing, even in the difficult situation. A social worker from the practice came out and met with Mrs. G, and was able to provide her with some therapy for her depressive symptoms and grief; she also helped her sign up for a senior center that would come and pick her up and provide transportation for events. Mrs. G says she feels better than she has in many years and has made new friends and increased her activity. She still receives visits from the House Call practice, but only in the winter months. In the summer she can use the senior transportation to go out to the clinic. Because of the house calls Mrs. G's health has improved, and not only her physical health, but her psychological and social well-being also. She still has her home and she still does not feel that it is possible to sell it, but she is making the best of her situation and hoping that the homes around her will be filled with new families soon.

The Suburban Elder Couple

Mr. and Mrs. M live a 1950s brick ranch in a suburban neighborhood. It is a safe neighborhood with homes on large lots. Most of the neighborhoods are dual professionals who are not home during the day. Mr. M has moderate dementia of the Alzheimer's type, and Mrs. M is his primary caregiver. They have two daughters in town, but their jobs require travel and they are often not available for support. Mr. M can be belligerent, and the last time Mrs. M drove him to a healthcare visit he balked and refused to get out of the car. His physical health is fair, with hypertension, an enlarged prostate, and mild diabetes his primary concerns. He is on six medications. He is a big man, and Mrs. M is having more and more trouble getting him to bathe. She must remind him to go to the toilet, and she shaves him with an electric razor when he will allow her to. Three weeks ago Mr. M fell in the kitchen. Mrs. M was not able to help him get up and she couldn't find anybody in the neighborhood who could help her. She had to call 911, and during the subsequent emergency department visit Mr. M was seen by a nurse practitioner. He had not suffered any serious injuries from the fall, but he was diagnosed with a urinary tract infection. The nurse practitioner recommended that Mr. M be seen by the house calls practice in follow-up.

Because of the severity of Mr. M's dementia he would meet the Medicare definition of homebound. A physician from the house calls practice made the initial visit and was able to help Mrs. M see just how functionally impaired her husband had become. To make her own life easier she had assumed some care for Mr. M that he may have been able to provide for himself. For example, she practically fed him all his meals because he took so long to eat them on his own. Having the opportunity to observe Mr. M in his own home, the physician could identify a number of health and safety concerns. Mr. M was prescribed several new medications and that, combined with his deconditioning due to lack of mobility, would require the skilled care that can be provided by home health agency services. Mrs. M was showing signs of caregiver stress, loneliness, and depression, but hadn't been able to reach out on her own for support. The social worker available from the agency would be able to work with Mrs. M to relieve at least some of her stress. An occupational therapist was able to work with both Mr. and Mrs. M to increase Mr. M's functional independence.

By the time the 60-day recertification for home health care was required, both Mr. and Mrs. M had improved quality of life and greater physical, mental, and social well-being. The skilled services of the home health agency were no longer necessary. Mrs. M learned that it was important to care for herself so that she could continue to care for Mr. M. She hired a health aide for 4 hours twice a week, and now she takes regular breaks from her caregiving responsibilities. The home health aide provides the care that used to result in battles between Mr. and Mrs. M. The occupational therapist had helped Mrs. M to identify some activities she could share with Mr. M that would be appropriate to his level of cognitive ability, so she can still enjoy his company in spite of his dementia. The house calls practice continues to provide primary health care and to monitor the overall health of Mr. M.

The Frail, Severely Impaired Elder

Mrs. S is a widow who suffered a severe stroke and has locked-in syndrome. While she is mentally alert, she cannot move anything except her eyes. Her grandson lives with her and is her primary care provider. Mrs. S has multiple chronic illnesses in addition to the severe impairment from the stroke. She is a diabetic, has high blood pressure, chronic kidney disease, high cholesterol, asthma, gastroesophageal reflux disease, and the list goes on. Her grandson was a medic in the military service and is hypervigilant in his care. Mrs. S cannot swallow and is fed through a G tube. Mrs. S and her grandson were in agreement that she wanted anything and everything done to sustain her life for as long as possible. This request was consistent with their spiritual beliefs, and in spite of the challenges that caring for his grandmother present, the grandson remains committed to this endeavor. Mrs. S is on both Medicare and Medicaid, and she is receiving skilled services covered by Medicare from a home health agency, as well as 8 hours of health aide services a day covered by Medicaid. If it weren't for the house calls practice she would rarely be able to see a primary care provider. A critical advantage in the care of Mrs. S is her grandson's hypervigilance. The ability of healthcare providers to be involved in the home made it possible to set up systems for the grandson to assess Mrs. S and follow guidelines that may prevent the need for a visit from the nurse or the primary care provider. When the grandson becomes concerned about a symptom, those providers who are familiar with the home can remind him which cupboard the medication he needs is located in, or where he can find the clean tubing for the suction machine. Without the support of the home health team, Mrs. S would not be able to remain in her home, and her end-of-life wishes could not possibly be honored.

References

Centers for Medicare & Medicaid Services. (2007). *Medicare and home health services 10969.* Baltimore: US Department of Health and Human Services.

Federal Interagency Forum on Aging-Related Statistics. (2008). *Older Americans 2008: Key indicators of well being.* Washington, DC: US Government Printing Office.

Fleming, K.C. (1995). Practical functional assessment of elderly persons: A primary care approach. *Mayo Clinic Proceedings, 70*(9), 890–910.

Landers, S. (2006, *Spring*). House calls and home care. *The Ohio Family Physician, 58*(1), 30–31.

Landers, S.H., Gunn, P.W., Flocke, S.A., Graham, A.V., Kikano, G.E., Moore, S.M., et al. (2005). Trends in house calls to Medicare beneficiaries. *Journal of the American Medical Association*, *294*(19), 1251–1252.

Levine, S.A., Boal, J., & Boling, P.A. (2003). Home care. *Journal of the American Medical Association*, *290*(9), 1203–1207.

Lundy, K.S., Utterback, K.B., Lance, D.K., & Bloxsom, I.P. (2009). Home health and hospice nursing. In K.S. Lundy & S. Janes (Eds.), *Community health nursing* (pp. 970–1001). Sudbury, MA: Jones and Bartlett.

McWhinney, I.R. (1997). The doctor, the patient, and the home: Returning to our roots. *Journal of the American Board of Family Medicine*, *10*, 430–435.

Meyer, G.S., & Gibbons, R.V. (1997). House calls to the elderly—A vanishing practice among physicians. *New England Journal of Medicine*, *337*(25), 1815–1820.

Moore, K. (1998). New options for billing for PA services. *Family Practice Management*, *5*(7), 23.

Ratner, E. (2002). *Myths about home care: Home care is only for the homebound*. Retrieved from American Academy of Home Care Physicians at http://www.aahcp.org/homebound.shtml

Unwin, B.K., & Jerant, A.F. (1999). The home visit. *American Family Physician*, *60*, 1481–1488.

World Health Organization. (2003). *WHO definition of health*. Retrieved from http://www.who.int/about/definition/en/print.html

Chapter 28

Teaching End-of-Life Care

Neil Hall

Why Teach End-of-Life Care?

Any curriculum for healthcare providers faces the daunting task of fitting in all that is mandated and that should be taught. Modifying allocations of curriculum time is often an arduous process, and there must be a strong case made to fit in a new area (Arnold, 2003). Often the impetus for change is a grant or a government mandate, and a skeptic might suggest that substantial change will come only by these means. But learning to manage end-of-life (EOL) care has some powerful emotional and statistical factors that might be helpful in pushing through a change. (The term *palliative care* often is used as a synonym for EOL care, but it can have multiple definitions. *EOL care* is without such ambiguities and will be used throughout this chapter.)

It is hard to dispute the emotional need for good medical and nursing care for the dying. There is no better demonstration of the worth of a fellow human being than tender administrations to ease one's passing from this world. And a healthcare provider who participates in this care lives the oft-repeated adage, "To cure sometimes. To relieve often. To comfort and support always" (Cerletty, 2000, p. 483). For many, there is nothing as meaningful or close to their reason for entering the healthcare field as this. Unfortunately, this is not enough to convince others to carve out some curriculum time. More practical and convincing arguments are needed.

The rationale for teaching end-of-life care is based on three facts:

- death and the dying process are common and important medical events;
- healthcare providers have a significant role in helping patients and their families through these events; and
- there is a substantial and important body of knowledge needed to provide this care well, but healthcare providers are not being taught adequately about it.

The Rapidly Growing Need for EOL Care

The only condition that every single person will suffer after birth is death. Usually there is a period of physical decline and suffering, known as dying, preceding it. Death affects proportionately more elderly, and the huge growth in the elder population and the consequent increase in chronic illness do not need to be reiterated.

But it is worth noting that the second-greatest killer of Americans is cancer, which usually has a long dying phase. Its incidence increases dramatically with age, and it is creeping up on heart disease as the number one killer in the United States. It already is substantially more common than heart disease as a cause of death in persons age 55–74 (Heron et al., 2009). Further, modern medicine has become very effective in keeping people alive longer. Persons with chronic lung disease, congestive heart failure, chronic kidney disease, degenerative brain and other neurologic disease, as well as those with cancer, survive longer, but in a debilitated state. Our technology has given them not just a longer life, but a prolonged dying course compared to previous generations. With the baby boomer bulge moving solidly into their senior years, we will see a major rise in the number of patients needing care during the dying process.

Much of the impetus for good EOL care can be traced to the hospice movement in our country, starting with the first formal hospice in 1974 in New Haven, Connecticut (Connecticut Hospice, Inc., n.d.). Hospices brought us the knowledge and techniques developed in England by Dame Cicely Saunders and St. Christopher's Hospice, founded in 1967 (St. Christopher's Hospice, n.d.). Their approach, using nursing and medical modalities, but also recognizing and responding to the emotional, social, and spiritual aspects of death and dying, caught on rapidly, with hospices springing up all over the country, supported by donations of time and money. With the approval of a Medicare benefit for hospice care in 1986 (National Hospice and Palliative Care Organization, 2010), which many health insurance companies adopted, hospices received a substantial source of revenue to support their missions. Since then, the growth of hospice and the number of formal hospices has ballooned (the majority now for profit), and the population of patients under the care of hospice increased threefold between 1995 and 2005 (Hospice and Palliative Care Association of New York State, n.d.).

Who Should Be Learning?

A case might be made that any person in the health field should have some basic knowledge of such an important medical event, and some rudimentary information could be built into any curriculum that discusses the roles of healthcare providers and the care of patients. The strongest and most logical learners, of course, are healthcare professionals who are likely to take care of dying patients.

Nurses, physicians, nurse practitioners and physicians assistants all have a high likelihood of having to make clinical decisions with dying patients and interacting with their families. Nursing assistants, despite receiving the least amount of health education, usually spend the greatest amount of time with the dying patients, and it is they who administer their most personal care. Social workers in healthcare settings often will be involved, and in hospice and formal long-term care settings will have a major role. Putting EOL care into the curriculum of these learners should be of the highest priority.

Other healthcare providers are not likely to have EOL responsibilities. The professions of dentistry, optometry, podiatry, physical and occupational therapy, speech pathology, recreation therapy, and others probably should have minimal curriculum time devoted to this subject. Nutritionists would fall into a category of needing some, but limited EOL education.

A brief review of any major textbook of palliative care will show that there is a substantial body of knowledge concerning EOL care that must be acquired to manage this care adequately. Given that physicians and nurses will need to apply this knowledge in some fashion in their professional work, it is surprising that this is not already a standard in their education. Anyone familiar with medical school and nursing curricula knows that certain topics are always included, even though many or even most graduates will rarely, if ever, deal with them again. Obstetrics is probably the most obvious example of an accepted part of the curriculum that is relevant to only the very small portion of physicians and nurses who manage pregnant patients. Surely the care of the patient at the end of life might be considered as important. It would seem difficult to disagree with the argument that anyone who will make important decisions about medical or nursing care, including EOL, should have preparation through knowledge and experience.

How Are We Doing?

Death and the dying process have always been with us, managed by individual families, physicians, nurses, and other providers. Unfortunately for patients, few US nurses and physicians receive anything more than rudimentary training in the management of the dying patient, even in primary care residency programs and oncology programs (Paice et al., 2006; Billings & Block, 1997; Oneschuk, Hanson, & Bruera, 2000; Herbert, Butera, Castillo, & Mega, 2009). It is commonly said that doctors especially, but probably also other professionals, avoid dying patients because they see them as personal failures. But to the extent that this is true, it is at least as likely that this is because they don't have much knowledge about the whole area of dying, or how to manage it as a provider.

When we don't know much about something we might be responsible for, we commonly avoid dealing with it as much as possible. If we can reduce this discomfort, learners may be more open to positive interactions with their patients, and therefore they may be more motivated to learn the facts and techniques needed.

Three state legislatures (California, Oregon, and West Virginia) have responded to the need and the absence of physician education with mandated, albeit minimal, education required for physician licensure (American Medical Association, 2009). Only Oregon has similar requirements for nurses, and that only in pain management (Law, 2006).

In sum, most people who have looked at this question believe that current medical providers are tremendously unprepared to deliver EOL care, and that the professional educational institutions overall, while improving, have not done enough to change that situation.

What Should We Teach?

The knowledge base in pain and symptom management is increasing, and the role of social and spiritual aspects of EOL care increasingly are recognized as areas physicians need to understand.

Because of the importance of hospice care, its professionals have placed great emphasis on educating providers. The original drivers of the US hospice movement were nurses, and they remain the core professionals managing the care of patients in hospice care and most other settings caring for dying patients. Nursing leaders recognized the importance of teaching nursing knowledge and techniques appropriate for EOL care and created the Hospice and Palliative Nurses Association (originally the Hospice Nurses Association) in 1986 (Hospice and Palliative Nurses Association, 2009). This organization offers many professional programs and resources for nurses interested in this field. The American Association of Colleges of Nursing administers an excellent educational program called ELNEC (End-of-Life Nursing Education Consortium) that helps nurses learn the elements of caring for this population. Nursing also offers special certification for nurses and advance practice nurses (nurse practitioners) through the National Board for Certification of Hospice and Palliative Nurses (2010).

Physicians traditionally were very involved in the management of dying patients, but with the advent of modern medicine their role often has focused on preventing death instead of managing the dying process. When Medicare made the hospice benefit a permanent program in 1986, it required that a physician medical director certify the need for care of all patients receiving the hospice benefit. This and the growth of academic and general physician interest in providing end-of-life care have caused hospices to increase physician involvement. The approval of a subspecialty in Hospice and Palliative Medicine by the American Board of Medical Specialties has further legitimized physician involvement in end-of-life care, and organizations such as the American Academy of Hospice and Palliative Medicine and the Center to Advance Palliative Care have become nationwide leaders in promulgating clinician education in this area (Portenoy, Lupu, Arnold, Cordes, & Storey, 2006).

There are many examples of curricula that can be used as resources to help create a curriculum adapted to any discipline. The nursing curriculum at ELNEC was mentioned earlier. The American Medical Association, with financial support from the Robert Wood Johnson Foundation and the National Cancer Institute, created a program in 1999 to teach physician educators what and how to teach other physicians about EOL care. This very successful program, now called Education in Palliative and End-of-Life Care (EPEC), has expanded to include a course dealing specifically with cancer care. Both programs are available online as credit-bearing learning modules. The American Academy of Hospice and Palliative Care Physicians has extensive educational materials available, including a nine-volume course (Unipac) that covers a very broad range of topics for physicians. Another widely respected resource is the Center to Advance Palliative Care, which has a wealth of information online. Putting "palliative curriculum" into your web search engine will generate more sites than one could explore in a lifetime.

It will be difficult to find faculty who feel comfortable in their mastery of the knowledge that will be taught. However, the educational resources noted previously can be used to educate faculty, and local hospices may be very interested in assisting in educational activities (in part because it may increase their referrals).

Although there will be tremendous variability depending on learners and curriculum time, it is likely that some or all of the following topics may be considered:

Introduction: This section prepares the student to learn by increasing awareness of the importance and relevance of EOL care and the role of that particular healthcare discipline. It provides background information, such as epidemiologic data, patient and family experiences at the end of life and the acute and remote effects of those experiences, the history of hospice, the philosophy of EOL care, and the profession's general approach to EOL care. It should also aim to decrease the common aversion to this topic and to interacting with dying patients.

Communicating with Patients and Families: Nurses generally learn a lot about communication with patients and families in their training. These topics are not as intensely taught in physicians' learning, and physicians are often faulted for avoiding communication that may be emotionally laden. This section would include basic information on the ethical and legal requirements of communication and approaches and techniques that can be used.

The Framework of End-of-Life Care: This section includes information about the various settings in which end-of-life care is provided, such as hospitals, long-term care facilities, patient homes, and of course inpatient hospice. It describes the professionals that participate in the care of dying patients in various settings, explaining their roles and also the team approach to managing these patients. It explains the different organizations that may be involved in providing care and their funding sources.

Pain and Pain Management: This is a huge topic that should be shaped to the particular needs of the discipline. In addition to information on the neurophysiology, detection, and assessment of pain, it should discuss nonmedicinal and medicinal management of pain. The former is particularly important because it is so commonly ignored. The concept of Total Pain, espoused by Dame Cicely Saunders, should be included. This concept is that there are four intertwining components of chronic pain—physical, emotional, social, and spiritual—and that until all are addressed, the pain cannot be relieved (Clark, 2000).

Other Symptom Management: This addresses the assessment and management of related symptoms such as nausea and vomiting, anorexia, fatigue, dyspnea, constipation, pruritis, hiccups, and any other problems likely to be managed by health care disciplines.

Emotional, Social, and Spiritual Aspects: Each of these aspects may be taught as separate modules, of course, depending on their importance to the learning discipline. Emotional aspects should address both patients and family members and should include at least anxiety, depression, and grief. Again, the pioneering work of Dame Saunders (who was trained as a social worker and a nurse before becoming a physician) is of tremendous help here. A more recent review of the emotional response to loss might also be helpful (Bonanno, 2009). Social topics might explain the important role of social interactions for patient comfort, family interactions at the EOL and after, and family discord. Spiritual topics could include the concepts of spirituality and religion, the importance of spirituality in EOL situations, and methods of assisting patients in addressing spiritual issues.

Special Populations: If the curriculum is relatively extensive or is geared to people expected to work with certain groups, this section could discuss in greater detail the care of pediatric patients, patients with HIV/AIDS, and specific medical illnesses, such as heart failure, chronic lung disease, dementia, and chronic kidney failure.

How Should We Teach It?

Teachers have individual tastes and styles of teaching, and this section is meant only to give a few thoughts that may be of use to those who are newer to the field, as well as some refresher points for the more experienced.

Some of the most helpful information for teaching adults comes from Malcolm S. Knowles, the "founder of androgogy" (defined as the teaching of adults, as opposed to pedagogy, the teaching of children) (Knowles, Holton III, & Swanson, 2005).

Knowles and his followers delineated six basic characteristics of adult learners, which can be summarized as shown in Figure 28-1.

---

1. Adults need to know why they should learn something.

2. All adults have a wide variety of past experiences that provide the foundation for their learning and can be tapped to improve results.

3. Adults need to be responsible for their decisions on education and involved in its planning and evaluation.

4. Adults learn best when the information to be acquired is seen as relevant to their current work or personal lives.

5. Adults want to learn how to solve problems, and not just memorize information.

6. The best motivation for adult learners comes from within themselves, not from external pressures.

Adapted from: M. W. Galbraith (2004).

Figure 28-1

TABLE 28-1 Teaching Methods at Different Levels of Learner Involvement

Outcomes Desired	Low	Medium	High
Affective	Lecture	Panel	Case Study
	Exhibit	Interview	Simulation
	Demonstration	Debate	Role Play
	Video	Computer-Aided Instruction	Group Discussion
Acquiring Information	Lecture	Panel	Field Trip
	Exhibit	Interview	Computer-Aided Instruction
	Video	Debate	
Psychomotor	Demonstration	Demonstration with Practice	
Problem Solving	Demonstration	Panel	Role Play/Simulation
	Debate	Interview	Case Study
	Video		Computer-Aided Instruction
			Group Discussion

Adapted from: M. W. Galbraith (2004, p. 109)

It takes only a little thought to create a curriculum or a single teaching-learning inter-action that fits these basic qualities, but doing so can be extremely beneficial to the learner and satisfying to the teacher.

It also is worth considering the outcomes desired. Should the learner to be able to do a new procedure, to mainly learn facts, to manipulate these facts to solve problems, to gain a new way of looking at something? The teaching approach should differ with the desired outcome. Gary J. Dean has suggested that a model for instructional design based on the desired outcomes may be helpful in creating a learning activity. For those who are used to thinking in terms of helping students acquire "attitude, knowledge, and skills," note that the outcomes are variations on these components (Table 28-1) (Dean, 2004).

By considering the characteristics of adult learners, the level of learner involvement desired, and the desired outcomes, one can quickly choose a teaching modality that should be effective. It is useful to remember that the greater the degree of learner involve-ment, the greater the success in achieving desired outcomes in adult learners. The size of the group being taught also may affect the teaching method, with discussions and role plays generally more suitable for smaller groups. The following example applies this teaching approach.

Teaching Plan for Healthcare Students

Topic: Approach to End-of-Life Care
Desired outcomes: Mainly attitude/affective, with knowledge as a secondary goal
Desired level of learner involvement: High
Teaching method: Case study with group discussion

After brief introductory remarks, each group member is asked to imagine that a family member or other beloved person has been diagnosed with terminal pancreatic cancer. Given their interest and involvement in medical care, the learners are asked to imagine that they become very involved in assisting with this person's last months of life, both helping the patient with the needs of a dying person and interacting with the medical establishment and family to improve the process. Focusing on the concept of achieving a "good death," learners are asked to think about areas they should or might need to address with the patient and others to achieve the best quality of life for the patient and family in this process and after. Learners then contribute their thoughts and ideas and expand them by discussing examples from their personal or professional experience. The teacher helps by encouraging, clarifying, repeating, and expanding on key concepts and facts and writes specific ideas on a whiteboard or other visual recording medium. These ideas are grouped as they are written, into five initially unlabelled categories—physical symptoms, emotional symptoms, social discomforts, spiritual concerns, and planning and preparation. After enough specifics are written in the category lists, the leader then labels the categories, adds to them as needed, and discusses the approach to EOL care that uses them as a framework for thinking about how such care should be given. In doing so, the teacher explains the concept of Total Pain described briefly earlier in the session, in terms of the role of the healthcare provider as a guide for the patient and family, expanding and discussing as seems appropriate for the group and as time allows.

This process uses a high level of involvement and draws on learners' previous knowledge to help them understand what is important in EOL care, giving them a framework to use in considering their own individual situations. It also allows them to learn from each other, as well as from the teacher, and gives a moderate amount of factual information that may be new to them. Most medical professionals have not been exposed to the concept of total pain, but they find it easy to understand and apply to their own situations. Because they are asked to think of someone important to themselves, they may be more open to accepting this information and approach as personally meaningful, which should facilitate the desired change in the learners' clinical actions.

Conclusion

With the baby boomer generation reaching their mid-sixties, our healthcare system faces a veritable onslaught of persons who will need care at the end of life. The Medicare hospice benefit has raised the expectations of patients and families, and we are likely to see continued increase in the percentage of dying patients receiving this care. There will be an inevitable need for much larger numbers of healthcare providers caring for dying patients.

A large amount of important knowledge of EOL care is readily available to medical providers, but unfortunately this area still has not claimed a place in professional curricula corresponding to its importance in people's lives. Widespread adoption of appropriate and substantial EOL education for those who should have it probably is still a long way off. Perhaps the power of the aging "boomers" will finally push leaders to make the needed curriculum changes. And the small but increasing numbers of educated EOL professionals may influence educational offerings on this topic in training programs. In the meantime, all healthcare educators have the opportunity to include EOL topics relevant to their disciplines in their teaching. For our patients' sakes (and possibly our own), it is worth doing.

References

American Medical Association. (2009). In *State Medical Licensure Requirements and Statistics, 2009* (pp. 54–56). Chicago: American Medical Association.

Arnold, R. (2003). The challenges of integrating palliative care into postgraduate training. *Journal of Palliative Medicine, 6*(5), 801–807.

Billings, J.A., Block, S. (1997). Palliative care in undergraduate medical education: Status report and future directions. *Journal of the American Medical Association, 278*(9), 733–738.

Bonanno, G.A. (2009). *The other side of sadness: What the new science of bereavement tells us about life after loss.* New York: Basic Books.

Cerletty, J.M. (2000). To cure, sometimes. To comfort, always. *Journal of Palliative Medicine, 3*(4), 483–485. doi:10.1089/jpm.2000.3.4.483

Clark, D. (2000, July/August). Total pain: The work of Cicely Saunders and the hospice movement. *American Pain Society Bulletin, 10*(4). Retrieved February 2, 2010 from http://www.ampainsoc.org/pub/bulletin/jul00/hist1.htm

Connecticut Hospice Inc. (n.d.). *About hospice.* Retrieved from http://www.hospice.com/cthospice/about.html

Dean, G. (2004). Designing instruction. In Galbraith, M.W. (Ed.). *Adult learning methods: A guide for effective instruction* (pp. 93–118). Malabar, FL: Krieger Publishing Company.

Herbert, H.D., Butera, J.N., Castillo, J., & Mega, A.E. (2009). Are we training our fellows adequately in delivering bad news to patients? A survey of hematology/oncology program directors. *Journal of Palliative Medicine, 12,* 1119–1124.

Heron, M.P., Hoyert, D.L., Murphy, S.L., Xu, J.Q., Kochanek, K.D., & Tejada-Vera B. (2009). *Deaths: Final data for 2006.* (National vital statistics reports, Vol. 57, No. 14). Hyattsville, MD: National Center for Health Statistics.

Hospice and Palliative Care Association of New York State. (n.d.). *A data book: Healthcare spending and the Medicare program, June 2008*. Retrieved February 16, 2010, from http://www.hpcanys.org/public_policy/June08MedPACReport_HospiceData%20(2).pdf

Hospice and Palliative Nurses Association. (2009). *History of Hospice and Palliative Nurses Association*. Retrieved from http://www.hpna.org/DisplayPage.aspx?Title=History%20of%20HPNA

Law, E. (2006). State-by-state guide for RN license renewal requirements. *Nursing, 36* (1) (Supplement: Nursing 2006 Career Directory), 30–33. Retrieved from http://www.nursingcenter.com

Knowles, M.S., Holton, E.F. III, & Swanson, R.A. (2005). *The adult learner. The definitive classic in adult education and human resource development* (6th ed.). Woburn, MA: Butterworth-Heinemann.

National Board for Certification of Hospice and Palliative Nurses. (2010). *Welcome*. Retrieved from http://www.nbchpn.org

National Hospice and Palliative Care Organization. (2010). *History of hospice care*. Retrieved from http://www.nhpco.org/i4a/pages/index.cfm?pageid=3285

Oneschuk, D., Hanson, J., Bruera, E. (2000). An international survey of undergraduate medical education in palliative medicine. *Journal of Pain and Symptom Management, 20*(3), 174–179.

Paice, J.A., Ferrell, B.R., Viriani, R., Grant, M., Malloy, P., & Rhome, A. (2006). Graduate nursing education regarding end-of-life care. *Nursing Outlook, 54*(1), 46–52.

Portenoy, R.K., Lupu, D.E., Arnold, R.M., Cordes, A., & Storey, P. (2006). Formal ABMS and ACGME recognition of hospice and palliative medicine expected in 2006. *Journal of Palliative Medicine, 9*(1), 21–23. doi:10.1089/jpm.2006.9.21.

St. Christopher's Hospice. (n.d.). *History*. Retrieved from http://www.stchristophers.org.uk/page.cfm/link=13.

Section VI

Promoting Personhood and Quality of Life in Elders

Chapter 29

Preserving Expression of Identity in the Face of Losses Associated with Aging

Sarah H. Gueldner

> Identity is the set of personal characteristics by which we are recognized or known, and that distinguish us from others. Likewise, our identity determines how we think about ourselves and how others think about us, influencing our self-image and our place in society. It is the base from which we are drawn to certain people, and from which others notice or do not notice us; it is also the base from which conversations start and friendships form. In this way, our identity is essential to our connection to the larger society. And at any age, self-identity is inextricably linked to pride and self-respect. (Gueldner, 2007, p. 3)

However, as outlined in Table 29-1, the losses associated with aging often challenge both our identity and our connection with society. Retirement marks the separation from our life work, with a likely reduction in income and circle of acquaintances, all of which could negatively affect identity. Changes over time may make us less attractive to some, and less capable of executing activities that once were accomplished with ease. Declining vision makes it harder to write letters and use the phone, and eventually may make it necessary to give up our driver's license, which in itself may represent a serious blow to one's identity. Hearing loss makes it difficult to talk with others; a stroke or dementia may diminish one's ability to speak or remember; stroke or a hip fracture may slow a once quick and sure gait; vertebral fractures may shorten stature (also an important aspect of identity) and make us stooped so we may not be able to see the eyes of others, nor they ours. Nor is incontinence easy to work into one's identity and social activities. Our family and cohort of longtime friends will of course be experiencing these same challenges, and over time we may lose our connections with those who knew our identity from an earlier time, at a time

TABLE 29-1   Areas of Loss Commonly Associated with Aging

Areas of Loss	Description

Biological decline	General health
	Decrease in vigor, strength, power
	Limited motility/mobility
	Compromised physiologic functions
	   Cardiovascular (compromised circulation)
	   Respiratory (less efficient oxygenation)
	   Genito urinary (frequency, nocturia, incontinence)
	   Gastrointestinal (loss of teeth, constipation)
	   Endocrine (lower metabolic rate, reduced calcium, diabetes)
	   Nervous (slowed reflexes, changes in sleep, less kinesthetic sense)
	   Integumentary (hair and skin changes)

Perceptual acuity due to sensory decrements	Vision Hearing Taste Tactile sensation Smell
Psychological losses linked to biology	Short-term memory, immediate recall ability Motor skills linked with reaction time Virility, libido "Looks," body image
Psychological losses centering around esteem (the need for self-respect and respect from others, and anxiety about being neglected, forgotten, needed, bypassed, retired out of usefulness)	Self-esteem Regard by others Influence, power Prestige positions, status, role confusion, rites of passage
Personal losses that focus on the need for affection from those who care out of love, duty, respect	Parents Spouse Children Siblings Extended family Friends Pets

TABLE 29-1   (Continued)

Areas of Loss	Description
Social losses that focus on the need for recognition, approval, and sense of worth	Friends, co-workers The everyday circle of friends, group (i.e., evening card game group) Memberships Social status (leader, advice giver in the community)
Loss of various social connections related to identity	Occupational status Reduced income Productivity, competition Driver's license Familiar place, home Familiar place of employment Familiar surroundings: contact with faces, places, landmarks, belongings Familiar routines Personal control
Philosophical losses that focus on the need to have one's life count for something, add up, make sense	Purpose in living Joy in living Will to live
Losses associated with religion or sense of spiritual connectedness that focuses on the need to believe that one's life has meaning, purpose, and a future	Physically unable to attend church Architecture of the church or environment makes it difficult to attend services or other gatherings Lack of transportation Financially unable to attend or donate to the church Attends alone; spouse ill or deceased Change from familiar services and congregations Decreased or absence of time with pastor may decrease symbolic presence and power of infinite life Composition of church membership may change Churches, like society, tend to build programs around couples or families, and may generate feelings of being lonely or out of place for those who have lost family members and are now alone.
Changes in body image	Organs or body parts may have been lost surgically, or through injury Sense of loss of the ability to control one's destiny Heightened awareness of mortality

Source: Adapted from listings developed by Donald Sanner, Chaplain, Bethany Home, Fargo, N.D., 1980, as cited in Steffl (1984) *Handbook of Gerontological Nursing*. Van Nostrand Reinhold Company, p. 45.

when it has become more difficult to meet and connect to establish new friendships. Eventually some elders may no longer be able to convey their sense of identity to others, or to deliver accounts of their accomplishments or feelings to their new and limited circle of acquaintances. Therefore, as caregivers of elders, it is important that we make every effort to facilitate and sustain a sense of identity in the elders we see, and that we create novel avenues for them to continue to express who they are, even in the face of loss that may seem to diminish identity (Gueldner, 2007). A guide for assessing actual or potential loss in older persons is provided in Table 29-2.

Portraits of Elders Who Were Able to Continue to Express Their Unique Identity

Lillian

Lillian, a "salt of the earth" country woman, was good with her hands. In fact, she had once won blue ribbons at the county fair for her needlework and canning. And she was known to make the best iced tea and cornbread in the hills of East Tennessee. She had learned to quilt by her mother's side, around a quilting frame set up in the living room of the person who had a quilt going. You could tell that she was an accomplished seamstress, just in the way she held the needle and used the thimble. Then one day, as she was cutting up a chicken to cook for supper, using the big butcher knife that Chart, her husband of 57 years, kept sharp with a whet rock, she had a gradual stroke. She didn't fall, so Chart didn't even realize anything was wrong until a neighbor came in and saw she couldn't talk. By the time she reached the hospital, the stroke had taken out Lillian's language capacity completely; she couldn't even make a sound, and the doctors thought she might never be able to speak again. The stroke also left her with right-sided weakness, and her visual field was affected so that she had trouble reading. Valedictorian of her high school class of 1930, now she had to look at a copy of her name in order to sign checks. Once very animated, she was now almost totally silent. Lillian's uncharacteristic quietness made it difficult for even her closest friends to spend time with her after the stroke. In fact, her longtime friends and neighbors would come in the back door saying they could only stay a few minutes, and then tell how they had to hurry off for another errand.

Then an unlikely quilt mending opportunity made it possible for Lillian to find expression. Just two weeks before she had the stroke, she had agreed to mend an out-of-town friend's tattered family quilt. Her daughter had picked up the quilt from her friend, but had not been able to get it to Lillian before she had the stroke. And now it was too late; it was clear that she could not mend the quilt now. But knowing what an avid quilter Lillian had been, her daughter took the quilt with her when she went to see her mother several weeks after the stroke, thinking she would enjoy at least seeing it. And since she still didn't talk, it would be a good way to spend the time during the visit. But when Lillian saw the friend's quilt, she took hold of it with great interest, as if trying to figure out a way to

TABLE 29-2   Guide for Assessing Actual or Potential Loss in Elderly Individuals

Assessment	Description
Actual or Potential Loss Related to Physiologic Dysfunction	Cardiovascular
	Respiratory
	Urinary
	Gastrointestinal
	Musculoskeletal
	Nervous
	Endocrine
	Integumentary
	Senses
	Vision
	Hearing
	Tactile
	Taste
	Smell
	General:
	Loss of organs/body parts
	Vigor, strength, power
	Motility, Mobility
	Awareness of mortality
	Mental Clarity
	Nutritional status
Loss of Significant Others Due to Death or Separation Due to Relocation	Spouse
	Child, grandchild
	Sibling
	Extended family
	Friends, including former co-workers
	Caregiver
	Physician
	Minister
	Pet(s)
	Frequency of contacts with others:
	Visitors
	Mail/email
	Telephone usage

(continues)

TABLE 29-2   (Continued)

Assessment	Description
Evidence of Psychological Loss	Body image
	Self-esteem
	Regard of others
	Sense of Influence/power
	Prestige/social status
Philosophical Status	Purpose for living
	Outlook, optimism
	Desire to live (i.e., something to live for)
	Adequate privacy (i.e., to allow meditation/reflection)
	Opportunity for life review
Financial Resources	Reduced income
	Inadequate fixed income
	Major expenditure or change in financial status (as may occur in association with admission to assisted living facility or nursing home)
	Significant loss of property or belongings (as in flim-flam incident, fire, or theft)
Sociological/Functional Status	Adequacy of transportation
	Adequacy of housing
	Proximity/access to essential services
	Physical safety of neighborhood
	Potential for neglect/abuse
	Access to news media
	Opportunity to be with friends (and to make new friends)
	Opportunity for intergenerational interactions
	Opportunity for interaction with enriched environment (entertainment, pets, cultural events, library)
Actual or Potential Loss of Identity	Productivity/leisure activities
	Familiar home or alternative abode
	Familiar surroundings (faces, places, landmarks, belongings)
	Familiar routines
	Personal control
	Territorial loss or change (i.e., reduced or shared life space)
	Altered life style, for any reason
Spiritual Resources	Able to attend church services
	Contact with minister or other spiritual leader

Source: Adapted from Table 2. Guide for Assessing Actual or Potential Loss in Elderly Individuals, in Gueldner, S.H. (1988). Grief and Loss. In S. Mcintire (Editor), *Nursing Series Update: The Older Adult*. A continuing education series offered by the North Carolina Nurses Association, Published by Continuing Professional Education Center.

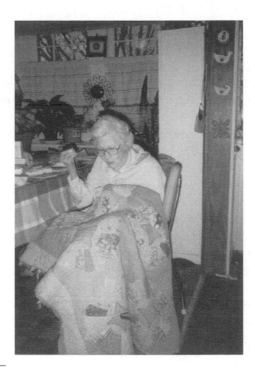

Figure 29-1 Lillian.

mend it. Her daughter, thinking she had misunderstood, quickly said, "No, Mother—Anne Carroll knows you have had the stroke, and that you can't repair it now. I just wanted you to see the quilt before I send it back to her." But Lillian continued to examine the quilt, and struggled to say, in broken, faltering language, "No . . . I . . . want to . . . do . . . it. Present." Her daughter finally realized that she was trying to say that she wanted to repair the quilt as a Christmas present for her friend. Her daughter and granddaughter found some quilt scraps in the attic, and sure enough Lillian could still sew! And what a blessing that turned out to be. The quilt project gave Lillian a way to visit with her friends without having to talk. Two or more of her neighbors would come one or two mornings almost every week, and they would sit for a while and replace a threadbare patch or two on the Dresden china quilt as they visited. Slowly the quilt began to look bright and new again. But the real magic was in the human healing factor. There, sitting quietly for hours with her friends around her mother's quilting frame, and listening to them speak even when she couldn't yet, Lillian eventually made a remarkable recovery from her stroke. In time she learned to speak again in sentences and to sign her name. And a highlight came when one of the women who came to quilt started bringing a pot of homemade soup, and they would send Lillian in to the kitchen to make the tea and cornbread to go with the soup for lunch (Gueldner, Hall, Asbury, & Jacobs, 2005)!

Janis

Janis, an accomplished piano player, taught piano lessons for most of her life. With the support of her family, 92-year-old Janis took her piano with her when she went to the assisted living facility. And despite a series of serious illnesses and setbacks, she still makes her way across the hall to the community room (now in a wheelchair) and plays her piano. And when she plays, other residents come from their rooms, some on walkers and in wheelchairs, to hear her play—and to sing along. They often ask her to play the songs they know, and she usually can. And everyone smiles and has a good time, like they used to. One wheelchair-bound resident requested that she play her favorite song, "You Are My Sunshine," and then she started singing along—she knew all of the verses, and she eventually had everyone singing with her. Then it was time to go to lunch, and the resident continued singing "You Are My Sunshine," and everyone in the lunchroom, including the staff, started singing along. It was as if Janis had spread sunshine throughout the facility. And when she plays, she absolutely beams with enjoyment. As I watched her, smiling and feeling happy and useful, I am reminded that humans have a multitude of talents and abilities, and that loss of ability in one area must not be casually generalized to signify the loss of others. It is important that society find ways for people to continue to express their identity as fully as possible. It would have been a tragedy if Janis Bible had been separated from her piano. Her gift of music is too precious to lose, and it continues to give her a way to continue to be who she has always been (Gueldner, Bible, & Miller, 2005).

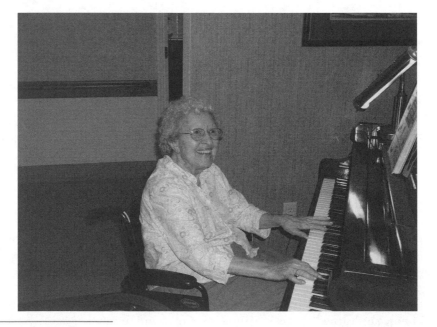

Figure 29-2 Janis.

Frances

Frances Hains was a young-hearted woman in her 90s who taught first grade for 37 years, then retired and enrolled in an art class with her relative. There were about a dozen "students" in the art class, most retired, and they became close friends and continued to take classes together when their instructor offered classes. That was more than 30 years ago, and during that time Frances and her artful friends painted their way across all seven continents as a way of keeping their lives vibrant and meaningful. Her favorite pieces were displayed on her wall in the assisted living facility, and she gave many to family and friends, but several hundred unframed pieces remained under her bed, stacked in large plastic bags. Assisted by a walker, she still met regularly with the group of friends who started out as an art class; they continued to get together and paint once or twice every month. The group became a support group to each other on their journey through the losses that accompany aging. Time took its toll, and only 6 of the original 15 members of the group still met. Several died, and others had to drop out due to health problems. One man developed macular degeneration and could no longer paint, but he still came sometimes, just for the company. Life had dealt other harsh circumstances, as well. One woman lost her husband, and her son was in prison. She found comfort in the group.

An all-time high point for the group came when Frances was invited to host an exhibit of her paintings and watercolors at the assisted living facility where she lived. A few days before the show, Frances was featured in a colored picture in the Sunday newspaper, and the turnout was amazing. And all of the five remaining members of the art class came to

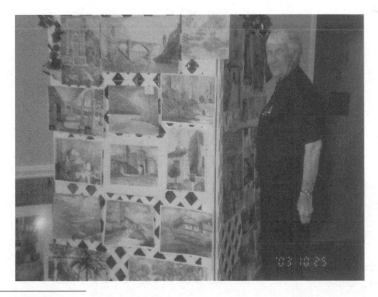

Figure 29-3 Frances.

the exhibit, to celebrate the remarkable accomplishment of their friend. When asked what it was that had kept them together all these years, the group offered, "It gets you out, and keeps you in touch." Being together transformed them, allowing them to leave reality behind for a while, and enjoy each other's talent and company. Frances passed away two years ago, on Valentine's Day, and those who knew her smiled, and thought that fitting (Gueldner & Bramlett, 2006).

Chart

Chart was a country farmer who knew how to grow things. He grew green beans, corn, tomatoes, sweet potatoes, and cucumbers to feed his family, and he gave them to other people who didn't have a garden. He also raised his own cattle and chickens. He plowed the garden with a mule, and was good at it. The rows were extra straight. But one day he went to his country doctor, with complaints that made the doctor think he had gallbladder trouble. So he was scheduled for gallbladder surgery. They went ahead and took the gallbladder out, but when he woke up, the surgeon told him that they had found a large aortic aneurysm that would have to be taken care of in 2–3 months, after he got over this surgery. Well, Chart also cut down trees to build houses and barns, and he had a project in mind, so while he was getting over the first (gallbladder) surgery, he and his friends cut down 13 trees, so they could be "curing" while he recovered from his aneurysm surgery. And then he went in for his surgery. But it didn't go well—the aneurysm ruptured during surgery, and he was in the operating room for more than 8 hours. In fact, his surgeon told his family that he had nearly died. And although he seemed to get over the surgery itself

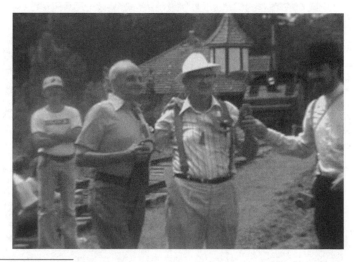

Figure 29-4 Chart.

better than expected, he seemed not to be able to get his usual energy and spirit back, and he seemed to lose interest in his usual activities. Finally, hoping to help him, his grown children entered him in the annual mule plowing contest at an authentic farm museum in south Georgia, a neighboring state! And do you know that he WON that mule plowing contest! In fact, he won over the local man who had won it almost every year. He won the blue ribbon, and the usual winner came in second (his row wasn't as straight as Chart's row was); but even the good-natured usual winner commended him on how straight his row was. Somehow getting back behind a mule and plowing, something that he had done well and enjoyed doing for so many years, picked up his spirits. His unlikely participation in that plowing contest offered him a chance to do something that he knew how to do better than almost anybody—plowing a row to plant corn or beans in. And in doing it, he was able to express his identity, which felt good again.

Chart's Friend, Kruger

Chart's friend Kruger was an absolutely delightful curmudgeon. He lived out in the country in a house with a porch wrapped all across the front, but you couldn't see any other houses, just land and a few cattle. His family had moved the house years ago from the next county, and put it back together again on the strip of land between the Maloneyville Road and the L&N Railroad track. The train went up in the morning and came back at night, hauling coal from the Kentucky coal mines. A two-person porch swing hung from the ceiling at one end of the porch, and Kruger sat in it almost all the time except in the winter. He kept his flyswatter in his hand, and he used it to wave at people he knew when they drove by and tapped their horns.

He was in his 80s and never married, so he lived there alone. He never had running water, but he did finally get someone to run a pipe from his spring house to the kitchen, and water just ran into (and out of) his sink all the time—it didn't even have any faucet handles. And of course he didn't have a phone, either. He did finally get light sockets put in some of the rooms, and a wall plug, so he could plug in his TV. In the late afternoons men would stop by after they came in from the fields, and sit on his porch for a while, and they'd talk politics with him and each other. Kruger had a high-pitched voice, especially if he got a little "riled up" over something. So they'd say things on purpose sometimes just to get under his skin, and he'd shake his head kind of sideways and take issue with them.

In his last years he had trouble with his knees, and it got to be hard for him to bring in coal to keep his stove burning in the winter time. So in cold weather his long-time friend Chart, who lived about a mile further on up the road, would drive down to Kruger's every night, often the last thing he did before he went to bed. Kruger would leave two empty coal buckets sitting just outside his front door before he went to bed at night, and Chart would take the buckets over to the coal pile and fill them up, and set them back by the door so Kruger would have coal in the morning to start his fire back up again, so he could keep warm.

Then one morning Chart got a call from Kruger's nephew, who lived in town, saying that they couldn't get Kruger to come to the door. They knew Chart would know how to get into his house by some secret way, because back then all country people knew how to get into each other's houses if they needed to. Chart, not a young man himself, grabbed his denim jacket and said quietly over his shoulder as he hurried out the door to his car, "Kruger's dead." His young grandson Charles went along, too, as he often did. Chart led the way into the house through the basement door, and sure enough, Kruger was dead. He hadn't made it all the way to bed the night before; he was lying across the foot of the bed, no life about him.

A while later, when his will was read at the county courthouse, Chart learned that Kruger had left him $1000—for gas, I'd say, to pay Chart back for all the errands he took him to do. Chart would drive him to get groceries, and to his doctor's appointments, and once in a while to do his business at the bank in town. But Kruger was skeptical about banks, and he was known to keep more money hidden in his house than he should have. Then near the end Kruger started to have episodes of passing out, and they made him go to a nursing home for several weeks to get his heart medicine "straightened out." Chart would stop by and see him at the nursing home pretty regularly, and one time Kruger asked Chart to take him to his barber to get his hair cut. Chart did, of course, and then Kruger said to Chart, "just take me on home." And that's what Chart did—he sprang Kruger out of the nursing home! What are good friends for, anyway? In his will, Kruger also left Chart his coal pile, and his dry kindling out in the woodshed.

When Chart's grandson Charles grew up, he got an "A" on a college freshman English paper he wrote about Kruger. Charles also played the guitar, and he and his young friends sang some nights at the Buffalo Nickel, a local nightspot in Buffalo, New York. Charles was the lead singer, and he wrote a song about Kruger; in fact, he burned it on a CD and gave it to all the family for Christmas that year. The song told about him sitting on the porch listening to his granddad and Kruger talk about their view of the world. Near the end of the song Charles, reflecting on Kruger's last night alive, sang, "and Kruger died alone that night . . . as all men really do." Kruger was a curmudgeon, and people respected him for that, and enjoyed him being that way. And a little boy who sat quietly listening to him on his porch remembered him, and wrote an essay and later a song about him, and burned it on a CD. Wouldn't you agree that makes Kruger immortal?

Endnote

I wrote this poem after the loss of our parents, who died two months apart when they were 81 and 83 years old, respectively. Despite many losses, they lived good lives, and were admired by everyone who had known them. It helped me deal with their loss to put their identity into words, to honor them, and to preserve their extraordinary "grit" (as their country friends would say) for future generations to learn from and aspire to. I offer it now as a way of grieving for others to consider.

The Magic of Longevity
by Sarah Hall Gueldner

All people who have lived a long time
Are remarkable.
They have been shaped by their life circumstances
Into extraordinary beings,
Unique and completely human.

Master survivors . . .
They have taken on the traits of long life.
They have seen so much,
And felt so much . . .
Both joy and crushing sadness.
They have lived where we have not yet,
And they have become wise,
As we are now becoming.

I marvel at them, all.
They have lived through an incredible slice of life—
Going from the days of horse drawn buggys
To space shuttles and
Computer superhighways, and . . .

> From diphtheria to AIDS, via typhoid fever, pneumonia, and polio;
> From radio to television without antennas;
> Through wars on many continents;
> Through the Depression.

They no longer claim to be perfect,
Nor expect perfection in others.
Right and wrong are no longer absolutes,
But principled living is paramount.
Tossed about by hardships,
But also sometimes riding the crest of happiness and success.
Compromised by age,
Weakened in some respects,
But siring fine children and reveling in their grandchildren
And great grandchildren,
Wherein may just lie their greatest joy and purpose in Life.

Life goes on . . .
One remarkable human being at a time.
Each makes their mark . . .
Each is a part of the Stream of Life . . .
And each is missed even before they are gone,
When it seems they may be leaving. (Gueldner, 2000, p. 39)

As a society, we must support and celebrate the unique identity of our elders, and help them to continue to pursue and express their passions that over a lifetime have become their identities. We must create ways for those disadvantaged by health problems or social decline to pursue their passions as well. The unique identity of each elder is their precious contribution to society, and we must not fail to take note of it, even in our frailest and quietest elders. We must continue to give them time on the center stage of Life, and help them connect with each other and with society in a way that fosters appreciation of the traits, talents, and memories that still define their being (Gueldner, 2007).

References

Gueldner, S.H. (1988). Grief and loss. In S. Mcintire (Ed.), *Nursing series update: The older adult.* Raleigh, NC: Continuing Professional Education Center.

Gueldner, S.H. (2000). Even before they are gone. *Wild Onions, XIV,* 39.

Gueldner, S.H. (2007, December). Sustaining expression of identity in older adults [Guest Editorial]. *Journal of Gerontological Nursing, 33*(12), 3–4.

Gueldner, S.H., Bible, J., & Miller, C. (2005). Music: A universal healing modality. In C. Wendler (Ed.), *The HeART of nursing* (2nd ed., pp. 83–84). Indianapolis, IN: Sigma Press.

Gueldner, S.H., & Bramlett, M.H. (2006). Frances Haines: Painting her way through loss. *Journal of Gerontological Nursing, 32*(9), 52.

Gueldner, S.H., Hall, D., Asbury, C., & Jacobs, K. (2005). Fixin' Anne Carroll's quilt. In C. Wendler (Ed.), The *HeART of nursing* (2nd ed., pp. 185–186). Indianapolis, IN: Sigma Press.

Chapter 30

Making Moments That Matter

Healthy Aging: Gerontological Education for Nurses and Other Healthcare Professionals

Kareen M. King

On September 1, 2005, the *Today Show* featured an interview with a family who survived the trauma of waiting out Hurricane Katrina because they chose not to leave behind their grandmother who was a wheelchair user and dependent on oxygen. When asked how the family dealt with the nightmarish events that unfolded around them, the adolescent grandson commented, "We tried to play games to get our minds off of drowning." I discovered this to be a profound metaphor for dealing with life's difficulties, a metaphor that captures the essence of my work as a registered drama therapist at a long-term care community.

I worked as Ulyssean Program Director/Activities Professional at Brookside Retirement Community, a long-term care community in the Midwest that offers skilled nursing care, assisted living, and catered living units. I oversaw the activity program at the Manor, which during my season of employment had a census of 70 residents, ranging in age from 52 to 100, who suffered from a variety of physical and mental limitations. My drama therapy training equipped me to introduce the value of play not only to the residents, but also to my coworkers. Conventional nursing home activities such as exercise and current events were transformed into theatrical productions. Quality of life for both residents and coworkers improved through drama therapy exercises that facilitated self-expression and played a significant role in facilitating a sense of community and belonging. I believe drama therapy played a role, along with many other contributing factors, in Brookside's earning the PEAK (Promoting Excellent Alternatives in Kansas Nursing Homes) award in both 2008 and 2009.

Introducing Drama Therapy

Drama therapy, as defined by the National Association for Drama Therapy, is the use of drama/theatre processes to achieve the therapeutic goals of symptom relief, emotional and physical integration, and personal growth. Among other things, drama therapy facilitates the client's ability to tell his/her story, to express feelings and achieve catharsis, and to strengthen their ability to perform personal life roles in a more flexible way. Within the context of elder care, drama therapy maximizes the older person's cognitive and communication skills, builds self-esteem, fosters creativity and individuality, encourages physical activity, and builds community.

As a drama therapist/activities supervisor in a nursing home setting, I saw the value of introducing theatrical elements into the everyday activities of the elders I worked with. Shakespeare asserts that "all the world's a stage, and all the men and women merely players. They have their exits and their entrances; and one man in his time plays many parts, his acts being seven ages." In the long-term care environment, we are privileged with the opportunity to participate as key characters in the story of our residents' lives. Most of them have already experienced the vital elements that make up story: a beginning, and a middle, which contains the bulk of the story—overcoming obstacles, working through conflict, and actively building momentum toward a climax, which in their case is likely the golden years of retirement. Now they have moved toward the completion of their story—resolution. Therefore, in the nursing home setting, why not let the last scene of all be the grand finale? Why not place seniors and their activity needs on center stage?

According to Centers for Medicare and Medicaid (CMS) Long Term Care Regulations, facilities are required to conduct a comprehensive assessment, and to provide a program of activities designed to meet the interests and the physical, mental, and psychosocial well-being of each resident. Activities refer to "any endeavor, other than routine ADLs, in which a resident participates that is intended to enhance her/his sense of well-being and to promote or enhance physical, cognitive, and emotional health. These include, but are not limited to, activities that promote self-esteem, pleasure, comfort, education, creativity, success, and independence." (p. 6) Research findings and the observations of positive resident outcomes confirm the importance of meaningful, enjoyable activities that contribute to a sense of community and belonging in the daily lives of residents.

Furthermore, the April 2006 Final Report of a groundbreaking study referred to as the *Creativity and Aging Study* (http://www.arts.gov/resources/Accessibility/CnA-Rep4-30-06.pdf) reveals that "actual stabilization and improvement apart from decline" is the result of powerful positive intervention effects of community-based art programs run by professional artists. Dr. Gene Cohen, author of *The Creative Age* and primary investigator of the report, maintained that, in regard to aging, "what has been universally denied is the potential. The ultimate expression of potential is creativity" (Cohen, 2000, p. 5).

Opportunities to unleash the creative potential of elders in long-term care communities are wide open. Shakespeare refers to the last of the seven ages as the "second childishness." In that context, drama therapy plays a pivotal role in nurturing the inner child that resides in all of us, but may be more easily accessible in our elders. When all else fails, what often remains are the songs, fairy tales, nursery rhymes, puns, games, and sayings that are learned in childhood. Unleashing them in a way that is person-appropriate, as opposed to age-appropriate, takes a bit of ingenuity and fortitude at times. But the results are often worth it. The following are some examples of introducing the element of drama into the nursing home setting and putting the spotlight on creative expression, improvisation, and play.

Theatricality in the Nursing Home Setting

I have discovered that in many ways, theater is a metaphor for life. For example, in the nursing home, like a theater director, an activity director should be the "eye of the audience," being keenly aware of the needs of the residents, both individually and corporately. As a drama therapist, I saw the importance of giving the residents something to look forward to, introducing magic into the mundane. For instance, a weekly activity that had been a coffee and news gathering became a platform for storytelling, puppetry, group poetry, sing-alongs, and improvisational theater games. Exercise, which normally consisted of nothing more than traditional stretching and strengthening, was transformed into a showcase of movement with streamers, colorful paper plates, rhythm instruments, balloons, and improvisational brain stretches. Typical bus outings became imaginative adventures (I called them "AdVantures"), exposing the residents to musicians, artists, actors, collectors, quilt-makers, singers, bakers, and storytellers. Each "performer" entered the "found space" that was the interior of the bus and transformed that space into an intimate showplace.

AdVantures

During our AdVantures, there was always room for serendipity. For example, one time we came across a gentleman riding his horse across his front lawn on a mission to retrieve his mail. I pulled over immediately, opened the side door, and introduced myself and our residents, inviting the man to poke his horse's nose through the door so that everyone could enjoy a close-up view of the horse's head. As a bonus, the man wound up becoming one of our regular guest musical performers! On another occasion, Alice, an incredibly flexible and spunky assisted living resident, offered to perform a stunt I've never been able to pull

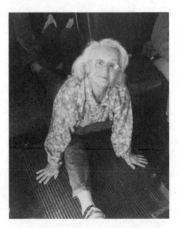

Figure 30-1   Alice does splits on an AdVanture.

off even as a teenager. On a playful whim, she exited the bus, walked across the parking lot, and did the splits on the grass just outside the windows of McDonalds where all the patrons looked out in amazement. It made everyone's day!

Movers and Shakers

Our daily exercise program, which I called Movers and Shakers, offered our residents opportunities for creative expression. Bertie, a stroke survivor who exuded positivity in spite of her physical limitations, asked to participate in this activity without fail. Creating a mini version of an arena stage in our dining room, I arranged the residents in a tight circle, placing myself on a medical stool, center stage. This allowed me to be both at eye level with the residents and to be able to maneuver quickly from resident to resident for more effective interaction. I would always begin each session with breathing exercises to pump more oxygen into the brain, allowing for more energetic participation. Bertie always asked to sit in the center of the circle with me so that I could hand her the microphone to let out the final dramatic exhale which, in her words, sounded like an "old goat." She knew it, but played along anyway, drawing chuckles from the entire room, corporately raising our endorphin levels, known to decrease our levels of stress and pain.

On one occasion, I was feeling less than enthused about facilitating Movers and Shakers because of the lethargy that remained from getting the flu bug earlier in the week. I was so focused on trying to create magic for the residents that I underestimated the potential of creating the magic for myself. I quickly discovered, however, the truth of the old saying, "Fake it till you make it." As everyone was joining the circle, I opened up a book called *Quotationary*, compiled by Leonard Roy Frank and published by Random House. I then asked how everyone was doing and one lady replied, "Lazy." "My sentiments exactly. Let's see what the book says about laziness," I announced serendipitously to the residents.

And so I recited a few quotes, including my favorite, "Laziness: the habit of resting before fatigue sets in," by Jules Renard. This led to a section on energy, which led to a section on enthusiasm. Just then, I recalled a fun exercise I'd seen demonstrated at theater camps. I thought it would be just plain goofy to try it out here. So I invited everyone to join me, with a smile on their faces, in the following chant:

> Look enthusiastic and you'll be enthusiastic!
> Look enthusiastic and you'll be enthusiastic!
> Look enthusiastic and you'll be enthusiastic!
> Boy are we enthusiastic!

Instantly the energy in the room increased. Did I feel ridiculous? Of course. But was it worth it? Most definitely.

At one point, Bertie was wheeled into the room. "Do you feel enthusiastic this morning, Bertie?" I inquired, expecting her to reply affirmatively. "No," she said, to my surprise. However, it wasn't long before she was calling out phrases while we moved our maracas to the music from a great CD called "Latin Fiesta." "Go cats, go!" she hollered. "Shake your bon bon!" she called out a while later. At the end of our activity, I asked if she had any more energy and enthusiasm. "I think so," she smiled.

As I went around giving each resident a hug, I knew that the residents had been touched by the efforts of my coworkers and me as I felt the return hugs and comments of appreciation. At the end of the day, as I hurried through the dining room to leave, I almost missed hearing Bertie's voice calling, "Hey!" I looked to my left to see Bertie seated at one of the dinner tables, looking my way. I rushed over to her and asked if she was calling for me.

"I wanted to see you," she announced matter-of-factly.

"Ahh, you are so sweet, Bertie," I replied. I then apologized for having to rush off and told her I'd be back in a couple of days.

"I'm glad I got to see you a little bit," she responded.

The nursing home is one place where if you don't keep your ears and eyes open, you could miss the magic.

Group Poetry

I discovered the beauty of group poetry during my drama therapy training at Kansas State University. On several occasions, I invited the residents, many of whom struggle with symptoms of dementia, to participate in this creativity-evoking exercise. One time, I arranged everyone in front of the large picture windows that faced a scenic pastoral setting. I invited them to call out everything they could see while I wrote their words and phrases on a dry erase board, acknowledging each contribution. After they had exhausted their ideas, with their assistance, I rearranged the words into a collective poem, inviting them to provide the title. I then typed the final product in large print and included each of their names as the authors, posting the poem throughout the facility. It was an enriching, rewarding, and validating experience for all. The following is the result of the creative endeavors of 10 individuals who interpreted a picture of a man swinging on his trapeze over a waterfall.

The Falls

Swinging free!
Hanging for dear life!
Colorado fun, Yellowstone, Niagara Falls, Hoover Dam, Camp Jayhawk, Cotton-
    wood Falls
I wanna go!
I'm goin' up my way in the flying trapeze
Pink flesh, white, green, light blue, yellow
You can exercise "in the nude" like Tarzan with the greatest of ease in the trees
Nice curves
Elated and beautiful

A similar process for this experience can be explored by visiting www.timeslips.org.

The Ulyssean Philosophy

I also developed the Ulyssean Philosophy (UP) training program which borrows its concepts from Dr. John McLeish (1976), author of *The Challenge of Aging*. The term *Ulyssean* is derived from the mythological hero, Ulysses of *The Iliad* and *The Odyssey*, known for a 10-year span of adventurous exploits in his old age. The program, which met 1 hour weekly for 12 weeks a session, was offered to Brookside's employees who were selected through an application process. The Ulyssean elements include (1) learning, insight, and creativity, (2) exploration of the self, (3) growth and development in the later years, (4) meeting change proactively, and (5) a zest for living. These were introduced through various drama exercises and assignments. The program, which incorporated a variety of theater games designed to enhance Ulyssean potential, produced several UP graduates who were transformed by the process. They not only experienced a higher level of vitality both personally and in the workplace, but also played a more significant role in contributing to the activity life of each resident.

One assignment in particular produced a beautiful testament to the value of collaboration between coworkers and residents. It occurred during preparations for a mini musical version of *The Sound of Music*. The assignment involved initiating individual conversations with each resident, asking them to share their favorite things in life. The answers were eventually submitted to me to incorporate in a parody of the song, *My Favorite Things*. The song was then performed by several coworkers for the residents, whose words were ultimately validated, adding meaning to their lives and empowering the staff.

Brookside's Favorite Things
(Based on conversations with the UP grads and the residents)
by Kareen King

Chocolate and cross-stitch and napping and ice cream
List'ning to music and reading and dancing
Being with family and watching t.v.
These are a few of my favorite things

Football and baseball and playing the piano
Knitting and baking and fruit and potatoes
Flowers and kites and trees budding in spring
These are a few of my favorite things

Children and puppies and painting and spelling
Christmas with relatives and Bible study
Love seeing my husband appear in my dreams
These are a few of my favorite things

Playing Bingo
Doing puzzles
Reading Danielle Steele
Living at Brookside and being with friends
I love how it makes me feel

Pepsi and cola and Diet Mountain Dew
Lilies of the Valley and red, white and blue
Baby back ribs, greens, and loving to sing
These are a few of my favorite things

Boston Red Sox
Country Music
Homemade rolls and pies
These are a few of my favorite things
I love life! Just ask me why!

Nonfiction Playwriting Principles Applied to Songwriting

Among the most unexpected, yet rewarding, perks of working in long-term care are the original songs that emerged as a result of my interactions with the elders. Borrowing concepts from the Playwriting class instructed by Sally Bailey at Kansas State University, I applied principles of nonfiction playwriting by capturing words and expressions from the elders and obtaining release forms from them and/or their durable powers-of-attorney to publish the songs. The result was a collection of story songs that were released in a CD entitled, *The Person in the Picture Ain't Me*. The purpose of the album, available at www .thegoldenexperience.com, is to empower current and potential caregivers to embrace the humanity and dignity of people who reside in long-term care facilities. The songs serve to increase the listener's role repertoire by inviting the listener to place him- or herself in the shoes of another.

Bertie, whose trademark was to request black coffee upon being wheeled into the dining room, inspired one of my favorite tunes. During one of Brookside's memorial services, Bertie sat quietly with her arm raised while the emcee conducted an open mic celebration of each of the residents' lives who had passed away. Expecting to have Bertie commemorate one of the residents, the emcee directed the mic to Bertie's mouth.

"I just want you to know that I'm here," Bertie announced.

The audience chuckled delightedly and the memorial service continued on.

Later, after everyone dispersed from the dining room, Bertie called for me.

"I just want you to know that I'm here," she declared again.

"I'm so glad you're here, Bertie," I affirmed.

"I want you to stay with me. I want you to take me with you wherever you go. I want to be with you," she maintained.

Her comments melted my heart, resonating in my mind from that moment on. I had to capture her spirit somehow. I knew that her words were representative of the cry of every human being. To be noticed, to be loved, and to be seen as valuable to the very end. This is the song I wrote to capture that human feeling, through Bertie's words:

Black Coffee
by Kareen King

Black coffee, please.
I like it straight.
Thanks, you know that you're such a dear.

I'm not hard to please.
I don't mind the wait.
I just want you to know that I'm here.

Why don't you stay
With me?
I wanna be with you.
Let's find a way
To be
Together
I just want you to know that I'm here.
Well, I had a stroke.
But not of luck.
I'm not giving up yet, that's clear.

And it ain't no joke.
That I'm kinda stuck.
And I just want you to know that I'm here.

© 2010 Kareen King

Note: "Black Coffee" will be included in a 2010 release of Kareen's CD, "Find Me."

My boss asked her what she thought of her song the first time I shared it at an in-service. "That's worth twenty-five dollars," she remarked. Well, Bertie was worth her weight in gold. And so is every elder entrusted to our care.

Dr. Gene Cohen's "Creativity and Aging" study provides evidence for the positive impact of creativity and the arts on aging. Dr. Cohen described his view as a new paradigm that sees older people in light of their potential rather than their problems. He promoted this view for the emerging field of creative aging. In his now landmark study on the impact of creativity and the arts on aging, Dr. Cohen found that seniors who participated in the arts had better health, fewer doctor visits, less medication usage, and increased activities and social engagement (Cohen, 2000). His findings have major implications for changing the experience of aging.

References

Cohen, G. (2000). *The creative age.* New York: Harper Collins Publishers, p. 5.

McLeish, J. (1976). *The Ulyssean Adult: Creativity in the middle and later years, Toronto; New York: McGraw-Hill.*

National Association for Drama Therapy, Available at http://www.nadt.org/upload/file/factsheet_elderly.pdf

The Creativity and Aging Study, The Impact of Professionally Conducted Cultural Programs on Older Adults, Final Report: April 1, 2006, p. 6. Available at http://www.arts.gov/resources/Accessibility/CnA-Rep4-30-06.pdf

TimeSlips: Creative Storytelling Project, http://www.timeslips.org

U.S. Centers of Medicare and Medicaid/Long Term Care Regulations. www.cms.gov

For booking information, inspirational blog, and samples of Kareen's music, visit her website at www.thegoldenexperience.com.

Chapter 31

Therapeutic Cooking Groups for Elders

Linda L. Buettner, Suzanne Fitzsimmons, and Nancy E. Richeson

One of the very nicest things about life is the way we must regularly stop whatever it is we are doing and devote our attention to cooking and eating.
—Luciano Pavarotti and William Wright, *My Own Story*

Introduction

The United States is facing a health care crisis as the nation's aging population swells due to the aging baby boomers. As older Americans live longer, they will also experience increasingly complex health needs. Currently the United States healthcare system is not ready to meet the needs of this aging population. Therefore, the Institute of Medicine has called for investments in preparing our healthcare system to care for older adults and their families. The timely and significant report *Re-tooling for an Aging America: Building the Health Care Workforce* (Institute of Medicine, 2008) points out that as the population of seniors grows to comprise approximately 20% of the population, they will face a healthcare workforce that is too small and critically unprepared to meet their health needs. Therefore, those who care for our elders must have the skills, knowledge, and attitudes to provide high-quality health care. Consequently, there is a need to: (1) enhance the geriatric competence of the entire workforce; (2) increase recruitment and retention of geriatric specialists and caregivers; and (3) improve the way care is delivered (Institute of Medicine, 2008). An innovative and fun way to develop these needed competencies among learners is involvement in therapeutic programs such as cooking. Participating in this everyday activity with elders provides potential health care workers the opportunity to gain basic professional skills in health promotion/wellness programming, biopsychosocial and risk assessment, healthcare management, and geriatric syndromes (see Figure 31-1).

Sociocultural Implications

Food, including the act of cooking, has powerful meaning to people of all ages. It defines culture, family history and traditions. For many, cooking signifies basic worth, self-image, and role identity. Food is also connected with feelings of love, pleasure, and enjoyment,

Figure 31-1 Basic professional geriatric competencies for health professionals.

Directions: The following is a list of basic professional skills; each is important for working effectively with and on behalf of older adults. This chart can assist students in assessing their skills. Place a check mark (✓) if you have familiarized yourself with this skill and/or have practiced the skill during the cooking intervention. Students may find it helpful to provide a narrative explaining their experiences.

Competency	I have familiarized myself:	I have practiced this:
Assessment		
Physical		
Functional		
Psychological		
Cognitive		
Psycho-social		
Geriatric syndromes		
Pathophysiology		
Atypical presentations		
Interventions & adaptations		
Risk assessment/Health promotion		
Assess Risks		
Apply 1°, 2°, 3° prevention		
Cultural diversity		
Health care management		
Individualized evidence-based plan		
Evaluate and modify plan		
Identify community support systems		
Empower self-control of care		
Advocate on behalf of older adult		
Interdisciplinary/team care		

Narrative:

holidays, celebrations, family, control, and spirituality. The product of cooking is generally regarded as something to share, as family recipes often have a history attached to them. In traditional cultures, cooking, as a practical art, is passed down from mother and grandmothers to daughter and granddaughters with great pride. This ritual creates strong family relationship bonds. For most of today's older adults, women were the traditional cooks and heads of the kitchen in the family. Due in part to an increase in single parenting, the male cook has evolved beyond the traditional outdoor cooking for barbecues, camping, or fishing or hunting trips. At any age, most people have fond memories or preferences for the home cooking of a loved one.

Cooking programs have the potential to increase appetite, calm and entice people to engage in appropriate social interactions, and motivate reminiscence. These programs may also be associated with feelings of self-esteem, identity, pride and mood. Social interactions and normalized cooking experiences provide older clients with opportunities to attain (or regain) self-esteem goals, a sense of purpose, and a state of improved well-being, independence, and quality of life. Engaging in meaningful activity has been shown to relieve stress, improve physical and cognitive function, reduce depression, and change behavior. Cooking programs for elders can provide familiar sensory stimulation through savory smells, textures, and tastes. They also provide cognitive stimulation and training in such areas as executive functioning, attention, planning, following direction, and interpreting sensory input. There is also physical stimulation: fine and large motor skills are also practiced under the guidance of the therapeutic recreation specialist. Cooking provides the opportunity to take pride in oneself and perform past roles. Providing cooking opportunities increases socialization, since preparing and eating foods is the most social of all activities of daily living (ADL) and is the glue of our social system. This makes cooking perfect for learning or reinforcing social skills, communication, and cooperation with others. The use of cooking as an intervention for a variety of conditions makes this a must-have facilitation skill for any care provider working with the elderly.

Definitions for the Cooking Group Facilitator and Clients

When you use cooking as an intervention, it is important to use pretested recipes adapted as needed for the specific clients, so that the participants can do as much as possible for themselves, while you offer systematic prompts. Cooking skills and terminology common to the art of food preparation should be used for the sake of clear communication. Some of the most common and widely used terms follow.

> *Recipe:* A set of instructions for making something from various ingredients.
> *Adaptation:* (1) The process or state of changing to fit a new environment or different conditions, or the resulting changes. (2) Something adapted to fit need: something that has been modified to suit different conditions or a different purpose.

System of least restrictive prompts: A hierarchy of prompts, beginning with less intrusive prompts and gradually proceeding to more intrusive prompts; used to encourage independence (Engleman, Mathews, & Altus, 2002).

Basic Food Prep Terms

Baste: To brush or spoon liquid fat or juices over meat, vegetables, or other foods during cooking.

Beat: To smoothen a mixture by briskly whipping or stirring it with a spoon, fork, wire whisk, or electric mixer.

Blanch: To boil briefly to loosen the skin of a fruit or a vegetable. After 30 seconds in boiling water, the fruit or vegetable should be plunged into ice water to stop the cooking action, and then the skin easily comes off.

Boil: To cook food in heated water or other liquid that is bubbling vigorously.

Braise: A cooking technique that requires browning meat in oil or other fat and then cooking slowly in liquid.

Chop: To cut into irregular pieces.

Core: To remove the inedible center of fruits such as pineapples.

Dice: To cut into cubes.

Dredge: To sprinkle lightly and evenly with sugar or flour.

Fold: To cut and mix lightly with a spoon to keep as much air in the mixture as possible.

Grate: To shred or cut down a food into fine pieces by rubbing it against a rough surface.

Knead: To work dough with the heels of your hands in a pressing and folding motion until it becomes smooth and elastic.

Mash: To beat or press a food to remove lumps and make a smooth mixture.

Pare: To peel the skin off or trim a food, usually vegetables.

Pit: Using a knife to take out the center stone or seed of a fruit, such as a peach or an apple.

Sift: To remove large lumps from a dry ingredient such as flour or confectioners' sugar by passing it through a fine mesh.

Skim: To remove the top fat layer from stocks, soups, sauces, or other liquids such as cream from milk.

Toss: To thoroughly combine several ingredients by mixing lightly.

Whip: To incorporate air into ingredients such as cream or egg whites by beating until light and fluffy; also refers to the utensil used for this action.

Zest: The thin, brightly colored outer part of the rind of citrus fruits. It contains volatile oils, used as a flavoring.

Summary

Food choices, cooking and eating are important in our family lives and cultures, and they often frame our traditions. Therapeutic cooking is perfect for teaching or reinforcing social skills, communication, and cooperation with others. Improved motor skills, ability to follow step-by-step directions, and the practice of good hygiene are additional therapeutic outcomes that can be attained during cooking interventions. In summary, preparing food can motivate and inspire creativity in older adults.

Theoretical Foundation

The sensation associated with the experience of hunger, preparing foods, and consuming food is one of our most basic needs, yet its impact on psychological, emotional, and social health is complex and far-reaching. Considering that food has a profound impact on health, it may be considered a strong motivator for positive health and wellness decisions and actions. Maslow's Hierarchy of Needs is one of the most often-cited theories for human motivation and one that supports the use of cooking for helping clients to meet goals and objectives (Maslow, 1943). Maslow's theory is that people have specific, unchanging needs, which are genetic in origin and are both physiological and psychological. The hierarchal nature of these needs indicates that some are more basic and more powerful than others. As basic needs are met, higher needs emerge. These needs are often described as a pyramid, with the first four defined as deficit needs and the fifth as a growth need.

Let's examine some examples of how food and/or the preparation and consuming of food can help meet these needs. Physiological needs include the basic life-sustaining requirements, including the body's need for water, protein, sugar, minerals, vitamins, maintaining a pH balance, the need to be active, to rest and sleep, and to avoid pain. Cooking programs can help teach the preparation of balanced meals, the importance of fluids, and the impact of food on rest and sleep. It may even help to divert one's attention from chronic pain. After physiological needs come safety and security needs. Persons whose security needs are not met have anxiety, phobias, insecurities, and fears. Well-planned and -executed cooking programs represent a familiar routine, a safe environment, structure, order, and a comfortable setting, and may lessen these psychological problems. The third layer of needs is the need for love and belonging. Clients whose needs are not met in this category may have poor self-identity, may be socially isolated or have poor social skills, and may have few friends; they may come from dysfunctional families or have disabilities that prevent their participation in community programs and events. A cooking program can provide that sense of belonging through being a part of a group with group goals. It can also provide individual friendships and the realization that there are others with similar problems and interests. The esteem needs are next. Maslow described two types of esteem needs. The lower esteem need is for the respect of others, the need for recognition, attention, appreciation, and for some dominance. The higher esteem need involves the quest for self-respect, confidence, competence, achievement, mastery, independence, and freedom. Persons lacking in this area have difficulty dealing with others, have low self-esteem and feel inferior. For many this shows up as apathy, avoidance, and depression. Cooking programs can provide feelings of accomplishment, control, mastery, self-esteem, and positive attention. And in some instances it can mean the difference between living independently and requiring assisted living.

According to Maslow's hierarchy, the highest need is self-actualization. This is the instinctual need to make the most of one's abilities. It is the acceptance of the realities of life rather than deny or avoiding them. It includes being creative and having problem-solving skills. It is a feeling of closeness to others and appreciation of life. It is reaching one's full potential based on one's given circumstances. It is possible that therapeutic cooking may provide opportunities to achieve some of these self-actualization outcomes as well.

Summary

Eating and preparing foods provide for many of the basic human and growth needs described in Maslow's Hierarchy. Carefully planned food preparation groups provide opportunities to take in food and fluids, meeting physiological requirements for life and providing time to practice ADL and community integration skills. The cooking group experience may provide improved social opportunities, the chance to build self-esteem and independence, and may even provide some self-actualization outcomes.

Literature Related to Effectiveness

Despite the common use of cooking programs in a variety of settings such as rehabilitation centers, nursing facilities, and psychiatric hospitals, there is very little research reported in the literature. Cooking programs can directly tie into one of the 10 goals of *Healthy People 2010,* which is a statement of national health objectives designed to identify the most significant preventable threats to health. Healthy People 2010 initiatives are a set of health objectives for the nation to achieve over the first decade of the new century, and they serve as the basis for the development of state and community plans (Healthy People 2010, 2007). Specifically, in this document therapeutic cooking falls under the category of Overweight and Obesity, but if the caregiver examines Figure 31-2, she or he can see how cooking programs for elders could fit into many of the highlighted areas.

Evidence of Effectiveness

As early as 1979, cooking groups have been recommended for older adults with various psychiatric problems, including dementia (Kretshmar, 1979). It has been found in older women that living a normal life means having the ability to perform food-related work, since cooking was almost certainly a central task in their past life (Gustafsson & Sidenvall, 2003; Gustafsson et al., 2002). A longitudinal study by Edstrom & Devine (2001) found that attitudes about food remain relatively unchanged across the life span, despite changes in health, social environment, and roles.

Cooking groups have been used in recreational and occupational therapy programs to help clients follow simple directions, socialize with each other, to plan and prepare snacks

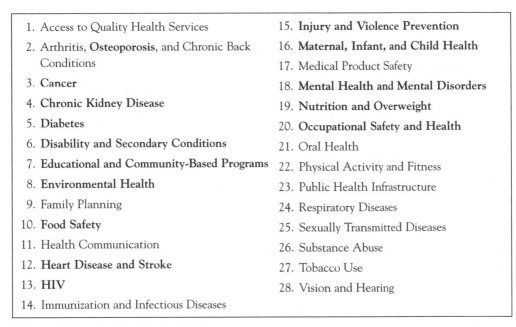

1. Access to Quality Health Services
2. Arthritis, **Osteoporosis**, and Chronic Back Conditions
3. **Cancer**
4. **Chronic Kidney Disease**
5. **Diabetes**
6. **Disability and Secondary Conditions**
7. **Educational and Community-Based Programs**
8. **Environmental Health**
9. Family Planning
10. **Food Safety**
11. Health Communication
12. **Heart Disease and Stroke**
13. **HIV**
14. Immunization and Infectious Diseases
15. **Injury and Violence Prevention**
16. **Maternal, Infant, and Child Health**
17. Medical Product Safety
18. **Mental Health and Mental Disorders**
19. **Nutrition and Overweight**
20. **Occupational Safety and Health**
21. Oral Health
22. Physical Activity and Fitness
23. Public Health Infrastructure
24. Respiratory Diseases
25. Sexually Transmitted Diseases
26. Substance Abuse
27. Tobacco Use
28. Vision and Hearing

Figure 31-2 Healthy People 2010 focus areas.

and meals, and to provide normalized sensory stimulation (Buettner, Lundegren, Lago, Farrell, & Smith, 1996; Merkle, 1994; Buettner & Fitzsimmons, 2003a; Buettner & Fitzsimmons, 2003b). The various cooking programs presented in these research articles have been field tested and present research-based evidence to support their use.

In a sample of individuals with brain injuries or strokes, it was found that those who participated in cooking programs achieved a greater positive impact on fine motor skills than those involved in tabletop activities such as puzzles (Neistadt, 1994a; Neistadt, 1994b). Two other studies compared the effectiveness of a variety of interventions, including cooking, for stroke rehabilitation (Logan, Gladman, Drummond, & Radford, 2003; Jongbloed, Stacey, & Brighton, 1989). Both studies found improvement, with no significant differences between the effects of ADL training, including cooking, and leisure activities or sensorimotor activities. This evidence indicates that in real-world settings, several options should be made available to improve skills, in order to accommodate client preferences.

A small study that implemented a cooking program for older adults with dementia and behavior problems found improvements in both levels of passivity and agitation, as measured using pre and post behavior scales (Fitzsimmons & Buettner, 2003a; Fitzsimmons & Buettner, 2003b). In a larger intervention study, each participant received two weeks of individually prescribed therapeutic recreation cooking, and biofeedback readings were

- Understanding of basic cooking terms and communication of these terms
- Understanding of food safety and hygiene issues
- Basic cooking skills
- Ability to select appropriate clients and group them in meaningful way
- Ability to select appropriate and obtainable goals for each client
- Ability to adapt recipes to client ability
- Ability to adapt recipes, tasks, and equipment for cooking

Figure 31-3 Skills needed by individuals implementing therapeutic cooking programs.

randomly taken three times during the 2-week intervention period to measure physiologic change. The predicted outcome was found between 79% and 91% of the time when treating passivity, and between 92% and 100% of the time for agitation (Buettner, Fitzsimmons, & Atav, 2007). Cooking interventions were found to be predictable and efficacious for reducing disturbing behaviors of dementia. Additionally, cooking was found to be one of the top leisure choices for older adults in a residential setting. Sadly, it was rarely offered to clients with dementia in the nursing homes used in the study (Buettner & Fitzsimmons, 2003b). Since nutrition, behavior, and social isolation are such important areas for clients with dementia, the use of cooking groups should be encouraged in long-term care settings.

Summary

The limited body of research provides some evidence that therapeutic cooking programs can foster improvements for elders with a variety of health problems. The programs included both male and female participants, and significant benefits were demonstrated in each study. Outcomes were both physiological and behavioral and fit into the Healthy People 2010 focus areas. Caregivers implementing therapeutic cooking programs should be familiar with the research to support cooking and develop the skills listed in Figure 31-3 before implementing a cooking program. Special considerations must be taken into account in cooking programs due to safety and hygiene issues; these matters will be addressed in the section that follows.

Special Considerations for Cooking Groups

Selecting Clients

Cooking and food-based programs can include persons of all ages, genders, and functioning levels. Figure 31-4 includes examples of disability groups that might benefit from

Male and female.

This list is merely a suggestion, there are many more.

Neurological disorders such as Parkinson's, Alzheimer's, Stroke, MS

Developmental disabilities such as autism, cerebral palsy, Down's syndrome, mental retardation, attention deficit disorder, learning disabilities

Sensory deficits such as vision, hearing loss

Eating and nutritional disorders

Psychiatric disorders such as depression, anxiety, paranoia

Trauma such as: traumatic brain injury, amputation, burns, MVI

Those with health management needs related to new diagnosis: diabetes, heart disease, cystic fibrosis, pregnancy, celiac disease, cancer, AIDS

Those with knowledge deficit related to lack of cooking skills and/or nutritional knowledge

Others: social isolation, need to help, poor self-esteem, self-identity disorder, poor coping, dysfunctional family, impaired physical mobility, activity intolerance, self-care deficits, pain, wandering

Figure 31-4 Clients/Conditions that may benefit from cooking programs.

cooking programs. Participants should be selected based on their individualized goals and objectives. For example, a person who needs to improve muscular endurance will probably not benefit from cooking, while a person with impaired fine motor skills may. It is important to tailor the program tasks to the specific clients' needs. For example, the client with impaired fine motor skills should be involved with tasks such as measuring, peeling, and chopping, while the client with anorexia might be involved in nutritional menu planning. Cooking programs can be useful with clients who have a need for dietary education, independence skills, cognitive stimulation, fine motor skills, socialization, and reminiscing. See Figure 31-5 for possible goals and objectives for cooking programs.

It is also important to consider who should not be invited to participate in cooking programs. Clients with destructive behavior or a tendency for unpredictable, violent behaviors should not participate until behaviors are manageable and safe. Clients with pica (i.e., the abnormal desire to eat substances not usually eaten) may participate with close supervision. Those with suicidal or cutting behaviors should of course not be invited or permitted to participate in programs with sharp instruments. Likewise, those with impaired swallowing will need close supervision and adherence to food consistency restrictions. Clients with socially deviant behaviors may threaten to spit or place inappropriate items into foods and would require close supervision. Clients with poor hygiene habits should be evaluated for appropriateness. These types of clients could participate in a one-on-one cooking program to ensure safety and to provide success experiences before joining a therapeutic cooking group.

- Improve or maintain ability to follow one-(two) three step directions
- Improved fine motor skills
- Improved behaviors
- Improved communication
- Increased knowledge of food hygiene, nutrition, diet, cooking skills
- Improve or maintain the ability to talk about favorite foods/recipes for the past
- Improve or maintain the ability to open, stir, pour, and serve foods
- Improved task completion
- Improved social skills as evidenced by using appropriate dining etiquette
- Maintained or improvement in reaching ideal body weight
- Increase in mood by facial expression or by verbal comments
- Decrease or prevention in target behaviors during and after program
- Improved food choices
- Decrease in non-aggressive behaviors, such as wandering during mealtimes
- Decreased vocalizing behaviors during mealtimes
- Increased involvement and participating in meals
- Improved ability to express self and emotions
- Improved self-feeding
- Increased social skills and social interaction with others
- Improvements in ability to communicate
- Improved attention to task
- Improved safety awareness related to feeding
- Improved sequencing skills related to feeding
- Improvements in upper extremity range of motion
- Increased fine motor abilities
- Maintenance or improvement of functional abilities
- Increased hydration and nutrition
- Improvement or maintenance of weight
- Increased socially appropriate behavior at meal times
- Increased self-esteem and sense of self-worth
- Decrease in non-aggressive behaviors, such as wandering
- Decreased vocalizing behaviors through participating in meaningful tasks
- Increased involvement and participating in daily events
- Improved ability to complete activities of daily living

Figure 31-5 Possible goals and objectives for cooking programs.

Hygiene Standards and Food Safety

Always check the facility's regulations, as well as local and state health regulations, prior to implementing a cooking program. The following list contains some general guidelines to follow in all situations.

- Disposable aprons or clean laundered aprons for all clients and staff should be available. Clients with respiratory, sinus, skin, ear, nose, eye, or intestinal infections should not participate. Clients with burns, cuts, scabs, ulcers, or any other type of open skin tears should have the wound covered with a waterproof dressing. If a client's wound is septic he or she should not handle food. A first aid kit should be available in the event of minor injury.
- Tie hair back or use a net if hair is shoulder length or longer.
- Fingernails should be cut short and clean.
- Clients and staff must wash hands with soap and warm water for 20 seconds, and use clean paper towels. Repeat washing after handling raw meats.
- It is preferable for each client to make and consume what he or she produced in the cooking class.
- Exceptions to this are items that are baked, such as cake or biscuits, or cooked with high temperatures, such as stews or soups.
- If preparing food that is to be eaten by others uncooked, such as tossed salad, gloves should be worn.
- Wash all fruits and vegetables well before using in cooking class and before eating.
- Cook all foods thoroughly.
- Store dry foods in clean, sealed containers, marking the date the item was opened.
- Taste foods only when thoroughly cooked. Use a clean spoon each time.
- Foods should be consumed as soon after preparation as possible.
- Use separate colored or marked cutting boards for meats, vegetables, and pastry foods.
- Clean surfaces with sanitizer after use and in between working with raw and cooked foods.
- All equipment used must be cleaned in very hot water and air dried or dried with disposable towels.
- Keep hot foods hot and cold foods cold. If food is allowed to remain at room temperature for 2 hours or longer, bacteria can multiply and cause food poisoning. Dispose of this food.
- Refrigerate all leftovers soon after meals.
- Hot food does not have to be cooled before placing it in the refrigerator.
- Keep refrigerated foods wrapped or sealed. Keep raw meats on the lowest shelf of the refrigerator.

- Refrigerator should be kept below 5° Celsius.
- Clean refrigerator each week, throwing out any old items.
- Don't buy or use food from dented, bulging, or rusted cans.
- If you have any doubt about the safety of the food, throw it out!

Guidelines: How Long Can Foods Be Stored?

- Refrigerated steaks and roasts should be used within 3 to 4 days after purchase.
- Ground meats, fresh poultry, and raw fish should be used within 1 to 2 days after purchase.
- Milk, cream, cottage cheese, and cream cheese are good for a week after opening.
- Hard cheeses that are tightly wrapped are good for 2 to 3 months.
- Eggs are good for 3 to 4 weeks. Keep them refrigerated.
- Cooked or uncooked vegetables are good in the refrigerator for 3 to 5 days.
- Berries are only good for about 3 to 5 days in the refrigerator before they mold or rot.
- Bread, cake, and cookies (anything made from a batter) should be used within a week to avoid mold.
- Baked goods will last longer (2 weeks) if refrigerated.
- Deli meats should be used within 4 days after opening the package.
- Leftover meats are good for 3 to 5 days.
- Leftover chicken, gravy, sauce, chicken, or tuna salads are only good for 1 to 2 days.
- Mustard, soy sauce, Worcestershire sauce, and other condiments should be used within a year of opening.
- Mayonnaise, once opened, is good for 2 months.
- Open bottles of salad dressing are good for 3 months.
- Ketchup, jams, jelly, and peanut butter are good for 6 months.
- Opened jars of salsa should be discarded after a month.
- Frozen food is good for a year if tightly wrapped and stored consistently at 0°F.
- If you cannot remember when a food was placed in the refrigerator, throw it out.

How Do I Know If Foods Are Cooked Thoroughly and Properly?

- Red meat should be cooked to 160°F. Use a food thermometer.
- Large cuts of red meat can be cooked to medium rare, 145°F.
- Ground meat and hamburgers should be cooked all the way through until the center is at least 160° to 165°F.
- Cook fish to 130° to 140°F, until the center looks opaque when tested with a fork.
- Cook pork to 155°F with no pink.
- Cook chicken to 170°–180°F or until the juices run clear.
- Eggs should be cooked until both the yolk and the white are firm.
- Heat leftovers to 165°F.
- When reheating sauces, soups, and gravies, bring them to a boil.
- Never allow clients to drink unpasteurized milk or dairy products.
- Do not allow clients to eat raw cookie dough that contains eggs.
- Do not use leftover marinades as they contain raw meat juices.

What Do the Various Dates on Food Mean?

"**Expiration**" is the last date on which a product should be used. If the date has passed, throw it away.

"**Sell by**" indicates the last day on which the product should be sold. You can keep the food 2 to 3 days longer than that if it is well-refrigerated.

"**Best if used by**" is the date by which the manufacturer guarantees the freshness and quality of the food. It is not dangerous to use the food after that date, but the food may not have top quality or top nutritional value after that date.

"**Packed on**" dates are sometimes found on canned and frozen food. This is not useful information unless you know when the food was picked and processed before the freezing or canning. As a rule of thumb, frozen foods can be kept for 3 to 4 months after that date. Canned goods can be stored for up to a year beyond that date. Foods stored and kept longer may lose their flavor and nutritional value. But they are not dangerous. Products may not necessarily be unusable after the date on the package. Examine the food carefully before using. To be safe, use common sense: If the food looks or smells unusual, don't use it.

Cooking With and Without a Kitchen

Many agencies can offer cooking groups despite the fact that they don't have a kitchen available. With the use of microwaves, hot plates, grills, blenders, and toaster ovens, many cooking groups prepare entire meals in a designated program area. It is also possible to prepare recipes that don't require cooking using a blender, or by simply chopping foods and mixing ingredients. The creative caregiver will develop recipes that can be prepared in a variety of settings with and without a full kitchen setup. See Figure 31-6 for basic cooking equipment and staple foods needed to start a therapeutic cooking program.

Facilitating

In all therapeutic interventions the goal is to engage the client to encourage him or her to complete tasks as he or she works toward a goal, and to be as independent as possible. Program staff in cooking groups should be taught the system of least restrictive prompts, which provides just enough cuing so the client completes the activity independently. Doing the task for the client must be avoided, because participants will only attain benefit if they are able to do it themselves.

Adapting recipes and tasks must be done well in advance of the program session. Either the day before the program or the hour just before the cooking group meets, the facilitator should prepare a sample of the recipe to display. This might be a completed fruit salad, a decorated cookie, a hot pretzel, or a small version of the recipe to be made.

The recipe must be tested, and each part of the recipe should be written in large print on a large index card that can be held up by a card holder. Most cooking groups can be broken down into the following basic tasks:

- Washing hands and washing food items
- Picking items from a garden or a grocery store
- Opening the packages of ingredients
- Measuring and pouring various ingredients that are needed
- Stirring, cutting, or chopping items
- Mixing and pouring the mixture into containers
- Plating and serving
- Cleaning up afterwards

An example of adapting one of these tasks might be if the client in charge of opening the milk container, the pudding boxes, and the other canned goods is not able to grasp and tightly grip them. The facilitator may simply preloosen the milk lid, lift a corner of the pudding box flap, or offer a gripper device or adapted can opener. Many adapted devices can be purchased to help with each category of tasks listed. If the client has a visual impairment, the recipe card should be enlarged and printed with large font on a yellow

Utensils
Mixing bowls (assorted sizes)
Measuring spoons
Glass or plastic cup for liquid measuring
1 set dry measuring cups
Wire whisk
Soup ladle
Grater
Potato masher
Long-handled fork
Can opener
Long-handled slotted and non-slotted
    spoons
2 flexible rubber spatulas
Wire-mesh strainers
Colander
Funnel
Vegetable peelers
kitchen timer
Pepper grinder
Plastic chopping boards
Thermometer

Knives
2 paring knives
1 serrated bread knife
2 butter type knives

Electrical equipment
Blender
Hand mixer
Toaster
Electric skillet
Electric frying pan
Crockpot
Double portable electric burner

Baking Equipment
2 8- or 9-inch round cake pans
1 square baking pan
2 loaf pans
2 baking sheets (rim less)
2 muffin tins
Rolling pin
Wire rack
Cookie cutters

Pots and Pans
3 pots (1 each of small, medium and
    large)
Stock pot with tight-fitting lid
Vegetable steamer
Ceramic baking dishes

Staple Food Items
Salt & pepper
Baking powder
Baking Soda
Garlic powder
Onion powder
Parsley
Cinnamon
Oregano
Basil
Granulated sugar
Brown sugar
Powdered sugar
Flour
Shortening
Vegetable Oil
White and red vinegar
Bullion

Figure 31-6 Basic cooking equipment and staple foods.

background. Recipes and instructions could also be given verbally or on tape if needed. For clients with cognitive impairment, it is best to provide simplified step-by-step tasks with only one or two steps per card.

Recipes often need to be done over 2 or 3 days. A recipe to make applesauce cake might be adapted to a 2-day project by having the clients use a crank-style apple peeler to peel and core the apples on the first day. The peeled and cored apples can be sweetened and quickly cooked in a nearby microwave. Make enough applesauce so that each person gets a sample that day, but also be sure there is enough to prepare the cake recipe on the following day. The applesauce can be refrigerated and used the next day to actually make the cake. Once the cake goes into the oven, the cleanup takes place, and clients may come together in a few hours to frost the cake for an evening party. The clients should be involved in all the steps of this process.

Simplifying, shortening, and clearly communicating the tasks involved in cooking groups are critical to successful experiences. Assigning tasks to group members, providing cuing as needed, and adapting equipment when required makes the process fun and positive for all involved.

The Program

When planning a cooking program there are several important considerations to think about and plan for. Consider the timing of the cooking group when establishing your cooking group time. Factors that you might need to take into consideration are energy level of the clients, meal times, fatigue due to other activities, behavior patterns, normal naps, pain medication times, and anything else unique to the client that might pose a problem.

The group size is determined based on the cognitive and functional abilities of the clients and how much assistance is needed. Compatibility of the clients in the group is another important aspect of planning. It is also important to be aware that billable therapy sessions cannot exceed a 1:4 staff-to-client ratio, but with challenging clients, it is wise to start with a ratio of 1:2. Make certain to have enough tasks planned so that everyone participates actively throughout the program. Although there are many different methods of designing a cooking program, one that includes planning, shopping or harvesting, and then ultimately preparing the food provides the most variety and skill-building opportunities. It is also the most realistic and normalized method of preparing food and cooking. This can be achieved in one longer session or two or three separate sessions during the week. Be sure to allow for time to discuss the program outcomes afterward, including what was accomplished, and how the group will proceed next time.

Planning

Set up a planning session and invite the clients to come. Participants are encouraged to greet each other by name in order to foster socialization and friendship opportunities from the beginning. Discuss and then select the types of recipes the group wishes to prepare. To stimulate ideas the facilitator might have the clients look through recipe cards, cookbooks, or cooking magazines to help make reasonable selections. Next the facilitator must select the version of the recipe most appropriate for the group and adapt a recipe to match their abilities. He or she will also need to determine how much of each ingredient will be needed for the size of the cooking group. The facilitator may order the supplies, harvest the produce, or plan to shop for the needed items, or he or she may involve members of the cooking group in these activities.

   The planning session should include a discussion of nutritional value, balanced meals, caloric needs, and other nutritional education tips. It might also be appropriate to discuss the pros and cons of fresh versus canned, packaged, or frozen ingredients, costs associated with each, selecting a store to make purchases, looking for coupons or other specials, and determining transportation options to the market or store. If possible, encourage one or two clients to record the shopping list of required ingredients, based on the recipes chosen. Between sessions, make copies of the recipes, adapted according to the needs of individual members of the group, for participants to follow on cooking day.

Shopping or Harvesting

Clients may spend time in a garden area to harvest berries, fruit, or vegetables for recipes. This activity provides an adjustment time and a change in environment that may foster helpful behaviors. Clients who take part in the community integration outing to obtain supplies for the cooking group should use the shopping list and stick to a budget to select and purchase items. Encourage them to compare prices of items, look for specials, and use coupons. It may be useful to ask the produce manager to help the group understand what to look for when selecting fresh fruits and vegetables, meats, or other items, but be sure to ask them ahead of time, so they can be better prepared.

Cooking

Each client should be provided with a simple large bold print copy of the recipe. Card holders or clips are useful so the recipe is held upright on the table. One client can be assigned to read the recipe step by step to the group before starting. Tasks like opening, cutting, and stirring can be assigned to various members of the group based on ability levels. (High ability level: Cut stems off of strawberries; Mid-level ability: Stir ingredients; Lower ability level: In a sealed container shake heavy cream into whipped cream or butter.)

Remind the staff and volunteer helpers about the following system of least restrictive prompts to cue clients.

System of Least Restrictive Prompts

Purpose

The system of Least Restrictive Prompts (LRP) (Engleman, Mathews, & Altus, 2002) was developed as an approach for the therapist to follow in order to maximize active involvement of the client and avoid feelings of failure.

Instructions

Familiarize yourself with the steps and method of giving the least amount of prompts so that this approach can be systematically used with all clients. The goal is to encourage active engagement and functional independence as much as possible. Selected appropriate prompts are:

1. Knock on the door before entering the client's room.

2. Greet the client, using the client's name (e.g., "Good morning Marion").

3. Introduce yourself each time ("It's Linda!"). "Let's go to cooking class."

4. Prepare the program area by eliminating disturbances and ensuring all necessary materials are available for step-by-step completion of the cooking tasks.

5. Identify the task to be completed (e.g., "It's time to cook our spring rolls").

6. Use at least two less intrusive prompts before giving physical assistance. Less intrusive prompts include verbal prompts, gestural prompts, and modeling.

7. Time prompts correctly. Wait 5 to 10 seconds between prompts to give sufficient time for response.

8. Use physical guidance correctly. As a last resort (e.g., after offering at least two less intrusive prompts), the interventionist should gently help clients to complete the current step of the activity.

The LRP system was developed as an approach for facilitators to follow in order to maximize the active involvement of clients (Engleman, Mathews, & Altus, 2002). When using the LRP system, first identify the task to be completed (e.g., "It's time to stir the batter"). Use at least two less intrusive prompts before giving physical assistance. Less intrusive prompts include verbal prompts, gestural prompts, and modeling (e.g., "Pick up the spoon" or "Stir the batter"). Always time prompts correctly, waiting 5 to 10 seconds between prompts to give sufficient time for a response. When resorting to physical assistance, gently assist the client to start the motion, using hand-over-hand help (e.g., place spoon in participant's hand, place your hand over participant's hand to gently start motion). Remove your hand if the participant responds by performing the current step of the activity.

Simple types of foods that can be prepared during a single cooking program include garden and fruit salads, vegetable soup, freshly squeezed lemonade, various types of pies (chocolate cream, banana cream, apple, cherry), cookies, bread, churned or shaken butters, homemade sherbet, pesto sauce, personal pizzas, and applesauce. Many other foolproof recipes can be found online and tested for usability in your group.

Evaluation

Figure 31-7 includes a detailed flow sheet for monitoring cooking groups that can be modified for your program. The best approach is to monitor each client during and after each session and make immediate changes that are needed. A change may be simply who the client sits next to, or it might be a revision in the tasks assigned. Another simple method of evaluation is to revisit the client's goal at least every 2 weeks. If progress is being made, make a progress note documenting exactly what has been observed. If the client is discharged from the group, follow-up sessions might be recommended in order to possibly find other settings. Finally, a client satisfaction scale or survey will help the facilitator gain insight into what the clients might recommend to improve the program.

Case Study: Memory Loss and Failure to Thrive

A very worried family member requested therapeutic cooking for her 86-year-old mother, Lisa, because of her anorexia, self-abusive behavior, lack of friends, symptoms of depression, and inability to interact socially with others in the continuing care retirement community (CCRC). Lisa had been moved to the CCRC assisted living unit 1 year ago. Prior to moving in, Lisa had lost her husband of 60 years. Lisa was unable to live alone due to moderate memory loss and left their apartment for an assisted living unit. She was always considered small framed, but over the past year she had lost 2 to 3 pounds each month, and was down to 85 pounds. In her CCRC she had no friends, refused to eat in the dining room, declined to participate in general activities, and was biting herself when in her room for extended periods of time. Over the past several weeks her biting behavior had led to serious wounds and infections. She is now being treated at as an inpatient in the skilled nursing unit. In addition to moderate memory loss, she was recently diagnosed with failure to thrive, due to the combination of her depression and poor nutrition.

Score	Objectives	Session date
	Client: _____ ID# _____ Diet Type _____	
	Program Title: _____ Day _____ Time _____	
	Favorite foods _____ Adapted equipment needs: _____	
6	Reads recipe card and follows directions to measure, mix, prepare	__ __ __
5	Reads recipe card/needs cuing to follow directions	__ __ __
4	Measures, mixes, prepares ingredients with verbal instructions	__ __ __
3	Measures, mixes, prepares ingredients with demonstration	__ __ __
2	Measures, mixes, prepares ingredients with physical assistance	__ __ __
1	Unable to measure but able to pour ingredients	__ __ __
0	Unable to measure or pour—spills or eats ingredients	__ __ __
	Name kitchen utensils used:_____	
6	Uses kitchen utensils properly	__ __ __
5	Uses kitchen utensils properly with step-by-step verbal cuing	__ __ __
4	Uses cooking utensils properly with demonstration	__ __ __
3	Uses cooking utensils properly with physical assistance	__ __ __
2	Holds utensils but unable to use purposefully	__ __ __
1	Unable to hold or use kitchen utensils	__ __ __
0	Refuses or unable to wash or clean up	__ __ __
6	Washes hands and cleans up area independently	__ __ __
5	Washes hands and cleans up area with step-by-step verbal prompts	__ __ __
4	Washes hands and cleans up area with demonstration	__ __ __
3	Washes hands and cleans up area with physical assistance	__ __ __
2	Washes hands with prompting but unable to clean up area	__ __ __
1	Washes hands with demonstration/physical assistance	__ __ __
0	Refuses or unable to wash or clean up	__ __ __
6	Initiates social conversation about foods, recipes, etc.	__ __ __
5	Engages in social conversation on topic when initiated by others	__ __ __
4	Engages in social conversation when asked direction questions	__ __ __
3	Converses with others with repeated phrases or questions	__ __ __
2	Speaks only occasionally but answers seem appropriate	__ __ __

Figure 31-7 Therapeutic food programs monitoring.

1	Speaks only occasionally and answers seem inappropriate	___ ___ ___
0	Moans, cries, unable to speak	___ ___ ___
6	Feeds self-prepared foods using spoon or fork	___ ___ ___
5	Feeds self-prepared foods with adapted equipment	___ ___ ___
4	Feeds self-prepared foods with considerable spilling	___ ___ ___
3	Feeds self-prepared foods with step-by-step verbal cuing	___ ___ ___
2	Feeds self-prepared foods with demonstration/physical assistance	___ ___ ___
1	Feeds self using fingers	___ ___ ___
0	Must be fed	___ ___ ___
	% of food consumed	___ ___ ___

Total score/30: (Comments on back)

___/   ___/   ___/   Therapist signature:_____

Figure 31-7   Therapeutic food programs monitoring (continued).

Source: ©LBuettner 1997.

Therapeutic Cooking Program

Lisa was referred to the therapeutic cooking program. During the first session Lisa joined the facilitator of the group and one other client named Mary for a tour of the berry garden and cooking areas. The clients were introduced, but did not verbally interact with each other. After the tour the facilitator discussed each person's favorite foods over a cup of tea. Lisa seemed genuinely interested in the daily time in the garden, and stated that she always wanted to learn how to make scones. She also stated she wanted to do this alone. The other client mentioned she loved blueberries and blackberries. The facilitator helped the clients decide that picking some fresh berries and making scones would be an excellent first project.

During the next three sessions Lisa and Mary spent 15 minutes in the garden picking berries. They worked separately and the facilitator used the system of least restrictive prompts to cue both clients to pick and sort the berries into plastic containers. The berries were collected daily and placed in the freezer for use when enough had been gathered. Both clients sampled the berries and joked about "never collecting enough for the recipe." They spent the remainder of the time during each session washing their hands, selecting cookbooks, and looking through cookbooks for recipes. Notes were made about appealing recipes that used berries, and the Berry Scones recipe was located. A large-print copy was made for each client, and a few extra copies were printed and laminated. Lisa and Mary were asked by the facilitator to look through the kitchen supply area to be sure that all the ingredients were available for the recipe. Mary was happy to start looking in the pantry, and found most of the supplies within 5 minutes.

Lisa did not initiate looking for supplies even when Mary asked for help. Lisa sat and simply yelled "Do it yourself"! The facilitator took Lisa aside and restated the object of looking for the supplies, and then provided a prompt to look for the flour, and then 15 seconds later she repeated the prompt. Lisa slowly reached up to the nearby supply closet and found the container of flour. Praise was given to Lisa for finding it, and the session closed with a reminder about the task for the next day. They would be making homemade butter for the recipe.

Session 5 involved making some homemade butter that would be used in the recipe the next day. A screwtop plastic container was filled with heavy cream and Mary and Lisa took turns shaking it until the yellow lump separated into butter. After draining off the watery fluid, the clients were encouraged to try some of the butter on a piece of bread. Lisa had two! The clients were talking about how good the butter tasted and how simple it was to make. The butter was drained once more and placed in the refrigerator in a closed container. The session closed with a discussion about the next day. There would be two groups tomorrow. One session would be held in the morning to prepare the scones for baking, and one session would take place later in the afternoon, to eat the freshly baked scones. Each person was encouraged to invite a guest for the 3:00 P.M. tea party the next day. Each client was then assisted in making choices and phoning a friend.

During session 6 in the morning, the Berry Scones dough was prepared, rolled, cut, and prepared for baking. The tasks were divided up into: (1) measuring flour and other dry ingredients, and (2) washing berries and measuring butter and cream. Then the clients wore latex-free gloves as they took turns stirring, rolling, and patting out the dough. Finally both clients cut the scones and placed them on baking sheets. Prompting was provided as needed throughout the session to remind the clients of the tasks and the steps to complete. At the end of the session Lisa stated, "I feel so proud of this cooking we did!" The facilitator told the clients that the scones would be baked during lunch, and then at 3:00 P.M. we would meet for tea and scones. Mary and Lisa were both talking about the afternoon event and what they would wear as the session ended. The discussion continued in the dining room during lunch, and several other residents asked if they could come at 3:00 P.M. (They of course were told that they were welcome to come.)

Session 7 was the culmination of a week of work. Lisa was dressed up in her best dress and eager to enter the program area just before 3:00 P.M. Mary also showed up and then the guests arrived. The facilitator had set up a "self serve tea and scones" table with a sign placed on the wall that said, "Thank you Lisa and Mary." Lisa's daughter attended this event, along with several residents and staff members. Everyone told the cooks what an excellent job they had done and asked for the recipe. Lisa and Mary were provided with large-print copies to distribute. Both clients had interacted with each guest and seemed to feel proud and good about the work they had done in their cooking class. In the next 7-day cooking program two new participants were added, and both Lisa and Mary were invited to continue in the group until they had met all their goals.

Summary

Lisa was provided with a therapeutic cooking program to help reduce her symptoms of depression, to motivate her to eat, and to help her connect with other people. An additional purpose of the program was to decrease her self-abusive behaviors. She successfully accomplished the following goals during the initial seven sessions:

- She interacted verbally with one other resident during the cooking activity each day
- With prompting, she completed two-step tasks during each session.
- She demonstrated an increased appetite and willingness to go to the dining room.

She will continue to be guided to work on increased appetite and improved nutrition, along with continued improvements in reports of self-abusive behavior over the next 30 days.

Professional Geriatric Competencies for Health Professions

Upon graduation, students in all health professions are expected to attain a standardized set of basic professional competencies for working with older adults. These competencies ensure that students learn the skills, attitudes, and knowledge to meet the basic standards necessary to provide quality care to older adults. Students can observe, assist, and/or facilitate in well-designed cooking programs for older adults, in turn gaining the competencies needed for graduation.

Figure 31-1 provides a checklist for students to use in assessing their level of professional competency while engaging in cooking programs for older adults. For example, clients will need to be assessed prior to entering cooking programs, then again at the end of each session, to evaluate which activities were used and how helpful they were in understanding the client's level of functioning. It is also important that personnel involved (including students) reflect on what types of syndromes the clients in the cooking group presented with, and how the intervention was designed and adapted to maximize the benefit for each client. For instance, how did a client's individual physiology play a role in his or her participation? Additionally, how were risks assessed and cultural diversity addressed? Was the cooking program a primary, secondary, or tertiary intervention? How was the intervention designed to empower each participant? What

416 ■ Chapter 31 Therapeutic Cooking Groups for Elders

professionals on the interdisciplinary team did you interact with, and what were their roles in making the cooking program successful for the members of the cooking group? Did you review the individualized care plans and identify any modifications of the plan? Lastly, how were the clients encouraged to interact with the community during the intervention?

As America continues to age, the increased demand for healthcare providers competent to provide health-promoting/self-empowering care is urgent. These competencies can provide healthcare professionals with a set of basic skills needed to enter the work force.

Conclusion

This chapter introduces small group cooking as a therapeutic modality. The use of the system of least restrictive prompts and simple preparation tasks involving fresh foods was highlighted to foster success experiences, motivation, opportunities for social interactions, and improved self-esteem. Therapeutic cooking focuses on the choices of the clients and establishes manageable tasks that can be accomplished together over a few sessions. The case study provided demonstrates the power of sharing the age-old activity of food preparation. In addition, the geriatric competencies checklist allows students to assess their readiness to enter the workforce.

Discussion Questions:

1. How is food related to control?
2. List five diagnostic areas from Healthy People 2010 that might benefit from therapeutic cooking.
3. Why would you pretest the recipe you will use in a therapeutic recreation session?
4. Name five safety concerns for therapeutic cooking.
5. What are the steps you would take from the system of least restrictive prompts to encourage a client to do the first step in a cooking task?
6. What are the primary findings of studies conducted using therapeutic cooking interventions?
7. Why would you maintain a ratio of 1:4 or less in a therapeutic cooking program?
8. What needs from Maslow's theory could possibly be met in a therapeutic cooking intervention?
9. Explain how the professional competencies checklist assessed your readiness for the workforce.

10. How could you offer therapeutic cooking if your hospital, clinic, or agency did not have a kitchen?

11. List three goals for older adults enrolled in a cooking intervention program.

Resources

Article

Fitzsimmons, S., & Buettner, L. (2003a). Therapeutic recreation interventions for need-driven dementia-compromised behaviors in community-dwelling elders, *American Journal of Recreation Therapy*, Winter, 17–32.

Internet

Connie Q Cooking: http://www.connieqcooking.com/
Real Simple Magazine recipes: http://food.realsimple.com/realsimple/recipefinder.dyn
Food Network: http://www.foodnetwork.com/
Using literature-related cooking experiences to foster the development of communication skills: http://www.highlightsteachers.com/archives/articles/using_literaturerelated_cooking_experiences_to_foster_the_development_of_communication_skills.html

References

Buettner, L., & Fitzsimmons, S. (2003a). Activity calendars for older adults with dementia: What you see is not what you get. *American Journal of Recreation Therapy,* Summer, pages 9–22.

Buettner, L., & Fitzsimmons, S. (2003b). *Dementia practice guideline for recreational therapy: Treatment of disturbing behaviors.* Alexandria, VA: American Therapeutic Recreational Association.

Buettner, L., Fitzsimmons, S., & Atav, S. (2006) Predicting outcomes of therapeutic recreation interventions for older adults with dementia and behavioral symptoms, *Therapeutic Recreation Journal*, XL(1): 33–47.

Buettner, L., Lundegren, H., Lago, D., Farrell, P., & Smith, R. (1996). Therapeutic recreation as an intervention for persons with dementia and agitation: An efficacy study. *American Journal of Alzheimer's Disease and Other Dementias, 11,* 412.

Edstrom, K.M., & Devine, C.M. (2001). Consistency in women's orientations to food and nutrition in midlife and older age: A 10-year qualitative follow-up. *Journal of Nutrition Education, 33*(4), 215–223.

Engleman K., Mathews R., & Altus D. (2002). Restoring dressing independence in persons with Alzheimer's disease: A pilot study. *American Journal of Alzheimer's Disease and other Dementias*, 17(1), 37–43.

Fitzsimmons, S. & Buettner, L. (2003a) A therapeutic cooking program for older adults with dementia: Effects on agitation and apathy. *American Journal of Recreation Therapy*, Fall, 23–33.

Fitzsimmons, S., & Buettner, L. (2003b). Therapeutic recreation interventions for need-driven dementia-compromised behaviors in community-dwelling elders. *American Journal of Recreation Therapy*, Winter, 17–32.

Gustafsson, K., Andersson, I., Andersson, J., Fjellstrom, C., & Sidenvall, B. (2003). Older women's perception of independence versus dependence in food-related work. *Public Health Nursing, 20*(3), 237–247.

Gustafsson, K., & Sidenvall, B. (2002). Food-related health perceptions and food habits among older women. *Journal of Advanced Nursing, 39*(2), 164–173.

Healthy People 2010. (2007). *Healthy people.* Department of Health and Human Services. Retrieved March 17, 2007, from http://www.healthypeople.gov

Institute of Medicine (2008). Retooling for an aging America: Building the health care workforce. Washington, DC: National Academy of Sciences Committee on Future Health Care.

Jongbloed, L., Stacey, S., & Brighton, C. (1989). Stroke rehabilitation: Sensorimotor integrative therapy treatment versus functional treatment. *American Journal of Occupational Therapy, 43*(6), 391–397.

Kretshmar, J.H. (1979). Intervention possibilities in the geronto-psychiatric department of a psychiatric hospital. *Z Gerontology, 12*(2), 141–148.

Logan, P.A., Gladman, J.R., Drummond, A.E., and Radford, K.A. (2003). A study of interventions and related outcomes in a randomized control trial of occupational therapy and leisure therapy for community stoke patients. *Clinical Rehabilitation, 17*(3), 249–255.

Maslow, A. (1943). A theory of human motivation. *Psychological Review, 50,* 370–396. Retrieved June 2001, from http://psychclassics.yorku.ca/Maslow/motivation.htm.

Merkle, R.B. (1994). Dementia activities should encourage self-expression. *Brown University Long-Term Care Letter, 6*(21), 8.

Neistadt, M.E. (1994a). A meal preparation treatment protocol for adults with brain injury. *American Journal of Occupational Therapy, 48*(5), 431–438.

Neistadt, M.E. (1994b). The effects of different treatment activities on functional fine motor coordination in adults with brain injuries. *American Journal of Occupational Therapy, 48*(10), 877–882.

Pavarotti, L., & Wright, W. (1981). *My Own Story,* New York, NY: Doubleday, p. 21.

Chapter 32

Gardening: A Natural Way for Elders to Exercise and Stay Engaged and Healthy

Martha Neff-Smith

> *A society grows great when old men plant trees whose shade they know they shall never sit in.*
> —Greek proverb

Introduction

Today there are unprecedented numbers of retirees and prospective retirees among the baby boomers. In America, the number of persons aged 65 years and older will double in the next 25 years to 72 million people (NIH News, 2006). The growth has caused a flurry in advertising retirement homes, travel, and insurance packages. People and organizations have become aware that retirement has more to offer than time. When as much as a third of our lives remains after retirement, there is the potential for new growth and to complete earlier plans that were put aside for work. There is now a need to "take charge of" this stage of our lives. Finishing a university degree, learning new skills, and reading all of the classics are now possible. The sentient "Third Ager" will, however, also consider this life stage a time to focus on health and fitness. While 80% of older adults have at least one chronic disease (King, Rejeski, & Buchner, 1998), there is evidence that exercise can prevent pain and disability and improve quality of life (Centers for Disease Control & Prevention, 2010).

Gardening offers a fantastic way to spend our older, healthy years without spending our life savings. Time can now be found for gardening projects that we postponed for years. The obvious benefit of gardening is the exercise it provides. The boredom associated with exercise can be beaten by the simple tasks of gardening, therefore making it more likable by the older adults.

Gardening is especially beneficial for people recovering from illness. Gardening uses creative abilities, strengthens muscles, promotes flexibility, improves range of motion, develops eye-hand coordination, improves motor skills, and increases self-esteem. With recent improvements in raised garden beds and unique tools, gardening is a hobby that can be enjoyed by almost everyone.

Regular exercise designed to raise the heart rate and build endurance and muscle mass is recommended for older adults. This regimen strengthens balance and flexibility and promotes maximum functioning. The exercise program recommended by most agencies is 150 minutes of moderate aerobic exercise each week and 2 or more days a week that work all major muscle groups (Agency for Healthcare Research & Quality [AHRQ] & CDC, 2002). Some geriatricians prescribe regular exercise (World Health Organization [WHO], 2002). The prescription should be simple, measurable, appropriate to the circumstances of the patient, and in a form that can be measured. Depending upon the client and the desired outcome, there should be variety in the prescription. As with many other regimens, there should be an emphasis on strengthening core muscle groups and reducing injury risk. A prescription should include the following components: Frequency, Intensity, Type, Time, and Progression (FITT-PRO) of exercise. The intensity and duration of exercise should depend upon an assessment of each person's health.

In our society where aging is generally associated with reduced physical activity, exercise is a powerful preventive prescription for many of the undesirable effects of aging. It benefits the elderly just as much as it benefits the young, and while our bodies document a lifetime of work, struggle, and ailments, there are benefits beyond our expectations. Seniors can get particular advantages from activities that are enjoyable and that use all of the motor skills. A single hour among the vegetables includes walking, bending, stretching, pushing, digging, and lifting. Endurance is easily improved since time goes by so quickly and pleasurably.

Regular physical activity provides substantial health benefits, reducing the risk of many chronic diseases (Centers for Disease Control & Prevention, 2010). Medical costs, especially for women, are reduced with regular exercise (AHRQ & CDC, 2002). Only 31% of persons 65 to 74 years of age report regularly engaging in moderate physical activity for 20 minutes or more 3 days a week; this rate drops to 20% by 75 years of age. Women are more likely than men to report engaging in no physical activity (AHRQ & CDC, 2002). Some loss of physical strength is seen as a normal part of the aging process. However, muscles respond to use, and those who have exercised throughout their lives suffer less decline when exercise is maintained. Seniors who have been more deskbound are more likely to have less muscle strength. Planning is important to successful gardening as we age, as with other areas of our post-retirement lives. There are many strategies we can adopt to deal with the effects of this loss of strength when gardening. Training and initial slow progress and the guidance of a professional may be useful to novices. As with any athletic pursuit, warming up and stretching are recommended.

Most of us will retire in possession of good health and a fair degree of strength. We can expect to live longer at retirement than any previous generation (AHRQ & CDC, 2002). Although we may have to be willing to make allowances for the osteoarthritis aches, we understand that gardening offers a pleasurable means of preserving and even enhancing our health and making a significant contribution to our quality of life. Everything that improves health requires personal participation and, as a means of exercise, gardening is no exception. If we hire help, we will not get the benefits of exercise by association.

The Consequences of a Sedentary Life

Unfortunately, life has become increasingly sedentary in the United States. The benefits of mechanization have brought many hours of leisure time. Many have used this time wisely, but others have become less active and suffer the consequences of inactivity. The World Health Organization states that 60% to 85% of citizens of the most industrialized nations live a sedentary life (WHO, 2002; Cherkas et al., 2008). Even in rural areas of developing countries, sedentary pastimes are becoming more and more popular. Inevitably, levels of diabetes, obesity, and cardiovascular disease have increased. In the entire world, with the exception of sub-Saharan Africa, chronic diseases are now the leading cause of death in the world. Data gathered on health surveys from around the world are remarkably consistent (WHO, 2002). Sedentary lifestyles increase mortality and double the risk of cardiovascular disease, diabetes, and obesity. The lack of exercise also increases the risk of hypertension, osteoporosis, colon cancer, depression, and anxiety.

Telomeres are repeat sequences of DNA that sit on the ends of chromosomes, protecting them from damage. Investigators (Mazzeo et al., 1998; Kraemer et al., 2002) found that telomeres shortened more quickly in inactive people. Examining white blood cells from the immune system, the researchers found that telomeres lost 21 component parts (nucleotides) every year. Conversely, the most active people had telomeres similar in length to those of inactive people who were up to 10 years younger. It is thought that inactivity may actually speed this process. Stress is also thought to have an impact on telomere length, and the researchers suggest people who exercise regularly may help to reduce their stress levels.

A common misleading metaphor is the comparison of the body to machinery, such as an automobile. This implies that the body wears out with use. In some instances, the human body actually becomes healthier with use. Only a small percentage of the population exercises to the point of overexertion or injury today. In today's world, many people just sit around. They spend endless hours watching TV, and they hold jobs that require them to sit behind a desk for 8 or 9 or 10 hours a day engaging in virtually no physical movement at all. As a result, they are being diagnosed with chronic diseases such as cancer, heart disease, diabetes, and respiratory ailments—all related to a lack of regular physical exercise .

In a study reported in the *American Journal of Epidemiology* (Leveille, Guralnik, Ferrucci, & Langlois, 1999) there was nearly a twofold increase in the likelihood of dying *without disability* among the most physically active group of persons 65 and older when compared with sedentary adults (adjusted odds ratio = 1.86, 95% confidence interval 1.24–2.79). The authors found encouraging evidence that disability prior to death is not an inevitable part of a long life, but that it may be prevented by moderate physical activity. Thus this study found physical activity to be a key factor in predicting nondisability before death.

Chronic Disease and Physical Activity

Looking at why physical exercise makes individuals so much healthier gives us an interesting perspective on how the human body really works. The human body is designed to move. And by moving the muscles, ligaments and limbs, you actually massage the underlying tissues and organs of the body, bringing them oxygen and enhancing their flexibility, and moving lymph fluid around the body. Outdoor physical exercise also exposes the body to the healing effects of natural sunlight, an essential nutrient for the human body that is deficient in most people. Getting enough sunlight on your skin can prevent and even reverse an astounding number of chronic diseases such as breast cancer, prostate cancer, osteoporosis, and more (Division of Nutrition, Physical Activity and Obesity and National Center for Chronic Disease Prevention and Health Promotion, 2008). Although there are recognized risks of skin cancer with sunlight exposure, an effective sunscreen applied judiciously will still permit vitamin D absorption. After age 70, vitamin D supplements are recommended.

If you put all of this together, you see that physical exercise is extremely beneficial to the human body, and that in fact the body won't live nearly as long without it. Studies also show that it doesn't take an enormous amount of physical exercise to achieve health-enhancing results (Cherkas et al., 2008; Werner et al., 2008; Brown, Burton, & Rowan, 2007; Bosomworth, 2009; Sattelmair, Pertman, & Forman, 2009). Only 30 minutes a day of walking, swimming, jogging, cycling, or other cardiovascular exercise can have astounding positive health effects.

Diabetes and Bone Issues

New research shows that moderate exercise can reduce the risk of death for people with Type 2 diabetes. A study followed over 3300 people and correlated their level of physical exercise with mortality, to find that moderate exercise reduced the chance of cardiovascular death by 9%, and more vigorous exercise reduced the total chance of death by 33% (Werner et al., 2008). Diabetics have long been advised to pursue physical exercise, especially cardiovascular exercise, in order to improve their overall health and reduce their chance of death. This study adds support to the notion that physical exercise is the number one way to enhance your health and avoid the downward health spiral associated with diabetes.

Osteoarthritis is common among persons over 55. Painful knees or hips can deter any activity. Many people experience morning stiffness and are perfectly able to exercise after an hour or so of stretching and slow activity. Exercise represents an excellent avenue for those with osteoarthritis to experience some relief of their symptoms, and it also offers an opportunity to improve their overall health. Those who suffer from arthritis often limit their activity and joint motion due to the pain they experience with movement of joints affected by osteoarthritis. Bosomworth (2009) states that inactivity may lead to muscle atrophy, loss of the ability to sense the position of joints, and reduced muscle strength and endurance. These factors may contribute to joint deterioration and diminished activity.

Osteoporosis is a common and frequently debilitating disease that affects mainly the elderly in our society. The discomfort of osteoporosis may be a deterrent to physical exercise of any kind. Bone loss that is the trademark of osteoporosis can lead to a loss in height and to curvature of the spine. Lower back pain, caused by ultrafine microfractures of the backbone, are responsible for much of the disfiguration associated with the disease. Bones thinned by osteoporosis are easily broken, and some may experience a fracture without any apparent trauma. Falls, common to the elderly, can do much more damage. Bone mass is at its highest level around age 30. As we age, both men and women lose bone mass. Nutrition, exercise, smoking, and alcohol consumption all affect the health of our bones. Weight-bearing exercises such as walking, stair climbing, dancing, and weight lifting help develop our bones to their maximum potential. Maximizing and maintaining our skeletal well-being during all phases of adult life through an adequate diet and regular weight-bearing exercise will help offset the effects of later bone loss. The walking and moving, carrying and carting that are a normal part of a gardening activity can play a significant role in guarding us against the deleterious effects of osteoporosis.

Gardening as Physical Exercise

The AHRQ and CDC (2002) recommend 2½ hours of moderate activity per week, along with strength training activities 2 or more days per week, or alternate equivalents for older adults. Gardening offers a variety of tasks, and activities change depending on climate and seasons. Tending to a garden can offer exercises such as digging holes, pulling weeds, carrying soil, and pushing a lawnmower, in addition to walking. Carrying a one-gallon sprinkling can of water in each hand is equal to eight-pound dumbbells. Lifting and pushing a wheelbarrow is a good bicep workout.

Developing endurance and cardiovascular health is very important to a longer life. Heart disease remains the major cause of death worldwide for persons over 65. The heart and circulation undergo changes as we age. Various constituent materials of the tissues are altered in a way that makes it more difficult to retain previous levels of strength and stamina. With training, however, our cardiovascular system responds and our heart and general circulation improve readily as we (carefully) increase our level of aerobic activities. Exercises for beginning gardening may be squats, bends, and arm rotations and lifting one-pound weights. Individuals who have been active joggers, swimmers, or bikers will have a higher beginning level of cardiovascular fitness and endurance. When diagnosed with cardiac disease, daily activities and gentle exercise may be safe, depending upon the advice of a physician. One of the safest choices for persons trying to recover strength can be gardening, which can be made rigorous or easy. With the help of professionals, a carefully designed regimen may be therapeutic.

Changes in the chemical components of the joints are an inevitable part of aging and may alter normal cushioning functions, causing pain and discomfort at the joint. Joint disease, particularly osteoarthritis, is extremely common in older people. It is estimated that 80% of people over 65 will have this form of arthritis. In addition, a significant number of older people have other forms of arthritis, resulting in a loss of flexibility, agility, and endurance. Flexibility requires continued use of muscles and joints. There are many examples of elderly musicians, such as Arthur Rubenstein, who continued to use their bodies well into old age. Andre Segovia was giving concerts on classical guitar at 92! Arthur Fiedler was conductor of the Boston Pops Orchestra for 50 years! The virtuoso cellist and composer Pablo Casals practiced 3 hours a day at the age of 93. Artist Georgia O'Keeffe continued to paint until only weeks before her death at age 98.

The effects of any training are highly specific, and a variety of activities is required in our daily routine to keep all muscles and joints healthy. Gardening, with its combination of gross movement (walking, bending, reaching up and out) and fine control (planting out, taking cuttings, sowing seeds) is an excellent means of achieving the desired variety in movement modes, thus maximizing our chances of retaining flexibility. However, those suffering from joint disease must take care not to aggravate the condition by overdoing, and a bit of a juggling act is necessary to balance the benefits of exercise against the dangers of excess.

Falls and Vision Changes and Outdoor Exercise

Among the most common reasons that older people fall are changes in vision and changes in blood pressure. Most home falls occur in transit areas such as garages, paths, and patios, and attention to safety in these areas is vital where older people are concerned.

Changes in the eye lens structure, loss of peripheral vision, and generally poorer eyesight may have an adverse effect on safety in the work of older persons who work outside. Vision changes occur in most older people. Presbyopia, or aging eyesight, may require the use of reading glasses for examining the contents of garden chemicals. While many will retain good long distance vision, some changes in our eyesight will affect us in an outdoor environment. Aging eyes may be slower when adjusting to different light levels, causing adaptation problems with sudden changes in lighting. Moving quickly into bright sunlight or deep shade can temporarily blind us. Some older people may have some center field vision loss, resulting in being able to only see in the periphery of their vision. The image formed will be blurred and lack strong color. This problem results, as with early cataract development, in increased light sensitivity. Reflective materials, such as stone walking paths, may reflect light and cause falls related to misinterpretation of depth or changes in level. Safety may be compromised unless there are adaptive measures or careful attention.

Another cause of falls associated with aging is the slower rate at which our blood pressure adjusts to a change in posture. Standing up too quickly can temporarily reduce the blood pressure in the brain, causing us to become dizzy or faint, and this potential problem needs to be taken into account when gardening.

Problems with balance are also a common cause of falls. As mentioned earlier, balance can be improved or maintained through exercise. Specific exercises can be prescribed to improve balance. There are many adaptations available to help prevent falls. Some of these are raised garden beds, the use of special lighting and materials, borders, and guides.

Temperature and UV Light

With aging, temperature regulation mechanisms change, and the body is slower to adjust to extremes of temperature and make the necessary physiological modification. This thermal deficit leaves us far more dependent on behavioral means of adjusting our body temperature, means such as putting on a sweater or moving inside. There should be family awareness of the potential for both hypo- and hyperthermia in aged persons, and time outdoors should be limited during poor weather.

Social and Mental Health

Outdoor exercise has many social, psychological, and emotional benefits (Infantino, 2004; Perrigrew & Roberts, 2008). Being outside makes us happy. Gardening can take your mind away from your worries, give you more interaction with your neighbors, and help you gain confidence. It also makes you look better. Meeting your exercise goals through pleasurable activity affirms your intelligence and tenacity.

It is no surprise that gardening is a wonderful activity for social health. Being in a garden is like walking a cute dog; everyone stops to comment, and conversations leading to friendships may begin. The elderly are often isolated because of geographic family separation, widowhood, or economics. When neighbors stop to talk, they ask about health and become involved in the welfare of the older gardener. They may benefit from horticultural advice, fresh vegetables, or shared flowers.

There are organized gardening classes and groups, the most notable of which are the Master Gardeners, trained and supported by land grant colleges and universities. Classes are generally small and last 6 weeks. It is possible to meet many other people who share interests in sailing, biking, or history in these groups. There are also groups that travel for the purpose of viewing beautiful gardens around the world. Gardening classes may be the source of a traveling companion.

Patients report that a walk or an exercise session helps in reducing their feelings of anxiety. Exercise can create a brief distraction, permitting a respite from anxiety-provoking thoughts. According to recent studies (Cherkas et al., 2008; Werner et al., 2008), regular exercise provides these same benefits and also lowers adrenalin levels, often decreasing the intensity of symptoms during future anxiety attacks.

Aerobic exercise has shown best results in reducing anxiety symptoms. Aerobic exercise improves sleep, improves the ability to cope with stress, and increases self-esteem. Exercise produces the best results in persons who are not physically fit and who experience initial high levels of anxiety. A perfect motivation to exercise when depressed is the immediate relief that results from only 10 or 15 minutes of exercise. Exercise can improve your mood for up to 12 hours. Doing something positive to manage anxiety or depression is a healthy coping strategy while drinking alcohol, dwelling on how badly you feel, or hoping anxiety or depression will go away on their own can lead to a worsening emotional state.

Growing and Creating

Caring for the world is the way we bring forth its fullest flowering potential. Some philosophers believe that gardening is a means to continue creative work and preserve life-sustaining order. Our traditions are to toil and keep the land as a means of service. The opposite of this tradition is narcissism and self-service.

Erikson (1950) used the word "generativity" to describe the stage in our psychosocial development when we feel a need to guide younger people, realizing that our legacy is this generation. Generativity is the seventh of the life stages in his theory. The opposite of generativity is self-absorption. This philosopher said that adults need to create or nurture things that will outlast them. Creative success generates feelings of usefulness and accomplishment, while failure results in shallow involvement in the world. When we garden, we are serving the earth, the next generation, and ourselves. In the last developmental stage, Erickson said that older adults need to examine their lives and feel a sense of fulfillment. A successful final stage of life offers feelings of wisdom, while failure brings regret and despair. Persons who are 65 and older ask the question "Have I lived a full life?" If we view our lives as unproductive, we become dissatisfied with life and may experience despair, which may lead to depression and hopelessness. If a review of one's life leads to the belief that one has led a happy and productive life, there will be contentment. Continuing to make contributions until the end of life supports the positive resolution of this developmental stage.

Stewardship is our spiritual heritage. Stewardship means thinking ahead seven generations. In caring for the earth, we must be more mindful of our great-great-great-grandchildren than we are of ourselves and our own wants and desires. What we do today impacts generations far into the future. The earth is a garden meant to bring delight and sustenance to all creatures past and present, and those yet to be born. Meaning is found in our relationships with the land that gave life, the creatures who inhabit the land with us, and the relatives who preceded us, who live with us, and who will follow us. Life is full of meaning when we look beyond ourselves to care and nurture others and the earth.

References

Agency for Healthcare Research and Quality, and Centers for Disease Control and Prevention. (2002). *Physical activity and older Americans: Benefits and strategies.* Retrieved from: http://www.ahrq.gov/ppip/activity.htm

Bosomworth, N.J. (2009). Exercise and knee osteoarthritis: Benefit or hazard? *Canadian Family Physician, 55*(9), 871–878.

Brown, W.J., Burton, N.W., & Rowan, P.J. (2007). Updating the evidence on physical activity and health in women. *American Journal of Preventive Medicine, 33*(5), 404–411.

Cherkas, L.F., Hunkin, J.L., Kato, B.S., Richards, J.B., Gardner, J.P., Surdulescu, G.L., et al. (2008). The association between physical activity in leisure time and leukocyte telomere length. *Archives of Internal Medicine, 168*(2), 154–158.

Centers for Disease Control and Prevention. (2010). Physical activity and health: The benefits of physical activity. Retrieved from: http://www.cdc.gov/physicalactivity/everyone/health/index.html

Division of Nutrition, Physical Activity and Obesity, and National Center for Chronic Disease Prevention and Health Promotion. (2008). *Growing Stronger—Strength Training for Older Adults.* Retrieved from http://www.cdc.gov/physicalactivity/growingstronger/why/

Erikson, E.H. (1950). *Childhood and society.* New York: Norton.

Infantino, M. (2004). Gardening: A strategy for health promotion in older women. *Journal of the New York State Nurses Association, 35*(2), 10–17.

King, A.C., Rejeski, W.J., & Buchner, D.M. (1998). Physical activity interventions targeting older adults. *American Journal of Preventive Medicine, 15*(4), 316–333.

Kraemer, W.J., Adams, K., Cafarelli, E., Dudley, G.A., Dooly, C., Feigenbaum, M.S., et al. (2002). American College of Sports Medicine position stand. Progression models in resistance training for healthy adults. *Medicine & Science in Sports & Exercise, 34,* 364–380.

Leveille, S., Guralnik, J., Ferrucci, L., & Langlois, J. (1999). Aging successfully until death in old age: Opportunities for increasing active life expectancy. *American Journal of Epidemiology, 149,* 654–664.

Mazzeo, R.S., Cavanagh, P., Evans, W.J., Fiatarone, M., Hagberg, J., McAuley, E., et al. (1998). American College of Sports Medicine position stand. Exercise and physical activity for older adults. *Medicine & Science in Sports & Exercise, 30,* 992–1008.

NIH News. (2006). Dramatic changes in U.S. Aging highlighted in new census, NIH report: Impact of baby boomers anticipated. Washington, D.C.: National Institute of Health. Retrieved from: http://www.nia.nih.gov/NewsAndEvents/PressReleases/PR2006030965PlusReport.htm

Perrigrew, S., & Roberts, M. (2008). Addressing loneliness in later life. *Aging and Mental Health, 12*(3), 302–309.

Sattelmair, J.R., Pertman, J.H., & Forman, D.E. (2009). Effects of physical activity on cardiovascular and noncardiovascular outcomes in older adults. *Clinics in Geriatric Medicine, 25*(4), 677–702.

Werner, C., Hanhoun, M., Widman, T., Kazakov, A., Semenov, A., Poss, J., et al. (2008). Effects of physical exercise on myocardial telomere-regulating proteins, survival pathways, and apoptosis. *Journal of the American College of Cardiology, 52,* 470–482.

World Health Organization. (2002). *Physical inactivity: A leading cause of disease and disability.* Retrieved from http://www.who.int/mediacentre/news/releases/release23/en/index.htm

Chapter 33

Seniors and Companion Animals

Mary Muscari and Kimberly Campbell

R are is the human who can resist the saucer-eyed look of a puppy or the playful antics of a kitten. In 2007, American households had 81 million cats, 72 million dogs, 11 million birds, and other animals as pets, and half of the pet owners surveyed considered their pets to be family members (American Veterinary Medical Association, 2007). Companion animals (pets) are an important part of human lives. They give unconditional love, act as surrogate children, provide exercise, and relieve loneliness.

When asked to identify the periods of their lives during which their pets were most important, respondents in one survey stated: when they were sad, lonely or depressed; when there was a temporary absence of a spouse; during childhood or adolescence; when there was a death or illness of a significant other; during a crisis, separation, or divorce, and during a childless marriage (Cain, 1985). Therefore it comes as no surprise that companion animals can enrich the lives of seniors. Pets can improve seniors' life patterns, emotional and physical responses, socialization, and general well-being. However, without proper support, companion animals can also cause negative effects for seniors, including falls, infections, and depression from pet loss. Pets can also become objects of abuse or neglect. Nurses and other healthcare professionals are in a key position to assure that companion animals remain positive influences by having a better understanding of human–animal interactions, and by working with animal care professionals, including veterinarians, veterinary technicians, shelter and rescue personnel, and animal control.

The Human–Animal Bond

According to the Center for the Human–Animal Bond at the Purdue University School of Veterinary Medicine (2000), the human–animal bond is defined as the dynamic relationship between people and animals whereby each influences the psychologic and physiologic state of the other. Human–animal interactions can have profound physiologic consequences, including a decrease in blood pressure, reduced anxiety, and a general feeling of well-being. Animals can be therapeutic to socially isolated persons in nursing homes, hospitals, hospices, and even prisons. By watching animal behavior, children can learn to be more nurturing, and perhaps will be better parents to their own children.

Theories on the human–animal bond have focused on pets as nonjudgmental members of social networks, as child substitutes, or as objects that help people define themselves (Horowitz, 2008). According to attachment theory, pets elicit an innate nurturing response, possibly accounting for those pet owners who view their pets as children. Self-object theory stresses the role of pets in defining a person's identity. Studies on human and dog interactions indicate that this interspecies partnership involves an increase in the neurophysiologic correlates of oxytocin (a hormone involved in affection, maternal behavior, and empathy); beta-endorphin; prolactin; betaphenylethylamine; and dopamine in both species, with a concomitant decrease in levels of cortisol in humans after positive interactions with animals (Fine & Belier, 2008; Horowitz, 2008; Odendaal & Meinties, 2003).

Morley and Fook (2005) noted that the human–animal bond is not only essential to those who are disabled, ill, or isolated, but also to any member of a community. Whether it is a cat, dog, or rabbit, the love, loyalty, and support that a companion animal provides is deemed to be immeasurable (Clements, Benasutti, & Carmone, 2003), and can go beyond other relationships in a person's life. Many clients find it easier to confide in an animal companion than in a human being because they are nonjudgmental and are always willing to lend a listening ear to their owners.

Pets help communities to feel safe, and may teach family members how to give and receive compassion. Studies show that owning a pet can lower blood pressure and levels of stress (Clements, Benasutti, & Carmone, 2003; Morley & Fook, 2005) and may provide emotional support to a person experiencing an illness (Toray, 2004). It has been shown that people who own pets tend to be more physically active and happy, and to display higher mental functioning and healthy emotional benefits (Clements, Benasutti, & Carmone, 2003; Morley & Fook, 2005). The presence of a pet may help to reduce feelings of loneliness or depression and increase self-esteem, and it may also be a source of laughter. Companion animals help people to feel that they are needed, act as surrogate children, and connect people to friends or relatives who have died (Toray, 2004).

Pets and Seniors

The Humane Society of the United States (HSUS) notes that companion animals can bring new meaning and purpose to the lives of seniors who are living a distance away from family and friends. Companion animals are associated with a sense of well-being, a sense of encouragement, and even a reason for living, because they enable seniors to be responsible for another life. Providing a loving home to a companion animal also helps seniors to remain active and stay healthy (HSUS, 2009).

The role of companion animals in the lives of seniors is well documented, particularly the role and effect of therapy animals (animal-assisted activity [AAA] and animal-assisted therapy [AAT]). Beck and Katcher (2003) described the immediate visual and emotional responsiveness of "deprived older people" to animals as one reason for the increase in AAT in facilities for seniors. Animals provide needed tactile contact and a sense of identity for seniors who have suffered losses of family, friends, career affiliations, and functioning. Animals facilitated social interaction and reduced agitation and aggression in patients with dementia, and watching fish in an aquarium stimulated residents to eat more and gain weight (Filan & Llewellyn-Jones, 2006). In a study of Medicare enrollees ($N = 938$), those with pets reported having fewer doctor visits over the course of a year than respondents who did not own pets. The researchers believed that pet owners were buffered from the impact of stressful life events associated with greater use of health services (Siegel, 1990). Elder participants in another study ($N = 58$) at a long-term care facility reduced their analgesic medication usage and pulse rate and reported improved overall quality of life as the result of contact with a therapy dog (Lust, Ryan-Haddad, Coover, & Snell, 2007).

It has also been shown that seniors who have Alzheimer's disease (AD) can benefit from companion animals, particularly dogs, provided that they live with a caretaker who can also care for the pet. The companion animal is constantly there for the senior, always willing to give and take affection. The pet does not care if the senior has deteriorated due to illness or if they repeat the same story time and again, and the senior-pet relationship can develop instantaneously. The pet may stimulate long-term memory, allowing for the recall of happy memories, enabling the senior to participate in conversations. Companion animals promote social interaction, allowing seniors to preserve their dignity and self-esteem, and they may provide the stimulation for vocalization for seniors who have not spoken in a long time. Pets also provide sensory stimulation through touch. Seniors can feel their heartbeat and cold nose, as well as the texture of their fur and the pads of their feet. Seniors can have intense physical contact with pets—hugging, kissing, and holding—that they may not have with humans. Companion animals allow persons with AD to have an increased sense of responsibility, promote relaxation, provide entertainment and humor, and create a nonthreatening environment. They can even provide diversion and relaxation for the caregiver, decreasing caregiver stress (Manor, 1991).

However, not all study findings have been positive. An Australian survey of 2551 individuals aged 60 to 64 years compared the sociodemographic attributes, mental and physical health measures, and personality traits of pet owners and non-owners (Parslow, Jorm, Christensen, Rodgers, & Jacomb, 2005). The researchers found that caring for a pet was sometimes associated with negative health outcomes, including more symptoms of depression, poorer physical health, and higher rates of use of pain relief medication. When they examined the personality traits of pet owners and carers, the researchers found that men who cared for pets had higher extraversion scores. A principal but unexpected finding, however, was that pet owners and caregivers reported higher levels of psychoticism (increased vulnerability to psychoses) as measured by the Revised Eysenck Personality Questionnaire. In another Australian study, researchers examined 32 community-dwelling older adults 60 years of age and older to determine attachment to pets in an older cohort. Results indicated limited support for a relationship between pet attachment and quality of life in the study group (Watt & Pachana, 2007).

Assisting Older Adults to Care for Their Companion Animals

Companion animals require food, shelter, veterinary care, and considerable love and attention. The complete care of pets is beyond the scope of this chapter, especially considering the different needs of different species and breeds. Interested caregivers can refer to the resources in Box 33-1 to learn more about pet care, and they can consult with their clients' veterinarians to be sure that their clients' pets are receiving quality care, which is important to the health of the owner as well as the pet.

Nurses and other health professionals can also assess whether the senior has the needed support to care for a pet by asking a few pet-oriented questions during the health interview:

- What type(s) of pet(s) live with you?
- Who is your veterinarian, and when was your pet's last wellness visit?
- Is your pet up-to-date on his/her immunizations (vaccines, "shots")?
- Where does your pet eat, sleep, and go to the bathroom?
- How often do you walk your pet?
- Do you need any assistance with pet care: financial, bathing, feeding, toileting, or exercising?
- Does your family help you with your pet?
- Who cares for your pet when you are ill?
- What plans have you made for pet care should your pet outlive you?

Healthcare professionals need not know how to intervene with pet issues; however, they should be able to assist the client in obtaining help from their family or veterinarian, from social services, or the local humane society.

Box 33-1: Pet Care Resources

American Association of Retired Persons Pet Page: www.aarp.org/family/love/pets

American Humane Association Adoption & Pet Care: www.americanhumane .org/protecting-animals/adoption-pet-care

American Society for the Prevention of Cruelty to Animals Pet Care: www.aspca.org/ pet-care

American Veterinary Medical Association Care for Pets: www.avma.org/care4pets

Humane Society of the United States Pets for Life: www.hsus.org/pets

---

Animal to Human Infections: Zoonoses

The migration of pets from the backyard to the bedroom can increase the risk for zoonoses, diseases that are transmitted from animals to humans. The modes of inter-species transmission include direct contact (ringworm from *Microsporum canis)*, scratches (cat scratch disease caused by *Bartonella hensela*), bites (rabies), inhalation of or contact with animal urine or feces (toxoplasmosis, giardia, leptospirosis), and vectors (Lyme disease). Children under five, elders, pregnant women, and immunosuppressed clients are most at risk for infection (Horowitz, 2008). Veterinarian Marty Becker, author of "The Healing Power of Pets," provides several preventive measures that can be added to client teaching to minimize the senior's risk of contracting infections from their pets (Becker, 2007):

- Choose pets from a reliable source, such as the local animal shelter. Seniors should refrain from choosing rodents or reptiles as pets, especially if they are immunosuppressed.

- Have the pet examined by a veterinarian at least once a year. The veterinarian can check stool samples for giardia, and make sure that the pet is up-to-date on vaccinations, especially rabies and leptospirosis.

- Keep the pet free of pests. Use veterinarian-recommended medications to protect against ticks, which can spread Lyme disease and Rocky Mountain spotted fever; fleas, which, in rare cases, transmit the plague bacterium; and mosquitoes, which can transmit such parasites as hookworms.

- Keep pets away from outdoor water sources and toilets. Always have fresh water available for them to drink.

- Practice good hand hygiene. Wash hands after discarding their waste, playing with them, or being scratched.

- Take special precautions. Cat feces sometimes contain a parasite, toxoplasma gondii, which can damage the brain and lungs of elders with weakened immune systems. Have someone else empty the kitty litter for them.

Supporting Seniors After the Loss of Their Pet

When an animal dies, seniors may be negatively affected. Pet death is given relatively little social recognition (Clements, Benasutti, & Carmone, 2003). As a result, society may view the loss of an animal companion as less important or less painful than when a person dies. When a senior loses a pet he or she may grieve similarly (or even more intensely) than when a family member or friend dies and may follow Kubler-Ross's stages of grief: denial, anger, guilt, bargaining, depression, and acceptance of the loss (Dunn, Mehler & Green-berg, 2005). Seniors who lose their pets may experience difficulties, such as sleep alter-ations, loss of appetite, persistent crying, sadness, and depression. They may also

---

Box 33-2: Techniques to Help Cope with Pet Loss

Have the pet cremated and keep the ashes in the pet's favorite room
Write a story, letter or poem about loss and how they feel
Write about the special moments they shared with the animal
Hold a memorial service for the pet
Open a scholarship fund in their pet's name
Plant a tree in the name of the pet
Create a scrapbook with memories that they have of the pet

---

experience cognitive changes such as hearing, smelling, and seeing their pet. Each person may go through the stages differently; for example, seniors who had their dog euthanized may experience anger or guilt over their decision. Their feelings of guilt may take longer for people to work through because elderly owners may feel that there was something that they could have done differently that would have kept their animal alive (Clements, Benasutti, & Carmone, 2003). Seniors who make the decision to euthanize a pet may experience a prolonged period of guilt because there are questions as to whether or not they made the right decision, or if the pet may have suffered more because of the decision that they made (Clements, Benasutti, & Carmone, 2003; Dunn, Mehler, & Greenberg, 2005).

Losing a pet can be a difficult time in a senior's life, but as a result of the lack of importance society places on pet loss, seniors may fear rejection or embarrassment when trying to talk about the overwhelming emotions that they have following the loss of their companion (Clements, Benasutti, & Carmone, 2003). Since clients may be reluctant to express their emotions, nurses and other caregivers may not know when they are experiencing grief and pain. Therefore, it is the caregiver's responsibility to perform a psychosocial assessment and inquire about possible pet loss. The caregiver should empathize with the clients and encourage them to talk about their loss and how they may be feeling as a result of the loss. Caregivers can also assist seniors in dealing with pet loss by using the techniques presented in Box 33-2. It may also be helpful to encourage seniors to express their feelings and to help them realize that what they are feeling is a normal part of the bereavement process.

Prevention of Animal Cruelty

Companion animals are most often treated like members of the family, but they may also become victims of abuse in violent households; animal cruelty may also be a sign of elder abuse. Animal abuse or cruelty is socially unacceptable behavior that intentionally causes unnecessary distress, suffering or pain, and/or death of an animal. Cruelty includes physical and sexual abuse, neglect, hoarding, and dog and cock fighting.

Hoarding, which is similar to neglect, occurs when a person accumulates a large number of animals, but provides minimal standards of nutrition, sanitation, and veterinary care, and fails to act on the deteriorating condition of the animals and/or the environment. Unlike most other perpetrators of animal cruelty, the majority of hoarders are female. Hoarded animals often suffer extreme neglect, including lack of food, proper veterinary care, and sanitary conditions. Hoarding also creates hazards for the human occupants of the home. Unsanitary conditions attract disease vectors such as insects and rodents, which can also threaten neighboring households. Homes involved in hoarding usually must be condemned by the health department due to unlivable conditions. Compulsive hoarding may or may not be part of another psychiatric disorder. It is most often associated with obsessive-compulsive disorder (OCD), an anxiety disorder characterized by intrusive thoughts and compulsive behaviors. Hoarding has also been considered a symptom of an impulse-control disorder (ICD), such as compulsive shopping or gambling, and it may be symptomatic of a neurodegenerative disease. Given that hoarding can appear in the absence of any other pathology, and that it can result in severe impairment, some believe that hoarding should be considered a syndrome or entity in its own right (Bohrer & Haynes, n.d.).

Although statistics are lacking, humane officers have sometimes found cases of elder abuse while responding to reports of animal cruelty—a dead dog in a dumpster led to their finding a neglected 90-year-old woman; whimpering from a closet proved to be a battered elder instead of suspected animal neglect. For complex reasons, abusive family members may also abuse the elder's pets. Perpetrators may abuse or neglect the elder's pet as a form of retaliation or control, a way to obtain the elder's financial assets, or as an act of frustration over their caretaking responsibilities. Extreme neglect can also indicate the elder's inability to provide self-care or care for the animal, signaling the need for assistance (Muscari, 2004; Muscari, 2005). Healthcare professionals who have the opportunity to observe their client's pets (e.g., home health nurses and social workers) should observe for signs of battered pet syndrome (Munro, 1999):

- Unusually subdued or fearful
- Openly frightened
- Fractures
- Bruising
- Eye injuries
- Burns and scalds
- Munchausen syndrome by proxy

Healthcare professionals who suspect animal neglect due to the senior's inability to care for the pet should talk to the elder and assess whether the elder is actually capable of caring for the pet. If not, the nurse can ask if there is a family member who can assist. If this is not possible, the care professional can enlist the assistance of the humane society

---

Box 33-3: Animal Assisted Activity/Therapy Organizations

Delta Society: www.deltasociety.org
Therapy Dogs International: www.tdi-dog.org
State by State Animal Therapy Organizations: www.activitytherapy.com/us.htm

---

or the senior's veterinarian. Suspicion of animal cruelty warrants reporting the situation to animal control; in addition, a thorough assessment should be conducted to ascertain if the senior may also be at risk for abuse. A report of suspected elder abuse should be prepared and submitted according to the agency protocol if there is any indication that the senior is also being abused.

Pet Therapy

Pet Therapy can provide contact with companion animals for those seniors who are not able to have their own pets. Pet Therapy encompasses two modalities: animal-assisted activity (AAA), casual visitation of pets, and animal-assisted therapy (AAT), a goal-oriented therapy process. These two types of activities are closely related. A study of eight Japanese elder females demonstrated six themes related to AAA: positive feelings about dogs; confidence in oneself; recalling fond memories about dogs; a break from the daily routine; interacting with other residents through dogs; and enhanced communication with volunteers (Kawamura, Niiyama, & Niiyama, 2009).

Even the frailest of seniors can benefit from AAA, since they would not be alone with an animal, and since the animals would be trained and accompanied by persons educated in pet therapy. Nurses can contact national pet therapy organizations to find a local group who will come to their agency (listed in Box 33-3), or they can encourage their organization to adopt a "pets in residence" program, whereby dogs, cats, birds, and/or other animals live in their institution's common areas for an overall human–animal bonding experience.

References

American Veterinary Medical Association. (2007). *US pet ownership—2007*. Retrieved from www.avma.org/reference/marketstats/ownership.asp

Beck, A., & and Katcher, A. (2003) *Future Directions in Human–Animal Bond Research American Behavioral Scientist, 47*(1), 79–93.

Becker, M. (2007). *Playing it safe*. The Pet Connection: VeterinaryPartner.com. Retrieved from http://www.veterinarypartner.com/Content.plx?P=A&A=2513&S=1&SourceID=28

Bohrer, G., & Haynes, L. (n.d.). *Compulsive hoarding: Sign of a deeper disorder*. Retrieved from www.nurse.com/ce/CE372-60/CoursePage.

Cain, A. (1985). Pets as family members. In M. Sussman (Ed.) *Pets and the Family*. New York: Haworth Press, 3–10.

Center for the Human–Animal Bond at the Purdue University School of Veterinary Medicine. (2000). http://www.vet.purdue.edu/chab

Clements, P., Benasutti, K., & Carmone, A. (2003). Support for bereaved owners of pets. *Perspectives in Psychiatric Care, 39*(2), 49–54.

Dunn, K., Mehler, S., & Greenberg, H. (2005). Social work with a pet loss support group in a university veterinary hospital. *Social Work in Health Care, 41*(2), 59–70.

Filan, S., & Llewellyn-Jones, R. (2006). Animal-assisted therapy for dementia: A review of the literature. *International Psychogeriatrics, 18*, 597–611.

Fine, A., & Beiler, P. (2008). Therapists and animals: Demystifying animal-assisted therapy. In A.L. Strozier & J. Carpenter, (Eds.), *Introduction to alternative and complementary therapies* (pp. 223–228). New York: Haworth Press.

Horowitz, S. (2008). The human–animal bond: Health implications across the lifespan. *Alternative and Complimentary Therapies, 14*(5), 251–256.

Humane Society of the United States (HSUS). (2009). *Older Americans and mature pets*. Retrieved from http://www.hsus.org/pets/pet_care/senior_partners_older_americans_and_mature_pets.html

Kawamura, N., Niiyama, M., & Niiyama, H. (2009). Animal-assisted activity: Experiences of institutionalized Japanese older adults. *Journal of Psychosocial Nursing, 47*(1), 41–49.

Lust, E., Ryan-Haddad, A., Coover, K., & Snell, J. (2007). Measuring clinical outcomes of animal-assisted therapy: Impact on resident medication usage. *Consultant Pharmacist, 22*, 580–585.

Manor, W. (1991). Alzheimer's patients and their caregivers: The role of the human–animal bond. *Holistic Nursing Practice, 5*(2), 32–37.

Morley, C., & J. Fook. (2005). The Importance of pet loss and some implications for services. *Mortality, 10*(2), 127–143.

Munro H. (1999). The battered pet. In F. Ascione & P. Arkow (Eds.), *Child abuse, domestic violence, and animal abuse*. West Lafayette, IN: Purdue University Press, 199–208.

Muscari, M. (2004, Jan./Feb.). Four-legged forensics: What forensic nurses need to know and do about animal cruelty. *Forensic Nurse*, 10–12, 23–24.

Muscari, M. (2005). Animal cruelty as a predictor of human violence. *Advance for Nurse Practitioners, 13*(4), 55–59.

Odendaal, J., & Meinties, R. (2003). Neurophysiological correlates of affiliative behavior between humans and dogs. *Veterinary Journal, 165*, 296–301.

Parslow, R., Jorm, A., Christensen, H., Rodgers, B., & Jacomb, P. (2005). Pet ownership and health in older adults: Findings from a survey of 2551 community-based Australians aged 60–64. *Gerontology, 51*, 40–47.

Siegel, J.M. (1990). Stressful life events and use of physician services among the elderly: The moderating role of pet ownership. *Journal of Personality and Social Psychology, 58*, 1081–1086.

Toray, Tamina. (2004). The human–animal bond and loss: Providing support for grieving clients. *Journal of Mental Health Counseling, 26*(3), 244–259.

Watt, D., & Pachana, N. (2007). The role of pet ownership and attachment in older adults. *Australian Journal of Rehabilitation Counseling, 13*(1), 32–43.

Chapter 34

Place, Reminiscence, and Interdisciplinary Gerontological Practice

Mary Ellen Quinn, Stacey Kolomer, and Jeffrey Burden

In the classic movie, *A Trip to Bountiful*, actress Geraldine Page plays Carrie Watts, an 81-year-old woman looking to make peace with her past. Striking out on her own in 1947 Texas, Carrie boards a bus headed toward her hometown of Bountiful. She forges a strong bond with a fellow passenger, Thelma, played by a young Rebecca DeMornay. Thelma helps "Mrs. Watts" along the way—listening to her stories of Bountiful while taking care of the older woman until the bus abandons them 12 miles short of Bountiful. Moved by Carrie's fierce determination "just to stand on the porch of her house again," the local sheriff takes Carrie on to Bountiful, even though he knows it is now a ghost town of empty houses and abandoned buildings. In the final scene of the movie, Page's Carrie Watts finally wanders alone through her childhood home, touching the architecture as if it were another character in the film, seeing Bountiful just as it was when she left it. For the first time in years Carrie Watts is truly happy, at peace with herself.[1]

Reminiscence and life review have long been recognized as phenomena of aging that can be healing (Butler, 1963), as well as providing the foundation for many reminiscence-based therapies. What *A Trip to Bountiful* so beautifully illustrates is how place, in this case the town of Bountiful, can be a vital catalyst for reminiscence and, intriguingly, assume the role of caregiver or nurse in that process.

The significance of place has its roots in the work of philosophers such as Heidegger and Bachelard (Heidegger, 1951/1993; Bachelard, 1958/1964). Fascinated by the places in which we dwell and "the meanings that they gather for us," place—as opposed to space—was

---

[1]Now referred to as an American treasure, the movie version of *A Trip to Bountiful* was produced in 1985. Directed by Peter Masterson, the film brought Academy Awards for actress Geraldine Page and screenwriter Horton Foote. In addition to the original television performance and this Academy Award-winning film adaptation, both written by Horton Foote, *Bountiful* has been performed on stage every year in America since 1947. In each adaptation, the fundamental relationship between Mrs. Watts, Thelma, and the town of Bountiful endures.

distinguished for these mid-twentieth-century thinkers by all of its human associations and inherent memories. Bachelard went so far as to propose a new way of dealing with the mind, *topoanalysis*, or the systematic psychological study of the sites of our intimate lives (Bachelard, 1958/1964, p. 8).

Contemporary theory in disciplines ranging from architecture to the broader humanities have built on the writing of these two thinkers to address an increasingly rootless modern society and its built environment (Jackson, 1994; Rappaport, 1994; Casey, 1996; Menin, 2003). For historians, reminiscence of place has become a tool in what is known as "oral history," or reconstructing the recent or living past through subject interviews (Perks & Thomson, 2006). As the practice of oral history spread, a distinctive phenomenon emerged: Vivid is the recall of research subjects, particularly older adults, when discussing home, particularly childhood homes and land or townscapes from their working past (Andrews, Kearns, Kontos, & Wilson, 2006).

This vivid recall of place, particularly in the older adult, initially presented a challenge for researchers who questioned the accuracy of oral history, emphasizing the mind's inclination to seek, not so much reality, but comfort in familiar places and what Brand (1997) described as the "lived aspects of the built environment" (p. 52). Oral history evolved from being just a tool for doing history to being a subject of study in and of itself, particularly in terms of place (Riley & Harvey, 2007). Geographers now refer to "emotional geography" when exploring the intersections between place, memory, and well-being, as well as a variety of other emotions (Smith, Davidson, Cameron, & Biondi, 2009). While the science of nostalgia continues to evolve, the recollection of place is now widely recognized as a powerful dynamic in the older mind.

Place-Based Reminiscence (PBR) in Gerontology

Working with reminiscence and specifically what he refers to as "Place-Based Reminiscence" (PBR), Chaudhury (1999) has opened new doors for research into the care of older adults and their care providers by looking at how place can be used to activate and steer the reminiscence process to positive outcomes. In reference to older adults, Chaudhury (2002b) characterizes PBR as a method to bring out the self "by tapping into recollections, of places lived and visited from the past sketched with rich colors and fine-grained texture along with idiosyncratic preferences and emotions" (p. 87).

Dementia and the long-term care facility have been the areas of his most concentrated study (Chaudhury, 2002a, 2002b, 2003a, 2003b, 2008). Because short-term memory is more impaired than long-term memory in older adults with dementia, Chaudhury (1999) makes a strong case for the use of reminiscence-based therapies in this population. He uses PBR to better connect with the personhood of the patient. Unlocking the mystery behind the behavior of an older adult with dementia is one method of preventing catastrophic behavior and its untoward consequences—a significant risk fact in older adults with dementia.

Chaudhury (2002a) developed a Place-Biosketch where places from the past became touchstones for reconstructing the older adult's history. Family members of nursing home residents with dementia made notes based on the questions about places in the residents' childhood and adulthood. The family members were then interviewed. Based on these interviews with the family members and pictures, the Place-Biosketch was developed as an instrument. Surveys of the nurse managers, nursing assistants, social workers, and activity directors indicated that the Bio-Sketch was a therapeutic activity tool, a conversation prompter, an empathy enhancer for staff, and a way of understanding residents' behaviors. As Chaudhury suggests, the Place-Biosketch should be incorporated into the nursing home setting, through care planning and practice. Although the respondents were family members of residents with dementia, the resident becomes a de facto participant in the Place-Biosketch process through the shared memories and understanding of the individual. Place is the lens for reconstructing the life of the patient. In many respects it is a bridge between the resident, family, and nurses and other staff.

In other studies, Chaudhury goes one step further, connecting directly with the older adult. Chaudhury (2002b) examined the ability of nursing home residents with dementia to remember places, as well as the dimensions and triggers of these memories. Building on Casey's (1989) concept of "reminiscentia" or prompts for reminiscence (Sherman, 1991, p. 127), Chaudhury found that personal photographs that included the residents' past home were more effective than generic photographs of the time period. Childhood homes were remembered at a greater frequency, as compared to adult homes. Chaudhury also found a theme of holding onto feelings that were emotionally charged with personal loss and yearning for homes from the past. While in one way this may seem difficult, many residents felt good discussing their past. Comments about the pride that a resident had in her past home and how much she enjoyed her activities in that home were noted.

In another study, Chaudhury (2003a) worked with cognitively intact and cognitively impaired nursing home residents and found both groups of residents were able to derive benefit from PBR. Themes of temporality were obtained and Chaudhury found that home was the physical context that threads together the many events that occur over the life span. The following data from a cognitively intact nursing home resident captures the rich meaning that home provides in the process of what Chaudhury terms self-evolution through self-reflection:

> Oh, mealtime was the only way you could see everybody. . . . Everybody was home from school or whatever activity they attended. You didn't have fast food and stop-off joints. Oh yes, I can see this—my mother is saying—come in, come in girls, Betty, Lucille, come in and set the table. It's time to do that. We come in and get the dishes out and set the places for everybody. Is so and so gonna be here tonight? (p. 93)

The participant goes on to describe how everyone had their own place at the long mahogany table with round corners and how plates were shifted if an unexpected visitor such as the preacher arrived. Based on the enthusiastic and poignant detail in this participant's narrative, Chaudhury found that he could almost "see" this home. The therapeutic power of place and home appears to be relevant for both cognitively impaired and cognitively intact older adults.

Many of Chaudhury's studies demonstrate that of all places in the life of an older adult, home or home place is the most resonant when it comes to reminiscence. While reminiscence is a recognized therapeutic process in the nursing care of older adults (Bramlett & Gueldner, 1993; Burnside, 1990; Haight & Webster, 1995; Puentes, 2002) and other disciplines, home is a trigger to this therapeutic process in Chaudhury's work. PBR may be particularly helpful due to the concrete nature of the reminiscence of home and place or what Chaudhury (1999) describes as a mnemonic anchor. For older adults with cognitive impairment and dementia, home is a simple construct to grasp and may ease the reminiscence process. In addition to promoting selfhood, PBR may be especially useful in addressing the safety and comfort needs in older adults with dementia and in all older adults.

At first glance, home may seem to be basic or mundane, but like water and food, its sheltering qualities are essential to existence. Clearly there are many variables to consider. We know that home is increasingly important to individuals as they age (Oswald & Wahl, 2005). Echoing the work with place in other disciplines, it is what Gouthro (2000) referred to as

> an evocative concept, the "homeplace" renders different images and memories for each person that are contextually dependent upon each individual's lived experience. The concept of the homeplace may be perceived more than an individual residence—it may be inclusive of extended family, community, and culture. (p. 66)

In Chaudhury's work, home takes on a richer meaning in old age. Together memory and home weave together the "disparate into a subjective unity" for the older adult (Chaudhury, 2003a, p. 93). In gerontological health care, particularly in nursing, home takes on significant meaning as often the role of the gerontological nurse is to help the older adult to age in place (Quinn et al., 2004). Aging in one's own home and living independently is the preference for the majority of older adults. Using the idea of home as a focal point for nursing interventions is ideal.

From a historical perspective, the reliability and validity of place memories in older adults may be a challenge. However, outside of obtaining information such as a health history in the context of gerontological nursing care, the accuracy of the older adult's memories may not have much relevancy. The patient is not remembering important health information, so much as connecting with self. It is the subjectivity of the process that is relevant. Home "embodies in its symbolic strength all that is meaningful" and remembering past places or remembering through place magnifies the "temporal transfusion or synthesis of self" (Chaudhury, 2003a, p. 93).

Chaudhury (1999) has brought place into the realm of gerontological research, demonstrating its effectiveness as what he calls a triggering mechanism for reminiscence— "anchoring, organizing and facilitating memories" (Chaudhury, 2002b, p.87). While it may not be a magic bullet in treating dementia, he has documented its effectiveness as an intervention in at least this aspect of gerontological care and as he points out, opens doors for further research in gerontology using place (Chaudhury, 2002b). As with any form of intervention, there are a variety of questions that will need to be addressed, which brings us to a closer examination of just how a PBR intervention might work. In addition to causal connections indicating that an intervention works, a causal explanation of how and why a PBR intervention is effective should also be explored (Burns & Grove, 2001, p. 334).

Nursing and PBR

First and foremost in constructing an operational model of PBR, we need to look at the nurse. The roles of the nurse in gerontological care are perhaps the most varied in all of nursing practice and the most integrated with other healthcare providers. Some nurses are solely gerontological in their practice, such as geriatric nurse practitioners and nurses in assisted living facilities, adult day health centers, and nursing homes. These nursing roles may be comprised of more direct care to the older adult or more of a supervisory/educational role supporting certified nursing assistants and other direct care workers.

Outside of these gerontological care settings, the recipients of nursing care are often older adults: In the hospital, other than obstetric and pediatric units (Mezey, 2007); in community nursing; and in home health nursing. The field of psychiatric mental health nursing is also increasingly addressing an aging demographic in areas such as depression. Nurses often play a pivotal role in chronic disease self-management programs (Lorig et al., 1999) and transitional care from acute care to home (Naylor et al., 2004). Even in programs that target children, such as the Healthy Grandparents Program(http://www.mcg .edu/son/grandparents.htm), nurses also provide care to older adults.

Agency of PBR

In many respects, it is the nurse who has the opportunity to open the critical pathway for reminiscence-based therapies in gerontological care. Often nursing care is the most intimate, including not only physical and mental health care, but also personal care and emotional care for both the patient and the patient's family. Puentes (1998) suggests that reminiscence-based therapies be part of acute care nursing practice. The provision of personal care, such as a bed bath, can be an opportunity for PBR by nursing staff. Nursing care in the home, such as home health or care management, provides another opportunity for PBR. The unseen and unsung tasks that nurses do in all realms of patient care, particularly in gerontology, are precisely the avenues where PBR may become most effective. Thus, nursing care provides a unique and powerful venue for reminiscence-based therapies and the integration of place. Nurses should be familiar with PBR not only because place is the most bountiful form of reminiscence with older adults, but because nurses are uniquely positioned due to the tasks they do to tap into that bounty.

Nursing care of older adults requires an interdisciplinary approach. Due to the increased heterogeneity of this age group (Maddox, 1987; Neugarten, 1968), the care of older adults is more complex. Additionally, the Joint Commission on Accreditation of Healthcare Organizations requires evidence of interdisciplinary collaboration in hospitals, nursing homes, and outpatient settings (Wexler & Siegler, 2007). It has been suggested that social work and nursing have many similarities (Gilgun, 2005). Often social workers and nurses work together in the gerontological system of health care. In many healthcare environments the nurse is the frontline provider who will open the door to reminiscence-based therapies. However, in evolving models of health care, nurses and social workers may share similar roles (Kolomer, Quinn, & Steele, in press). In addition to services such as care/case management and care planning, nursing and social work both provide reminiscence-based therapies. While other disciplines do reminiscence-based therapies, nursing and social work may be the ideal therapeutic agents for PBR.

Some reminiscence-based therapies may be done in isolation, but the therapeutic listener is important to consider (Haber, 2006; Haight, Coleman, & Lord, 1995) and should be part of PBR. Being able to listen without judgment and with a caring demeanor is vital to therapeutic listening. Much like the Thelma in *Bountiful*, the nurses, social workers, or others may serve in this capacity. Nurses and other clinicians refer to this as the "therapeutic use of self" and are trained in therapeutic listening techniques.

Context

The culture of the healthcare environment is another consideration that is always important in all of health care, but particularly in the case of PBR. It is not just the identity of the therapeutic listener, so much as the therapeutic listener is working in a culture of therapeutic listening. A culture of place provides the context for nursing, social work, and other disciplines to provide age-appropriate care to older adults. Nurses, social workers, and other healthcare providers can work together to create an environment that embodies place. Creating a culture of therapeutic listening is needed at the micro level for individual clinicians in facilities, as well as at the macro level for the healthcare system.

A model for interventions using PBR is illustrated in Figure 34-1. Together, the older adult and the nurse, social worker, and other care providers harness the power of place and home memories as a triggering mechanism to impact successful aging outcomes. In our model, place and home memories form a mediator variable; it is not only the triggering and steering mechanism for the reminiscence process as Chaudhury (2008) suggests, but the ideal tool for all of these healthcare providers to use in working together. A culture of therapeutic listening is an important contextual or environmental variable in our model. A PBR intervention has many potential positive outcomes, and in order to encompass them all, we use the term *successful aging outcomes*. Even in dementia and other chronic diseases without a cure, older adults can be viewed as successful agers by using

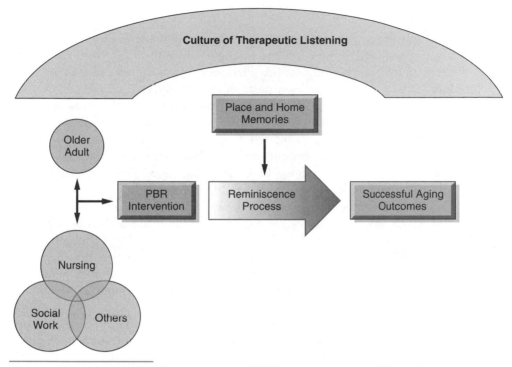

Figure 34-1   A place-based reminiscence (PBR) intervention model.

all of their capabilities to live to their greatest potential. Place and home memories, properly cued, are a key to that world.

Applications for the Place-Based Reminiscence Intervention Model

While a focus on function rather than cure for older adults is not new to nursing, this needed focus is often overshadowed by fast-paced, high-technology components of the healthcare system (Quinn et al., 2004). In contrast to the "medical model" focus on treatment and cure, Quinn and colleagues suggested that function and maintenance be a significant focus of gerontological health care. PBR requires a personalized approach and as such provides a foundation for the quest for patient-centered care and the appropriate healthcare needs of older adults. Developing an "inner ear" (Clark, 1997) is vital to gerontological nursing care (Quinn et al., 2004) and to PBR. Let's examine how nurses can harness PBR in gerontological care.

Nursing Home

One potential application is expanding PBR in the nursing home environment. In addition to providing staff with a better understanding of the resident, applications directed at the resident might be expanded for other therapeutic uses. Reminiscence-based therapies for older adults with dementia show great promise (Woods, Spector, Jones, Orrell, & Davies, 2005). There is a growing literature on reminiscence-based therapies leading to improved cognition in older adults with dementia (Nawate, Kaneko, Hanaoka, & Okamura, 2008; Tanaka et al., 2007; Wang, 2007). In addition to cognitive improvement, Tanaka and colleagues also found an improvement in blood flow as indicated with single photon emission computed tomography. PBR may enhance reminiscence when it is used as a cognitive rehabilitation strategy for older adults with dementia.

Agitation and catastrophic behavior can be a challenge for the older adult with dementia, as well as nurses, other care providers, and family. Redirecting is one nonpharmacological method to prevent agitation and catastrophic behavior (Zec & Burkett, 2008). Home may play an important role in redirection. For example, when a resident with dementia cries "Mama, Mama" for a mother who died decades ago, the nurse might redirect the resident by talking about happy memories of mother and home (L. Wright, personal communication, February 21, 1996)

Promoting independence in the care recipient is a basic premise of nursing, as proposed in Orem's theory of self-care (Foster & Bennett, 1995, p. 100), and this includes individuals with dementia. Using PBR in this regard may yield positive outcomes in the nursing home environment. Although nursing home programs that promote a more homelike environment, such as the Eden Alternative (1999) have emerged, there is much work yet to be done. Allowing a nursing home resident's room to be "translated" based on a resident's PBR may improve the quality of life and other health outcomes of residents. While the potential exists to implement a PBR program in this way, many nursing homes do not operate on nursing models, but on models replete with rules that often preclude personalized care such as PBR. Programs are needed to improve the quality of life of the residents, and the use of PBR may have many uses in the nursing home setting.

Community Nursing

PBR may also be a vital tool for gerontological nurses practicing in the community. Alzheimer's disease and dementia and the associated cognitive decline are an increasing challenge for older adults, their families, and our healthcare system. Considerable work has been done in the area of the prevention of dementia (Centers for Disease Control and Prevention & The Alzheimer's Association, 2007). The focus of this body of literature is on the modification of risk factors and cognitive stimulation. PBR may be a form of cognitive stimulation that promotes brain health and the prevention of dementia.

Reminiscence-based therapies have been used as interventions to help older adults cope with the many transitions that come with age (Magee, 1988), many of which relate to home and place. Relocation from a home of many years to either a child's home, a senior community, or a long-term care facility can be challenging for both the older adult and the family. PBR may be useful in this transition by helping the older adult to remember the original home and subsequently trying to find positive similarities in the new home, thus making for a smoother transition. Or perhaps remembering negative characteristics of the original home may be useful. For example, a memory of what one older adult called the "singing toilet" may bring a smile, but also the insight that absence of the irritating drips in the plumbing may make the new home seem not so bad.

Promoting self-care and chronic disease self-management is another area where PBR may be very therapeutic in community nursing. While PBR serves as an organizing process in the promotion of selfhood (Chaudhury, 1999), this organizational quality may translate to problem solving that is required of older adults as they manage their lives, including chronic disease self-management. Emotional management, or the management of stress and depression, is an essential component of chronic disease self-management (Lorig, 1999), and reminiscence-based therapy increases chronic disease self-management skills (Kralik, Koch, Price, & Howard, 2004). As many older adults have a chronic disease, PBR may be an even stronger intervention to promote self-care and chronic disease management, and subsequently may reduce health care expenditures.

Working with Caregivers

In addition to being helpful for nursing staff in nursing homes (Chaudhury, 2002a), PBR may be instrumental in other caregiving relationships. Family caregiving is growing at a staggering rate (National Alliance for Caregiving [NAC], 2004). For spousal or adult children caregivers, evoking the memory of life shared together through PBR may be very supportive and may help both the caregiver and the care recipient with the transition to their new roles or a rejoined family. Early in the caregiving trajectory, PBR may serve to strengthen the bonds between the family caregiver and the care recipient. If the care recipient is cognitively impaired, PBR may be a means of helping the caregiver to reconnect with their loved one. As the caregiver role continues, caregivers are at higher risk for adverse health outcomes and significant health crises due to the strain and stress of providing care and their neglect of their own healthcare needs (NAC, 2006; Toseland, Blanchard, & McCallion, 1995). The age of caregivers is increasing (NAC, 2009) thus an aging spouse may often be the family member who assumes the caregiver role, along with any associated stress. Reminiscence is thought to be an important part of the stress and coping process (Puentes, 2002), and with the meaningful relevance of place and home to aging individuals, PBR may be effective in preventing the deterioration of the caregiving relationship, as well as promoting the health of the caregiver.

Acute Care Nursing

Nursing care in the acute care environment is another venue for reminiscence-based therapies (Puentes, 1998), including PBR. Older adults undergoing surgical procedures who received the Life Challenges Interview and the Life Experience Interview had significant improvements in coping and anxiety (Rybarczyk, 1995). However, there was no significant difference in secondary benefits of the intervention, such as nurse-rated adjustment during the procedure, pain perception during the procedure, post-procedure medication use for pain, length of stay after the procedure, and maintenance of psychological adjustment 30 days after the procedure. PBR might be another approach that is more tailored for the hospitalized older adult. By mentally or emotionally transporting the patient from hospital to home, PBR may tap into what Wong (1995) describes as escapist reminiscence. This type of reminiscence is defined as seeking comfort from people and events that are part of one's "memory landscape," and it is considered a defense mechanism that can be used as a "source of happiness and a buffer against present stress" (Wong, 1995, p. 27). An even greater focus on home through PBR may be particularly effective. On the other hand, Cappeliez, O'Rourke, and Chaudhury (2005) found that the use of reminiscence to reduce boredom was associated with lowered life satisfaction. This study was based on surveys of older adults' reasons for reminiscing, which can include conversation and intimacy maintenance, but apparently without a therapeutic listener. The inclusion of a therapeutic listener may mitigate the potential negative outcomes and actually promote adaptation and coping. This highlights the essential role of the therapeutic listener. By eliciting memories of home and place, PBR may promote a feeling of safety and comfort, as well as promoting other health outcomes in hospitalized older adults or those undergoing medical procedures.

PBR has primarily been used to help older adults with dementia (Chaudhury, 2008). However, many applications are possible for older adults in general. The unseen and unsung things that nurses do in all realms of patient care, particularly in gerontology, are precisely the avenues where PBR can become most effective.

Implications for Practice, Education, Policy, and Research

The future of PBR has great potential, thus research, translation, and dissemination is needed. Much work is required in order to harness the power of place and home in gerontological nursing and health care in general. Next, we will outline suggestions for practice, education, policy, and research.

Practice

The first step is starting PBR. Visiting the older adult's homestead is one prop for stimulating the reminiscence process. If it is not possible to visit the old homestead, Magee (1988) suggests the following:

> Older adults can facilitate their recall by drawing the ground plan of their home with as much detail they can. By locating windows accurately, they may recall the views that these windows faced and their own activities that could be seen from that viewpoint. By locating furniture precisely, they may remember whose favorite chair that was, and think back on the quality of their interaction with that person. (pp. 41–42)

Graphics and art play a role in reminiscence-based therapies. Chaudhury (2003b) found that art was an effective strategy in nursing home residents with dementia. Sherman (1991) found that cherished objects, such as old photographs of the home, were helpful in reminiscence-based therapies (p. 128). Personal pictures of one's past places and home are more useful than generic pictures in older adults with dementia and should be considered with all older adults (Chaudhury, 2002b).

The PBR process is important to consider. Specific steps for the role of the therapeutic listener in PBR might include the process described by Chao, Chen, Liu and Clark (2008) as entrée, immersion, withdrawal, and closure. Concluding with some sort of evaluation in the closure is recommended (Chaudhury, 2008, p. 115; Haight, Coleman, & Lord, 1995, p. 181). Integrative reminiscence promotes an acceptance of self and others, conflict resolution, a sense of meaning and self-worth (Wong, 1995) and should be part of this evaluative component. Haight also suggests ending on a positive note. Including adapted items from Haight's (1979) Life Review and Experiencing Form (Haight, Coleman, & Lord, 1995, pp. 189–192), such as "what was the happiest time in your home?" or "what about your home made you proud or feel special?" might be part of PBR.

There are risks with any reminiscence-based therapy, and the nurse and others conducting PBR should be aware of them. As life is not always a happy affair, sometimes sad or difficult memories rise to the surface in reminiscence-based therapies. In most cases, home seems to be a warm and positive memory. Thus using home as a benchmark and foundation for this process may in and of itself extend and overtake difficult memories. But what if PBR does evoke sad or difficult memories? Trying to find one specific memory about the place that prompts a feeling of happiness may be helpful. Once a specific place memory is obtained, one can use it to reshape the difficult memories or focus on the specific place memory. Determining what was positive may help with coping. Recalling a happy place or room within the home is one possible strategy. Perhaps it is the couch where a mother patiently helped her child learn to read or the living room where a father carried his child who awoke in the middle of the night with an earache. The keys to avoiding problems may be embedded in the memories of the older adult.

However, if even happy memories do not prevent a descent into sadness or if there are few or no happy memories, the gerontological nurse must be aware of the risks. Magee (1988) recommends that clinicians be aware of what Butler (1963) identified as individuals who are at risk for depression, such as individuals who "(a) have consciously exercised the human capacity to injure others; (b) are categorically arrogant and prideful; and (c) tended throughout their life to live for the future" (pp. 13–14). If the nurse or other staff member lacks advanced practice preparation, he or she must know when to refer an older adult with these characteristics to clinicians such as an advanced practice psychiatric-mental health nurse, a licensed social worker, a psychiatrist, or another therapist. Other hazards exist, such as obsessive reminiscence, which is described as ruminating about negatives from one's past Wong (1995, p 27). Puentes (2008) points out that obsessive reminiscence should not be ignored and that it provides an associational trends framework within which gerontological nurses and other clinicians can address mental health problems.

Education and Policy

The role of educator is part of gerontological nursing, and it may be particularly relevant in PBR. While the gerontological nurse is often the PBR interventionist, this may not always be the case. Often nursing staff, such as certified nursing assistants or others unfamiliar with PBR, may serve as interventionists. Thus the gerontological nurses should provide reminiscence-based therapy training or continuing education for nursing staff. Issues do arise if any type of reminiscence-based therapy is conducted by lay people, including family members or those without adequate preparation. Haber (2006) suggested that a certified training program be implemented for nonclinicians, to promote safe and effective use of reminiscence-based therapies. Policy might be needed to address this concern.

The Institute of Medicine (2008) reported that in addition to a need for increasing licensed gerontological healthcare professionals, there is a critical need to promote the education and competency of certified nursing assistants and other direct care workers. Policy might address the role of the nurse in educating those for whom they have supervisory responsibility, such as certified nursing assistants and other direct care workers. Place-based strategies might be a critical component in these educational programs. While an interdisciplinary approach is needed, nurses should at least be part of the team leading this initiative in order to ensure that the basic concerns of nursing are included. Place is an ideal tool for teaching nursing staff how to do reminiscence-based therapy in general, in addition to making reminiscence-based therapies work better.

While it is clear that reminiscence is an important nursing intervention (Bramlett & Gueldner, 1993; Burnside, 1990; Haight & Webster, 1995; Puentes, 2001), there are challenges to including it in the education of nurses. Reminiscence-based therapies can be an important way to teach therapeutic communication to nurses and nursing students (Puentes, 2000). Place and PBR may be the ideal way to bring reminiscence-based therapies into the curriculum in nursing schools. In addition to the importance of home in an older adult's life, nursing care of the older adult is increasingly occurring in the community and home. As health care moves from the acute care environment to the community environment, innovative strategies are needed to prepare future clinicians. Maintaining older adults in the least restrictive environment is beneficial for older adults, their families, and society. PBR addresses the needs of the older adult, and if included in curricula, simultaneously addresses the need to produce a gerontologically prepared nursing workforce. However, only 34% of BSN programs even have a gerontological nursing course in their curricula (Mezey, 2007). Furthermore, it remains unclear how reminiscence-based therapies and interventions, such as PBR, are included in the curriculum or in the existing gerontological nursing courses. Sense of place may be just the tool to bring metrics to pedagogy, and PBR may be an ideal tool for teaching future nurses how to conduct reminiscence-based therapies in general. Nursing programs struggle to adapt their curricula to include ever-growing content requirements. However, because of current demographic trends, gerontology should be required in all nursing programs. It is important to stress the importance of aging in the context of human development, and because of their effectiveness, reminiscence-based therapies should be part of nursing education. In programs for licensed nurses that are of short duration or do not include this content, continuing education is necessary.

Nurses who are knowledgeable about geriatrics may advocate more effectively with legislators to support community-based programs so that older adults may be sustained in their own homes. Where PBR is not already in place, nurses and social workers can advocate to make senior centers, assistive living facilities, adult health centers, and nursing homes more "PBR-friendly" environments. Policies aimed at the more general purpose of creating more appropriate environments can also use tools such as PBR.

Interdisciplinary and interprofessional issues are an important part of gerontological health care (Kolomer, Quinn, & Stelle, in press). To address the diverse needs of an aging population, professionals across a broad spectrum need to collaborate with one another and therefore be familiar with other disciplines. Other than Chaudhury's work, very little interface between the environmental and geographical reminiscence literature and the health care reminiscence literature exists. The concepts and applications in this chapter were born from the nontraditional interdisciplinary union of the environmental disciplines with the healthcare disciplines. As there is very little in the literature about interdisciplinary education among allied health professionals, it is not surprising that this union is also not captured in the literature. This phenomenon demonstrates the importance of broad interdisciplinary research, education, and practice.

Research

Based on some of the issues we have brought up here, additional research is needed in the area of PBR. The PBR Intervention Model described in this chapter requires testing, as do any of the suggested applications. Much of Chaudhury's research used qualitative methods. Mixed methods research that includes quantitative research designs is also needed. Open-ended questionnaires are useful tools in reminiscence-based therapies. Chaudhury (2008, pp. 110–111) has developed a set of questions to conduct a PBR with family members of older adults with dementia. His finding of the saliency of the childhood home (Chaudhury, 2002b) as compared to the adult home may also exist in cognitively intact older adults. Adapting Chaudhury's (2008) PBR questions for use in the general older adult population should be examined. This intervention tool may be useful in many other venues of nursing, and it might be adapted for use with cognitively intact older adults to promote their self-identity, mental health, self esteem, and overall social well-being (Birren & Deuthchman, 1991; Bohlmeijer, Smit, & Cuijpers, 2003). Addressing the cultural sensitivity of the PBR tool would also be helpful.

In addition to the applications we have already proposed, other applications of the PBR Intervention Model might be tested. The inclusion of PBR in health assessments in nursing care management and social work case management should be explored. For example, having knowledge of the homeplace might provide valuable information about environmental safety issues. Older adults residing in assistive living facilities might benefit from the PBR intervention as a way to promote a family culture in this shared living environment. Reminiscence-based therapies are helpful in end-of-life care (Jenko, Gonzalez, & Seymour, 2007), and capitalizing on home may be particularly helpful as an image of finally "going home." Journaling has been shown to be an effective mental health intervention (Pennebaker, 1997). Having older adults write about their home and place and subsequently share the writings with the gerontological nurse or other therapeutic listeners may be an effective strategy to promote PBR. Research is needed to examine how Pennebacker's and others' research might be translated to PBR.

While evidenced-based practice is critical, innovative interventions are an important step in gerontological care. The next generation of older adults, the baby boomers, are uniquely different from the older adults who came before them. They are large in number and strong in voice. What has worked in institutional and community-based health care and services before probably will not be effective with the next cohort of older adults. New approaches will need to be tried to better serve this population. Thinking "outside of the box" with new partners will be important for all professions to consider. In addition, as money will have to stretch farther, small studies may have more significance in the future.

Conclusions

When Horton Foote penned *Bountiful* more than 60 years ago, it is safe to say that he was not writing an allegory for one of today's emerging trends in gerontological care. Yet the similarities between his screenplay and our model are striking. In the literary piece Thelma does not go to Bountiful, yet she is critical to Mrs. Watts getting there, as are others. In much the same way, the nurse and other care providers may not physically go to the place or home that a patient remembers. But by working together the nurse and other care providers are critical to the older adult's journey to these place and home memories, as well as the potential of positive outcomes from this journey. It is journeys such as PBR that capture the essence and the potential of nursing, and it is the shared journey that makes gerontological care so rewarding.

What our model stresses is this team approach to gerontological care by nurses, social workers, and other care providers in a context of therapeutic listening and reminiscence structured around place. While human relationships are certainly a focus in reminiscence-based therapies, place and home have an implicit importance and presence in the process that those interested in gerontological care, research, and education need to recognize: place matters, particularly in healthy aging.

As individuals age and move though life transitions, home is where they start and where they are going—even if home is only in their minds. The suggested applications, as well as research and policy recommendations that capitalize on the PBR intervention are a significant vehicle for the promotion of the health and well-being of older adults—with the nurse, the nursing staff, and the rest of the healthcare team working together with the older adult to get there.

References

Andrews, G.J., Kearns, R.A., Kontos, P., & Wilson, V. (2006) 'Their finest hour': Older people, oral histories, and the historical geography of social life. *Social and Cultural Geography, 7*, 153–177.

Bachelard, G. (1964). *The poetics of space* (M. Jolas, Trans.). Boston: Beacon Press. (Original work published 1958.)

Birren, J.E., & Deutchman, D.E. (1991). *Guiding autobiography groups for older adults: Exploring the fabric of life.* Baltimore: Johns Hopkins University Press.

Bohlmeijer, E., Smit, F., & Cuijpers, P. (2003). Effects of reminiscence and life review on later life depression: A meta-analysis. *International Journal of Geriatric Psychiatry, 18*, 1088–1094.

Bramlett, M.H., & Gueldner, S.H. (1993). Reminiscence: A viable option to enhance power in elders. *Clinical Nurse Specialist, 7*, 68–74.

Brand, S. (1997). *The architecture of ecology.* London: Architectural Design Press, p. 52.

Burns, N., & Grove, S.K. (2001). *The practice of nursing research.* Philadelphia: W.B. Saunders Co.

Burnside, I. (1990). Reminiscence: An independent nursing intervention for the elderly. *Issues in Mental Health Nursing, 11*, 33–48.

Butler, R. (1963). The life review: An interpretation of reminiscence in the aged. *Psychiatry, 26*, 3–14, 65–76.

Cappeliez, P., O'Rourke, N., & Chaudhury, H. (2005). Functions of reminiscence and mental health in later life. *Aging & Mental Health, 9*, 295–301.

Casey, E.S. (1989). *Remembering: A phenomenological study.* Bloomington: Indiana University Press.

Casey, E.S. (1996). *The fate of place: A philosophical history.* Berkeley: California University Press.

Centers for Disease Control and Prevention & The Alzheimer's Association. (2007). *The healthy brain initiative: A national public health road map to maintaining cognitive health.* Retrieved from: http://www.cdc.gov/aging/healthybrain/roadmap.htm

Chao, S.Y, Chen, C.R., Liu, H.Y., & Clark, M.J. (2008). Meet the real elders: Reminiscence links past and present. *Journal of Clinical Nursing, 17*, 2647–2653.

Chaudhury, H. (1999). Self and reminiscence of place: A conceptual study. *Journal of Aging and Identity, 4*, 231–253.

Chaudhury, H. (2002a). Place bio-sketch as a tool in caring for residents with dementia. *Alzheimer's Care Quarterly, 3*, 42–45.

Chaudhury, H. (2002b). Journey back home: Recollecting past places by people with dementia. *Journal of Housing for the Elderly, 16*, 85–106.

Chaudhury, H. (2003a). Quality of life and place-therapy. *Journal of Housing for the Elderly, 17*, 85–103.

Chaudhury, H. (2003b). Remembering home through art. *Alzheimer's Care Quarterly, 4*, 119–124.

Chaudhury, H. (2008). *Remembering home: Rediscovering the self in dementia.* Baltimore, MD: The Johns Hopkins University Press, pp. 110–111.

Clark, P.G. (1997). Values in health care professional socialization: Implications for geriatric education in interdisciplinary teamwork. *The Gerontologist, 37*, 441–451.

Eden Alternative. (1999). Retrieved from http://www.edenalt.org/

Foster, P.C., & Bennett, A.M. (1995). Dorothea E. Orem. In J. B. George (Ed.), *Nursing Theories: The Base for Professional Nursing Practice* (pp. 99–123). Norwalk, CT: Appleton & Lange.

Gilgun, J.F. (2005). The four cornerstones of evidence-based practice in social work. *Research in Social Work Practice, 15*, 52–61.

Gouthro, P. (2000). Globalization, civil society, and the homeplace. *Convergence, 33*(1–2), 57–77. (Quote, p. 66).

Haber, D. (2006). Life review: Implementation, theory, research, and therapy. *International Journal of Aging and Human Development, 63*, 153–171.

Haight, B.K. (1979). *The therapeutic role of life review in the elderly.* Unpublished master's thesis, University of Kansas, Kansas City, Kansas.

Haight, B.K., Coleman, P., & Lord, K. (1995). The linchpins of a successful life review: Structure, evaluation, and individuality. In B.K. Haight & J.D.Webster (Eds.), *The art and science of reminiscing: Theory, research, methods, and applications* (pp. 179–192). Washington, DC: Taylor & Francis Publishers.

Haight, B.K., & Webster, J.D. (Eds.). (1995). *The art and science of reminiscing: Theory, research, methods, and applications.* Washington, DC: Taylor & Francis Publishers.

Heidegger, M. (1993). Building dwelling thinking. In D. Farrell Krell (Ed.), *Martin Heidegger: Basic writings* (pp. 347–363). London: Routledge.

Jackson, J. B. (1994). *A sense of place, a sense of time.* New Haven: Yale.

Jenko, M., Gonzalez, L., & Seymour, M.J. (2007). Life review with the terminally ill. *Journal of Hospice and Palliative Care, 9*, 159–167.

Kolomer, S., Quinn, M.E., & Steele, K. (in press). Interdisciplinary health fairs for older adults and the value of interprofessional service-learning. *Journal of Community Practice.*

Kralik, D., Koch, T., Price, K., & Howard, N. (2004). Chronic illness self-management: Taking action to create order. *Journal of Clinical Nursing, 13*, 259–267.

Lorig, K.R., Sobel, D.S., Stewart, A.L., Brown, B.W., Bandura, A., Ritter, P., et al. (1999). Evidence suggesting that a chronic disease self-management program can improve health status while reducing hospitalization: A randomized trial. *Medical Care, 37*(1), 5–14.

Institute of Medicine (2008). *Retooling for an aging America: Building the health care workforce.* Retrieved from http://www.nap.edu/catalog/12089.html

Maddox, G.L. (1987). Aging differently. *The Gerontologist, 27*, 557–564.

Magee, J.J. (1988). *A professional's guide to older adults' life review: Releasing the peace within.* Lexington, MA: Lexington Books.

Menin, S. (Ed.). (2003). *Constructing place: Mind and matter.* London: Routledge.

Mezey, M. (2007, September). *Geriatric resources.* Presented at the Hartford Geriatric Nursing Institute Geriatric Nursing Education Consortium Faculty Development Institute, Atlanta, GA.

National Alliance for Caregiving (NAC). (2004). *Caregiving in the U.S.* Retrieved from http://www.caregiving.org/04finalreport.pdf

National Alliance for Caregiving. (2006). *Evercare Study of Caregivers in Decline.* Retrieved from http://www.caregiving.org/pubs/data.htm

National Alliance For Caregiving (2009). *Executive Summary Caregiving in the U.S.* Retrieved from http://www.caregiving.org/

Nawate, Y., Kaneko, F., Hanaoka, H., & Okamura, H. (2008). Efficacy of group reminiscence therapy for elderly dementia patients residing at home: A preliminary report. *Physical & Occupational Therapy in Geriatrics, 26*, 57–68.

Naylor, M.D., Brooten, D.A., Campbell, R.L., Maislin, G., McCauley, K.M., & Schwartz, J.S. (2004). Transitional care of older adults hospitalized with heart failure: A randomized, controlled trial. *Journal of the American Geriatrics Society, 52*, 675–684.

Neugarten, B.L. (1968). *Middle age and aging.* Chicago: University of Chicago Press.

Oswald, F., & Wahl, H.W. (2005). Dimensions of the meaning of home in later life. In G.D. Rowles & H. Chaudhury (Eds.), *Home and identity in late life* (pp. 221–45). New York: Springer Publishing Co.

Pennebaker, J.W. (1997). Writing about emotional experiences as a therapeutic process. *Psychological Science*, 162–166.

Perks, R., & Thomson, A. (Eds.). (2006). Critical developments. *The oral history reader* (2nd ed., pp. 1–14). London: Routledge.

Puentes, W.J. (1998). Incorporating simple reminiscence techniques into acute care nursing practice. *Journal of Gerontological Nursing, 24*, 14–21.

Puentes, W.J. (2000). Using social reminiscence to teach therapeutic communication skills. *Geriatric Nursing, 21*, 315–318.

Puentes, W.J. (2001). Coping styles, stress levels, and the occurrence of spontaneous simple reminiscence in older adult nursing home residents. *Issues in Mental Health Nursing, 22*, 51–61.

Puentes, W.J. (2002). Simple reminiscence: A stress-adaption model of the phenomenon. *Issues in Mental Health Nursing, 23*, 477–482.

Puentes, W.J. (2008). Using an associational trends framework to understand the meaning of obsessive reminiscence. *Journal of Gerontological Nursing, 34*, 44–49.

Quinn, M.E., Berding, C., Daniels, E., Gerlach, M.J., Harris, K., Nugent, K., et al. (2004). Shifting paradigms: Teaching gerontological nursing from a new perspective. *Journal of Gerontological Nursing, 30*, 21–27.

Rappaport, A. (1994). A critical look at the concept of "place." In R.P.B. Singh (Ed.), *The spirit and power of place. Human environment and sacarality* (pp. 31–45). Varanasi, India: Banaras Hindu University Press.

Riley, M., & Harvey, D. (2007) Talking geography: On oral history and the practice of geography. *Social and Cultural Geography, 8*, 345–351.

Rybarczyk, B. (1995). Using reminiscence interviews for stress management in the medical setting. In B.K. Haight & J.D. Webster (Eds.), *The art and science of reminiscing: Theory, research, methods, and applications* (pp. 205–217). Washington, DC: Taylor & Francis Publishers.

Sherman, E. (1991). *Reminiscence and the self in old age.* NY: Springer Publishing Co.

Smith, M., Davidson, J., Cameron, L., & Biondi, L. (2009) Geography and emotion-emerging constellations. In M. Smith, J. Davdison, L. Cameron, & L. Biondi (Eds.), *Emotion, place and culture* (pp. 1–18). London: Ashgate.

Tanaka, K., Yamada, Y., Kobayashi, Y., Sonohara, K Machida, A., Nakai, R., et al. (2007). Improved cognitive function, mood and brain blood flow in single photon emission computed tomography following individual reminiscence therapy in an elderly patient with Alzheimer's disease. *Geriatrics & Gerontology International, 7*, 305–309.

Toseland, R., Blanchard, C., & McCallion, P. (1995). A problem solving intervention for caregivers of cancer patients. *Social Science Medicine, 40*(4), 517–528.

Wang, J.J. (2007). Group reminiscence therapy for cognitive and affective function of demented elderly in Taiwan. *International Journal of Geriatric Psychiatry, 22*, 1235–1240.

Wexler, S.S., & Siegler, E.L. (2007). Models of care and interdisciplinary care related to complex care of older adults. Module from the Hartford Geriatric Nursing Institute.

Woods, B., Spector, A.E., Jones, C., Orrell, M., & Davies, S.P. (2005). Reminiscence therapy for dementia. *Cochrane Database of Systematic Reviews, 2*. Retrieved February 7, 2010 from http://wf2dnvr1.webfeat.org/3OoZN12160/url=http://search.ebscohost.com/login.aspx?direct=true&db=cin20&AN=2009822712&site=ehost-live .

Wong, P.T.P (1995). The process of adaptive reminiscences. In B.K. Haight & J.D. Webster (Eds.), *The art and science of reminiscing: Theory, research, methods, and applications* (pp. 23–35). Washington, DC: Taylor & Francis Publishers.

Zec, R.F., & Burkett, N.R. (2008). Non-pharmacological and pharmacological treatment of the cognitive and behavioral symptoms of Alzheimer disease. *NeuroRehabilitation, 23*, 425–438.

Chapter 35

Social Dimensions of Late Life Disability

Eva Kahana, Jessica Kelley-Moore, Boaz Kahana,
and Jane A. Brown

We report on the development of the Burden of Disability Scale (BDS) to assess experiences of personal and social burden among elderly persons living with chronic illness and functional disability. Based on a sample of 627 community-dwelling elders, the nine-item, single-factor scale had an inter-item reliability of .89. Through a series of regression analyses, we explored health-related and social correlates of the BDS. Of the three models tested, the final regression model predicted 60% of the variance in burden of disability. While a substantial portion of the explained variance was from functional limitations, prevalent morbidity, and cognitive impairment, manifestations of ill health such as falls and level of pain were also significant. Notably, demographic characteristics did not impact burden of disability. Furthermore, appraisals of general life satisfaction and satisfaction with social life significantly diminished perceived burden of disability. The BDS offers a reliable measure of the social experience of the burden of illness and disability among community-dwelling elders. It conceptually parallels indicators of caregiving burden in the gerontological literature, but emphasizes patients' perspectives. Findings regarding social construction of the burden of disability support our prior results about social influences on a disability identity (Kelley-Moore, Schumacher, Kahana & Kahana, 2006).

Introduction

Chronic illness, physical frailty, and attendant functional disabilities are among the normative stressors of aging (Pearlin & Mullan, 1992; Kahana & Kahana, 2003). Although the cascade of late life disability has been extensively documented (Verbrugge & Jette, 1994), there is far less data available in the literature on the social experience of disablement in late life. Medical sociologists have identified the importance of stigma for those experiencing disabling illness and the threats to identity posed by feelings of social exclusion and marginalization (Charmaz, 2000; Goffman, 1997). While these experiences often unfold in the stories of individuals struggling with illness and disability, quantitative research must also capture this critical dimension of the illness experience.

The Burden of Disability Scale (BDS) we developed and discuss in this paper has addressed this important gap in relation to elderly persons with disabilities. Specifically, we report on the psychometric properties and health and social correlates of the newly developed Burden of Disability Scale. Scholars interested in the subjective experience of illness and disability have increasingly emphasized suffering, stigma, and marginalization (Frank, 1995; Sontag, 1997). In this research we consider the relationship between burden of disability and mental and physical health, manifestations of ill health, personal and social resources, and demographic characteristics among community-living old persons.

Our prior work, based on our ongoing longitudinal study of adaptation to frailty (Kahana & Kahana, 2003), has identified the critical importance of social factors for developing a self-concept of being a disabled person (Kelley-Moore, Schumacher, Kahana, & Kahana, 2006). Specifically, we found that having a dense social network slowed the rate of labeling oneself as disabled. In this paper we expand consideration of self-reported disability to diverse indicators of burden due to health conditions and symptoms of illness. We report on the development of the Burden of Disability Scale (BDS), which allows social scientists to capture the degree to which elderly persons attribute social costs to their illness experiences.

Some older adults cope well with illness-related normative stressors and continue to maintain high levels of social functioning and psychological well-being, even in the face of physical impairment. Others succumb to the stresses of illness and experience a dramatic decline in their quality of life. The Burden of Disability Scale (BDS) was conceptualized in the context of research on the cascade from chronic illness to physical impairment to activity limitations and, ultimately, to diminished quality of life (Verbrugge & Jette, 1994).

Within the gerontological literature there has been extensive focus on social and psychological burdens experienced by caregivers (Weitzner, Haley, & Chen, 2000). It is widely recognized that being responsible for the care of a frail or cognitively impaired relative often results in appraisals of disruption in quality of life. The BDS provides a useful conceptual parallel to prevalent indices of caregiving burden (Zarit, Todd, & Zarit, 1986; Kahana & Young, 1990). It could also help caregiving researchers to recognize and compare the burdens of illness experienced by older caregivers and their care receivers.

Even as researchers and theorists show great interest in the disruption and costs associated with being a carer for the frail elderly, there has been little research attention paid to the costs incurred by the care receiver, the elderly person suffering from illness and frailty. In a recent conceptual paper we explored this imbalance and advocated for greater research attention to the patient's lived experience coupled with the burden of disability close to the end of life (Kahana, Kahana, & Wykle, 2007). In this paper we direct empirical attention to appraisals of elderly persons who live with normative stressors of illness with regard to the social and personal disruptions that those stressors create. It is important to note that patients' appraisal of the impact of their illness on their lives has been referred to in the medical literature as a "blind spot" of quality-of-life assessments (De Geest & Moons, 2000).

A major contribution of the present paper is a description of the psychometric properties of the BDS and consideration of health-related, social and personal resource–related, and demographic antecedents of BDS. Accordingly, we examine to what extent chronic illnesses, physical impairment, and illness-related health events affect the reporting of burden of disability. We also consider demographic predictors and social appraisals such as coping, general life satisfaction, and domain-specific life satisfaction as they influence burden of disability in the aged.

Methods

Sample

The data for this study are taken from a panel study of older adults living in retirement communities in Clearwater, Florida. Baseline interviews were conducted in 1990 on 1000 adults aged 72 or older who lived in Florida at least 6 months out of the year. Respondents were interviewed annually. Those who moved to another location or went into a nursing home or other long-term care facility continued to participate as long as their health would allow. Death was the primary source of attrition for this sample. Loss to follow-up for other reasons (e.g., moving with no forwarding address) accounted for only 7% of annual attrition. The Burden of Disability Scale was first included in the interviews at W4. Thus, the effective *N* for these analyses is 627. Since the dependent and independent variables are drawn from the fourth annual interview, we adjust estimates for potential selection bias due to nonrandom attrition.

Measurement

Table 35-1 presents the variables for each domain with their coding, mean, and standard deviation. The outcome for this study is the Burden of Disability Scale, a nine-item scale capturing perceptions of the social and personal consequences of health problems and disability. The final scale ranges from 0, meaning that the respondent reported no social or personal difficulty due to health problems, to 36, reporting a great deal of difficulty with each item. The inter-item reliability for the scale is .89.

The independent variables fall into four categories: physical and mental health, manifestations of ill health, personal and social resources, and demographic characteristics. Measurement of each domain will be discussed in turn. Physical and mental health indicators include functional limitations, total prevalent morbidity, total incident morbidity, and cognitive impairment. Functional limitations were measured by combining two scales: Activities of Daily Living (ADL; Katz, Ford, Moskowitz, Jackson, & Jaffe, 1963) and Instrumental Activities of Daily Living (IADL; Lawton & Brody 1969). Respondents were asked about their level of difficulty performing five ADL tasks (washing and bathing; dressing and putting on shoes; getting to or using the toilet; getting in/out of bed unassisted; and eating without assistance) and six IADL tasks (getting from room to room,

TABLE 35-1 Variables, Coding, and Descriptive Statistics

Variable	Coding	Mean (Standard Deviation)
Burden of disability	Ranges 0 (none) to 36 (high)	4.42 (5.99)
Functional limitations	Ranges from 0 (no limitations) to 33 (unable to perform any domains)	2.68 (5.03)
Total prevalent morbidity	Range 0 conditions to 10 conditions	1.80 (1.15)
Total incident morbidity over 3 years	Range 0 conditions to 10 conditions	.30 (.59)
Errors on MMSE	Range 0 to 10 errors	.64 (1.41)
Stopped driving in past 2 years	1 = Yes; 0 = Other	.06
Level of pain	1 = Not at all; 5 = A great deal	2.65 (1.19)
Experienced fall in past year	1 = Yes; 0 = Other	.19
Number of medications	Range 0 to 18	2.06 (2.06)
Number of hospitalizations	Range 0 to 4	.20 (.50)
Active coping	Continuous factor	$2.25\ e^{-10}$ (.85)
Life satisfaction	1 = Strongly disagree; 5 = Strongly agree	3.52 (.87)
Satisfaction with social life	1 = Not at all; 5 = A great deal	3.75 (.92)
Female	1 = Female; 0 = Male	.66
Age	Ranges from 71 to 98	79.35 (4.81)
Education	1 = Less than HS; 6 = Graduate degree	2.88 (1.30)
Widowed	1 = Widowed; 0 = Other	.46

Standard deviations not reported for binary variables. Effective N = 627.

going outdoors, walking up or down stairs, doing own housework, preparing meals, and shopping for groceries). Response categories range from never having difficulty (0) to having difficulty all of the time (3). All 11 items were then summed, creating a single measure of limitations ranging from no limitations (0) to limited on all items (33).

Chronic illness is measured by summing the prevalence of 10 health conditions at baseline: arthritis, asthma, emphysema, heart trouble, cancer, stroke, Parkinson's disease, hypertension, diabetes, and kidney disease. These were selected from among health conditions included in the larger OARS Multidimensional Functional Assessment (Fillenbaum & Smyer, 1981). The potential range of the variable is 0 to 10. We also measured the incidence of these same 10 conditions over the previous 3 years. Cognitive impairment was assessed using Pfeiffer's (1975) mental status questionnaire, which consists of a series of 10 questions, such as the current date and the current president of the United States. Incorrect answers were summed, creating a single measure ranging from 0 wrong to 10 wrong answers.

Manifestations of ill health are those outward indicators of poor health that may not be directly associated with a specific health condition or physical limitation but are likely to limit activity or social interactions. There are five such manifestations in this study: stopped driving in past 2 years, level of pain, experienced one or more falls in past year, number of medications, and number of hospitalizations in past year. Those who reported a permanent cessation in driving in the past 2 years are coded as 1 and all others are 0. Level of pain is a five-category scale ranging from not at all (1) to a great deal (5). Those who reported at least one fall in the past year were coded 1 and all others were coded 0. Number of medications and number of hospitalizations in the past year are a self-reported total.

Personal and social resources captures an orientation toward life that may influence how one perceives his/her health problems. In these analyses, we use three: active coping, life satisfaction, and satisfaction with social life. Active coping is a factor of eight strategies used to cope with challenges. Respondents indicated whether (yes or no) they engaged in specific items such as "I asked people with similar problems what they did" and "I get advice on what to do." Reliability for this factor is .67. Life satisfaction is the level of agreement with the statement: "In most ways, my life is close to ideal." Responses ranged from strongly disagree (1) to strongly agree (5). Satisfaction with social life ranges from not at all (1) to a great deal (5).

Finally, we include several demographic variables as controls. Age is measured in years and ranges from 72 to 98. Females are identified in a binary variable where 1 equals the name of the variable and 0 equals all others. Education level is a categorical variable that ranges from less than 12 years (1) to a graduate degree (6). Those whose current marital status is widowed are identified with the value of 1 and all others are coded 0.

Analysis

The purpose of this paper is to demonstrate the psychometric properties of the BDS and estimate a series of regression models to determine what health and social characteristics best predict the burden of disability. We estimate three stepwise regression models. In model 1 we entered the indicators of physical and mental health: functional limitations, prevalent morbidity, incident morbidity, and errors on MMSE. Model 2 adds the manifestations of ill health: stopped driving, level of pain, experienced a fall, number of medications, and number of hospitalizations. Finally, model 3 adds the personal and social resources active coping, life satisfaction, and satisfaction with social life. All models control for demographic differences. Improvement in model fit is estimated with the difference in the F test across models per degrees of freedom. Models were adjusted for potential selection bias due to nonrandom attrition with the Heckman two-stage selection equation.

TABLE 35-2 Burden of Disability Indicators with Mean and Standard Deviation and Factor Loading

Indicator	Mean (Standard Deviation)	Factor Loading
To what extent do . . .		
. . . your health conditions prevent you from doing social activities?	2.08 (1.33)	.81
. . . your health problems interfere with your daily activities?	2.08 (1.30)	.83
. . . you consider yourself disabled?	1.56 (1.04)	.79
. . . have people turned away from you because of your health problems?	1.06 (.36)	.50
. . . people view you negatively because of your health problems?	1.05 (.32)	.47
. . . you view yourself negatively because of your health problems?	1.28 (.74)	.69
. . . your health problems make you feel anxious or depressed?	1.62 (.97)	.77
. . . your health problems rob you of the joy of living?	1.49 (.99)	.82
. . . your health problems make you angry with the world?	1.20 (.63)	.59

Each item is coded: 1 = Not at all; 2 = A little; 3 = Some; 4 = Much; 5 = Very much. Effect N = 627.

Results

Each of the nine individual indicators for the Burden of Disability Scale is presented with its mean and standard deviation in Table 35-2. All items had five possible responses ranging from not at all (1) to very much (5). The highest means were for the two items capturing the impact of health problems on social life and daily activities. The average score was 2.08 for both items. The lowest means were for the two items capturing the social stigma of health problems: people have turned away and people view you negatively.

In exploratory factor analysis, all of the indicators loaded well into a single factor. The highest factor loadings (.81 and .83, respectively) were for health problems limiting social activities and daily activities. The lowest factor loadings were for the two items that capture social stigma: people have turned away (.50) and others view you negatively (.47). The inter-item reliability for the scale is .89, indicating a high agreement among all of the indicators of burden of disability. We tested the inter-item reliability without the two social stigma items, but it dropped substantially (.72).

We now turn to the stepwise regression models predicting the burden of disability. These results are presented in Table 35-3. In model 1, where we entered just the physical

TABLE 35-3   Stepwise Regression Models Estimating Burden of Disability

	Model 1	Model 2	Model 3
Functional limitations	.78 (.04)***	.72 (.04)***	.65 (.04)***
Total prevalent morbidity	.69 (.16)***	.39 (.18)***	.38 (.17)*
Total incident morbidity over 3 years	−.10 (.27)	−.03 (.27)	−.004 (.26)
Errors on MMSE	.30 (.12)*	.28 (.13)*	.27 (.12)*
Stopped driving in past 2 years	—	1.51 (.59)*	.73 (.58)
Level of pain	—	.70 (.15)***	.61 (.15)***
Experienced fall in past year	—	.93 (.43)*	.85 (.41)*
Number of medications	—	.19 (.10)	.12 (.09)
Number of hospitalizations	—	−.39 (.35)	−.42 (.33)
Active coping	—	—	−.13 (.19)
Life satisfaction	—	—	−.50 (.20)*
Satisfaction with social life	—	—	−1.44 (.20)***
Female	.28 (.38)	−.02 (.38)	−.06 (.37)
Age	−.06 (.04)	−.07 (.04)	−.04 (.04)
Education	−.10 (.13)	−.06 (.13)	−.07 (.12)
Widowed	.37 (.36)	.36 (.36)	.21 (.34)
Constant	5.73	4.80	10.88
R^2	.52	.55	.60
F (df)	85.26 (8)	57.21 (13)	56.30 (16)

* $p < 0.05$; **$p < 0.01$; ***$p < 0.001$. Effective $N = 627$.

and mental health indicators and control variables, we predicted 52% of the variance in the BDS. Those with greater functional limitations and more prevalent health problems rated their burden of disability much higher. Incident morbidity, which is measured as new conditions in the past 3 years, was not related to burden of disability. Those with more errors on the Pfeiffer mental status test also reported higher burden of disability. None of the control variables were significant.

In model 2, we added manifestations of ill health to the model. Those who stopped driving in the past 2 years rated their burden of disability higher than those who did not cease driving. Those with a higher level of pain, independent of actual diagnosed health problems, were more likely to perceive a burden of disability. Finally, those who experienced one or more falls in the past year have a higher burden of disability. Number of medications and hospitalizations were not associated with burden of disability. Functional limitations, prevalent morbidity, and cognitive impairment continue to be significant and positive, even with the addition of illness symptoms. In model 2, 55% of the variance was explained.

In model 3, we added three indicators of personal and social resources, including general life satisfaction, satisfaction with social life, and active coping dispositions. Those who are generally satisfied with their lives, and more specifically with their social life, tended to rate their burden of disability lower, independent of actual health status and symptoms. Contrary to expectations, active coping was not significantly associated with burden of disability. Functional limitations, prevalent morbidity, cognitive impairment, level of pain, and experiencing a fall continue to be significant. Stopping driving was no longer significant with the addition of personal resources in the model, likely due to the significantly lower life satisfaction among those who do not drive. In model 3, 60% of the variance is explained.

Discussion

The purpose of this paper was to demonstrate the strong psychometric properties of a new scale that measures the perceived social and personal burden of health problems and disability among older adults. The nine-item scale has a high reliability (.89), and the individual items have moderate to high factor loadings. Although the two items that capture social stigma of health problems loaded at a level somewhat lower than the other items (.47 and .50), there was not sufficient evidence to confirm that the scale was a two-factor solution. Rather, we argue that social stigma is a subscale of the larger burden of disability concept.

Our second purpose in this paper was to identify key predictors of burden of disability to better understand who is likely to consider themselves troubled by their health problems. Not surprisingly, we found that those with more functional limitations rated their burden of disability lower. In addition, the existence of prevalent health problems was also strongly associated with perceived burden. These two indicators continued to hold even after we controlled for symptoms of ill health and personal resources.

Indeed, we hypothesized that it was not the diagnoses per se that influenced one's perception of health burden but the daily reminders of those health problems such as an inability to drive and level of pain. These symptoms transcend specific, named, health problems and could even be caused by a vector of health problems. Most importantly, pain, inability to drive, and falling can directly affect one's ability to pursue desired social and daily activities. Of particular note, the final regression model predicted 60% of the variance in burden of disability. While a substantial portion of the explained variance was from functional limitations, prevalent morbidity, and cognitive impairment, manifestations of ill health such as falls and level of pain were also significant. Furthermore, appraisals of general life satisfaction and satisfaction with social life significantly diminished perceived burden of disability.

Our findings thus indicate that the BDS is a reliable indicator of the social experience and burden of illness and disability among community-dwelling elders. All items are based on a single factor, suggesting that there is substantial commonality among scale items that capture the personal and social experience of being burdened. These items cut across appraisals of psychological distress and social stigma. These findings suggest a symbolic interactionist view that disabled and frail older adults internalize negative views by significant others and society at large (Goffman, 1997; Blumer, 1969).

Our findings regarding antecedents of burden of disability among the aged underscore the powerful and anticipated influences of chronic illness and functional disability, including cognitive impairment, on the social experience of burden. The lack of significant demographic influence is notable and merits discussion.

The concept and measurement of the burden of disability applies to persons living with illness and disability across the life course. Nevertheless, we recognize that individuals are likely to attach different meanings to their disability as they encounter different role expectations in old age from those present at earlier periods of life. Thus, it is possible that in old age when illness and disability become normative, the social burden of stigma may be reduced. Alternatively, with shrinking social resources of the aged who may have experienced losses of spouse, siblings, and close friends (Kahana & Kahana, 2003), living with illness may pose greater social burdens due to feelings of helplessness or loneliness, compounding problems of ill health.

Similarly, it is important to consider the differential social meaning of disability and illness for men and women. It has been argued that, in American culture, being female and disabled is viewed as "redundant," whereas being male and disabled is seen as posing a contradiction (Asch & Fine, 1997). Such gender differences have been generally proposed in the context of young people dealing with illness and disability. Data from our research suggest that old age may serve as a gender equalizer in terms of the social meaning of disability. This observation is consistent with early gerontological theorizing about greater psychological androgyny that is arrived at in old age (Neugarten & Guttman, 1958). These data are also consistent with observations in the stress literature suggesting that while illness-related stress exposure increases in later life, adaptation to illness is also enhanced, possibly due to stress inoculation (Kahana & Kahana, 1998).

The second model we report explored the influence of illness- and disability-related health events (e.g., falls) and social limitations (e.g., driving cessation) and found that these illness-related stressors also contribute to the subjective burden of disability. Inclusion of these antecedents helps us refine elements of the illness and disability experience that collectively contribute to social and psychological burden. These findings help us recognize that the illness experience and attendant disability cascade often involve significant health events such as falls, and may limit social activities due to pain (Kahana, Kahana, & Wykle, 2007).

In our final model, we considered the role of general psychological resources such as life satisfaction and coping strategies as shaping one's interpretation of illness and disability as burdensome. Our findings suggest that general life satisfaction and domain-specific satisfaction with social life may dispose individuals to interpret their illness and disability as less burdensome. In contrast, active coping strategies had no significant impact on burden of disability. These findings are notable for their confirmation of the role of social attribution and the social construction of burden of disability. They support our prior findings based on longitudinal data about social influences on the assumption of a disability identity (Kelley-Moore, et al., 2006).

In future research, the role of social and psychological disposition may be more fully explored through inclusion of personality and dispositional factors such as optimism and locus of control. Additionally, having established the reliability and appropriate external correlates of the BDS, we plan to extend future analyses to consideration of the sequelae of burden of disability, particularly as it influences social participation and functioning of old-old adults. Use of longitudinal data will also help to more conclusively establish causal ordering of predictor and outcome variables.

Beliefs, commitments, and motivations have been described as important underpinnings of appraisal of threats to one's self, attendant to illness and other stressful life situations (Lazarus & Folkman, 1984). In instances of illness and disability, salient beliefs relate to one's ability to deal with pain and incapacitation, while preserving a satisfactory self-image (Moos & Tsu, 1977). To the extent that individuals feel stigmatized for their disability and feel prevented from performing important social functions, they reflect beliefs about lack of controllability of their situation, and hence may experience negative adaptational outcomes. The concept and measure of burden of disability contributes a promising avenue for further understanding mechanisms by which chronic illness and disability translate into diminished quality of late life for older adults.

References

Asch, A. & Fine, M. (1997). Nurturance, sexuality, and women with disabilities. In L. Davis (Ed.), *The disability studies reader* (pp. 241–258). New York & London: Routledge.

Blumer, H. (1969). *Symbolic interaction: Perspective and method.* Englewood Cliffs, NJ: Prentice-Hall.

Charmaz, K. (2000). Experiencing chronic illness. In G.L. Albrecht, R. Fitzpatrick, & S.C. Scrimshaw (Eds.), *The handbook of social studies in health and medicine* (pp. 277–292). Thousand Oaks, CA: Sage Publications.

De Geest, S., & Moons, P. (2000). The patient's appraisal of side-effects: The blind spot in quality-of-life assessments in transplant recipients. *Nephrology Dialysis Transplantation, 15,* 457–459.

Fillenbaum, G. & Smyer, M. (1981). The development, validity, and reliability of the OARS multidimensional functional assessment. *Journal of Gerontology, 36*(4), 428–434.

Frank, A. (1995). *The wounded storyteller: Body, illness, and ethics.* Chicago, IL: University of Chicago Press.

Goffman, E. (1997). Selections from stigma. In L.J. Davis (Ed.), *The disability studies reader* (pp. 203–215). Florence, KY: Taylor & Frances/Routledge.

Kahana, B., & Kahana, E. (1998). Toward a temporal-spatial model of cumulative life stress: Placing late life stress effects in life course perspective. In J. Lomranz, (Ed.), *Handbook of aging and mental health: An integrative approach* (pp. 153–178). New York: Plenum Publishing Co.

Kahana, E., & Kahana, B. (2003). Contextualizing successful aging: New directions in an age-old search. In R. Settersten (Ed.), *Invitation to the life course: A new look at old age* (pp. 225-255). Amityville, NY: Baywood Publishing Company.

Kahana, E., Kahana, B., & Wykle, M. (2007). (In submission to *The Gerontologist* [being considered for special section 2007 GSA Social Gerontology Theory Award winner and finalist papers]). "Caregetting": A missing link to completing the life cycle in social gerontology.

Kahana, E., & Young, R. (1990). Clarifying the caregiver paradigm: Challenges for the future. In D.E. Biegel & A. Blum (Eds.), *Aging and caregiving: Theory, research, and practice* (pp. 76-97). Newbury Park, CA: Sage Publications.

Katz, S., Ford, A.B., Moskowitz, R.W., Jackson, B.A., & Jaffe, M.W. (1963). Studies of illness in the aged. The index of ADL: A standardized measure of biological and psychosocial function. *Journal of the American Medical Association, 185*, 914-919.

Kelley-Moore, J., Schumacher, J., Kahana, E., & Kahana, B. (2006). When do older adults become "disabled"? Acquiring a disability identity in the process of health decline. *Journal of Health & Social Behavior, 47*, 126-141.

Lawton, M.P., & Brody, E.M. (1969). Assessment of older people: Self-maintaining and instrumental activities of daily living. *The Gerontologist, 9*(3), 179-186.

Lazarus, R.S., & Folkman, S. (1984). *Stress, appraisal, and coping.* New York: Springer Publishing Company.

Moos, R.H., & Tsu, V.D. (1977). The crisis of physical illness: An overview. In R.H. Moos (Ed.), *Coping with physical illness.* New York: Plenum.

Neugarten, B., & Gutmann, D. (1958). Age-sex roles and personality in middle age: A thematic apperception study. *Psychological Monographs 72*: 1-33.

Pearlin, L.I., & Mullan, J.T. (1992). Loss and stress in aging. In M.L. Wykle, E. Kahana, & J. Kowal (Eds.), *Stress and health among the elderly* (pp. 117-132). New York: Springer Publishing Company.

Pfeiffer, E. (1975). A short portable mental status questionnaire for the assessment of organic brain deficit in elderly patients. *Journal of the American Geriatrics Society, 23*, 433-441.

Sontag, S. (1997). AIDS and its metaphors. In L. Davis (Ed.), *The Disability Studies Reader* (pp 232-238). New York & London: Routledge.

Verbrugge, L.M., & Jette, A.M. (1994). The disablement process. *Social Science and Medicine, 38*(1), 1-14.

Weitzner, M.A., Haley, W.E., & Chen, H. (2000). The family caregiver of the older cancer patient. *Hematology/Oncology Clinics of North America, 14*(1), 269-281.

Zarit, S.H., Todd, P.A., & Zarit, J.M. (1986). Subjective burden of husbands and wives as caregivers: A longitudinal study. *The Gerontologist, 26*(3), 260-266.

Section VII

Cultural Perspectives on Aging

Chapter 36

The Experience of "Healthy Life" in Rural Dwelling Elders

Amy Shaver

Context

"Just let me plant my feet under my own table and I'll be happy." Words such as these spoken by a 94-year-old woman sitting outside her senior apartment building may be idle conversation to those who were there at the time. Her peers all laugh, as does she as she looks at them to note the effect of her statement, then moves on to another topic entirely. The depth of a simple statement such as hers may not be grasped while in the moment of the interaction. In the context of one's latter years or even days of life, however, the statement takes on new meaning. A lifetime of experiences has perhaps led to this saying, which is an indicator of one elder's perception of being healthy.

As a growing segment of the US population, elders residing in all areas encounter a variety of challenges to having a healthy life. Those elders residing in rural areas have similar issues to those of others in growing old. At the same time they have specific cultural characteristics and unique qualities that make their experience of growing older distinct from those of their urban and suburban counterparts. These characteristics may help move them toward healthy life but may also present barriers to health. Knowing how rural elders perceive being healthy could influence the practices of healthcare professionals as they try to meet the challenges of healthcare provision for this special population.

The goal of this chapter is to provide one perspective of healthy life perceived by rural elders as revealed in a narrative analysis qualitative research study. Topic areas in the chapter are: *healthy life, rural elders, research needs, healthy life research and findings, quality of study methods and practice imperatives.*

Healthy Life

Life Expectancy

Life expectancy in the United States has increased significantly during the past century (Healthy People 2010, 2000). Those who are now 65 years old can expect to be living 15 years from now. Likewise, a person who is now 75 years old can expect to have an average of 11 more years of life. According to the National Center for Health Statistics (NCHS,

2007) the average life expectancy overall in the United States is now 77.8 years. In the year 2000, 13% of the population was over the age of 65, and the expectation is that by the year 2030, 20% of our US population will be more than 65 years of age. This is the year when all "baby boomers" will officially reach that age (US Census Bureau, 2008). Healthy People 2010's goal to achieve health promotion and disease prevention in older adults may be more difficult to reach, due to the longer span of years that they may have been practicing a particular lifestyle.

Quality of Life and Healthy Life

Although statistics show that years of life have increased in the past century, years of life and quality of life may have different meanings. Healthy People 2010 (2000) refers to quality of life as a "general sense of happiness and satisfaction with our lives and environment" (p. 10). The Healthy People 2010 report recognizes that health-related quality of life is more subjective, as individuals rate their own health and ability to perform daily activities. Ratings of poor, fair, good, very good, or excellent can be reliable indicators of one's perception of their own health status. Peters and Rogers (1997) note that one's perception of health may actually affect one's mortality rate. Self-report of the number of healthy days is another measurement of quality of life, based on an estimate of number of days of poor health during the past 30 days. Years of healthy life is the most recently developed indicator used to measure quality of life (Healthy People 2010, 2000). This number is measured by taking the difference between life expectancy and average amount of time spent in less-than-optimal health. This number could be related to both acute and chronic illnesses. Based on this knowledge, discovering the meaning of healthy life or optimal health for elders may produce better indicators than statistical figures for predicting health promotion needs.

Health Promotion

Access to health care includes health education programs, which include individual health teaching as well as community-based health promotion and disease prevention activities. Promoting health has been a health delivery concept since the early days of nursing when Lillian Wald promoted the health and welfare of mothers, children, and families through active teaching in the community (Backer, 1993). There has also been an increased recognition of lifestyle habits that contribute to chronic disease risks (Glanz, Lewis, & Rimer, 1997; Haber, 2007). This awareness has led to a growing interest in preventing problems before they occur by increasing the public's general knowledge of risks and healthy lifestyle practices. The Lalonde Report (Morgan & Marsh, 1998), published in response to criticism of the biomedical model of health care, was released in 1974 in Canada. This report presented the view of a person's health as including not only biological and physical aspects of health, but also environmental and social lifestyle. A shift in healthcare focus was made from the perspective of disease treatment to disease prevention. Health promotion in the United States places most of its emphasis on lifestyle change. This is thought to be related to the strongly individualist tenor of American culture, in which people are expected to be responsible for their own actions. The increasingly accepted focus on quality of life as well as longevity has resulted in more research and theory related to health promotion methods across health-related disciplines. Still, over time the tendency has grown to use medical interventions as the primary way to deliver health care to Americans. Improved technology, new pharmaceutical discoveries, and new surgical procedures make these products and services easier to access. Healthcare reform initiatives (United States Department of Health and Human Resources, 2009) may provide a new opportunity to refocus on health promotion and primary prevention programs in the United States.

Rural Elders

What Is Rural?

Rural is classified by the United States Census Bureau (2008) as consisting of "all territory, population and housing units located outside of urbanized areas or urban clusters" (para. 7). The Office of Management and Budget defines non metro populations as areas other than metropolitan statistical areas or a county with fewer than 50,000 persons, not adjacent to an urban county (Rosenthal & Fox, 2000). Boyd and Quevillon (2007) note that rural communities are as diverse as urban communities economically, religiously, educationally, and so on. Knowing and understanding the differences and similarities of people living in these areas will help us to provide appropriate care.

Rural Characteristics

Haber (2007) writes that while Americans living in rural areas of the United States are highly dispersed throughout the country, they account for only 17% of the total population, whereas 23% of elders in the United States reside in rural communities. This means that the proportion of people 65 years and older living in rural areas is higher than in metro areas. The number of older people living in rural areas is expected to continue to increase as the overall population of those over age 65 continues to grow. The proportion is also expected to grow as rural elders tend to age in place, while younger residents migrate out, and those that stay have fewer children (Beale & Fugitt, 1992).

Fewer nonmetro elderly have high school educations, and more are likely to be poor and have lower monthly Social Security benefits. Nonurban elders are more likely to own their own homes, although the home is more often described as substandard (Rosenthal & Fox, 2000). Rural elderly are more likely than urban-dwelling elders to rate their health as poor and to have at least one functional problem (Rogers, 1993; Healthy People 2010, 2000). Likewise, elderly people are part of the rural culture, and they may possess some of the characteristics of that culture. For instance, Lee (1998) concludes in her study of rural people that they demonstrate a great degree of hardiness, self-reliance, and devotion to work.

Access to Healthy Life

Access to health care is conceptualized primarily as access to primary care, access to health insurance, and access to emergency medical care. Access to health care in rural areas is influenced by a number of factors, including geography, income, insurance status, health beliefs, and the supply of healthcare facilities and workers in a given location (Ricketts, 1999). Rural elderly residents have barriers to accessing health care in many of these areas, and they are likely to encounter additional challenges related to chronic disease and functional deficits (Rosenthal & Fox, 2000). As pointed out by Lee (1998), rural characteristics may also lead to internal barriers that prevent rural community dwellers from seeking health care, even when it is available. The characteristic of independence may cause them to put off seeking health care as a primary prevention measure and wait until tertiary interventions are necessary.

Health Promotion for Rural Elders

A discussion of the health promotion attitudes and practices of rural elderly people needs to be approached from a number of perspectives. One perspective would be that of generational cohorts. Knapp (2005) has found in his research that being brought up in a particular decade has an impact on that cohort of people. Many elders alive today were alive prior to and during World War I, and many lived through the Depression. Many were immigrants who came to the United States for a variety of reasons that may have influenced their worldview (Rowley, 1996). Those born in 1940 were alive during World War II. The oldest of the group has lived through all of these events and times.

Life in the rural United States during those years must also be considered. The elders who have aged in place know of a very different life than those who are younger. Many were brought up on farms. Their livelihood most likely came from farming, fishing, forestry, or mining (Rowley, 1996; Tisdale, 1942).

Rural elderly are open to health promotion programs when these are presented in a culturally competent manner. Care given in the home by rural home care nurses can provide an environment and an opportunity for teaching and learning for elders (Congdon & Magilvy, 2001; Lee, 1998). Nurses' use of creative strategies, their cultural sensitivity, and their skills are important in providing care (Lee, 1998; Shreffler, 1999).

Research Need

Gaps in Research

Searching the literature for *rural elders* and *wellness* produces little current research that is relevant to rural elders and healthy life. Searching the terms *elders, rural*, and *nursing* revealed only 62 articles over a span of 20 years, with at least one third of these studies conducted prior to the year 2000. Likewise searching the terms *elders, rural*, and *health promotion* led to just 14 studies from between 1995 and 2008. Only one article surfaces when looking for *elders*, *rural*, and *wellness* in an occupational health journal. Lastly, searching the terms *elders*, *rural*, and *healthy life* revealed one research dissertation (which is the one explained in this chapter).

Much of the research that has been conducted concludes with reported findings about how far it is to get to the physician, and about how many hospitals, physicians, nurses, dentists, and other healthcare professionals exist in rural areas. Southwest Rural Health Research Center, School of Public Health, and the Texas A&M University System Health Services Center (2003) conducted an extensive survey to identify specific areas of importance for rural people. This survey gives their top 10 issues, which includes access to health care. The report emphasizes that part of health care access is having access to knowledge that will enable people to make good health decisions.

Few current studies, however, have addressed the attitudes that rural elders themselves have toward attaining health. A single method of healthcare delivery does not fit all elders, nor does one method of healthcare delivery fit elders in all geographic locations. Although health promotion models have been developed for 30 years, none have been specific to rural community-dwelling elders. Further research in the area of rural elderly and health-related activities will lead to more effective health promotion programs for this unique population and increased sensitivity to educational approaches. These data-based programs may in turn help them to attain longer and healthier lives.

Public Health Nurses' Role

Nurses working in rural health care are the primary vehicle for disseminating health promotion education programs. It is not enough to know the demographic aspects of a population in order to help them adhere to a healthy life. Parse (1992) notes that it is important for nurses to understand the meaning their particular clients assign to health when attempting to illuminate possibilities for them.

Healthy Life Research

Recognizing the importance of health practices on overall health and the lack of understanding related to this area for rural elders prompted research questions. The gold standard of health care provision stemming from evidenced-based practice created a research imperative (Alexander, O'Malley, & Androwich, 2008). Knowing the thoughts and perceptions that rural elders have about a healthy life became a research quest that led to the narrative-based study, *Attaining Healthy Life as Perceived by Rural Community Dwelling Elders: A Narrative Analysis*. This study captured the essence of past life practices for certain elders, and the coinciding effects that these practices have had on their current healthy lives. The strengths they developed from hardships earlier in life, the contentment in having lived a satisfying lifetime, and the belief in the goodness of others were all important to uncovering the diverse meaning of the healthy life for rural elders. The findings of this study demonstrate the depth of wellness within each that motivates them to move forth each day. *Attaining Healthy Life as Perceived by Rural Elder Community Dwelling Elders* focused on participants' perceptions of: (a) "healthy life," (b) practices leading to healthy life, (c) resources that facilitate attaining healthy life, and (d) barriers that may hinder attaining healthy life.

Description of the Research Method

Mode of Inquiry

Polkinghorne's (1995) narrative analysis was the mode of inquiry used for this research. Narrative tradition is situated within the human realm, which in turn leads to the search in narrative research for understanding the meaning of human experience. Telling stories is a natural way of expressing the everyday happenings in our lives (Atkinson, 1998; Mishler, 1986; Riessman, 1993). The researcher interprets the story as a narrative. This process becomes a "constructive and reconstructive" process (Aranda & Street, 2001). Within this context, the researcher is part of the narrative making. As the teller is telling the story, she or he is constructing and placing meaning of their own into it. The researcher is hearing it and becoming part of it, reconstructing. The second construction or reconstruction brings a challenge to the researcher to reconstruct and interpret the story without losing the elements that are the truth of the teller. A third construction places new meaning on the story through the new interpretations of future readers. This process demonstrates a fundamental part of qualitative research, in that it is not seeking to find an absolute truth in repetition, but new meaning.

The process began with collection of descriptions of accounts or events related to the focus of the research (Polkinghorne, 2005). The inquiry began as the participants used the natural process of reminiscence to recall past events (Butler, 2005). Important to this study was the precept that "interpretive schemes from the narrative can be used to establish the significance of past events and to anticipate consequences of possible future actions" (Polkinghorne, 1995, p. 162).

The goal of narrative analysis is to create the story or storied episode. This is a key difference between analysis of narrative that begins with stories and evaluates them to produce categories that are common across the data base. The knowledge in narrative analysis comes through the emplotted stories. The researcher in this study was called upon to first listen to the narratives of life events that related to "healthy life." The final product would be a collection of individual stories in which "thought moves from case to case instead of from case to generalization" (Polkinghorne, 1995, p. 11).

Philosophical Underpinnings

Parse's (1992) human becoming theory was the guiding philosophical perspective for this study. A basis of Parse's theory is that of freely choosing meaning of situations and bearing responsibility for those choices. Congruent with Polkinghorne's (1988, 1995) view, Parse believes that the choices a person makes are influenced by the past and have an effect on the future. Subconcepts of the human becoming theory are useful in explaining how one's story is always connecting them to the past while at the same time their present condition exists, metaphorically distinguishing them from their past. Healthy life practices may be enabling a person to have quality of life while at the same time current practices may be limiting their ability to attain a healthy life. Freely choosing is a concept of Parse's that also allows one to determine his or her own meaning of health and wellness as the nurse "illuminates" possibilities of action for them.

Process

Participant Selection

Of concern for myself as the researcher was my "outsider" status. Recognizing this, efforts were made to help potential participants feel comfortable with me. Permission and support was obtained from the local Offices for the Aging directors and meal site attendees in each county to attend their senior programs. Once I had spent time with people at the senior centers and made them aware of the research intent, individuals were invited to consider participating in the study. All of those who agreed met the inclusion criteria. Participant selection then began with purposive and "snowball" methods to access elders who live in two rural counties, one in West Virginia and one in upstate New York. Thirteen participants ranging in age from 75 to 90 joined the study, nine women and four men. Eight others joined focus groups, making a total of 21 participants in all. Each signed an informed consent prior to being interviewed. Confidentiality of the narratives has been maintained.

Gathering Information

Methods triangulation (Denzin & Lincoln, 2003; Patten, 2005) was used to collect accounts, including participant observation, individual interviews, and focus groups. Although the primary accounts of experiences gathered were from individual narratives, each method's special features helped to clarify the "healthy life" perceptions of these elders.

The first step in collecting information was through participant observation at the senior program sites. Participant observation is a method of watching the behaviors of people to supplement and clarify information in many cases (Polkinghorne, 2005). This method comes from anthropologic tradition (Morgan, 1997; Speziale & Carpenter, 2003), wherein the observer joins in the activities of the group. In this case, the researcher was able to meet with the seniors at the meal site in the morning, when many came to socialize by playing games and cards. During this time I was able to get acquainted with the potential participants in the study and to observe relationships and interactions among the elders. I was readily accepted during this time. I also joined them in having lunch, and many days I helped to set up for lunch and clean up after. This method of getting to know the participants is a culturally sensitive way of respecting the rural elders. It is also consistent with Parse's (1992) concept of the researcher as an integral part of the experience, as well as Polkinghorne's (1995) view of the narrative forming out of the natural conversation of people.

Individual interviews between the researcher and the participants constituted the next part in the process of gathering accounts (Mishler, 1986). Each participant chose the place for the interview where they felt comfortable. Semi structured questions were asked, and the ensuing narratives were audiotaped. A great deal of flexibility was applied to when to change, add, or delete questions from any one interview, based on the researcher's reasoning and intuition at the time.

The last method for gathering accounts of healthy life perceptions was through focus groups (Morgan, 1997). Three focus groups were conducted with between three and eight individuals participating in each. They were held about 2 months after the original interviews were completed. Two of the focus groups included some who had already completed individual interviews and some newcomers; one group was made up of all new participants. Focus group information confirmed perspectives that were shared in the individual interviews, and sometimes presented fresh views.

Analysis and Understanding

Analysis Method

Polkinghorne's (1995) narrative analysis approach was used to analyze the information. Narrative cognition attempts to find the diverseness of the individuals' experiences, rather than seeking common themes or generalities. The goal is to look at each case as having its own unique information.

Polkinghorne's (1995) five phases for this analysis were followed: (a) audiotaped interviews were transcribed; (b) reading of transcripts and listening to tapes offered a naïve understanding of the whole; (c) for each interview, an outcome was specified, data elements were put into chronological order, elements were identified that contributed to the outcome, and causes and influences among past events were sought; (d) stories were written; and (e) a comparison report of the storied cases was written.

Analysis Process

Each interview was first transcribed and then read several times for a first understanding of the person's perceptions of "healthy life." The original audiotapes of each interview were listened to at this time and throughout the analysis process. The second part of the process was completed by reviewing each written narrative to identify the potential outcome of the story and important story elements that might affect that outcome. During this process each transcribed narrative was reduced significantly (deconstructed) to a product that reflected the necessary elements for story completion. It was at this point in the process that a decision was made to write stories using the narratives of seven of the participants. These seven narratives stood out as having elements that would demonstrate a unique perspective to the meaning of "healthy life," and they possessed the necessary elements that could be drawn together into a coherent whole. Writing (reconstruction) of each story was an iterative process that consisted of movement back and forth between the constructed story and the narrative elements. This process validates the story as being true to the narrative elements and clarifies the plot as plausible. Layers of understanding emerged during this process.

Findings

Three layers of meaning of healthy life unfolded throughout the analysis process: (a) initial understanding, (b) cognitive understanding, and (c) interpretive understanding. Meaning came from participants' views and researcher's insights.

Initial Understanding

The initial understanding of the narratives came after repeated listening to each tape and repeated reading of the narratives. Cultural and historical commonalities of the participants gave a sense of linkage to their stories. For example, the majority came from farming backgrounds, and gardens were a main source of nutrition when they were growing up. Each also had knowledge of poor health choices, such as smoking, drinking too much alcohol, and eating high-fat diets, and good health choices such as eating fruits and vegetables.

This understanding was at the surface level, as though reliving the actual interview. The researcher's concentration at the time was on remembering the actual situation, what the people looked like, how they were dressed, and how well the interview process flowed. Prior conceptions of rural lifestyle that had been gained from a review of related literature and experiences were compared to the settings encountered during the interviews. It was easy at this point to view the participants from a global perspective and as a group. Reflection upon possible researcher influences on narratives took place at this time also.

Cognitive Understanding

Cognitive understanding of healthy life was evident as participants reminisced about childhood injuries, biomedical issues, or physical abilities. They revealed knowledge they had of health and health practices, resources and barriers. Cognitive understanding for the researcher came during story development. It was an important function of the analysis that separated the individuals from their common backgrounds by searching for the elements that made each plot unique. The following are excerpts from three stories that demonstrate their diversity.

Ninety-year-old Jenny, who is aging in place in her rural home, describes a healthy life as:

> Oh, dear. Well, every day's get up to the Vedallion and usually I get an egg sandwich. Today, I got a biscuit and gravy and come up here [the senior center] and help, you know, eat a good lunch and go home. On Sunday I usually go to church down around the corner. It's not too far from where I live, but I still have to drive my car

to that. I got this old car and I can, I'm, so glad I can get around. My beauty shop I go to is right there, 1/2 block, so I can walk up with my cane.

For Rebecca, healthy life is:

Having people that care for us. I have a first cousin, lives over in Larsons. And I used to spend a lot of my younger years with her, growing up. And she told everyone I'm her sister; I'm the only sister she ever knew. Yeah, and we've always gotten along good. I go over and visit her. I went over last weekend and spent two nights with her. But, so, when she and I gets together we talk about old times and things, you know, when we were younger.

For George, healthy life is about keeping mentally active:

Well, I really think more mental attitude than maybe anything else, because [refers to a time in the hospital] I talk to all these people coming through, there was a steady stream of doctors and nurses and all sorts of people through there, and this one lady doctor was telling me that she'd talked to a patient and asking how he was and he swore at her and says, "I'm in the hospital." But if you have a bad attitude it's hard to get everything to work right. But it is important, of course, to eat a reasonably healthy diet. But it's probably more important to keep active mentally.

Interpretive Understanding

Synthesis of the stories revealed diverse meanings of "healthy life" for each person. A deeper understanding of each story emerged when viewing the person within their cultural and social world and within the historical context of their lives (Denzin, 2001). Denzin also calls this the emotional or authentic understanding that comes from the interaction and sharing of the experience. Parse (1992) sees this as having "true presence." It is through this lens that we can understand the actions taken by one person that differ from those of another.

For example: Jenny's healthy life is enmeshed with her community. She has had this routine for 30 years. Her reference points are community locations, activities, and people. For Rebecca, healthy life is being where her "roots" are. Contentment emanates from her as she sits on her porch three miles out on a one-lane dirt road, surrounded by land owned by other family members. George's meaning of healthy life is a positive mental attitude. He values mental attitude over physical abilities as most important.

Commentary

A commentary section, following the stories and interpretations, is thought by Polkinghorne (1995) to bring to light the similarities and differences among the stories or cases. He suggests use of White's (1975) study of three lives as an exemplar for narrative analysis and use of a commentary. White emphasizes the importance of cultural, historical, and generational influences, which are helpful in understanding the healthy life perspectives of the rural elders who participated in this study.

TABLE 36-1 Commentary: Similarities Among Participants' Perceptions	
Perceptions	**Descriptions**
Perceived healthy practices	Rural upbringing, knowledge of healthy habits such as no smoking, limited alcohol consumption, eating fruit and vegetables, staying physically active—exercise.
Perceived barriers to healthy life	Aging process, chronic illness, turning point incident such as a fracture or fall, own negligence at seeking health care or follow-up screening.

The information provided in this table represents a summary of healthy practices and resources as well as the barriers or hindrances to a healthy life as perceived by the participants. These similarities were discovered in the early phases of the analysis within the narratives of all 13 participants.

Similarities

The stories of seven of the participants are about people who have much in common with each other, fitting the descriptions above. Historically they have lived through many of the same major national and global events. As part of the same generation they tell of times that the others in the group understand, having lived and experienced similar things. Culturally their stories tell of times in the lives of people who have lived many or in some cases all of their years in a rural area. A visual summary of these similarities is found in Table 36-1.

Differences

When comparing people who have common backgrounds with similar influences, it is much easier to see their likenesses (White, 1975). In the present study of rural elders this was also found to be true. With this understanding, it is easy to see why when reading George, Charlie, Irene, Genette, Jenny, Rachel, and Alice's narratives, the similarities stood out, rather than the unique differences that they had to offer on the topic. Seven stories written about these people recognize their remarkable contribution to this study. A visual summary of these differences is provided in Tables 36-2 and 36-3.

Quality of Study Methods

Assurance of Rigor

Rigor in a qualitative study, according to Macnee (2004), is a "strict process of data collection and the associated analysis and a term that reflects the overall quality of that process" (p. 163). Components necessary for rigor are trustworthiness of data collection, confirmability or consistency of data collection, analysis and interpretation, transferability of findings, and credibility (Lincoln & Guba, 1985; Macnee, 2004;

TABLE 36-2   Commentary: Uniqueness Among Selected Participants: Healthy Life and Resources

Participant	Unique Wellness Quality
Rebecca	Loyalty to family with reciprocated caring
Alice	Care for her cats
George	Mental attitude
Genette	Strength through faith in God, trust in others at church to be supportive.
Jenny	Reliance on the concrete aspect of familiar community: people, places, and things.
Charlie	Seeing the silver lining of having a stable life and security of his home and wife.
Irene	Staying productive, enjoying what she has.

The information provided in this table presents a summary of the uniqueness among the participants in their perceived healthy life and resources. The differences were revealed during the latter phases of the analysis.

TABLE 36-3   Commentary: Uniqueness Among Selected Participants: Hindrances and Barriers

Participant	Unique Hindrances
Rebecca	Grew up on the mountain, childhood accidents and injuries, coping with a child who had Wilms' tumor
Alice	Long work hours in a plant with cement floors, poor shoes, chronic illness
George	Colon cancer
Genette	Postpartum depression
Jenny	Fractured hip at 88 > loss of mobility
Charlie	Visual decline > giving up drivers license > leaving job of over 60 years
Irene	Worry about husband's health

The information on this table provides a summary of uniqueness of hindrances to a healthy life as perceived by the participants.

Morse, 1991). Polkinghorne (1995) recommends using *plausibility* and *accuracy* also for judging the credibility of the stories written as part of the analysis. Lastly, important to the quality of the study is the reflective thought of the researcher (Burns & Grove, 2009; Morse, 1991). All of these methods were used to assure rigor in this study.

Ethical Considerations

Informed consents were presented to and signed by participants prior to the individual interviews and focus groups. Confidentiality of the narratives was met by keeping the data in a secure place, under lock. Names of the informants were not used in the original dissertation study document, nor will they be used in any other publications. Likewise, the actual names of the counties and the sites were not used. Participants who decided to have their individual interview at the senior sites were informed that others present may become aware of their participation in a study. Also, those who were part of the focus groups obviously knew of the others who were in the group. Rules of etiquette were given prior to the beginning of each focus group session, specific to confidentiality. As it turned out two people chose to have individual interviews at the centers.

Three people assisted in transcribing the interviews. They, along with me, took the human subjects online self-learning module and test. This test was submitted to Binghamton University's Human Subjects Review Board. A form was completed and they were added to the study. One of these people also was added as an observer and note taker for the focus groups.

Practice Imperatives

Overview

A humanistic approach was taken to gaining rural community dwelling elders' perceptions of healthy life. Assessing the meaning of "healthy life" was a subjective endeavor. Therefore the findings of the study were subjective in nature. Lessons learned from this study were (a) healthy life perceptions are unique to each individual, (b) healthy life perceptions reflect personal experiences, (c) perceived hindrances to healthy life may lead to self-limiting potential of reaching healthy life goals, (d) perceived resources may lead to healthy life practices that lead to reaching healthy life goals, (e) perceived resources may actually become hindrances to healthy life, (f) perceived hindrances may actually become resources to healthy life. Based on these findings the following types of implications will be discussed: Implications for nursing practice, implications for nursing education, and implications for nursing research.

Implications for Nursing Practice

The findings of this study should affect the practice attitudes of nurses who are working in rural public health institutions, rural acute care settings, or rural clinics. The findings could also influence the attitudes of nurses who work in urban healthcare settings that service those from the rural population. Most importantly, clinicians should assess each person they care for with attention to cultural and generational characteristics. Health promotion activities are important to helping people to reach their potential to have a healthy life. With these concepts in mind, public health nurses are most likely to utilize the findings from this study. As healthcare providers and specifically as providers of health education, public health nurses need to find these unique qualities in each of their clients and especially, in light of this study, in rural elders. As the elders in this study reflected on their past lives, they came to recognize their own beliefs about the resources needed for a healthy life.

Nurses working with this population can help them to reach their potential by tapping those resources. Some of the unique resources found in the rural elders in this study can be used as building blocks for health promotion initiatives. Such resources were (a) empowering of self by being productive, (b) building strong family ties, (c) accepting the things you cannot change while changing the things you can, (d) caring for someone, and (e) having a passion.

Implications for Nursing Education

Nurse educators have the challenge of preparing future nurses to be culturally competent practitioners. The diversity of the US population makes it increasingly difficult to teach student nurses about every cultural group for whom they may someday provide care. Educators do not want to presume that their knowledge base can be completed primarily through exposure to information in a text or other literature.

The findings in this study promote a perspective of attentiveness in nursing practice that will view each person individually within the context of cultural influences. To instill this attitude of practice in future nurses, healthcare educators must teach students from an affective perspective. Just as it is important for them to know the biophysical needs of elders and specific cultures, it is equally important for them to participate in activities that promote reflection on the individuals' own perceptions of their needs. This study focused on rural elders, but the concepts are important to think about when teaching students about all cultures.

Implications for Future Research

Many questions remain about rural elders and healthy life. Implications for future research would be to continue studies of this sort with rural elders as follows:

1. Conduct a similar study related to healthy life in other rural areas.
2. Conduct a similar study with rural elders who are homebound.
3. Use narrative analysis to study other research questions related to rural elders.
4. Conduct a quantitative research study exploring the same questions.
5. Develop health promotion education initiatives for the specific purpose of discovering the potential within the participants, and help them to recognize and use their potential.

Narrative analysis is a method that allows the participants to reveal the information they wish to reveal, tell stories as they remember them, and be viewed as individuals. This qualitative study addresses the important issue of understanding "healthy life" perspectives of rural elders. The stories written using descriptive elements found in narratives of the participants demonstrate the personal aspect of healthy life for each individual. As we age, "healthy life" takes on new meaning. It is important that research of this type continue with rural elders so that we can provide them with the best resources to recognize and reach their own potential for healthy life.

Summary

The thoughts, beliefs, and values of rural elder community dwellers were captured in this study as the participants spoke of their past experiences with health, and of their efforts to attain health in their lives. The process of sharing life events is perceived as the beginning of "knowing" for the elder storytellers. As they narrated instances about their own actions related to attaining health, these actions became more meaningful and significant (Polkinghorne, 1988). The telling of their healthy life events provided an opportunity for reflection on past times when they were stronger and perhaps more productive. In reflecting on their own strengths, each of the elders in this study recognized healthy life for themselves. In many cases this recognition was the basis of hope in spite of less-than-perfect conditions associated with aging. Faced with decisions that represented change in the world as they knew it, these elders were able to maintain their feelings of wellness. It is "knowing" that Parse (1992) believes is most significant in mobilizing one to move forward.

References

Alexander, R., O'Malley, A.A., & Androwich, I.M. (2008). Evidence-based health care. In P. Kelly (Ed.), *Nursing leadership & management* (pp. 110–126). Florence, KY: Delmar Thomson.

Aranda, S., & Street, A. (2001). From individual to group: Use of narratives in a participatory research process. *Journal of Advanced Nursing, 33*(6), 791–797.

Atkinson, R. (1998). *The life story interview*. Thousand Oaks, CA: Sage.

Backer, B.A. (1993). Lillian Wald: Connecting caring with activism. *Nursing & Health Care, 14*(3), 122–128.

Beale, C.L., & Fugitt, G.V. (1992). Nonmetro population older than metro: Relatively fewer working age adults. *Rural Development Perspective, 8*(2), 37–39.

Boyd, B., & Quevillon, R.P. (2007, September). Effects of trauma. *Rural Clinician Quarterly,* 2–3.

Burns, N., & Grove, S.K. (2009). *The practice of nursing research, conduct, critique & utilization*. Philadelphia: Saunders.

Butler, R. (2005). *The nature of memory: Life review and elementality*. Speech presented at the International Longevity Center, Rio De Janeiro, Brazil, November 17–18.

Congdon, J.G., & Magilvey, J.K. (2001). Themes of rural health and aging from a program of research. *Geriatric Nursing, 22*(5), 234–238.

Denzin, N.K. (2001). *Interpretive interactionism* (2nd ed.). Thousand Oaks, CA: Sage.

Denzin, N.K. & Lincoln, Y.S. (Eds.). (2003). Collecting and interpreting qualitative materials (2nd ed.). Thousand Oaks, CA: Sage.

Glanz, K., Lewis, M.L., & Rimer, B.K. (1997). *Health behaviors and health education* (2nd ed.). San Francisco: Jossey-Bass.

Haber, D. (2007). *Health promotion and aging: Practical applications for health professionals* (4th ed.). New York: Springer.

Healthy People 2010. (2000). *Understanding and improving health* (2nd ed.). U.S. Department of Health & Human Services. Washington, DC: U.S. Government Printing Office.

Knapp, J.L. (2005). *Understanding the generations.* San Diego, CA: Avenue Press.

Lee, H.L. (1998). *Conceptual basis for nursing.* New York: Springer.

Lincoln, Y.S., & Guba, E. G. (1985). *Naturalistic inquiry.* London: Sage.

Macnee, C.L. (2004). *Understanding nursing research: Reading and using research in practice.* Philadelphia: Lippincott Williams & Wilkins.

Mishler, E.G. (1986). *Research interviewing: Context and narrative.* Cambridge MA: Harvard University Press.

Morgan, D.L. (1997). *Focus groups as qualitative research* (2nd. ed.). Thousand Oaks, CA: Sage.

Morgan, I.S., & Marsh, G.W. (1998). Historic and future health promotion contexts for nursing. *Journal of Nursing Scholarship, 30*(4), 379–383.

Morse, J. (1991). *Qualitative nursing research: A contemporary dialogue.* London: Sage.

National Center for Health Statistics. (2007). *Health United States with chartbooks on trends in the health of America.* Hyatsville, MD.

Parse, R.P. (1992). Human becoming: Parse's theory of nursing. *Nursing Science Quarterly, 5*(1), 35–42.

Patten, M.L. (2005). *Understanding research methods: An overview of the essentials* (5th ed.). Glendale, CA: Pyrczak.

Peters, K., & Rogers, R.G. (1997). The effects of perceived health status and age on elders' longevity. *International Journal of Sociology and Social Policy, 17*(9/10), 117–143.

Polkinghorne, D.E. (1988). *The narrative knowing and human sciences.* Albany, NY: State University of New York.

Polkinghorne, D.E. (1995). Narrative configuration in qualitative analysis. In J.A. Hatch & R. Wisniewski (Eds.), *Life history and narrative* (pp. 5–23, 162). London: The Farmer Press.

Polkinghorne, D.E. (2005). Language and meaning: Data collection in qualitative research. *Journal of Counseling Psychology, 52*(2), 137–145.

Reissman, C.K. (1993). *Narrative analysis.* London: Sage.

Ricketts, T.C. (Ed.). (1999). *Rural health in the United States.* New York: Oxford University Press. Rogers, C.C. (1993). More nonmetro elderly rate their health as fair or poor. *Rural Development Perspectives, 9*(3), 32–37.

Rosenthal, T.C., & Fox, C. (2000). Access to health care for the rural elderly. *Journal of the American Medical Association, 84*(16), 2034–2036.

Rowley, T.D. (1996). The value of rural America. *Rural Development Perspectives, 12*(1), 2–28.

Shreffler, M.J. (1999). Culturally sensitive research methods of surveying rural/frontier residents. *Western Journal of Nursing Research, 21*(3), 426–435.

Southwest Rural Health Research Center, School of Public Health, & the Texas A&M University System Health Services Center. (2003). *Rural Healthy People 2010.* College Station, TX

Speziale, H.S., & Carpenter, D.R. (2003). *Qualitative research in nursing* (3rd ed.). Philadelphia: Lippincott, Williams, and Wilkins.

Tisdale, H. (1942, March). The process of urbanization. *Social Forces, 20,* 311–316. United States Census Bureau (2008). Table 10: Resident population projections by sex and age: 2010 to 2050. Retrieved from www.census.gov/prod/2008pubs/09statab/pop.pdf. *Census 2000 urban and rural classification.* Retrieved from TIGER/LINE October, 2003.

United States Department of Health and Human Services. (2008). Health Reform. Retrieved from http://healthreform.gov.

United States Department of Health and Human Resources (2009). *Health Reform.* Retrieved from http://healthreform.gov.

White, R.W. (1975). Lives in progress: A study of the natural growth of personality. New York: Dryden.

Chapter 37

The Need to Have Roots: A Philosophical Discussion

Ryutaro Takahashi

> *Roots are the essence of life. They are our life line; our connection to Life. Without roots we cannot live. . . . Without roots, we will become lifeless—which is what growing old sometimes looks like. It is essential that we as a society help elders to stay connected to their unique roots, so that they can experience and participate in Life even as they pass away.*
>
> —Ryutaro Takahashi, 2010

To Have Roots

As the certainty of death approaches, it is natural for older people to think deeply about and sometimes even dwell on the meaning of life and death. Life and death are not two separate entities opposed to each other, but rather they are closely associated. The title of this chapter was consciously written as "the need for roots," as discussed by Simone Weil (Weil, 2009). Roots are not only available to people with special experience or those who are in a particular situation; they are available to all people as they lead their normal lives, including the experience of death. The difference is that while people may consciously do something "to have roots," the ordinary experiences of life and death are also dimensions of the feeling recognized as "having roots." For elderly people who are exceeding the average life expectancy, the topic here might seem to be an unexpectedly simple and plain discussion. If possible, I hope this essay can capture the variety of experiences that emerge when death is becoming unavoidable.

Insights Revealed While Growing Old

Function Declines

What does "getting old" or "aging" mean? I have come to think that it is a process whereby capacities that living organisms have in common appear gradually. As humans, we are members of the elite community of living creatures that inhabit the earth. Plants, animals, and we humans are all living creatures. Although newborn infants already have the basic abilities recognized as life, the "function" to be a human in society is not yet fully acquired, and at first newborns appear to have an animal-like existence, without language facility. They will acquire knowledge, skills, and experience from their schooling, and from their employment. They will gradually come to wear the masks and develop the integument recognized as social humans, and it is expected that they will live for decades thereafter.

After entering old age, some will still work, enjoy taking part in society, or plow a field, and a number of them will be active up to 90 or even 100 years of age. However, at each point, they come to notice that the physical and mental functions that sustained their adolescence and midlife do not work in the same way as before. Although human traits such as intelligence or wisdom provide convenient and reliable function for a long time, eventually these traits become less useful in terms of the usual meaning of usefulness. Furthermore, some functions, including perception and motor functions that humans have in common with animals, and mental functions that capture the nature of objects and circumstances, and move the individual to action, become increasingly difficult to perform in old age. For instance, it gradually becomes more difficult to perform delicate operations with hands, and recognizing the nature of objects and ordinary daily situations becomes less clear.

Common Attributes of Life That Are Shared with Plants

What will our lives be like if we exceed average life expectancy? Plantlike functions remain, and will become more prominent as we age. At earlier ages these functions may receive little attention, but as people grow older, a diminished ability to perform these functions may gradually become apparent to both the elders and those around them. Plantlike aspects of our body include those functions associated with life itself, such as respiratory and circulatory functions, nutrition intake, digestion, and excretion. These functions are controlled by the autonomic nervous system, sometimes referred to as the vegetative nervous system. The purpose of this vegetative nervous system is to control the daily activities that sustain life, including excretion after eating, breathing fresh air and circulating blood, and those basic activities essential to living organisms. In old age, as other functions decrease (i.e., some cells degenerate and become extinct), these vegetative functions gradually come to predominate.

An ultimate factor in growing older is the gradual predominance, phase inversion, and manifestation of plantlike functions; the most important thing becomes how well the plantlike function works, or how well the person can live comfortably from the viewpoint of those who assist him or her. Consider a recent television documentary (Nippon Hoso Kyokai, 2006) about the four seasons of giant trees, including some more than 100-year-old beech and *Quercus crispula* that grow deep in the Waga Mountains, located in the secluded district between Akita Prefecture and Iwate Prefecture in the interior forest of Japan. The documentary was filmed by a fixed-point camera. In order to live, these giant trees, each having 200,000 leaves, shed all of their leaves in autumn, so that they can survive through the winter; it is necessary that they "cut off" those leaves that functioned to support their lives. If that is not done before the onset of snowing, branches may be broken by the weight of accumulated snow. The giant trees also protect themselves by making scab-like knots to prevent bacteria from entering from wounded sites on the branches. Like these giant trees, we humans may also be maintaining the condition of old age and surviving by "defoliating" many of the "functions" that were useful in youthful days.

Comfort or Discomfort Beyond Willingness and Intention

Elders often cannot convey their experience in words. The words may not come out due to dementia, or the person may simply be unable to describe his own declining physical condition coherently. If an elderly person wants to express something (and if a welcoming atmosphere can be created), or if the person can be helped to feel comfortable with us, it is possible that signs of what he really wants to convey will become apparent, giving the observer a chance to understand what the person is trying to express.

A traditional saying among elders in Japan is, "Meals taste great and bowel movement is great, so I am in a good condition." Comfort or discomfort is not what the heart feels or the head thinks; rather, it is a plantlike reaction. It might be said that the aging of humans is such that the vegetative aspects remain after the outer skin fails. This way of thinking was inspired by what was described about humans' vegetative side in the classic *De Anima* by Aristotle, and in *Human Body*, by Shigeoo Miki (1997).

The relation between aging and plantlike function hits on what I have been thinking may be the cause of sudden death while bathing that often occurs in elderly people in Japan (Takahashi, Asakawa, & Hamamatsu, 2007). In consideration of why those sudden deaths during bathing occur more often in elderly women, who are less likely to be carelessly bathing, or in elderly who are independent, I reached the conclusion that one of the causes may be related to the fact that the autonomic nervous system, or vegetative nervous system, may become unbalanced by aging and may be easily overtaxed due to weakness (Takahashi, 2005). There is a risk that the gap between activation during the bath procedure and its return to normal after the bath may cause a significant fluctuation in terms of the vegetative functions of daily living. Subsequently, I have thought of other examples in addition to bathing, including mealtime and the physiological event of excretion. Within this context, it seems appropriate to think of the experience of old age as an existence, such as a tree, that has both life and death existing together.

Gerontological Aspects of Medical Care in Japan

Unfamiliarity with Gerontology in Japan

While there are many programs of study in gerontology in universities in Europe and the United States, no faculty or department in universities in Japan offers educational programs in gerontology, except for a few universities that include sessions majoring in gerontology. On the other hand, medical care for the elderly or geriatric gerontology is recognized as an area in medical science, and some of the faculty of medicine in Japan's universities would like to see geriatric/gerontology and medical care for the elderly become a specialty. However, very few of those universities seem to have been successful in integrating gerontological concepts systematically into the course of training for medical students. In fact, in spite of a rapidly aging society, the number of universities that offer sessions in gerontology is gradually decreasing. Even in European countries, while some schools are increasing the number of gerontology sessions, other schools are rapidly decreasing sessions specific to aging clients (Michel, Huber, & Cruz-Jentoft, 2008). We healthcare professionals who have been engaging in gerontology have a responsibility to correct this situation. Although there are great numbers of physicians and other health-care professionals who work in geriatric settings or see primarily elderly patients, I doubt that we fully understand how important the gerontological aspect is in providing care for the elderly.

The Basis of Medical Care for the Elderly

One might question how gerontology can emphasize the aspects of human living in a society that is aging. For example, my nursing colleague and I have previously reported about the feelings in regard to the social life of elderly who are living in a nursing home, or how they felt when they experienced urinary incontinence for the first time (Takahashi & Liehr, 2004, 2007). Care is about focusing on elderly people as humans living in a society that values their personal history. Perhaps this point should be the main theme in sociology and anthropology among academic fields. How can this point be actualized in clinical practice? The answer can be seen in what Marjory Warren (Matthews, 1984), a pioneering British doctor, was able to achieve.

The stage was Britain in 1935. In those days, medical care for the elderly was in a similar situation to the previous nursing homes in Japan, which tended to be facilities for the poor, just putting the patients down on the beds and leaving them there for years, until their death. Little aggressive medical intervention was performed; meals and showers or baths were provided, and the patients lingered, some for years, receiving basic care from care workers or nurses. Dr. Warren came to see that it was impossible to maintain the vitality or motivation for life among the elders when they only received monotonous, everyday care. As she visited the patients in the wards every day, she observed them according to the two standards she considered most important. One standard was whether the patients had the ability to be able to control their excretions by themselves, and the other was whether they maintained perception or awareness of their surroundings. From those results, she classified patients into the following categories: (1) those who needed to strengthen their rehabilitation, with a goal of returning to their homes if their condition became better; (2) those who should be helped to find another place to live for a short time, if staying home was not currently possible but might be possible at a later time, and (3) those who would need care for a long time (Matthews, 1984).

Experience in Japan

This way of classifying elderly patients has received widespread adaptation since that time; for instance, examples are seen in Japan in the development of care plans based on the assessment performed when nursing care insurance (long-term care insurance) is available to provide care services for elderly individuals. But 70 years ago this idea of classification was unique, though it was later adapted by others, as seen in the widely accepted method for classifying plants by counting the number of stamen and pistils, which was developed by Swedish naturalist Carl von Linne (Nishimura, 1997). Likewise, the body of science has come to respect classification for its power to explain other concepts (such as aspects of the human condition of becoming old) with a simple principle. Finding a viewpoint from which to understand and classify the "human characteristics" of elderly people with disease and expressing them in a common language that will provide a basis for change is certainly not an easy task. But it is a task we must continue to undertake to improve life for the at-risk elders who reside in our world.

Compared to my previous experience, I realize that understanding this concept is very difficult. In 1994, comprehensive assessment wards that followed the idea of Dr. Warren (it can be thought so now) were established in the Tokyo Metropolitan Geriatric Hospital (Itabashi ward, Tokyo). Becoming the person in charge there, I began the discussion, "What can we do to improve the ward?" with the other doctors, nurses, and social workers. We engaged in this discussion over and over, but at the time even I could not understand enough; therefore nobody was able to answer this question (Ozawa, Eto, & Takahashi, 1999). Then nursing care insurance began a decade after that. As described earlier, you might say that now everyone in health care knows about the procedure that determines the care plan after the detailed assessment. However, is it true? It remains doubtful whether consensus can be reached that gerontological aspects are of high importance in medical care for the elderly.

Death Certificate of a Man: A Personal Encounter

This story is about an 82-year-old man who happened to visit our outpatient clinic recently, hoping to participate in a rehabilitation program. At the moment he entered my office, I thought I had seen him before. His name was Mr. S, and he noticed me, saying, "Hello doctor, long time no see." He was the vice president of a diabetes patients association which I had been engaged in more than 10 years ago. He is a patient with diabetes, 50 years since onset, and came here to participate in a rehabilitation program, this time due to a weakening of his legs and back since being hospitalized for heart failure a short time ago. He asked to be in the rehabilitation program, and I said, "Let's do it." At the last moment, Mr. S asked me, "By the way, what would you say if I asked you to write down a death certificate that said "died at home"? I answered, "Well, I have had a few patients ask for that before, so I will do that for you. Feel free to ask me if you do not have another doctor to ask." Then he murmured, "It is hard to ask Dr. X, who is currently my physician in charge, because he always escapes from my request."

In case of death at home, a different type of procedure documentation is needed from the hospital. One of the requirements is a death certificate, and Mr. S knows it will be troublesome if no doctor can be found who is available or willing to write one. I wondered why he asked me, in spite of the fact that we met for the first time more than 10 years ago. I didn't think he let his guard down because of feelings of nostalgia. He lives with his family at home and in a community, and he has a lot of problems; nevertheless his request cannot be ignored. Among other problems, his heart failure and renal failure are advanced, and if dialysis is started, then the patient eventually dies. I imagine he doesn't want to explain such a complicated private circumstance, when it isn't yet an urgent or imminent matter. He probably trusted me from our previous relationship, and felt comfortable asking the question. However, I feel there may be different reasons for why he had this conversation with me.

Although the conversation sounded "heavy," since the contents are about life and death, Mr. S neither talked about a "heavy" topic as if it was a "light" thing, nor did he consider it as a "light" matter. Therefore, I guess he spoke to me with the understanding that I would neither take it "heavy" nor "light" when I listened to his story. Whether it is heavy or light, since life and death are very close to us, such stories may emerge within our daily lives.

A Trifling Matter and an Important Matter

As a physician, I hear a lot of stories, and many are sensitive in nature. For instance, in speaking with a patient who I have seen for a few years, I learned what kind of inheritance he has and how much it is worth; I heard a tale about a daughter-in-law who does something in secret; and I was touched to learn that a man wanted to start rehabilitation soon, because he was going to help radio gymnastic exercises for the "Kids Circle" during the summer vacation. Certainly, doctors working in hospitals or as local general practitioners (as well as other healthcare providers) must have similar experiences. If there are any differences, their stories range from trifling matters such as table talk to important matters such as death certificates, happening at the same places, and based in their daily lives. Almost all of the stories concerning living in a society are trifling, and most are generally perceived as unimportant to others. It might be difficult to answer when a patient asks permission to buy a manju (Japanese-style bun usually filled with sweet paste) at a mall on the way home from the hospital. However, I don't think of these comments as either heavy *or* light. Even though it is important to respond when health problems occur, such as when an individual has a pain or feels ill, our patients understand that we are there for more than just pains and illnesses. We are there to hear their other light or heavy thoughts, as well.

I would say that the importance of the gerontological aspects of caregiving means accepting the person's "historical problems" that are scattered in his life and measured not by the general standards of the world, but by the person's own standards, then pointing out directly to the person what a doctor can offer in between the general category and the individual category (realizing that it may be limited). When setting the care plan after assessment, there is a point that should be a clear priority, which is often referred to as the "nitty gritty." Once that is understood, it is almost always possible to discuss other issues, even when those issues concern life and death, and to understand each other as two human beings who are connected, and who care about each other's well-being.

The Truth Is Not One

One Half of Each of Me

By the way, Mr. S, as described before, continuously spoke as follows: "Improvement of current dialysis and hemodialysis is very fast. I anticipate that the time when I will need dialysis will be 3 years from now, and it would be much more comfortable to receive then, since the dialysis technique will be more advanced in 3 years." Immediately after a serious conversation during which he's been looking for a doctor who can sign his death certificate because he wants to die at home, he anticipates the improvement of dialysis technique over the next 3 years, then at his present age of 82 years, thinks about the chronic renal failure that will likely lead to his death. I thought, at that moment, that this is the point. Although we tend to presume that we know what a person must be thinking, the thoughts of elderly people are always swaying (as are our own), and their range of fluctuation may be wide. But it is important to remember that all of their accounts reveal an aspect of the truth.

We have a somewhat puzzling word, ambiguity, which speaks to this issue of fluctuation. What we do or judge to be is full of ambiguity. It may sway from one extreme to the other. Concerning death, it can happen to anyone. It is important to accept ambiguity as a fact that is continually swaying from "possible" to "likely." Daijiro Hashimoto, former governor of Kochi Prefecture, wrote of Asahi Shinbun, "When I felt that the roadwork widening the construction at Shimanto river can be a destruction of nature, rather than needed for the convenience of the roads, I realized that nature oriented is a view of people in urban areas; on the other hand, when I heard a visitor who said Kochi is wonderful, my local way of thinking came to my mind, tempting me to ask the visitor, 'If you love nature, why don't you live here?' I am frequently aware of myself as one half of each of me." (Hashimoto, 1993, p.15)

Opportunism Regarding Death

We have a problem concerning the recruitment of doctors for remote areas, including Iwate Prefecture, where I have worked before. This problem is currently spreading among the local governments. A mayor has said to me, "Any doctors will be okay, anyway." We might say it is really an honest opinion, but it would be impossible to attract a doctor to our area with such a comment. Nevertheless, it is also difficult to hide the real opinion without saying it. The medical specialist system has been widely adopted within the doctor's world. It means that people need both local medical facilities that are available on holidays, and high-level medical organizations for more serious medical problems. Much of what we think of as morality may actually be opportunism that is strongly influenced by the special interests of those who stand to gain from a specific situation. For instance, if your finger was accidently amputated by a sharp-edged tool, you would need a medical specialist nearby who can suture your nerves and vessels. If you do not have such a specialist nearby, you will almost certainly think, "Why don't they have such a specialist here?" It is a fact that the view of the problematic issue "collapse of local medicine," which is being widely discussed in Japan, differs from the ordinary person's experience or needs. Rather, Japanese people consider themselves as the exception in most cases. However, it is impossible for people (particularly elders) to accept their increasing potential for death.

All-Aroundness in Old Age

The meaning of most of our "digital information" (or possibly digitalized information) disappears when we become older than the average life expectancy. It is thought that these people are living in the world where the detail of the parts and the whole become nested together as one. Shunsuke Tsurumi wrote, "It is difficult to realize the all-aroundness when getting older. In childhood, it is easily realized. Can you realize it again in the old age?" (Tsurumi, 2007, pp. 10–15) All-aroundness may aspire to the freeness that deals with specifics without being bothered by details. At least a part of the people will be able to accomplish death in all-aroundness. It is important that healthcare professionals make every effort to help each of those under our care to achieve all-aroundness.

References

Hashimoto, D. (1993, January 8). Opinion. *Asahi Shinbun*, p. 15.

Matthews, D.A. (1984). Dr. Marjory Warren and the origin of British geriatrics. *Journal of the American Geriatrics Society, 32*, 253–258.

Michel, J.P., Huber, P., & Cruz-Jentoft, A.J. (2008). Europe-wide survey of teaching in geriatric medicine. *Journal of the American Geriatrics Society, 56*, 1536–1542.

Miki, S. (1997). *Human body: Consideration under the biological history*. Tokyo: Ubusuna Shoin.

Nippon Hoso Kyokai. (2006). [*Giant tree: A mystery of life in Waga mountains*]. Retrieved from http://www.nhk.or.jp/special/onair/060305.html

Nishimura, S. (1997). [*Linne and his apostles*]. Tokyo: Asahi Shinbunsha.Ozawa, T., Eto, F., & Takahashi, R. (1999). *Guide for comprehensive geriatric assessment* [Japanese]. Tokyo: Ishiyaku Pub. Inc.

Takahashi, R. (2005). Prevention of accidental falls by the aged. *Nippon Naika Gakkai Zasshi (Journal of Japanese Society of Internal Medicine), 94*, 2400–2406.

Takahashi, R., Asakawa, Y., & Hamamatsu, A. (2007). Deaths during bathing in Japan. *Journal of the American Geriatrics Society, 55*, 1305–1306.

Takahashi, R., & Liehr, P. (2004). His-story as a dimension of the present. *Journal of the American Geriatrics Society, 52*(9), 1594–1595.

Takahashi, R., & Liehr, P. (2007). Nutritional improvement through an alternative perspective. *Geriatrics and Gerontology International, 7*, 201.

Tsurumi, S. (2007). Special topics: Tsurumi Syunsuke, talking about poem. *Gendaishi Techo (Modern Poetry Journal), 50*, 10–12.

Weil, S. (2009). *The need for roots*. (Y. Yamazaki, Trans.). Tokyo: Shunjusha.

Chapter 38

Telenovelas and *Cafecitos*
Culturally Sensitive Intervention Strategies
Janice D. Crist and John B. Haradon

The Intended Population

Latino elders have higher rates of hypertension, diabetes, heart disease, and death than their non-Latino counterparts (Laditka, Laditka, & Drake, 2006). The Latino population in America is expanding seven times faster than the population as a whole, and Latino elders are the fastest-growing minority group in the United States. Although many of one Latino subgroup, Mexican-American elders, could benefit from home care services, some of their traditional cultural beliefs, such as familism, have made many Mexican-American elders resistant to using these services (Crist, Kim, Pasvogel, & Velázquez, 2009).

Chronic illnesses also begin to occur among Mexican-American elders at earlier ages than in older persons of other ethnicities. While home care services provide low-cost and supportive care so that elders can age in place, these services are used less frequently by Mexican-American elders.

The Interventions

We tested two focused interventions, the *telenovela* and the *cafecito*, separately as initial pilot studies. Our research questions were: (1) Does the *telenovela* intervention increase the use of home care services among Mexican-American elders and their family caregivers? (2) What are the attitudes and practices of older Mexican-American elders and their caregivers about using home care services? (3) Does the *cafecito* intervention increase the use of home care services among Mexican-American elders and their caregivers?

The *Telenovela*

Latino people report that they are most likely to learn about health issues from *telenovelas*, the Spanish version of "soap operas" (Mayer, 2003; Spader, Ratcliffe, Montoya, & Skillern, 2009; Wilkin, Valente, Murphy, Cody, Huang, & Beck, 2007). This chapter describes a dramatized videotape intervention (a transcultural *telenovela*), including the process of scripting and producing its pilot version by members of a Mexican-American community advisory council drawn from the intended demographic audience. Presented as an exemplar, the method could easily be adapted to other cultures for other health promotion efforts, such as increasing consumer use of other available services, or for promoting healthier lifestyles, such as increasing physical activity.

The project's *telenovela* promotes an intra-audience dialogue that results in learning about available services. It provides familiar examples to facilitate this dialogue. The plot, presented in Spanish and English versions, includes an elder, her sister, and daughter-caregiver protagonists.

The *Cafecito*

Prior to developing the *telenovela*, Mexican-American elders and family caregivers were invited to participate in *cafecitos*, traditional small and informal get-togethers over coffee and *pan dulces* (pastries). During the *cafecitos*, elders and family caregivers discussed their needs, their attitudes about whether home care services should be brought into the home to assist the elder and support the caregiver, and any actual or potential barriers to using the services. The purpose of the cafecito was twofold: to gain new data and understanding about attitudes and practices, and to create a forum for exchanging perceptions and beliefs, nurturing possibilities for collaborating toward the creation of new solutions.

The culturally sensitive strategy of using the medium of the *telenovela* and the forum of the *cafecito* illustrates a method and model for achieving successful client outcomes, and is applicable to other interventions that are both culturally sensitive and specific.

The Cultural Context of Familism

Although it is also found in other cultures, familism (a traditional norm throughout Latino culture) has been documented as the most important distinguishing characteristic of Mexican-American culture (Kao & Travis, 2005; Romero, Robinson, Haydel, Mendoza, & Killen, 2004). Familism has been an important asset to the Mexican-American culture, providing for cohesiveness and the continuity of family values. Familism promotes "positive interpersonal familial relationships, high family unity, social support, interdependence in the completion of daily activities, and close proximity with extended family members" (Romero et al., 2004, p. 34), and is especially strong in Mexican-American families (Im et al., 2007; Weiler & Crist, 2007). A central component of familism is the expectation that children will be the primary caregivers for their parents and elders (Kao & Travis, 2005).

Besides being a positive tradition of Latino culture, familism can also present a barrier to elders' use of home care services. This perceived reluctance to use home care services may be because of the expectation by elders and family caregivers that family members "should" be able to provide all the care that is needed, that their family caregivers can give better (and more personal) care than outsiders, and that elders are safer being cared for by their children than by paid home care services providers. However, many Mexican-

American caregivers today, usually daughters, are not always able to provide for all needs of the elder, due to competing demands for their time (Romero et al., 2004); they would perhaps welcome some form of home care services, yet feel guilty and depressed if they do use them (Valle, Yamada, & Barrio, 2004; Scharlach et al., 2006; Im et al., 2007).

In our study, we considered the construct of familism to be a strong, positive, contextual aspect of the Latino culture. It was not seen as something likely to change; thus our aim was to challenge the cultural assumption that familism prohibits or inhibits a Mexican-American family from using any home care services that can assist with supporting elder family care in the home. The *telenovela* intervention (described later in this chapter) supports the perspective that elders can maintain their links with their informal family caregiver networks while still taking advantage of available professional resources (Ruiz, 2007). Traditional familism can be perceived as being supported, preserved, and honored when home care services supplement and complement existing family care, rather than those services being perceived as attempting to replace it (Morano & Bravo, 2002).

The effect of watching a videotape or DVD can be enhanced and strengthened by a follow-up dialogue among the elder, the primary caregiver, and other family members (Losada et al., 2006; Agree, Freedman, Cornman, Wolf, & Marcotte, 2005). Thus, *telenovela*-based studies should include guided dialogues following each presentation. In this study those guided dialogues were the *cafecitos*, also described later in this chapter. Though the dialogues were "guided," sometimes the principal investigator (PI) took field notes while the participants talked among themselves.

Other Challenges

Service Awareness and Confidence in Home Care Services

In previous studies, we have identified two strong barriers to the use of home care services (Crist, Kim et al., 2009). They were: (1) not knowing about the services that are available (lack of service awareness), and (2) lack of confidence in home care services. Service awareness is defined as knowing about home care services, how they can help the elder, and how to access them. Confidence in home care services is defined as trust that the elder will be safe and receive quality care while using them.

Designing the Intervention

We proposed that the interventions would promote service awareness and increase confidence in home care services to the point that the services would be accepted and used as referring primary care practitioners had suggested or prescribed. Table 38-1 provides an overview of the theoretical basis of the intervention.

Although many Mexican-American elders and their families still view the duty of caregiving through the traditional cultural lens of familism, some of today's Mexican-American caregivers also report varying levels of caregiving burden (Crist, McEwen et al., 2009). These caregivers often work full-time jobs outside the home, while still providing care to other family members as well as their elder loved ones. Unlike their elders, the care-givers often report they would welcome the extra support of home care services.

The purpose of the intervention was to increase the utilization of home care services by decreasing family resistance to those services. To achieve this goal, we designed a cultur-ally sensitive intervention using the *telenovela* and *cafecito* to inform family participants

TABLE 38-1   **Theoretical Framework: Narrative Pedagogy Synthesized with Components of the Intervention**

Theoretical Component Learning by:	Intervention Theoretical Construct	Intervention Modality	Application to *Telenovela* Intervention
Identifying with role models	Confidence in home care	Recognition of like plot family	***Confidence in home care services*** (2 dimensions): confidence/trust in services characters home care services and fear/worry about home care services. An elder, sister, and daughter are role models for family members in the story of an elder deciding whether to use home care ser-vices. Familism promoted in plot.
Social dialogue	Service awareness	Dialogue based on similar situation within family context	***Service awareness*** (3 dimensions): knowing that services exist, how home care services apply, and ability to access services. Family watches the *telenovela* together to learn information. Guided dialogues promote collaborative, comprehensive learning within a family context.
Multiple perspectives	Familism	Recognition of familism	The story models and the dialogue invite sharing of multiple views to support ***familism:*** home care services support, not replace, fam-ily (i.e., they promote, through teaching and support of all family members, positive familial rela-tionships, family unity, social support, and interdependence in meeting elders' daily needs).

about services and to encourage them to create new solutions (Diekelmann, 2001; Ironside, 2006). Learning is dynamic, social, based on dialogue, and takes place through identification with familiar people (role models) and contexts. An intervention framed or phrased in the familiar symbols of a culture is more likely to be effective than if it is perceived as being externally imposed (Diekelmann & Mendias, 2005).

The Plot of the *Telenovela*

A *telenovela* is the Spanish-language version of a soap opera. *Telenovelas* are traditional and popular sources of entertainment in the Mexican-American community. The script for a *telenovela*, "Todo Ha Cambiado," ("Everything Has Changed") was developed from an original story by the second author and videotaped in partnership with the ENCASA Community Advisory Council. (ENCASA, which literally translates as "in home," is an acronym for Elder aNd Caregiver Assistance and Support At-home). This original *telenovela* lasted 8 minutes and was staged in four acts: (1) the introduction of a *nana* (grandmother) with uncontrolled diabetes, and her daughter, who is concerned about her mother's health; (2) at a family party, the *nana's* sister's sharing about her own improved health outcomes following knee surgery and urging her to try home care services; (3) a home care services visit by a nurse who employs culturally competent *respeto* and *personalismo* in getting to know the *nana*; for example, in addition to treating the *nana* with deference and *respeto*, the nurse notices and comments on the *nana's* family photographs in a friendly manner; (4) a telephone conversation with a friend, during which the *nana* exclaims "*¡Todo ha cambiado!*" ("Everything has changed!"). Now she feels well enough to attend her grandchildren's soccer games.

This first *telenovela* was previewed by the ENCASA advisory council members, who then helped to publicize future public showings in four settings. Table 38-2 shows the scenes of the *telenovela*.

TABLE 38-2   Intervention: Telenovela

Telenovela Script				
Act 1: 1–2 min.	**Act 2:** 3–4 min.	**Act 3:** 5–7 min.	**Act 4:** 8–9 min.	**Summary:** 10th min.
Caregiver (daughter) visits mother, concerned about mother's health	Party, elder's sister and friends encourage her to use home care services	Elder at home with caregiver: culturally competent home care services visit	Telephone, elder: feels healthier and positive about home care services	Bullets: How to access home care services

Samples and Settings of the *Telenovela*

The *telenovela* was tested with four mostly Mexican-American samples in four settings, as follows:

Telenovela 1:
A *nanas* group (N = 12). Some of the same *nanas* had also participated in the first *cafecito* previously described.

Telenovelas 2 and 3:
The samples in settings 2 and 3 were members of two neighborhood associations (N = 12 and N = 13, respectively), of mixed ages and genders, and primarily Mexican-American.

Telenovela 4:
Small audiences throughout the day at a neighborhood association's arts and crafts fair held on a Saturday (N = 18, mixed ages and genders, and primarily Mexican-American).

Telenovela Evaluation:
Viewers were encouraged to comment on, react to, and evaluate the *telenovela* verbally to the PI at the end of the showings in settings 1 through 3, and by completing questionnaires in setting 4.

Samples and Settings of the *Cafecitos*

Cafecitos were tested with three Mexican-American samples in three different settings, as follows:

Cafecito 1:
A group of *nanas* who gathered at a local community family wellness center twice a week for prayer, activities, and lunch (N = 20). The *nanas* spoke mainly Spanish during the *cafecito*.

Cafecito 2:
Older women who regularly gathered at a local community center for exercises and lunch (N = 20; 2 groups of 10 each). The *cafecitos* were conducted in Spanish and English.

Cafecito 3:
Two men and one woman (N = 3), residents of a predominantly Mexican-American neighborhood, had voluntarily agreed to arrive 1 hour early before a monthly neighborhood association meeting. The three participants mainly spoke English during the *cafecito*, but they also spoke Spanish when a word or phrase could not be translated. The three participants were either 55 years of age or older, or were family caregivers of elders 55 or older. The principle investigator (PI) facilitated the *cafecitos* and was aided by bilingual members of the bicultural/bilingual advisory council in settings 1 and 2.

Data Collection and Analysis

All of the *telenovela* participants in setting 4 at the Saturday arts and crafts fair completed identical one-page, pre- and post-test, 12-item questionnaires about their knowledge, attitudes, and use of home care services, in Spanish or English. To test whether there were significant differences between their knowledge and attitudes about using home care services before and after viewing the *telenovela*, the chi-square test was used. The *cafecitos* were audiotaped (settings 1 and 3) or recorded by handwritten field notes (setting 2). Inductive content analysis was used to identify themes from the taped or handwritten narratives (Neuendorf, 2001).

Results

Watching the *Telenovela*

After the *telenovela* showings, anecdotal comments from some of the viewers revealed that they had identified with the story. For example, a son-caregiver said, "That was exactly the story of my mother!" Other viewers seemed to have opened up to learning about home care services, to be able to "hear" about what they are. One of the elders insisted that he had not known these services were available, although he had previously attended neighborhood association meetings where the PI had described home care services and how to access them. Although the overall pilot sample was too small to derive statistical significance, comparisons of the pre-and post-test results in setting 4 showed a trend toward increased knowledge about home care services and the propensity to use them (Crist, 2005).

Changes in Knowledge and Attitudes at the *Cafecitos*

In setting 1, themes emerged from the *nanas* indicating that their participation in *cafecitos* increased their knowledge that home care services even existed. For example, one *nana* told the group, ". . . they sent a nurse to the house. If it had not been for this nurse, my mother would have lost her leg; because she was so good, so conscientious, so very human you know, she just felt the compassion for my mom, and she would clean that leg that was so horrifying . . ." (Crist, 2005, p. 231). Thus, the group of *nanas* learned about home care services through hearing a peer describe a compelling example. Also, they agreed that these services could be beneficial, indicating attitudinal change. However, an advisory member who had been designated as a cultural advisor told the PI afterwards that a *nana* sitting next to her had confided that she still did not want anyone other than her daughters to care for her. The *nana* probably felt shy about sharing with such a large group. Therefore, although overall, knowledge was improved, some elders' attitudes were not addressed and remained unchanged.

In setting 2, the community center participants reported increased knowledge about services. In addition, they reported that they appreciated the positive opportunity to share their experiences of receiving family care, using home care services, and of caring for loved elders.

In setting 3, the themes emerging from the three participants revealed a strong expectation of traditional familistic values by Mexican-American elders and family caregivers.

Also, some additional attitudes and perceptions evolved during this smaller *cafecito*. This evolution was seen in participants who had an initial hesitation to use home care services. As they discussed their various points of view and heard about some of their long-time neighbors' willingness to use home care services, the services were understood better, and seemed to be more carefully considered, and sometimes incorporated, into their own attitudes. However, that sample's willingness to show up an hour early might also indicate they had strong preexisting personal opinions of their own, which they wanted to express. Another explanation is that the participants' personal acceptance or support of the PI prompted their willingness to attend.

Nevertheless, setting 3 is evidence that small *cafecitos* can yield valuable qualitative data as well as attitudinal or behavior change. Additionally, *cafecitos* may be a more effective forum than larger, more structured and thus more intimidating discussion groups because of their smaller group size and comfortable informality.

Discussion: Lessons Learned

Telenovelas and *cafecitos* are promising, innovative, culturally sensitive strategies for increasing Mexican-American elders' and caregivers' knowledge about, and willingness to consider using, home care services. Through these pilot tests, we learned how to improve the process of these interventions.

After watching the *telenovela*, viewers showed increased knowledge of, and more willingness to consider using, home care services, because use of home care services had been demonstrated in a culturally familiar venue, by way of a story with which they could relate and identify. The *telenovela* facilitated dialogue, and many participants reacted positively to its message. The group viewing of a *telenovela* may be a good way to facilitate dialogue afterwards in *cafecitos*. There are also advantages to holding *cafecitos* both pre- and post-*telenovela*; thus another possible future strategy would be to begin the *cafecito* for social purposes, break for the 10-minute *telenovela*, and then return to the *cafecito* for discussion.

During the *cafecitos*, at setting 1, the *nanas* frequently spoke to one another, but more often they spoke directly to the PI. In setting 2, the groups were scheduled to end after 45 minutes, because of other planned events at the community center. Unfortunately, the women were just beginning to express their authentic attitudes, and they may have talked more if there had been more time, according to the cultural advisor (an ENCASA advisory council member). In setting 3, the three members of the group spoke to each other directly, rather than addressing the PI, and in that instance they were evidently better able to express their true attitudes to one another, including their hopes and doubts about family caregiving and the use of home care services. In general during the *cafecitos*, diverse views were expressed; and some participants who had previously been resistant to the prospect of using home care services seemed to have gained some learning and acceptance.

Recommendations for the future structuring of *cafecitos* are: to keep the size of the groups small and, if groups are large, to budget at least 1 hour to be able to include initial formalities, small talk, and exchanges of stories and experiences, as well as providing time for the group's comfort level to grow. When the group is larger, sharing of genuine beliefs and attitudes is more likely to occur during a more informal setting.

Possible limitations of the pilot study included: (1) the *nanas* who had previously participated in one *cafecito* may have been positively influenced in their reactions to the showing of the *telenovela*; (2) whether and how much the presence of the Anglo PI, rather than a Mexican-American facilitator, may have impeded the flow of the *cafecitos*, is unknown.

The Ongoing Study: Present Research

We are now professionally producing and testing an expanded version of the home care *telenovela*, as well as producing an attention control (placebo) *telenovela* on a different topic (senior health screening). This project, the *telenovela/cafecito* intervention, is currently funded by a grant from the National Institute of Nursing Research (1R21NR010901-01A2). The ENCASA Community Advisory Council has continued to provide consultations regarding each step of the research process and intervention development. The procedures will be more controlled in the hospital setting, to test for efficacy before we test in the community for effectiveness (Whittemore & Grey, 2002). We will present the combined *telenovela* and follow-up guided dialogue (*cafecito*) intervention two times in the hospital setting using a randomized control design. We will thus determine to what extent these types of culturally sensitive strategies actually increase Mexican-American elders' use of home care services.

The *cafecito* will be a structured "guided dialogue" based on the pilot *cafecitos*. Table 38-3 shows the facilitative questions and prompts of the planned 50-minute session.

TABLE 38-3　Cafecito (Guided Dialogue) Components

	Cafecito (Guided Dialogue)			
	First 5 minutes	**Minutes 6–25**	**Minutes 26–44**	**Minutes 45–50**
Topics:	Introductions, small talk; goal: dialogue, not certain answers	Barriers to using home care services? How did the elder/caregiver view the visit? Your experience? What made the elder/caregiver change their mind? What else did you see this time?	What is the role of the caregiver if home care services come to help the family? How does it affect the elder? Does using home care services show support or disrespect for the family? Elder? Caregiver?	New scenarios; summary; conclusion

Summary

"Culture care negotiation" (Leininger, 2001) can be accomplished through showing *telenovelas* and then discussing them afterwards in *cafecitos*. Future studies are needed to determine whether these strategies may be useful in influencing healthcare practices within other cultural groups, for example, Asian immigrants, Latino farmworkers, First Nations groups, and Black American and Anglo American subgroups.

Future uses of the intervention could be as part of a regular literature and DVD handout in hospital and ambulatory care settings, to increase knowledge and utilization of home care services. The ENCASA community partnership that has been a sustained reality during the 10 years of this program of research continues to ensure the success of its endeavors (Crist & Escandón-Domínguez, 2003). The more the community, perceived by some outsiders as a vulnerable population, owns the research question, proposed solutions, methods of intervention, testing of outcomes, and dissemination (Crist, Parsons, Warner Robbins, Mullins, & Espinosa, 2009), the more its members will be receptive to new behaviors and innovative programs designed to improve healthcare resource utilization, in order to maximize and prolong their active well-being.

References

Agree, E.M., Freedman, V.A., Cornman, J.C., Wolf, D.A., & Marcotte, J.E. (2005). Reconsidering substitution in long-term care: When does assistive technology take the place of personal care? *Journal of Gerontology: SOCIAL SCIENCES, 60B*(5), S272–S280.

Crist, J.D. (2005). Cafecitos and telenovelas: Culturally competent interventions to facilitate Mexican-American families' decisions to use home care services. *Geriatric Nursing, 26*(4), 229–232.

Crist, J.D., & Escandón-Domínguez, S. (2003). Identifying, recruiting and sustaining Mexican American community partnerships, *Journal of Transcultural Nursing, 14*, 266–271.

Crist, J.D., Kim, S.S., Pasvogel, A., & Velázquez, J.H. (2009). Mexican American elders' use of home care services. *Applied Nursing Research, 22*(1), 26–34.

Crist, J.D., McEwen, M.M., Herrera, A.P., Kim, S.S., Pasvogel, A., & Hepworth, J.T. (2009). Caregiving burden, acculturation, familism, and Mexican American elders' use of home care services. *Research and Theory for Nursing Practice, 23*(3), 165–180.

Crist, J.D., Parsons, M.L., Warner Robbins, C., Mullins, M.V., & Espinosa, Y.M. (2009). Pragmatic action research with two vulnerable populations: Mexican American elders and formerly incarcerated women. *Family and Community Health, 32*(4), 320–329.

Diekelmann, N. (2001). Narrative pedagogy: Heideggerian hermeneutical analyses of lived experiences of students, teachers, and clinicians. *Advances in Nursing Science, 23*(3), 53–71.

Diekelmann, N., & Mendias, E.P. (2005). Being a supportive presence in online courses: Attending to students' online presence with each other. *Journal of Nursing Education, 44*(9), 393–395.

Im, E., Chee, W., Guevara, E., Liu, L., Lim, H., Tsai, H., et al. (2007). Gender and ethnic differences in cancer pain experience. *Nursing Research, 56*(5), 296–306.

Ironside, P.M. (2006). Using narrative pedagogy: Learning and practising interpretive thinking. *Journal of Advanced Nursing, 55*(4), 478–486.

Kao, H.F., & Travis, S.S. (2005). Development of the expectations of filial piety scale—Spanish version. *Journal of Advanced Nursing, 52*(6), 682–688.

Laditka, S.B., Laditka, J.N., & Drake, B.F. (2006). Home- and community-based service use by older African American, Hispanic, and non-Hispanic white women and men. *Home Health Care Services Quarterly, 25*(3/4), 129–153.

Leininger, M.A. (2001). *Cultural care diversity and universality: A theory of nursing.* New York: National League of Nursing.

Losada, A., Robinson Shurgot, G., Knight, B.G., Márquez, M., Montorio, I., Izal, M., et al. (2006). Cross-cultural study comparing the association of familism with burden and depressive symptoms in two samples of Hispanic dementia caregivers. *Aging & Mental Health, 10*(1), 69–76.

Mayer, V. (2003). Living telenovelas/telenovelizing life: Mexican-American girls' identities and transnational telenovelas. *Journal of Communication, 53*(3), 479–495.

Morano, C.L., & Bravo, M. (2002). A psychoeducational model for Hispanic Alzheimer's disease caregivers. *Gerontologist, 42*(1), 122–126.

Neuendorf, K.A. (2001). *The content analysis guidebook.* Thousand Oaks, CA: Sage.

Romero, A.J., Robinson, T.N., Haydel, K.F., Mendoza, F., & Killen, J.D. (2004). Associations among familism, language preference, and education in Mexican-American mothers and their children. *Developmental and Behavioral Pediatrics, 25*(1), 34–40.

Ruiz, M.E. (2007). Familismo and filial piety among Latino and Asian elders: Reevaluating family and social support. *Hispanic Health Care International, 5*(2), 81–89.

Scharlach, A.E., Kellam, R., Ong, N., Baskin, A., Goldstein, C., & Fox, P.J. (2006). Cultural attitudes and caregiver service use: Lessons from focus groups with racially and ethnically diverse family caregivers. *Journal of Gerontological Social Work, 47*(1/2), 133–156.

Spader, J., Ratcliffe, J., Montoya, J., & Skillern, P. (2009). The bold and the bankable: How the Nuestro Barrio Telenovela reaches Latino immigrants with financial education. *Journal of Consumer Affairs,43*(1), 56–79.

Valle, R., Yamada, A.M., & Barrio, C. (2004). Ethnic differences in social network help-seeking strategies among Latino and Euro-American dementia caregivers. *Aging & Mental health, 8*(6), 535–543.

Weiler, D.M., & Crist, J.D. (2007). Diabetes self-management in the migrant Latino population. *Hispanic Health Care International, 5*(1), 27–33.

Whittemore, R. & Grey, M. (2002). The systematic development of nursing interventions. *Journal of Nursing Scholarship, 34*(2), 115–120.

Wilkin, H.A., Valente, T.W., Murphy, S., Cody, M., Huang, G., & Beck, V. (2007). Does entertainment-education work with Latinos in the United States? Identification and the effects of a telenovela breast cancer storyline. *Journal of Health Communication, 12*, 455–469.

Acknowledgments

Funding for this study was provided from the Dean's Research Award, Jan 02–Jan 03; NINR, 1R21NR010901-01A2; 1 R15 NR009031-01; grateful acknowledgement is also extended to the ENCASA Community Advisory Council; Sunnyside and Elvira Neighborhood Associations, Pueblo High School Media Class, and Stevens Production Company.

Chapter 39

Mother Wit and Self–Health Management
Learning from African-American Elders

Cheryl M. Killion

"My mother still drinks dandelion tea and she's 94."

"Well I still take cod liver oil, 'cause I think, well I think it's good. It's good for a lot of things."

"I feel so good and relaxed after my Reiki session!"

"When she gets pain in her legs or something, she always used ice on that part, the bottom part and then after using the ice, she turns around and uses the heat pad and then she believes in rubbing Vicks salve."

"I like to just sit and watch nature."

"Just open the Bible to any verse and it helps."

"I work with my doctor and try to follow his instructions."

Groups of older African Americans who reside in a large Midwestern city were convened to gain a keener understanding of their approaches to self–health management. Particular focus was on the extent to which they integrated complementary and alternative medicine (CAM) with conventional health practices as they engaged in self-care. Group participants demonstrated vast knowledge about health and revealed that they used a wide range of health practices. Additionally, their responses, filtered through a lens of spirituality, reflected health wisdom, or "mother wit," that had been molded by history, personal experience, cultural identity, and reactions to adversity.

Since the era of slavery, African Americans have endured poorer health than the general population and have experienced marginalized health care. During enslavement and even now, African Americans have used ingenious ways to manage their health in order to survive. They often improvise, titrate, adjust, or create "new therapies" from what is available to them in their immediate surroundings (Fletcher, 2000). Rarely do African Americans voluntarily disclose these tactics to their health providers (Chao, Wade, & Kronenberg, 2008). The safety and efficacy of a number of approaches they use are not known. While the goal of clinicians is to support and encourage the use of measures that apparently work and are harmless, there is also concern that health conditions may worsen as a consequence of some self-invented health actions. African Americans over the age of 55 are particularly at risk as they seek ways to alleviate their symptoms. Older African Americans have greater rates of disease and death than the general population and are more likely to be afflicted with comorbidities, to have multiple prescriptions, and to be poor. This chapter provides a glimpse into the health practices of an often misunderstood and underserved population and offers lessons that may be particularly useful for those who seek to enhance the management of chronic illness among older African-American adults.

Taking Health into Their Own Hands

Historically, African Americans have always used health products, practices, and healthcare systems in conjunction with and in lieu of conventional medicine (Baer, 2001; National Center for Complementary and Alternative Medicine, n.d.; Brown, Barnes, Richards, & Bohman, 2007). Use of a parallel system of health care for this ethnic group has been a necessity since slavery. After being forcibly captured from their countries of origin, African slaves had to alter and adapt their strategies for healthful living in accordance with their new environment. The flora and climate in the Americas, for example, were unfamiliar and not conducive to growing their usual medicinal plants. As African health traditions were externally thwarted, however, remnants of cures were retained and privately practiced. Slaves were actively and ingeniously inventing strategies to cope with the harshness of their captivity and to devise new ways of healing, also often borrowing from, and sharing, with American Indians (Puckrein, 1981; Savitt, 2002).

The experience of slavery and the subsequent sequel of oppression further sculpted a distinct modus operandi for seeking and maintaining health and treating illness, as versions of conventional medicine were simultaneously employed. During the post-Reconstruction and Jim Crow eras, African Americans received health care in separate, substandard facilities, and were compelled to use parallel healthcare systems since they were denied access to healthcare institutions and services available to the general population (Byrd & Clayton, 2000). Centuries later, racial integration of healthcare services has allowed for exposure to mainstream health care. Instances of racism, unequal access and treatment, and discrimination persist, however.

Although African Americans in the United States are certainly heterogeneous, their common heritage is foundational to their health beliefs and practices. This historical backdrop is the basis of a distinct perspective on health among African Americans, though seldom given credence. Instead, differences in approaches to health are often viewed as merely a diluted and/or deficit version of mainstream medicine that needs to be corrected or brought in line with biomedicine (Baer, 2001).

The Health Status of African-American Older Adults

Focus on the health self-management or health practices of African Americans is essential. In 2006, the US Census Bureau estimated that there were 39.5 million African Americans in the United States (Williams, 2005; National Center for Health Statistics, 2009). African

Americans, nationally and locally, experience poorer health status than the general population and suffer disproportionately from heart disease, diabetes, stroke, and cancer, all leading causes of death in the United States (Williams, 2005; U.S. Department of Health and Human Services, Agency for Healthcare Research and Quality, 2006). These diseases are the major causes of decreased longevity, diminished quality of life, long-term disability, and poor treatment outcomes. African Americans have a life expectancy of 73.1 years as compared to 78.3 years in the general population (Arias, 2007).

The health status of African Americans is likely to be improved by building upon and incorporating their personal repertoire of self–health management tactics. In this paper selected dimensions of the approaches used by older African Americans to manage their health are described.

Methodology

The study's original and primary intent was to convene focus groups to elicit help from older African Americans in constructing a survey that would yield culturally specific data about African-American older adults' use of complementary and alternative medicine (CAM). CAM encompasses nonconventional approaches to health that are derived from whole medical systems, such as traditional Chinese medicine; mind-body medicine such as meditation and prayer; biologically based practices, including herbal products; manipulative and body-based practices, such as chiropractic, and energy-based medicine such as qi gong and therapeutic touch (National Center for Complementary and Alternative Medicine, n.d.). Home remedies and folk medicine are not included in this CAM definition. Although a survey has been developed and its description and associated methodology are detailed elsewhere (Killion, 2009), this chapter is centered on one of the themes that emerged from the focus group findings: Lessons Learned from Older African Americans about Health.

After informed human subject consent protocols were approved through the university Institutional Review Board, three focus groups were convened. Each group was comprised of five to seven African Americans, with an age range of 55 to 87. With the exception of one, all of the participants were female. Sample members were recruited from senior recreation centers, churches, and agencies that provide service to older adults. Focus group meetings took place in these respective settings. Participants, all of whom were managing at least one chronic illness, were asked about their own use of CAM therapies and their knowledge of use by family members, acquaintances, and others in the community. In addition, the study participants were asked to identify practices, products, systems of care, and beliefs about health and sources of healing specific to African Americans in the community, about which inquiries, in the survey, should be made. The focus groups were audiotaped and transcribed verbatim. Participants were modestly compensated for their involvement.

Responses were analyzed by using content analysis. In addition, a thematic analysis was performed. The Atlas ti qualitative software (Version 6) was used to store, sort, and assist with both analyses. Demographic and background information were summarized by using descriptive statistics.

Findings

Although data were not organized around CAM use and any particular health conditions, several domains were identified that provided the core constructs of the survey under development. The domains included Healers/CAM Providers; Health-Related Locations; Health Events; Health-Related Activities; and Health Products. In addition, two major themes emerged from the data: (1) The Legitimacy of African-American Health Practices and (2) Lessons Learned from Older African Americans about Health. The latter theme is the focus of this chapter.

Lessons Learned from Older African Americans about Health

Four major lessons were learned from this study: (1) Strategies for self–health management are derived from multiple sources; (2) Decisions about using self–health management approaches are based on multiple factors; (3) Cultural influences on self–health management are often subtle, yet powerful; and (4) Reminiscing is an effective means for eliciting and understanding health practices and patterns.

Strategies for Self–Health Management Are Derived from Multiple Sources

In this pilot study, the data revealed a common, though diverse core of beliefs and practices among older African Americans. A pattern of self-management, beginning at home, then spiraling out to other sources was found. Responses from the focus groups indicated that initially, health solutions were dealt with at home, and self-care approaches were used for as long as possible. These first actions were often "trial and error," though participants also had distinct ways of preventing illness and maintaining health. This approach is consistent with findings from other investigations related to self-care and health-seeking behavior (Saint Arnault, 2009).

The majority of health actions were self-administered; prayer was the overarching mode of self–health management. Other self-administered approaches to health included exercising, fasting, hugging someone, and engaging in expressive writing. Home remedies were widely used. Some practices had been used since childhood, and many participants remembered and continued to use remedies that had been passed down from generation to generation. Garlic continues to be used for hypertension. Various recipes for "hot toddies"(usually a mixture of brandy, honey, lemon, and tea) were presented, and an array of teas (sassafras, blessed thistle, ginger, golden seal, and peppermint) were described. Mogen David wine, in particular, was used for "low blood." A number of remedies used in the past had been adapted to include one or two additional ingredients. Also, red clay, used decades ago, primarily in the South, for skin disorders, can now be ordered online and shipped in packaged bricks directly to one's home. Household items, such as turpentine ("to cut coughs"), soot or spider webs (to stop bleeding; to heal wounds); and food products, such as the skin from egg shells (to "dry up bumps or boils") were remembered, but no longer used by the participants. A host of vitamin and mineral supplements were listed, as were salves, ointments, and oils. Vicks VapoRub was a staple in everyone's medicine cabinet. Study participants used what was immediately available to them and relied upon their own inclinations and past experiences:

> I had a great uncle who used to do a lot of work for my mother, and he was much older than she was. He was a carpenter, and my mother would call him and ask him to do some work for her, and he said, "I can't work anymore. I had to stop working because my hands, you know, I have arthritis really bad." And so then he came by one day and told my mother that he was back able to work and so she asked him what had he done to get his arthritis under control. He has this concoction that he mixes up . . . I now use it all the time. I keep a bottle of it at my house. It's Bayer's aspirin, vinegar, wintergreen alcohol, and cayenne pepper.

Others acknowledged the importance of the mind-body-spirit connection. A participant who had survived cancer stated:

> The mindset is basic. The mindset is that, I will be all right! I will prevail! I talk to my body, ask it for help, apologize to it when I've done something stupid and move on! The mindset, and just faith. You've got to take your health into your own hands, and then let God do the rest!

Outside of the home, participants engaged in a number of health actions in conjunction with others. For example, three of the participants had been involved in healing circles. Four exclaimed about their experience when they participated in a drumming circle. The majority of health actions involving others, however, centered on the activities with the participants' churches. Rituals, such as foot washings, were mentioned, as well as praise dancing. Prayer partners were valued. Even celebrating historical legends, such as Martin Luther King and Malcolm X, were construed by group members as having an individual, as well as collective, healing effect.

Findings revealed that study participants moved back and forth from their home remedies, health actions derived from family, friends, spiritual leaders, and community and their conventional medical sources: their nurse practitioner, physician, physical therapist, or pharmacist. Aside from these sources, many sought help from known healers in the community, depending on the severity of symptoms. For others, CAM approaches were used.

Participants identified health approaches that were administered exclusively by CAM providers. Reiki, massage, biofeedback, laying on of hands, therapeutic touch, music therapy, and reflexology were among other approaches used by participants as they sought help from CAM providers. A former dancer in one of the focus groups now used yoga and meditation to enhance her well-being. Two participants had experienced acupuncture, and one participant remarked about her encounter with a local Chinese herbalist: "She looks at your tongue and then writes something down. They then blend herbs and give you a tea. . . . All I know is, it works!"

Clearly, the findings reveal that the participants used a wide array CAM health actions as they simultaneously used conventional methods. Examples of the range of approaches and practices used are presented in Table 39-1.

Decisions About What Health Approach to Use Are Based on Multiple Factors

Self–health management or self-care in this study refers to self-initiated, deliberate, and purposeful activity, on behalf of oneself, to manage illness, improve functioning, and maintain wellness (Saucier, 1984; Frey & Fox, 1990; Orem, 1997). Self–health management is a problem focused, active, and proactive process that is based on an individual's perception of his/her health status and needs (Schilling, Grey, & Knafl, 2002; Lorig & Homan, 2003). One's lifelong experiences and values enable individuals to recognize and understand factors that must be controlled and regulated to promote optimal functioning and development (Fawcett, 2000). Use of CAM and indigenous approaches presumes independent health decision-making and reflects taking responsibility for one's own health.

The precise mechanism by which the focus group participants made decisions about using specific health strategies cannot be discerned from the data. Statements made by the participants, however, suggest that health-related decisions were based on the meanings and interpretations formed in response to a particular symptom or illness episode, or to achieve a particular health goal. In essence, meanings associated with health and illness generally focused on the individual's perception of the etiology, onset of symptoms, pathophysiology, course of illness, and treatment. According to Kleinman (1980) this process is consistent with one's explanatory model of health. Each person has a unique perspective on health that reflects social class, cultural beliefs, education, religious orientation, and past experiences with illness and health care (Kleinman, 1980).

One participant, for example, in seeking a treatment for her health condition, likened her body to a machine and stated that she occasionally used WD-40 oil for her arthritis. "That little small can of WD-40 used to put in your locks to make your lock work? Well, sometimes I hurt, so I use it. Instead of putting it on the lock, I put it on me." Surprisingly, another participant had done the same thing, and neither of them confessed to having any untoward effects.

In another situation a woman relied solely on her faith for healing:

> I used to work with a lady named Helen (pseudonym). That lady, she prayed for everyone. She was a good support to all of us there in the office, especially those who believed in God and Jesus Christ. And faith, I mean, for Helen, was a kind of detriment to her. Helen liked to eat. She liked to eat a lot and she liked to eat everything. The doctors found that she was seriously diabetic. They recommended that

TABLE 39-1 Complementary and Alternative Medicine (CAM) Health Practices of Older African Americans

	Self-Administered			Administered By/With Others	
Health Actions/Habits	Homemade Concoctions	Purchased/ OTC Items		Facilitated By/In Concert with Others	Rendered By Cam Provider
Prayer	Salt & water rinse/gargle	Salts (epsom)		Healing circle/network	Acupuncture
Reading the Bible	Hot toddy	Salves/ointments		Drumming circle	Reiki
Exercise	Vinegar/cranberry juice	Oils		Foot washings	Qi gong
Water/steam	Aspirin mixture	Spices		Speaking in tongues	Tai chi
"Eating right"	Wine/Wine mixture	Herbs		Music therapy	Drumming circle
Being in nature	Asfidity	Teas		Prayer partners	Biofeedback
Gardening	Teas	Vitamins/Minerals		Confiding in friend	Therapeutic touch
Not worrying	Soups	Food products		Libations	Massage
Fasting	Food products	Household products		Family gatherings	Laying on of hands
"Having the right mindset"	Household products			Praise dancing	Music therapy
Self therapy/ Self-evaluation	Dirt/red clay			Celebrating our forefathers	Reflexology
Hug someone	Mustard plaster			Martial arts	Herbs
Engage in distracting activities				Storytelling	
Listening to music					
Expressive writing					

she take a medication. So, Helen felt like she didn't need that medication because God was going to bring her through. I tried to explain to her how God was in this. He gave those doctors that knowledge. He gave the people that created that medication the knowledge to help her. But she refused and it worked out that she eventually had to have a double amputation. Both of her legs were amputated because she avoided facing her condition and then it had gotten to that point.

In this case Helen's perception of her condition and the appropriate course of treatment caused an unfortunate delay with a tragic consequence. In contrast, meditation, family support, and especially prayer undoubtedly enhanced a positive outcome in another scenario:

When I had surgery, I was 79 years old, and for them to cut on me and take a tumor off of my colon, I thought at my age I would never pull through, but I prayed. My daughter, my son-in-law, all of them, were standing around me. I didn't even think I was gonna come out of it, but I prayed, and I would meditate before I went under surgery, and I really believe that God will heal.

Although lay explanations of illness may not be fully articulated, tend to be less abstract, may be inconsistent, and even self-contradictory, they nonetheless are comparable to scientific interpretations as attempts to explain clinical phenomena (Kleinman, 1980). These explanations of sickness and treatment guide the choices made about available therapies and therapists and provide personal and social meaning to the experience of sickness. Healthcare professionals also have explanatory models of care, which are guided by scientific principles. These explanations about health determine what is considered relevant clinical evidence and how that evidence is organized and interpreted to rationalize specific treatment approaches. Hence, explanatory models are the main vehicle for revealing the cultural specificity and historicity of socially produced clinical reality, regardless of whether it is based upon scientific medical knowledge (Kleinman, 1980). Having a clear understanding of the patient's perspective on their condition sets the stage for a partnered plan of care.

Cultural Influences on Self–Health Management Are Often Subtle, Yet Powerful

Culture is a pattern of living and involves the way people experience, perceive, and interpret their world. It constitutes a shared system of meaning, though it is dynamic and ever-changing. African Americans are bicultural. While African Americans have a distinct culture, with its own history, concepts, rules, and social organization, this group also coexists within the larger American context, often adhering to principles and engaging in practices that overlap between the two cultures. African Americans may adhere to standards specific to their group, such as particular values associated with self-care practices, while at the same time espousing values of the larger society (Becker, Gates, & Newsom, 2004).

The findings of this report suggest that many of the self-health management approaches of African Americans emerged from strategies for survival, long-term efforts to overcome adversity, and struggles with a dual identity. Responses from the focus group participants revealed strategies centered on spirituality, and God was viewed as the ultimate healer. They embraced holism, but acknowledged contextual factors that framed daily life situations that could potentially hinder their full focus on, and access to, health and well-being. Whenever possible the respondents sought and used an eclectic approach to health. Because of past experiences and lack of trust with providers in general, respondents indicated that they were less likely to disclose their range of health practices to conventional health providers. Respondents were resentful because many of the approaches they used in the past had become commercialized and presented as if they were newly discovered products. Their responses revealed that they were not only concerned about their own individual health, but were also concerned about the health of the African-American community:

> This has always bothered me: Why is it that it always seems like us, African Americans have the most problems that the doctors or statistics always find? I read a pamphlet and. . . . It's like the Black people have TB. Oh, we have the most of cancer or we have the most of this, or we have the most of that, and I don't understand why sickness is always pointed in a direction of us, . . . of my people. . . . I've been reading history. We were the healthiest people on earth before we came here from Africa.

Responses from the focus groups reflected ambivalence about wholeheartedly embracing conventional medicine as practices derived from African-American culture were simultaneously devalued, denigrated, and discarded. Moreover, a number of the respondents lamented that African Americans were losing their culture.

> "We let all our history just fade away."
>
> "No, actually, some of it was stripped away from us."
>
> "But we have played a part. You know our African forefathers had these remedies and we thought we were too sophisticated to do these things any more. Rather than thinking that what we were doing was "country" we probably should have continued with it all.

During the process of data collection, numerous references were made about grandmothers. The manner in which individuals developed their explanatory models of health and ultimately their self-care tactics were greatly influenced by mothers and grandmothers, who usually are the primary individuals engaged in socializing the family for good living and good health.

Reminiscing Is an Effective Means for Eliciting and Understanding Health Practices and Patterns

By engaging older African Americans in a discussion about health practices in the community, important domains and related data were uncovered. Members in each focus group were eager to discuss this topic and actually had not thought deeply about patterns in their own health actions prior to the focus group discussions. The process of eliciting the data was as important as the actual data.

The reminiscing that occurred called up details of a rich heritage that had been forgotten and often misinterpreted. In addition to discussing their own health habits, all of the participants gave specific examples of health actions from their own families. One half of the participants had the same health conditions, such as diabetes, heart disease, or cancer, as their parents. Recalling illness episodes within their families laid the groundwork for viewing their own conditions and comparing their own health tactics with health strategies of others. The majority of comments, however, centered on the childhood experiences of the focus group members and their current health actions. For example, the participants acknowledged that important changes in healthcare delivery had occurred. The reminiscing helped the focus group members to validate their ability to cope with their own health and to make appropriate decisions regarding their own care. Moreover, from listening to others in the group, their sense of cultural pride was enhanced after revisiting health memories of the past and current concerns. Reminiscing about health with older African American adults was an effective way to encourage them to see the relevance of their own experiences (Housden, 2007).

In addition to the rich dialogue, vivid examples, and thoughtful reflections, very perceptive views about health were articulated, and group support and concern for each member were evident. An appropriate label for the content and process rendered from the focus groups may be collective "mother wit." Although this term was used as a code word during slavery, the dictionary definition of "mother wit" is simply "common sense" or sound judgment (Dundes, 1973; Kinnon, 1997). This phrase, however, has a much deeper meaning, particularly among African Americans, today and is considered a cipher for the knowledge one must have to survive and thrive. According to author and Nobel Prize Laureate Toni Morrison (1985, p. 230), mother wit is "a knowing so deep" representing life lessons indelibly inculcated from one's mother or otherwise respected, caring individual (Kinnon, 1997) and passed down from one generation to another.

When the term "mother wit" is applied to health, its meaning is much broader in scope than mere beliefs about health. Rather, this term encompasses decision making and strategies used to obtain, preserve, and transmit whatever is necessary for optimal health and healing. The individual and collective insight garnered from the focus groups may be mimicked by those for whom the elders serve as models and can be tapped by clinicians from whom the elders seek care. As African-American older adults are approached about health maintenance and care, it is critical that clinicians and health educators take the time to learn about who they are, where they have come from, and what they already know and believe as the starting point. African-American older adults possess a wealth of knowledge about health and the human condition. Let's listen and take heed to the lessons they live!

References

Arias, E. (2007). United States life tables, 2004 (National vital statistics report 56). Hyattsville, MD: National Center for Health Statistics.

Baer, H. (2001). *Biomedicine and alternative healing systems in America: Issues of class, race, ethnicity, and gender*. Madison: University of Wisconsin Press.

Becker, G., Gates, R., & Newsom, E. (2004). Self-care among chronically ill African Americans: Culture, health disparities, and health insurance status. *American Journal of Public Health, 94,* 2066–2073.

Brown, C., Barnes, J., Richards, K., & Bohman, T. (2007). Patterns of complementary and alternative medicine use in African Americans. *Journal of Alternative and Complementary Medicine, 13,* 751–758.

Byrd, M., & Clayton, L. (2000). *An American health dilemma: A medical history of African Americans and the problems of race.* New York: Routledge.

Chao, M.T., Wade, C., & Kronenberg, F. (2008). Disclosure of complementary and alternative medicine to conventional medical providers: Variation by race/ethnicity and type of CAM. *Journal of the National Medical Association, 11,* 1341–1349.

Dundes, A. (1973). *Motherwit from the laughing barrel: Readings in the interpretation of AfroAmerican folklore.* Mississippi: University Press of Mississippi.

Fawcett, J. (2000). Orem's self-care framework. In J. Fawcett (Ed.), *Analysis and evaluation of contemporary nursing knowledge: Nursing models and theories* (pp. 259–361). Philadelphia: F.A. Davis Co.

Fletcher, A.B. (2000). African American folk medicine: A form of alternative therapy. *Association of Black Nursing Faculty Journal, 11,* 18–20.

Frey, M., & Fox, M. (1990). Assessing and teaching self-care to youths with diabetes mellitus. *Pediatric Nursing, 6,* 597–599.

Housden, S. (2007). Forward into the past. *Adult Learning, 19,* 12–13.

Killion, C. (2009). *Complementary and alternative healing among older African Americans: Developing a culturally tailored survey* (Unpublished document). Franes Payne Bolton School of Nursing, Case Western Reserve University, Cleveland, Ohio.

Kinnon, J. (1997, March). Mother wit. *Ebony Magazine, 23,* 31–33.

Kleinman, A. (1980). *Patients and healers in the context of culture: An exploration of the borderline between anthropology, medicine, and psychiatry.* Los Angeles: University of California Press.

Lorig, K.R., & Homan, H.R. (2003). Self-management education: History, definition, outcomes, and mechanism. *Annals of Behavioral Medicine, 26,* 1–7.

Morrison, T. (1985, May). A knowing so deep. *Essence Magazine, 29,* 5, 230.

National Center for Complementary and Alternative Medicine. (n.d.) *What is CAM?* Retrieved on January 14, 2010 from http://nccam.nih.gov/health/whatiscam/overview.htm.

National Center for Health Statistics. (2009). *Health, United States, 2008* (p. 155). Hyattsville, MD: Author.

Orem, D. (1997). Views of human beings specific to nursing. *Nursing Science Quarterly, 10,* 26–31.

Puckerin, G.A. (1981). Humoralism and social development in colonial America. *Journal of American Medical Association, 245,* 1755–1757.

Saint Arnault, D. (2009). Cultural determinants of help seeking: A model for research and practice. *Research, Theory and Nursing Practice, 23,* 259–278.

Saucier, C.P. (1984). Self concept and self care management in school-age children with diabetes. *Pediatric Nursing, 10,* 135–138.

Savitt, T. (2002). *Medicine and slavery: The diseases and health care of blacks in antebellum Virginia.* Urbana and Chicago: University of Illinois Press.

Schilling, L.S., Grey, M., & Knafl, K.A. (2002). The concept of self management of type 1 diabetes in children and adolescents: An evolutionary concept analysis. *Journal of Advanced Nursing, 37,* 87–99.

U.S. Department of Health and Human Services, Agency for Healthcare Research and Quality. (2006). *National healthcare disparities report.* Rockville, MD: Author.

Williams, D.R. (2005). The health of US racial and ethnic populations. *The Journal of Gerontology, 60B*(Special Issue II), 53–62.

Chapter 40

Care of the Elderly in Botswana, Africa

Ditsapelo M. McFarland

Introduction

In this chapter, I will first describe the living environment for the elderly in African countries, and the close relationship between African elders and their families. I will also comment on the traditional network of care for African elders, both at home and at the societal level. The challenges faced during the care of the elderly will also be highlighted. Finally, I will close by sharing the tribute that I had written and read during my grandmother's funeral. The tribute highlights the multiplicity of roles that the elderly continue to play in most African societies.

Living Arrangements of the Elderly Within the Botswana Context

In order to understand care of the elderly in Botswana, one needs to understand the traditional family structure. As in most African countries since time immemorial, the elderly, particularly the grandparents, have been a revered part of the Botswana nuclear family right up to their death and beyond. Unlike in most developed counties, there are no boundaries between the children, grandchildren, and grandparents. The decisions that are made regarding the family revolve around grandparents as a major source of wisdom and custodians of tradition and custom.

Children, grandchildren, and grandparents live in the same home of origin, which is commonly referred to as the ancestral home. The ancestral home is where the elderly like to be cared for when they are sick and where they want to be buried when they die. Children may go to urban areas to seek employment or work, but during holidays and vacations, and after retirement from work, they return home to their roots to join their parents and extended family members. Cities are considered places of work, and they get abandoned when children return home to connect with their parents.

As members of the nuclear family, the elderly, in particular the grandparents, contributed significantly to raising and caring for their children and grandchildren. Apart from the caring, the elderly also have a major role in guiding young generations, and in transmitting the wisdom, culture, and traditions of the ages.

Care of the Elderly at a Family Level

In Botswana, as it is in most developing countries, care of the elderly is done by the family. When the grandparents grow older, weaker, and sicker, it becomes the responsibility of the children and grandchildren to take care of their aged relatives. The African society expects children and grandchildren to take care of the older people. Unlike in Western cultures, institutions for the elderly, such as nursing homes, are nonexistent in Botswana and are also considered to be not part of the Setswana culture. This absence of nursing homes in Botswana in particular could be explained by the desire of the elderly to be taken care of by their families in their ancestral homes, as well as by societal (i.e., village or community) expectations. Further, it would be culturally inappropriate for an older person to be placed in an institution for care. Rather, it would be considered a disgrace to the family for an elderly person to be cared for in an institution such as a nursing home. Similarly, it would also be against societal expectations for older people to be removed from their ancestral homes and families when they cannot take care of themselves anymore. The few nursing homes that were developed and operated in some African countries were generally unused and subsequently closed. This resistance to using nursing homes for elders is a sign of social unacceptability by African society.

Apart from fear of violating the older person's wishes and societal expectations, our conscience would not allow us to place a grandparent in an institution where they would be taken care of by someone other than their family members. In most African societies, people derive power and direction from their ancestral spirits as well as from societal norms and expectations. The elderly are looked up to and revered as *Badimo ba rona,* which means "Our Ancestors." They mediate between us and *Modimo* (God) and are highly respected. It is believed that going against the wishes of the ancestors might bring misfortune to the family. In Botswana in particular, illness is associated with having made the ancestral spirits angry (Staugard, 1985).

Most fortunately, perhaps due to strong support systems, most elderly in Botswana, as well as in other parts of Africa, do not suffer from dementing illnesses such as Alzheimer's or Parkinson's disease. Therefore their care at home is to a larger extent manageable. For the most part the aged are afflicted by physical conditions associated with aging, such as poor eyesight and respiratory infections (Department of Printing and Publishing Services [DPPS], 2005).

It should be noted that not all families in Botswana have children of their own. In case of older adults who were not blessed with children, care of such individuals becomes the responsibility of close relatives. The African society expects close relatives to take care of others who are not able to care for themselves because of age and illness.

As a point of illustration, it was difficult and unacceptable for the author of this article to place her husband, who was Caucasian and from the United States, in a nursing home when he became terminally ill. The author's cultural values related to care of a family member and her conscience as his wife were strong influencing factors. As such, she moved him from a developed country to Botswana, her country of origin, for care. Here, in her homeland, her husband was cared for by her entire family until he passed away (McFarland, In press).

Care of the Family at the Community Level

While there are virtually no nursing homes in Botswana, some institutional mechanisms have been put in place to support families and provide some daytime respite from the burden of care. For example, in Botswana the Botswana Retired Nurses Society (BORNUS) was formed by the retired nurses of Botswana to relieve families of the 24-hour burden of care at home. This society is nongovernmental and not for profit, and it caters to clients of all ages and conditions. Clients may be picked up from their homes and returned by the center vehicle, or families may drop their sick relatives off at the center in the morning and pick them up later in the day. At this center, all the needs of the clients are met by the nurses and community volunteers, including their physical, nutritional, and recreational needs. Community Home-Based Care (CHBC) is another organization that was developed to relieve families in regard to the burden of care. This is a public program that is managed by the local government clinics. It also caters to clients of all ages and conditions who are nursed at home. The care at home is provided by nurses and family welfare educators from the local clinics.

Challenges Related to Care of the Elderly at Home

Care of the elderly at home in their African villages is not without challenges. Among the challenges are the effects of urbanization, weakening of the extended family and traditional systems, nonexistence of programs for the elderly, and limited research related to care of the elderly. These challenges affect the families and the healthcare providers as well.

> **Urbanization.** The rise of urbanization and industrialization in most African societies has led to greatly increased migration of younger people from rural areas to urban areas to seek employment. In Botswana in particular, living conditions in urban areas may not be suitable to accommodate care of the elderly. Therefore, the majority of the elderly live in rural areas, and their care is left largely to hired help, which may be costly, unreliable, and unacceptable to both the older person and family members. Furthermore, rural-urban migration and urbanization have to some extent weakened the extended family and traditional systems, from which the family derives most of its support.
>
> **The Nonexistence of Programs for the Aged.** The nonexistence of society-based programs to support care of the elderly is highlighted as both a positive and a negative influence on elder care in Africa (Shaibu & Wallhagen, 2002). It poses a major challenge, particularly to working families. While African families try to stay connected as much as possible, the distance between some urban and rural areas is too vast, separating the families from their parents for longer periods. Additionally, nurses who provide care in the home may be faced with the daunting challenges of inadequate supplies and

equipment. Thus plans that are culturally sensitive and appropriate need to be put in place to both improve the care of elders and to lighten the burden of care for families.

Limited Research. Care of the elderly in Africa has not yet been fully explored, and thus is not fully appreciated (Shaibu & Wallhagen, 2002). Although Botswana has a lower proportion of older population than some developing countries, the percentage of the elderly has been projected to rise somewhat by 2010 (Kinsella & Ferreira, 1997). Therefore there is a critical need to strengthen the research base to better inform health workers about the care needs of elders and possible alternative ways to meet those needs within a climate fueled by urbanization associated with development in African countries.

A Tribute to My Grandmother: Mme Koorapetse Maifhala Sabokone

Born in 1902. Died in 2004 at 102 Years of Age.

I am writing to say how blessed we are to have had you as our grandmother.

Not many children have had the opportunity to experience the warm and tender love of such a grandmother.

You raised us since we were young when our parents were working; you were a mother, a provider, a caretaker, a friend, and a disciplinarian for unruly behavior.

You raised our children as well when we went to work, and for this you never asked for any payment.

You instilled in us the importance of respect, in particular, of the older person. Furthermore, you instilled in us the importance of sticking together as a family at all costs.

You also taught us the importance of abiding by the cultural norms and societal expectations. For this, you leave us responsible and well-respected citizens.

You raised us in the Anglican Church faith. Together with other members of the Anglican Church Mother's Union, we stand proudly around your coffin saying, ***Good bye and thank you ever so much for this gift you left for us.***

To your brothers and sisters, you raised them when your mother died at an early age. You raised their children and grandchildren, and they are highly respectful and thankful for that.

To the community, you were looked up to as a "Matriach." You were revered and highly respected for your wisdom and good sense of humor.

Your friends nicknamed you "Darlie" for a good reason. Indeed you were a darling to everyone who knew you.

To your church, what an honor that your priest would cut his overseas trip short to come and officiate at your funeral, when other priests would have done it!

The support you got from the family, relatives, friends, the community, and the church, was unsurpassed.

Although we are sad to see you go, we should be happy that we lived with you for many years and during these years you guided us through the right path.

You did a wonderful job in guiding and influencing generations throughout the life span. The legacy you left for us will be passed through generations to come.

May your Soul Rest in Peace, Darlie!

References

Department of Printing and Publishing Services. (2005). *Health statistics report 2003*. Gaborone, Botswana: Central Statistics Office.

Kinsella, K., & Ferreira, M. (1997). *Aging trends: South Africa* (Issue Brief No. 97-2). Washington, DC: US Department of Commerce.

McFarland, D.M. (In press). A journey through Pick's disease with a loved one: A personal account. *International Nursing Review*.

Shaibu, S., & Wallhagen, M.I. (2002). Family caregiving of the elderly in Botswana: Boundaries of culturally acceptable options and resources. *Journal of Cross-Cultural Gerontology, 17*(2), 139–154.

Staugard, F. (1985). *Traditional medicine in Botswana: Traditional healers*. Gaborone, Botswana: Ipele-geng Publishers.

Chapter 41

The Power of Life Story Books
Irish Stories

Mary Rose Day, Teresa Wills, Geraldine McCarthy,
and Joyce J. Fitzpatrick

Stories have been described as threads that weave together the life of an older adult and are the raw material from which the sense of self emerges (Hirst & Raffin, 2001). Life story work (LSW) is one of the methods used in the reminiscence process. It originated in the United Kingdom within foster care services and was used to help create a sense of identity for foster children in care (Ryan & Walker, 1985, 1993). Life story work has been described as a range of activities that could include biography, life history, and life stories (Murphy, 1994; Murphy & Moyes, 1997). McKeown, Clarke, and Repper (2006) defined LSW as "... a term given to biographical approaches in health and social care settings that gives people time to share their memories and talk about their life experiences" (p. 238). Life story books can consist of photographs, written accounts in peoples' own words, materials relating to a person's life, and life history (Heathcode, 2005). There is a growing interest in the recording of life stories, biography, and history (Hecht & O'Brien Tyrell, 2007).

Life Story Methods

There are a number of life story methods that have been used with older people; these include reminiscence, life review, and LSW. Reminiscence is a psychosocial intervention that involves discussion about past activities and events using prompts such as old music, photographs, and antique memorabilia (Woods, Specter, Jones, Orrell, & Davies, 2005).

Life review is another method used in the reminiscence process that usually involves individual sessions through which participants are guided chronologically through experiences both positive and negative. Life review includes recent and past experiences and may produce a life story book (Woods et al., 2005). While reminiscence tells the story, life review not only focuses on the story but also analyses and dissects the stories, seeking meaning in what is happening. LSW uses a biographical approach in the reminiscence process, giving people the opportunity to tell their stories chronologically. The terms *reminiscence*, *life review*, and *LSW* have been used interchangeably in the literature. A key commonality between these methods is that they are therapeutic interventions, and the sharing of past memories is a common denominator.

Reminiscence and life review have been used to create life story books across a variety of settings, with a diverse range of people, including people with intellectual disabilities (Hewitt, 1998, 2000), older people with mental health problems (depression, dementia), persons in continuing care (Haight, Gibson, & Michel, 2006; Plastow, 2006), older people in residential care (Hansebo & Kihlgren, 2000; Wills & Day, 2008), and older people on medical wards (Clarke, 2000; Clarke, Hansen, & Ross, 2003). The life story books have been developed with the support of nurses, speech and language therapists, research assistants, care staff, and family carers (Day & Wills, 2008; Wills & Day, 2008; Haight et al., 2006; Hamilton & Atkinson, 2009) on an individual basis and by using small group processes.

There is considerable research to support the use of these interventions. Guse et al. (2000) used reminiscence as the approach to complete life albums with residents ($n = 13$) in a long-term care setting over an 8-week period. Research assistants were given training and development on interpersonal skills and role play, and they developed a group life album for the project. The research assistants then helped residents individually to complete albums capturing their unique chosen life events and memories. Residents valued the completed albums, and family members were enthusiastic and engaged with the residents in the creation of the life albums. Staff members were also interested in life albums; however, they identified time and staffing issue as barriers to completion of the life albums. Guse et al. (2000) concluded that the life albums gave the residents a sense of accomplishment and enhanced communication with staff, families, and residents.

Elford et al. (2005) explored the benefits of engaging nursing home residents ($n = 5$) in writing their life stories and sharing memories using a series of booklets containing prompts. Each completed booklet was typed up by the researchers and given to the participants. The activity provided residents with a meaningful purpose, it and gave them an opportunity to share memories and stories with others and to maintain their skills in writing. The authors suggest that the process can improve the psychological well-being of older people.

Similarly, Haight, Gibson, and Michel (2006) examined a life review/life story book intervention with 30 people with dementia residing in an assisted living facility in Northern Ireland. The investigators focused on the production of a life story book based on an individual structured life review; the process was facilitated by care assistants. Carers enjoyed engaging in the process, and families felt that it improved the mood of their relatives. The process was seen as a low-cost, low-risk, brief intervention that could enhance care. Likewise, Plastow (2006) explored the use of life history books with residents who were depressed ($n = 3$) and living in a care home. Residents were involved in a process of creating their own life history books. Themes that emerged from the study related to reviewing the past, accepting the present, and dreaming of an alternative future. Creating the life history books provided the residents with a regular, goal-directed, and meaningful opportunity to cope with the losses they had experienced in their lives. The process provided a safe environment for the residents to explore past emotions and to share personal events with family members and staff, thereby improving relationships.

Wills and Day (2008) engaged residents ($n = 5$) and family carers ($n = 3$) in developing life story books in a nursing home setting, and they explored the narratives and life story books with residents and their families. The central themes that emerged related to the social construction of people's lives, social roles, and relationships, influences of religion, and sense of self. The researchers concluded that creating the life story books provided a holistic view of the older adult and offer the potential to enhance person-centered care. In a similar study, Day and Wills (2008) facilitated the development of life story books with family carers and described the value of the life story books. Eight family carers attended a series of six workshops, where they were actively engaged and supported in developing a life story book. Three key themes emerged from the experience: carers' perspectives on life story books, relationships and life story books, and seeing and understanding the person. The life story book captured the uniqueness of each person's story and promoted awareness of the person's identity, personality, values, and relationships. Day and Wills concluded that creating the life story books was an innovative therapeutic activity for family carers. It gave carers the opportunity to bring to life the person's life story and fostered connectivity with the person's past and present life.

A characteristic feature of all the research conducted is that compiling life story books is an activity that shows the uniqueness of the individual, and that can be an integral factor in providing person-centered care. The challenge for healthcare professionals is to get to know the individual as a person, to uncover what makes that person unique, and to individualize the care provided. As the researchers have identified, the life story books have the power to advance the well-being of older adults as stories help healthcare professionals and family members to understand the experiences of older people. The life story books can open up possibilities for improved communication between individuals and their families, and they serve as a way to engage them in meaningful conversations.

Developing Life Story Books in Practice

Before introducing life story books, managers and staff need to set up a policy and guidelines for the development of life story books in practice. A facilitator needs to be appointed who will coordinate the project; the facilitator needs to have good understanding, knowledge, and training on the different life story methods, along with good interpersonal skills (McKeown et al., 2006). People need to feel safe and supported to participate and engage in life story work. This is very important since sad memories, traumatic life events, divorce, suicide, or unwelcome family secrets may come to the fore during the process (Haight et al., 2006).

Based on the authors' experiences, any person who is engaging individuals or groups in the development of life story books needs to understand the different life story methods, as well as the potential barriers and difficulties that can arise with each method. The following is an example of a difficulty that arose in practice. A facilitator was engaged with an older person in developing a life story work when a secret was disclosed in confidence to the health professional. The person lacked knowledge on how to manage the issue, policy and guidance were not in place, and there was no supportive clinical supervision available. This left the facilitator feeling overburdened, as she could not share what was disclosed. Therefore, clinical supervision and identifying support structures are critical before engaging in life story work. The facilitator will need to decide on the best approach to use, and from experience there is consensus that the individual approach is best suited to those who have cognitive or communication difficulties. This allows the facilitator to support the person and write down their story in their own words. Facilitators also need to be aware that engaging people in life story work is not for everyone. The life story book can give people an opportunity to pay tribute to the older person by sharing a story or memory. However, this can be difficult for some people, depending on the nature of relationships and family history. Sensitivity and awareness of issues of privacy is also critical throughout the process. Reminiscence and life review can be used to create life story books (Haight et al., 2006); however, it is important that these methods be facilitated by skilled professionals such as clinical nurse specialists, occupational therapists, counselors, therapists, or social workers (Hargrave 1994; Jones, Lyons, & Cunningham, 2003; Plastow, 2006).

Life story books can be developed on the basis of one-to-one conversations with the person, listening to their story and documenting that story (Gibson, 1994; Wills & Day, 2008). Most life story books have been collected by engaging people in a series of supported workshops over a 6- to 8-week period, with the support of the older person, friends, care staff, and professionals (Hepburn et al., 1997; Caron et al., 1999; Clarke et al., 2003; Haight et al., 2006). Family carers also have a wealth of knowledge about the elder, and engaging them in developing the life story books is critical when the older person is cognitively impaired (Reichman, Leonard, Mintz, Kaizer, & Lisner-Kerbel, 2004). Participants need to be selected carefully, and our experiences have taught us that group membership should be kept at fewer than 10 people. McKeown et al. (2006) also suggested that life story work is a complex activity that is not suitable with large numbers. Potential participants can be invited to attend an information session on life story books. Consent, confidentiality, and ownership of the life story book need to be agreed upon with the individual, family, or group at the outset of the process. The literature supports the view

- Before engaging in life story work, facilitators need knowledge and training on life story methods.
- Think through any possible problems, and talk these over with your manager.
- Draw up a project plan for developing life story books, to include materials required, resources, supports, and costs.
- Select participants carefully with the support of colleagues and manager.
- Develop an information leaflet for stakeholders outlining the uses of the book and its benefits for the person, family carers, and health professionals.
- Carefully discuss with group members issues about the ownership and uses of the life story book, and discuss confidentiality issues.
- Ask group members to complete a consent form agreeing to the guidelines on group function and membership.
- Decide and allocate times for individual sessions/group work or both.
- Set goals on what is to be achieved and time frames with person/family carers.
- Have a good understanding of group processes, and set ground rules with group members.

Figure 41-1 Suggested checklist for facilitator.

Source: Day, M.R., & Wills, T. (2008). A biographical approach. *Nursing Older People*, 20(6), 24–26.

that ownership of the life story book remains with the older person and his or her family (Hewitt, 1998, 2000; McKeown et al., 2006).

Guidance on best practice for the introduction of life story work has been published in different formats; one of the most popular forms is DVDs (Murphy 1994; Mitchell & Chapman, 2007; Dementia Services Development Centre, 2007). A range of steps need to be considered by the facilitator before introducing story book activity. A suggested checklist is outlined in Figure 41-1.

Showing a completed life story book to individuals or groups will give them ideas about the information and memorabilia that could be included. Supporting materials, such as a ring-bound photograph album and guidelines on headings for inclusion in life story books, need to be provided to each person. The aim is to collect and gather information, stories, and photographs about the person with a view to compiling a unique life story book. Participants' life books can include family trees, photographs, documents, certificates, recipes, songs, poems, old newspaper clippings, family tributes, stories, and biography. From the authors' experiences, life story books have most often been concentrated on the positive aspects of people's lives, both past and present, and interestingly did not include anything on ill health or illness. Support groups create a forum for exchange of ideas, and while people feel challenged in creating life story books, the benefits outweigh the challenges. Engaging in developing life story books increases socialization for those involved through communicating, sharing, and listening to stories. As the life story book develops, it will provide insights into the uniqueness of each person's life and life experiences consistent with that described by Caron et al. (1999). The facilitator's skills are key to creating a supportive environment.

Barriers to Life Story Book Development

It is important to be aware that barriers may exist that can inhibit the development of life story books. For instance, a philosophy of care or organizational culture that does not see the benefits of life story work in the provision of quality care can be a barrier to implementing life story work approaches (Hepburn et al., 1997; Kunz, 2006). Past personal experience, the private nature of people, and ethical issues in relation to consent for older people with cognitive problems can also be prohibiting factors (Clarke et al., 2003). Barriers that have been put forward by older people and their families for not engaging in life story work include the timing of the process, emotional difficulties, poor support, and lack of time (Hepburn et al., 1997).

Memorabilia That Can Be Included in a Life Story Book

Showing a completed life story book to individuals or groups will give them ideas about the types of information and memorabilia that could be included. Suggestions are to find out about a person's life—childhood and school experiences, favorite games played, parents, siblings, relationships, work life, family life, hobbies, spiritual beliefs, routines, preferences, attitudes and values, and personality (Gibson & Burnside, 2005). Other types of memorabilia that have been included in life story books are birth/marriage certificates, personal recollections, old electricity bills, personal letters, personal objects, birthday cards, mortuary cards, old newspaper cuttings from the 1930s, recipes, and photographs (Wills & Day, 2008).

From the authors' experiences, Box 41-1 lists some areas of *significant life events* that could be used to guide the development of a life story book.

It is important that the items and stories to be included in the book are selected by the older person if at all possible (Haight et al., 2006), and professional ethics dictates that the story is accurately portrayed and presented (Hecht & O' Brien Tyrell, 2007). Collecting life stories and deciding what to include in a life story book can be challenging for all involved, but most would agree that it is worth the effort.

Benefits of Life Story Books for Relatives

Life story books have also been found to be beneficial for family members. The process of creating life story books can enhance relationships between the older person, family mem-

---

Box 41-1   Suggested Themes

Family Early Years
Childhood Days
Memories Growing Up
School Days
Relationships and Family Life
Holidays
Hobbies Now and in the Past
Likes & Dislikes
Stories, Heirlooms

    Day, M.R., & Wills, T. (2008). A biographical approach. *Nursing Older People*, *20*(6), 24–26.

---

bers, and carers, and can help unite families in the face of illness. Family members can assist in a variety of ways by providing photographs, stories, memorabilia, poems, and reflections. These photographs and memorabilia can bring the person's story alive, evoking memories for many people as they view the book, and allowing people to see the person behind the illness. From the authors' experiences, creating the life story books enabled family members to tell their stories about living with the illness, as well as providing autobiographical information on their relative. It created the opportunity for family members to reflect on their parents. The books can be used as a method of communication for people and can offer family, friends, and professionals a greater insight into the person through that person's life and history.

Boxes 41-2 and 41-3 are reflective extracts taken from a life story book written by a son for his father and mother.

Life Story Books as a Means of Promoting Person-Centered Care

There is an increasing need to meet the needs of older people and to enhance their quality of life in the context of the delivery of nursing care for older people. Patient, client, or person-centered care reflects the emergence of new approaches to work with older people in a range of care environments (Nolan, Davies, Brown, Keady, & Nolan, 2004). Key components of person-centered care are knowing the person as an individual and being responsive to individual and family characteristics, and providing care that is meaningful to the person in ways that respect their values, preferences, and needs (Talerico, O'Brien, & Swafford, 2003). The creation of a life story book is an important component in a person's identity and in the promotion and maintenance of self (Surr, 2006). Mitchell and Chapman

Box 41-2   Reflective Extract from a Son's Life Story Book

My Father
Fragile as life
We walked to the edge
Remembering diamonds that shimmered in sand
Remembering words we spoke through a glance.
Moments we missed
In times that were lost
And chords that we played on whispering nights.
All glories dissolve
As shadows we jumped
Rich in resolve, yet numb in defeat
Like death that meant loss
Of feelings on fire
And pain that meant fear
Of ghosts from the past.

My Dad like all Dads, is to me an extraordinary man. If I can trace one constant in his life it would be his love, kindness, and an admirable respect for others. He is hugely innocent and vulnerable, immensely complex and proud. A perfectionist and incredibly hard working. His life has been almost entirely about work and providing his family with the chances that sadly had never been available to him. As a family we were rich in cuddles and laughter and yet faced all the pain and hurdles that trying to bring up five children entailed.

His ethic was to provide and in order to do this he worked every God-given hour that each day could allow. Overtime and sacrifice; duty and dedication, that's what put bread on the table and kept us all in warmth and comfort. As a child I remember a determination in him to get us all to the top . . . of course this slowly changed and diluted into different realities as we grew up and realized our own determinations. . . . And like every teenager gallantly challenged his reign over us.

I have always felt a need to protect my Dad and often wonder why? He has adapted to every situation thrown at him over the years, largely I suppose because we all guarded him from the complexities of life. His relationship with my mother his only constant, and now the mark by which he tries to measure his current situation. They have a huge and enduring love. There has only been one person and one experience in each of their lives and that has been each other. Thus it seems understandable that he now tries to clutch to his only certainty, as his mind increasingly eludes him of the most basic cognitive functions.

Dad is a man of dreams, and I believe his mind often soars to places where only untarnished minds can go. I sometimes watch him trying to reason and see the confusion in his eyes . . . the helplessness and frustration of ineffective judgment clouding his mind and draining his insight. It is heartbreaking to observe, and all one can do is reach out to touch him and reassure him in whatever way he will allow at the time. He asked me tearfully about 2 years ago if something was wrong with him because he was aware of some significant change, and I told him the truth, explaining that Alzheimer's would make him forget even what I was explaining to him, but the one thing I begged him never to forget is that we love him dearly and will always be there to support him. He listened nobly and with dignity and thanked me for being honest and caring and said that he would do his best to stay well for as long as possible. He questioned that there must be a cure of some kind . . . sadly I told him no. His slide has been rapid and sustained, but I hope these days that in his aloneness he still holds on to the fact that he is loved and means more than he can ever imagine to all of his family.

If I trace a quality which he has given to me in abundance it must be a quiet gentlemanly charm. I am always conscious of manners and etiquette . . . this was drummed into me by both Mum and Dad from an early age, but even now in Dad's nebulous mind these traits are innate to his personality and character. I am incredibly proud of him and see him as both challenging and adorable. He responds best to cuddles and affection; never overly demonstrative in his life, he now yearns for our love and affection above all else. He is a private man and has only ever exposed his true nature to us at home. Even his own brothers and sisters he has kept at arm's length and has always refused to become too involved in their lives . . . choosing instead to surround himself with his wife and five sons. We are close because we respect one another and all lead independent lives. Dad has immense patience and understanding and allows us all the freedom that we need, but always insists that he is there with support and kindness if we ever need him.

I left the nursing home recently where he now lives and completely broke down in tears. The angst and horror of being with him and realizing that he wasn't quite sure of who I was; too much to bear. His life now quiet and noble has still been a huge success. I look at the marvelous work that he has done . . . the attention to detail and utter perfection which was always his benchmark. He has no bills left unpaid, no castles to bestow . . . just a legacy of hard work, sacrifice, and love. What more could I ask of the man that I am so lucky to call Dad and whom I shall love dearly and proudly forever.

Box 41-3   Reflective Extract from a Son's Life Story Book

My Mother
Take all my loves, my Love
Yea take them all.
What hadst thou then
More than thou hadst before?
No love, my Love
That thou may'st true love call
All mine was thine
Before thou had'st this more.
    —William Shakespeare

In my life of 50 years I have met and known many great women, most of whom were special and some of whom have been extraordinary in a host of diverse ways. I know a handful who are a cut above the rest and are as charismatic and radiant in their character as they are inspirational and magnetic in their aptitude and approach to life. My observations have taught me that women by and large have a far better overview of the human condition and have cognitive intuitions which are far superior and more immediate than those of their male counterparts. One woman who has been the soul of my world and counts among the best of all that I value in women has been my mother.

She has a selfless and enduring love which has been the driving force of her entire life. There was never a precise moment when Mum first realized that Dad was ill . . . just a growing catalogue of events and moments when she was puzzled by his lack of insight and growing failure to recall the most basic events from his short-term memory. He asked her one day if Princess Diana was still married to Prince Charles after the lady had been dead for many years. A visit to Mum's aunt whom he had known for a lifetime left him asking: who is that woman? Mum put all this down to getting old and forgetful and could never have foreseen the far more sinister undercurrent which lay ahead. Dad's personality almost changed overnight, it seemed, and suddenly she was a prisoner in her own home with a man she no longer knew. She was bullied and threatened, told to get out and go back to her own house, told never to use the phone and not even to speak to me when I rang. Her world was turned upside down . . . the misery and stark reality of living with a mid-term Alzheimer's patient became her only reality . . . not able to go outside . . . not able to talk . . . not able to summon help . . . not able to sleep in case Dad would try to climb out of a window . . . not able to have the washing machine or central heating fixed (Dad would not allow anyone into the house) . . . not able to get her hair done . . . not able to talk to Dad . . . not able to share with him . . . not able to breath calmly because his temperament could change so rapidly . . . torment and suffering . . . her eyes swollen from crying morning, noon, and night. The depth of despair made her feel unable to share her plight or even to seek outside help. Evenings seemed worse than days when Dad would often go through a morbid change of personality, and then we waited fearfully, wondering what lay ahead for the night and whether he would eventually fall asleep or not. Intense loyalty and love kept her by his side and looking after him during those dreadful 2 or 3 years. Despite the abuse and fear of a stranger with whom she now shared a home, she clung to the hope that Dad would get better and perhaps one day all would be well again. At one meeting with Dad's general practitioner, he introduced me as Ita's brother and at this juncture Dr. Hearty realized that something significant had changed in his mind and the ball started to roll . . . help from a variety of sources finally started to flow in. An exhausted and fragile Mum watched wearily as though from inside a mirror out upon a world where nothing made much sense anymore. The unpredictable had become the norm, and the fine line between sanity and insanity was often pushed way beyond acceptable boundaries. She maintained a dignity and selflessness throughout all this suffering and even on her 50th wedding anniversary had to acknowledge the fact that a celebration could never be possible . . . just the heartache that had now become the fabric of her daily life.

The nursing home and the quality of staff there have helped her immeasurably. Her tensions and sorrows have eased significantly in the past 3 months as she has witnessed love and care and individualism on a profoundly professional scale. For once during this terrible affair she knows that when she walks away from Dad the staff at the nursing home truly recognize him for the man that he was and understand his inconsistencies and confusion. They see what she sees; a lost soul in a beautiful mind from which even Alzheimer's cannot rob the dignity. Her heart is now more at peace as she waits for four buses every day. Her life has been hard and her sorrows many, but she has triumphed over all adversity and met every challenge. Like the words from Shakespeare that I quoted at the start of this reflection, she has always given all of her love . . . if we were to take more from her it would not increase the measure because we have always had everything from her in the first place. Mum is the most extraordinary, deep, intelligent, spiritual, hard working, selfless, and inspirational woman that I have ever known. She pushes the boundaries on every front and is the most loving soul that I have ever known. I am inordinately proud of her and realize what a great blessing and privilege it has been to be able to call her Mum . . . only five of us can do this (six in fact . . . including Dad) . . . and we all feel exactly the same way about her. An amazing woman, an amazing mother, an amazing human being . . . that's my Mum . . . who I love dearly.

(2007) suggest that a clearer understanding of what older people want or need in the present can be gained if their lives are seen in the context of their past. Life story books can give people a sense of identity and can provide a more holistic view of older adults for staff, helping them to get to know the person, and they offer the potential to enhance person-centered care (Clarke et al., 2003). Life story books contain details beyond what is included in care plans or health needs assessments, and they provide a basis for personalized care that can be used therapeutically to enhance communication (Hansebo & Kihlgren, 2000). Records or care plans in most care settings do not hold this type of biographical detail, yet that information is important in the delivery of quality, person-centered care (Wills & Day, 2008). The process can be therapeutic and beneficial in building and enhancing relationships with older people, family, and health professionals, thus improving quality of care (Caron et al., 1999).

Conclusion

Life story work or personal narratives have the potential to provide a greater insight into a client's needs and behaviors (Clarke, Hanson, & Ross., 2003; Johnson, 1976) and may help challenge ageist attitudes about later life (Meininger, 2006). Life story books are valuable tools and need to be seen "as a core activity in the forming of intimate family like settings" (Kunz, 2006, p. 12). Elford et al. (2005) stated that "encouraging older people to write stories provides a way of preserving a valuable historical resource of memories for future generations" (p. 313).

Education, knowledge, and guidance are critical to developing and understanding the importance of life story books in practice. The support of management and health professionals is important to creating opportunities to support older people/family members in developing a documentary of their life story. Clinical supervision, policy guidelines, ownership, and confidentiality need to be addressed before engaging in the process. Life story books are not for everyone, and facilitators need to have good interpersonal skills. Research on life story work is at a relatively early stage of development, but the findings thus far support it as a pleasant way to connect elders and those who care for and about them with their past, in order to enrich their present. The technique merits further study to provide additional evidence-based support for the potential of life story books in the realm of practice (McKeown et al., 2006).

References

Caron, W., Hepburn, K., Luptak, M., Grant, L., Ostwald, S., & Keenan, J. (1999). Expanding the discourse of care family constructed biographies of nursing home residents. *Families, Systems and Health, 17*, 323–335.

Clarke, A. (2000). Using biography to enhance the nursing care of older people. *British Journal of Nursing, 9*(7), 429–433.

Clarke, A., Hanson, E.A., & Ross, H. (2003). Seeing the person behind the patient: Enhancing the care of older people using a biographical approach. *Journal of Clinical Nursing, 12*(5), 697–706.

Day, M.R., & Wills, T. (2008). A biographical approach. *Nursing Older People 20*(6), 24–26.

Dementia Services Development Centre. (2007). *Switching on the light: An introduction to life story work* [DVD]. England: University of Sterling.

Elford, H., Wilson, F., McKee, K.J., Chung, M.C., Bolton, G., & Goudie, F. (2005). Psychosocial benefits of solitary reminiscence writing: An exploratory study. *Ageing and Mental Health, 9*, 305–314.

Gibson, F. (1994). What can reminiscence contribute to people with dementia? In J. Bornat (Ed.), *Reminiscence reviewed: Perspectives, evaluations, achievements* (pp. 46–60). Buckingham, UK: Open University Press.

Gibson, F., & Burnside, I. (2005). Group goals and contracts: Assessment and planning. In B. Haight & F. Gibson (Eds.), *Working with older people* (pp. 73–95). Sudbury, MA: Jones and Bartlett Publishers.

Guse, L., Inglis, J., Chicoine, J., Leche, G., Stadnyak, L., & Whitbread, L. (2000). Life albums in long term care: Resident, family & staff perceptions. *Geriatric Nursing, 21*(1), 34–37.

Haight, B.K., Gibson, F., & Michel, Y. (2006). The Northern Ireland life review/life storybook project for people with dementia. *Alzheimer's & Dementia, 2*, 56–58.

Hamilton, C., & Atkinson, D. (2009). A story to tell: Learning from the life-stories of older people with intellectual disabilities in Ireland. *British Journal of Learning Disabilities, 37*(4), 316–322.

Hansebo, G., & Kihlgren, M. (2000). Patient life stories and current situation as told by carers in nursing home wards. *Clinical Nursing Research, 9*(3), 260–279.

Hargrave, T.D. (1994). Using video life reviews with older adults. *Journal of Family Therapy, 16*(3), 259–268.

Heathcode, J. (2005). Part two: Choosing and individual reminiscence approach. *Nursing and Residential Care, 7*, 78–80.

Hecht, A., & O'Brien Tyrell, M. (2007). Life stories as heirlooms: The personal history industry. In J. A. Kunz & F. Gray Soltys (Eds.), *Transformational reminiscence: Life story work* (pp. 103–122). New York: Springer Publishing.

Hepburn, K.W., Caron, W., Luptak, M., Ostwald, S., Grant, L., & Keenan, J.M. (1997). The families stories workshop: Stories for those who cannot remember. *The Gerontologist, 37*(6), 827–832.

Hewitt, H. (1998). Life story books for people with learning disabilities. *Nursing Times, 94*, 61–63.

Hewitt, H. (2000). A life story approach for people with profound learning disability. *British Journal of Nursing, 9*, 90–95.

Hirst, S., & Raffin, S.R. (2001). Contemplating, caring, coping, conversing: A model for promoting wellness in later life. *Journal of Gerontological Nursing, 30*, 16–21.

Johnson, M.L. (1976). That was your life: A biographical approach to later life. In C. Carver & P. Liddiard (Eds.), *An ageing population* (pp. 98–113). Sevenoaks: Hodder and Stoughton.

Jones, C., Lyons, C., & Cunningham, C. (2003). Life review following critical illness in young men. *Nursing in Critical Care, 8*(6), 256–263.

Kunz, J.A. (2006). Using life-story circles to change the culture of LTC. *Ageing Today, 1*(1), 11–12.

McKeown, J., Clarke, A., & Repper, J. (2006). Life story work in health and social care: Systematic literature review. *Journal of Advanced Nursing, 55*(2), 237–247.

Meininger, H.P. (2006). Narrating, writing, reading: Life story work as an aid to (self) advocacy. *Journal of Advanced Nursing, 34*, 181–188.

Mitchell, R., & Chapman, A. (Eds.). (2007). *Dementia skills starters. Booklet 6: Understanding the importance of life story work.* Sterling, UK: Dementia Services Development Centre.

Murphy, C. (1994). *It started with a sea-shell: Life story work with people with dementia.* Sterling, UK: Dementia Services Development Centre.

Murphy, C., & Moyes, M. (1997) Life story work in state of the art in dementia care. In M. Marshall (Ed.), *State of the art in dementia care* (pp. 149–153). London: Centre for Policy & Ageing.

Nolan, M.R., Davies, S., Brown, J., Keady, J., & Nolan, J. (2004). Beyond 'person-centered' care: A new vision for gerontological nursing. *International Journal of Older People, 13*(3a), 45–53.

Plastow, N.A. (2006). Libraries of life: Using life history books with depressed care home residents. *Geriatric Nursing, 27*(4), 217–221.

Reichman, S., Leonard, C., Mintz, T., Kaizer, C., & Lisner-Kerbel, H. (2004). Compiling life history resources for older adults in institutions: Development of a guide. *Journal of Gerontological Nursing, 30*(2), 20–28.

Ryan, T., & Walker, R. (1985). *Making life story books.* London: British Agencies for Adoption and Fostering.

Ryan, T., & Walker, R. (1993). *Life story work: A practical guide to helping children understand their past.* London: British Agencies for Adoption & Fostering.

Surr, C. (2006). Preservation of self in people with dementia living in residential care: A socio-biographical approach. *Social Science and Medicine, 62,* 1720–1730.

Talerico, K.A., O'Brien, J.A., & Swafford, K.L. (2003). Person-centered care: An important approach for 21st century health care. *Journal of Psychosocial Nursing and Mental Health Services, 41*(11), 12–16.

Wills, T., & Day, M.R. (2008). Valuing the person's story: Use of life story books in a continuing care setting. *Clinical Interventions in Ageing, 18*(3), 547–552.

Woods, B., Spector, A., Jones, C., Orrell, M., & Davies, S. (2005). Reminiscence therapy for dementia. *Cochrane Database Systematic Review, 18*(2), CD001120.

Chapter 42

Care of the Elderly in South Korea

Yong Hae Hong

Introduction

The aging population in South Korea has increased dramatically (from 3.8% of the total population in 1980, to 9.1% in 2000, and 10.7% in 2009) and demographic changes have occurred, including a sharp decrease in the labor forces (Korean National Statistics Office, 2006–2009). In addition, the traditional family system in South Korea has changed due to changes in the industrial structures. Extended families have turned into nuclear families, and many of the elderly parents now live alone. To meet the challenges associated with these rapid demographic changes, it became necessary for the South Korean government to establish the Elderly Welfare Act and the Elderly Long-Term Care Insurance (Hyun, 2009).

The Elderly Welfare Act

Its Definition

The Elderly Welfare Act prescribes the government's policy on the specifics of welfare benefits for the elders in Korea (Elderly Welfare Act, 2009a,b). The objectives of the law are as follows:

1. to prevent illnesses among the elderly population,

2. to discover their illnesses early by medical check-ups and institute proper treatments,

3. to maintain their mental and physical health,

4. to take stringent measures that lead to stable lives for the elderly, contributing to the promotion of their health and welfare, and

5. to meet the demand for better quality of life for elders.

Background of the Establishment of the Elderly Welfare Act

Changes in the Elderly Population

The population of persons over 65 years of age was approximately 820,000 in 1960, comprising 3.3% of the country's total population; there were 1,460,000 people over age 65 in 1980, which was 3.8% of the whole. However, over the next two decades the elderly population increased by 77%. In 2000, 7.2% of the whole population was over age 65. Elders accounted for 9.1% of the total population in 2005 (Population estimates, population projections, 2006), and 10.7% in 2009; the elderly are expected to account for 14% of South Korea's population by the year 2018. It took just 18 years to turn an aging society to an aged society (Choi, et al., 2006). Korea has become one of the fastest-aged countries, which has resulted from a rapid decline in fertility rates and an increase in the average life expectancy. In 2008 the average length of life was 79.4 years; the average life span of men was 76.5 years and that of women was 83.3 years (Population estimates, population projections, 2006; Korean National Statistics Office, 2009; 2008 Life table, 2009).

Perception Change in Supporting the Family

Rapid industrialization and urbanization have caused South Koreans to change their perceptions about supporting their families. In the past, the eldest son was expected to support his parents and hold a memorial service for his ancestors, and in turn he would inherit his parents' property. However, under amendments to the Civil Code in 1977, not only the eldest son alone, but also any direct descendants could inherit their parents' property. Then both the eldest son and any direct descendants were expected to support their parents. Since that time it has been expected that the eldest sons would share their responsibility of supporting their parents with other direct descendents. The proportion of the population aged 65 years or older living alone was 8.9% in 1990, but increased to 18.8% in 2005; the proportion of elders doubled in the course of just 15 years (2005 Population and housing census, 2006). Almost one third (29%) of the elderly population is comprised of elderly couples who live together. Quality of life was found to be lower in single households than in elderly married couples (Ann, 2005).

Necessity of the Elderly Welfare Act

The number of nuclear families in Korea is getting larger, and people have tended to change their perception of supporting their family. There have been increasing issues related to poverty among the elderly, a housing shortage, loss of their social status and roles, and loneliness. These issues aroused the public's attention about the welfare of their elderly. It became apparent that old-age income security needed strengthening, and that public aid to the elderly should be extended. Furthermore, the elderly expected a better quality of life with welfare services given by nursing homes, senior citizen centers, and schools of senior citizens. To solve the issues and meet these demands of the elderly, the Elderly Welfare Act was established.

Characteristics of the Elderly Welfare Act

Since its enactment in 1981, the Elderly Welfare Act has been amended several times (Choi, et al, 2006; Hyun, 2009). The main purposes of the law are: implementing a home care nursing program; enforcing the National Pension Policy; implementing the National Healthcare Policy; providing the Old-Age Pension and jobs for the elderly; providing a variety of welfare facilities for the elderly; designating the Day of the Elderly (Oct. 2) and the Month of the Elderly (every October); and preventing elder abuse (Elderly Welfare Act 2009a,b).

The Elderly Welfare Act guarantees income security, housing, and medical treatment. Aside from these guarantees, there are also other welfare services for the elderly, as described in point 4, below.

1. Income security: To alleviate poverty among the elderly, the National Pension and Old-Age Pension is provided and jobs are offered.

2. Housing: Many residences have been established and are provided for the elderly.

3. Medical treatment: Health care is provided to prevent illnesses among the elderly and to solve problems with long-term care and isolation from the larger society.

4. Other welfare services: A variety of welfare services are provided by nursing homes, senior citizen centers, and schools of senior citizens. Other services exist to provide opportunities for leisure activities (Korean Ministry of Health & Welfare, 2008; Elderly Welfare Act, 2009a,b).

Welfare Facilities for the Elderly

The welfare facilities help the elderly and their families to stay healthy and enjoy the rest of their lives, provided with a variety of services and resources.

Activities of Welfare Facilities for the Elderly

1. Helping the elderly to participate in social activities
2. Supporting the business of the elderly
3. Giving discounts to the elderly
4. Providing medical check-ups
5. Organizing counseling and arranging with the elderly to be admitted to the facilities
6. Managing businesses relating to dementia
7. Managing businesses relating to medical rehabilitation for the elderly

Types of Welfare Facilities for the Elderly

There are two forms of welfare facilities for the elderly:

Admission facilities, which the elderly are actually admitted to, and

Use facilities, which the elderly use, but are not admitted to as a place to live.

There are two kinds of admission facilities: residential welfare facilities for the elderly, and medical welfare facilities for the elderly. Depending on people's mental and physical conditions, the facilities are divided into elderly housing facilities and nursing homes.

1. Admission facilities—According to the cost, the admission facilities are divided into:
   A. Complimentary
   B. Low-cost, and
   C. Charged.

2. Use facilities—There are two kinds: Welfare facilities for the elderly in home, and recreational welfare facilities for the elderly.

In all, there are five types of welfare facilities for the elderly: (1) residential welfare facilities for the elderly, (2) medical welfare facilities for the elderly, (3) welfare facilities for the elderly in home, (4) recreational welfare facilities for the elderly, and (5) specialized institute for protecting the elderly. (See Table 42-1.)

1. *Residential Welfare Facilities for the Elderly*

   Complimentary Elderly Care Facilities: The elders are admitted to these facilities and provided with meals and services 24 hours every day, free of charge.

   Low-Cost Elderly Care Facilities: The elders are admitted to these facilities and provided with meals and services 24 hours every day at low cost.

   Charged Elderly Care Facilities: The elders are admitted to these facilities and provided with meals and services 24 hours every day; the elders cover all the expenses.

   Low-Cost Elderly Housing Facilities: These housing facilities are offered at low cost to the elderly whose income is below the minimum amount that is set by the Minister of Health. These housing facilities are rented to the elderly by a lease contract or sold in lots to them. The elderly can get the benefits of residing in the facilities, counseling, and safety management.

   Charged Elderly Housing Facilities: This type of housing facilities are rented to the elderly by a lease contract or sold in lots to them. The elderly pay for the facilities, and get the benefits of residing in the facilities, counseling, and safety management.

TABLE 42-1   Types of Welfare Facilities for the Elderly

| Welfare Service Policy for the Elderly | | | | |
| System of Admission Facilities | | System of Use Facilities | | |
Residential Welfare Facilities	Medical Welfare Facilities	Welfare Facilities in Home	Recreational Welfare	Relevant Policy
1. Complimentary elderly care facilities	1. Complimentary nursing home	1. Home care nursing	1. Welfare centers for the elderly	1. Old-age pension
2. Low-cost elderly care facilities	2. Low-cost nursing home	2. Day custody	2. Schools of senior citizens	2. Supporting business of the elderly
3. Charged elderly care facilities	3. Charged nursing home	3. Short-term custody	3. Senior citizen centers	3. Giving preferential treatments
4. Low-cost elderly housing facilities	4. Specialized nursing home		4. Recreation centers for the elderly	4. Providing jobs
5. Charged elderly housing facilities	5. Charged specialized nursing home			5. Giving medical check-ups
	6. Specialized hospital for the elderly			

2. *Medical Welfare Facilities for the Elderly*

This type of facility provides residences as well as medical services.

Complimentary Nursing Home: The elderly are admitted to the home and provided with meals and medical services 24 hours a day, free of charge.

Low-Cost Nursing Home: The elderly are admitted to the home and provided with meals and medical services 24 hours a day at low cost.

Charged Nursing Home: The elderly are admitted to the home and provided with meals and medical services 24 hours a day; the elderly cover all the expenses.

Specialized Nursing Home: The elderly with severe illnesses such as dementia or stroke are admitted to the home and provided with meals and medical services 24 hours a day free of charge or at low cost.

Charged Specialized Nursing Home: The elderly above age 65 with severe illnesses such as dementia or stroke are admitted to the home and provided with meals and medical services 24 hours a day; the elderly cover all the expenses.

Specialized Hospital for the Elderly: The majority of the patients are the elderly. The dying elderly or those who suffer from senile disorders get treatments from the hospital.

3. *Welfare Facilities for the Elderly in Home*

The elderly reside in their own homes but get necessary services 24 hours a day from the facilities. Three types of services are offered:

Home Care Nursing: Recipients of this service are those who can't live without the aid of others, due to mental or physical disabilities.

Day Custody: Recipients of this service are those who need day care due to mental or physical disabilities or weakness.

Short-Term Custody: Disabled elderly or those over age 60 in frail health, whose families cannot take care of them due to unavoidable circumstances, are admitted and cared for short-term.

4. *Recreational Welfare Facilities for the Elderly*

The recreational welfare facilities provide the elders with a variety of services so that they can stay healthy and participate in leisure activities. There are four types:

Welfare centers for the elderly
Schools of senior citizens
Senior citizen centers
Recreation centers for the elderly

Income Security for the Elderly

1. The Income Security Policy for the Elderly (see Table 42-2)

2. Structure of the Income Security Policy for the Elderly (see Table 42-3)

3. Main Contents of the Income Security Policy for the Elderly

The National Pension

The National Pension Policy has been implemented since 1999, and Koreans from 18 to 60 residing in Korea are obligated to join the National Pension Plan (Hyun, Cho, Yun & Kim, 2006).

TABLE 42-2   The Income Security Policy for the Elderly

Direct Income Security Policy		Indirect Income Security Policy	
Methods	Programs	Methods	Programs
Public pension	Civil Servant Pension (1960)	Reduction of fees	Free or Fee Reduction of Public Facilities (1980)
	Military Pension (1963)		Distribution of Bus Tickets (1990)
	Teaching Staff of Private School (TSPS) Pension (1975)		
	National Pension (1988)		
Public aid	Livelihood Security (1961)	Employment promotion	The Elderly Bank (1981)
	The National Basic Livelihood Security Act (2000)		The Elderly Work place (1986)
	Old-Age Allowance (1991)		The Center for the Elderly Employment (1992)
	Old-Age Pension (1997)		
	Affiliation with the Elderly (1989)		
	Distribution of Transportation Allowance each month		
Social benefits	Benefits of supporting old parents (1986)	Supporting business of the elderly	Giving priority to open a government-run shop (1989)
Personal pension	Severance Pay (1953)	Tax relief	Inheritance Tax Deduction (1986)
	Personal Pension Trust		Income Tax Deduction (1986)

TABLE 42-3　Structure of the Income Security Policy for the Elderly

Classification	Average Income Bracket			Low Income Bracket	
3rd	Civil servants/ Teaching staff of private schools (TSPS)/ Soldiers	Employees	Self-employed	Low income over the poverty line	Below the poverty line
	Personal Pension				
2nd	Civil servant pension TSPS pension Military pension	Severance pay (company pension)	—	—	—
		National pension	—	—	Old-age pension (about 620,000 people)
	The Lowest: Poverty Line				
1st	—	—	—	Exemption of tax payment (about 4.3 million people)	Basic livelihood security policy (about 1.37 million people)

Under the National Pension Policy, an insured person turning age 60 can receive a pension benefit. In 2004, 582,000 people (13.9% of South Korea's elderly population) were beneficiaries of public pensions such as the National Pension, Civil Servant Pension, TSPS Pension, and Military Pension.

The National Basic Livelihood Security Act

The family receives the amount that subtracts income from the minimum cost of living per household as the National Basic Livelihood Pension. In 2006, the minimum cost of living for a family of one person was $358, and the family received a maximum of $306.

Figure 42-1 The old-age pension system in South Korea.

Per-capita income below $530 / Property below $56,000

- Amount of the government fund: $365,782,100
- Number of recipients: 1,257,155 people
- Amount of benefits
  - National Basic Livelihood Security beneficiaries
    - Under age 80: $38.5
    - Over age 80: $42.8
  - The Elderly with Low Income
    - No spouse: $29.9
    - Co-recipients with his/her spouse: $26.18

Source: 2004 Korean national survey on living profile and welfare needs of the elderly. (February 18, 2005). The Ministry of Health, Welfare and Family Affairs (2004). Retrieved March 15, 2010 from http://mw.go.kr./front/jb/sjb030304vw.jsp?PAR_MENU_ID =03030304&BOARD_FLAG=03&CONT_SEQ=32392&page=1.

For a family of four, their minimum cost of living was $1,000 and the family received a maximum of $856 (Introduction to health and welfare services for the elderly, 2006).

The Old-Age Pension

According to official statistics from the Ministry for Health, Welfare and Family Affairs (MIHWFA) in 2006, the Old-Age Pension is offered to 1,257,155 of the elderly in South Korea who have less than $56,000 worth of property and less than $530 per capita yearly income (see Figure 42-1) (Introduction to health and welfare services for the elderly, 2006).

Income Sources of the Elderly

Income sources of the elderly are the Public Pension, National Basic Livelihood Pension, Old-Age Pension, and Transportation Allowance. Earned income, income from a business, and other social insurance benefits are calculated into their income sources (2008 Korean national survey on living profile and welfare needs of the elderly, 2009).

The Elderly Long-Term Care Insurance

The Elderly Long-Term Care Insurance System aims to offer Medicare services and home-visit care for senior citizens who have difficulty performing the activities of daily living (ADL) because of chronic degenerative diseases. This insurance system has been implemented since July 2008. The elderly long-term care insurance fee is 4.78% of the National Health Insurance (NHI) fee individually (equal to 0.2547% of the employee's monthly income) (The elderly long-term care insurance Act, 2010).

The beneficiaries of the insurance are senior citizens over age 65 who have difficulty in performing ADL, or those under age 65 with chronic degenerative diseases. The Elderly Long-Term Care Insurance Program is funded by national health insurance at 60%, with government and out-of-pocket payments each set at 15 to 20%.

Within grade 3, senior citizens and chronic degenerative disease patients are given home care services such as home visiting, bathing, and health aid equipment. They can also get long-term care and medical treatments in nursing home or hospital settings. In the home care setting, the elder pays 15% of expenses for care services, whereas in an institutional setting the elder pays 20% of the cost (The elderly long-term care insurance Act, 2010).

Senior citizens who are not within the grade 3 category receive care from the community health center in the area of their residence. If senior citizens are admitted to the specialized hospital for the elderly, their medical service expenses are covered by national health insurance. Those who live in remote areas such as rural fishing and agricultural villages can also receive a cash reimbursement, with which they can receive home care provided by family members. Family members having a national license of Personal Care Assistance can also have cash back when they provide care for an elderly family member at their home in the city. The government plans to expand the program to provide coverage for medical expenses and home care services for all of the elderly and chronic degenerative disease patients.

Conclusions

1. Elders who live in South Korea get income security from the National or Public Pension, Old-Age Pension, National Basic Livelihood Pension, free or reduced-fee public facilities, or from their jobs.

2. Health care is provided in order to prevent illnesses of the elderly, and to avoid problems related to long-term care and being isolated from society. The service expenses are covered by national health insurance and elderly long-term care insurance.

3. Residential care is provided by elderly care facilities, elderly housing, nursing homes, home care nursing, day custody, and short-term custody.

4. The elderly can receive a variety of services through recreational welfare facilities such as welfare centers for the elderly, schools of senior citizens, senior citizen centers, and recreation centers for the elderly.

References

Ann, K. S. (2005). Study on the quality of life and social support of married couples and single households elderly. *Journal of the Korea Gerontological Society. 25*(1). 1-19.

Choi , Y. H., Shin, K. R., Ko, S. H., Kong, S. J., Kong, E. S., Kim, M. A., et al. (2006). *Elderly and health.* Seoul: Hyunmoonsa.

Elderly Welfare Act. (2009a). Center for National Law and Information. Retrieved February 20, 2010, from http://law.go.kr/IsSc.do?menuid=o&p1=&query.

Elderly Welfare Act. (2009b). The Ministry for Health, Welfare and Family Affairs, Retrieved February 20, 2010, from http://mohw.go.kr/front/jb/sjb04011s.

Hyun, O. S., Cho, C. Y., Yun, E. K., & Kim, Y. Y. (2006). Textbook about Korean elderly welfare. Seoul: Yupoong Public company.

Hyun, Oye-Sung (2009). Seeking for 'Science of the Elderly Welfare'—Study trend and task of the elderly welfare. *Journal of the Welfare for the Aged. 44.* 279-302.

Korean Ministry of Health & Welfare. (2008). Elderly policy. Retrieved from: http://english .mw.go.kr/front_eng/jc/sjc0105mn.jsp?PAR_MENU_ID=1003&MENU_ID=100305

Korean National Statistics Office. (2006). Estimation on future populations. Retrieved from: http://kosis.kr/eng/e_stat_OLAP.jsp?org_id=101&tbl_id=DT_1B35001&stts_nm=Population %20Projections%20and%20Summary%20indicators%20for%20Korea&vwcd=MT_ETITLE& listid=&olapAt=Y&itm_id=&lang_mode=eng

Korean National Statistical Office. (2009). Vital Statistics 2004-2009. Retrieved from: http://kosis.kr/eng/e_stat_OLAP.jsp?org_id=101&tbl_id=DT_1B8000F&stts_nm=Vital%20 statistics(number%2C%20rate)&vwcd=MT_ETITLE&listid=&olapAt=Y&itm_id=&lang_mode=eng

Population estimates, population projections (November 21, 2006). Korea National Statistical Office. Retrieved February 25, 2010, from http://www.Kostat.go.kr /board_notice/Board Action.do?/method=view&board_id=144&seq=14&Num<news_attach>.

The elderly long-term care insurance Act (2010). Retrieved March 8, 2010 from http://law .go.kr/lsSc.do?menuId=0&p1=&query=%EB%85%B8%EC%9D%B8%EC%9E%A5%EA%B8%B0%E C%9A%94%EC%96%91%EB%B3%B4%ED%97%98%EB%B2%95&x=27&y=12#liBgcolor0.

2006 Introduction to health and welfare services for the elderly (February 10, 2006). The Ministry for Health, Welfare and Family Affairs, Retrieved February 20, 2010, from http://mw.go.kr ./front/jb/sjb030301vw.jsp?PAR_Menu_ID=03&Menu_ID=03030301&BOARD_ID=1003& BOARD_FLAG=02&CONT-SEQ=36825&page=1.

2008 Korean national survey on living profile and welfare needs of the elderly. (February 13, 2009). The Ministry for Health, Welfare and Family Affairs. Retrieved March 15, 2010 from http://mw.go.kr./front/jb/sjb030301vw.jsp?PAR_MENU_ID=03&MENU_ID=03030301& BOARD_ID=1003&BOARD_FLAG=03&CONT_SEQ=217530&page=1.

2008 Life table (December 9, 2009). Korea National Statistical Office. Retrieved February 25, 2010 from http://www.Kostat.go.kr/board_notice/BoardAction.do?/method=view&board_id=144&seq =89&Num<news_attach>.

Chapter 43

Physiologic Aspects of Frailty in Aging and Possible Interventions

Gee-youn Kwon, Soo-kyung Kim, and Yeonghee Shin

Frailty in the elderly is a very serious matter because it not only reduces their quality of life, but it also shortens their life expectancy. In recent years, researchers and gerontologists have recognized frailty as a promoting factor of the aging process. There are a number of physiological factors associated with cellular aging throughout the human life cycle. For instance, according to the mitochondrial theory of aging, leakage of reactive oxygen species (ROS) from the mitochondrial respiratory system causes damage to DNA, protein, and lipids; chronic accumulation of such damages exhausts the homeostatic reserve, resulting in cellular aging. This cellular damage can induce telomeric erosion during chromosomal duplication, resulting in telomeric shortening of differentiated cells as well as stem cells. Frailty is indirectly linked to factors other than physiologic effects, including psychosocial stress. The authors' purpose is to give an overview of frailty and how it relates to aging, to offer the physiologic correlates to frailty, and to identify the risk factors and propose interventions that nurses and other healthcare professionals can utilize in the care of the elderly.

Background

The improvement of socioeconomic conditions, medical care, and the quality of life during the last several decades has brought a reduction of overall morbidity and mortality, resulting in increasing life expectancy in all industrialized countries (World Health Organization [WHO], 2002). As people age and lose functional capacity, often succumbing to disabling disease, it becomes important to understand the role of frailty in the aging process. Because people age at different rates, it is difficult to evaluate these trajectories. Frailty is expressed as a balance between biomedical and psychosocial components, and it is important to recognize the special needs of frail elderly people (Rockwood, Fox, Stolee, Robertson, & Beattie, 1994). The CSHA (Canadian Study of Health and Aging) Clinical Frailty Scale was developed for clinicians. The CSHA Clinical Frailty Scale is both predictive and easy to use (Rockwood et al., 2005; Mitnitski, Graham, Mogilner, & Rockwood, 2002).

Frailty is not a medical term, but rather is a commonly used word to refer to a state of fragility, delicacy, and weakness. We often use the term when referring to someone's state of health, such as, "she still looks frail after her long illness." Until recently, the medical profession has tended to think of frailty as a general descriptor rather than a medical concept. It wasn't until the early days of space travel, when the young and fit astronauts returned from space and complained about their sense of frailty, that the term began to be taken seriously. We now know that weightlessness in space causes: (a) a decrease in muscle strength and work capacity; (b) loss of calcium and phosphate from the bones, as well as loss of bone mass; and (c) a decrease in maximum cardiac output, and in the capacity of other body systems (Guyton & Hall, 2000). Thus space medicine drew attention to frailty as a scientifically important concept for the first time.

Nowadays, geriatric clinicians and researchers recognize frailty as an unmistakable and critical parameter of the terminal aging process, and frailty has become an emerging clinical entity. On a review using a MEDLINE or NCBI (National Center for Biotechnology Information) search it was found that frailty was cited in over 1000 articles from 1989 to 2005. Frailty is now defined as a multidimensional syndrome of loss of reserves (energy, physical ability, cognition, and health) that gives rise to vulnerability (Mitnitski et al., 2002). Frailty is a valid and clinically important construct that is easily recognizable by clinicians, and even by family members and acquaintances. Frailty can yield valuable predictive information in terms of both service and research on aging. Frailty, sarcopenia, falls, and aging are very familiar concepts among nurses, physicians, and other healthcare professionals. Sarcopenia, weakness of muscle and physical ability, is a major syndrome of frailty. Currently, a number of experimental studies have reported that frailty along with sarcopenia is associated with mitochondrial dysfunction (Ku, Brunk, & Sohal, 1993).

Frailty and Sarcopenia

The causes of human aging are complex, and sarcopenia is one of the most critical syndromes associated with frailty (Nair, 2005; Kujoth, Leeuwenburgh, & Prolla, 2006). Mechanisms of sarcopenia are also complex at the cellular and molecular levels. Human aging is associated with muscle atrophy, so-called sarcopenia, with weakness and functional impairment. It starts in the fourth decade of life with a rate of strength loss of about 1% per year, accelerating with each passing decade (Hadley & Dutta, 1995; Doherty, 2003). Progressive sarcopenia in old age is ultimately central to the development of frailty associated with impairment in the ability to perform activities of daily living. Mechanical force on bone is essential for modeling and remodeling of bone tissue, processes that increase bone strength and mass. Body weight and weight-bearing exercise provides a direct mechanical force on bones; the largest voluntary loads on bone come from muscle contractions. Changes in bone mass and muscle strength correlate over the life span (Frost, 1997). The extent and duration of any period of immobilization or inactivity stemming from illness or aging is dramatic: only 50% of patients admitted to an intensive care unit return to work within a year (Bams & Miranda, 1985), and over 50% of women older than 65 who sustain a hip fracture never walk again (Cooper, 1997).

However, a growing body of evidence suggests that mitochondrial dysfunction is a major contributor to sarcopenia (Nair, 2005). Association between mitochondrial dysfunction and sarcopenia has been observed in a number of single skeletal muscle fibers from mammalians, including humans (Kujoth et al., 2006; Zhan et al., 2006).

Mitochondrial Theory of Aging

To understand frailty, it is important to understand the pathophysiology of human aging. Currently, numerous experimental studies support the association between mitochondrial dysfunction and cellular aging, linking indirectly but ultimately to frailty. Within the cell, mitochondria are the sites where the accumulative products of respiration are exchanged, as well as the sites of energy production in the form of adenosine triphosphate (ATP). Accordingly, mitochondria have a high rate of both oxygen consumption and ATP production. However, only a small proportion of this oxygen (less than 3%) generates free radicals (so-called reactive oxygen species, ROS) which are toxic to DNA, protein, and lipid. Studies have demonstrated that cellular aging is associated with a significant accumulation of such markers (free radicals and ROS) of oxidative stress, and accumulation of oxidized proteins in many tissues is considered a hallmark of aging (Harper, Monemdjou, Ramsey, & Weindruch, 1998). The more tissues overwork, the more free radicals will accumulate; consequently, a commonly held paradigmatic view for the mitochondrial theory of aging was "live fast, die young." This view was based on the observation of the inverse relationship between mitochondrial ROS production and longevity in mammalian species (Harper, Monemdjou, Ramsey, & Weindruch, 1998). However, we have to remember that human cells are also equipped with enzymes defending against oxidative damages, minimizing mitochondrial DNA mutation and cellular apoptosis, as well as an anti-aging protein, SIRT (Harper et al., 1998; Harman, 1972; Miquel, 1992).

The "mitochondrial theory of aging" seems to be able to explain a variety of experimental investigations, clinical observations, and interventional studies on aging. In his seminal paper, Harman (1972) states the critical role of mitochondria within the context of his "free radical theory of aging." The mitochondrial theory of aging is supported by a large number of experiments related to cellular aging, such as neurons and muscle cells, and the renewing cells, as well as clinical intervention studies showing the effects of calorie restriction and physical exercise on aging.

Aging of Permanent Cells

Theoretically, organismal aging is associated with cellular aging. Human tissues and organs consist of terminally differentiated nondividing cells and renewing cells. The terminally differentiated cells, having been generated in appropriate numbers in the embryonic stage, are retained throughout adult life. Almost all nerve cells and skeletal muscle cells seem never to divide, and they cannot be replaced if lost; thus they are known as permanent cells. However, it is clear that permanent cells maintain and renew their organelles; nerve cells have to renew organelles such as synapses to keep the continuous informational flow, and heart muscle cells have to continuously adjust and distribute the blood load throughout an individual's lifetime. Their life cycles are metabolically active, driven by aging-sensitive cellular and molecular mechanisms that are susceptible to oxidative stress and death (Toescu, 2005).

The aging of a normal brain is not, as previously thought, associated with a decrease in neuronal numbers, but instead is associated with a small decline in cognitive and memory functions, at the level of synaptic activity (Toescu, 2005). In the aged nervous tissue, mitochondria are chronically depolarized. This mitochondrial depolarization affects their capacity to produce adenosine triphosphate (ATP) and their ability to reduce their production of free radicals. The ATP content in the brain slices of old animals was about 50% lower than that of younger animals, indicating decreased functional reserve. Such changes in the metabolic status would decrease the homeostatic reserve of the neurons and increase their susceptibility to injury. Toescu summarized normal brain aging as a decrease in the neuronal homeostatic reserve, which is equivalent to frailty (Rockwood et al., 2005).

The majority of skeletal and heart muscle cells are terminally differentiated permanent cells, and loss of muscle mass occurs as a result of the aging process. As mentioned previously, the term sarcopenia has been adopted to describe this loss of muscle mass. Sarcopenia involves significant alteration in the architecture that originates from the loss of some myofibers and the remodeling of the remaining myofibers. An exaggerated loss of contractile proteins and overall decreased muscle size seen with aging are believed to be due to a decreased rate of muscle protein synthesis; however, the mechanism of sarcopenia is not yet completely understood (Nair, 2005).

Replicative Senescence of Stem Cells and Renewing Cells

Most tissues and organs consist of multiple tissue-specific cell types. The size and function of tissues and organs are maintained by progeny cells of tissue-specific stem cells. Those progeny cells are produced from stem cells through multiple steps of differentiation, and are called renewing cells. Their rates of renewal vary widely from tissue to tissue. Very long-lived renewing cells such as liver, blood vessel, and pancreas cells renew by simple duplication, whereas other families of renewing cells such as blood cells, bone cells, skin cells, and others undergo complex differentiation steps from stem cells during cell renewals. Those renewing cell populations have an aging problem. Historically, Leonard Hayflick (1965) demonstrated that normal primary fibroblasts could not be maintained indefinitely in serial culture, and he proposed a concept of limited life span. The impact of aging on hematopoietic stem cells has also been studied by using numerous assays, including colony-forming unit-spleen (CFU-S) activity, bone marrow transplantation, and serial transplantation (Bryder, Rossi, & Weissman, 2006; Wobus & Boheler, 2005). The phenomenon of the replicative senescence (loss of proliferative capacity) of normal human cells occurs after a number of population doublings in vitro or in vivo (Hayflick, 1965). Replicative senescence is known now to be caused by a DNA-damage response that is triggered by uncapped telomeres of the chromosomes (von Zglinicki, 2002), which in turn result from replication-driven loss of telomere repeat sequences in the absence of telomere extending polymerase, telomerase. Telomere shortening rate and replicative life spans of cells can also be greatly accelerated by DNA-damaging oxidative stress (von Zglinicki, 2002). In summary, telomeres are regions of repetitive DNA, located at the ends of chromosomes (much like the tips at each end of shoelaces), which protect the ends of the chromosome from deterioration (and thus from loss of the chromosome's memory of DNA). Telomere shortening in length is associated with the processes recognized as aging (i.e., frailty and longevity), and with some types of cancer. Scientific and public interest in telomeres recently increased when three scientists (Elizabeth Blackburn, Carol Greider, and Jack Szostak) were awarded the 2009 Nobel Prize in Physiology or Medicine for their discovery of how chromosomes are protected by the telomeres and the enzyme telomerase.

Stem cells replenish tissues and organs throughout life. Tissue-specific stem cells have the ability to self-perpetuate through a process known as self-renewal, as well as to produce a daughter cell that will undergo differentiation and expansion. In general, stem cells are believed to have slow turnover and reside in specialized niches, so that only a few are activated at a time. Existence of tissue-specific stem cells has been amply demonstrated in many tissues and organs, including nervous, muscular, cardiac, hepatic, hematopoietic, and vascular systems (Bryder et al., 2006; Wobus & Boheler, 2005). Still unclear has been the effect of aging on the stem cells themselves; endothelial and hematopoietic stem cell aging seems to be due to the telomeric shortening described previously (Kurz, Decary, Hong, Trivier, Akhmedov, & Erusalimsky, 2004; Allsopp, Morin, DePinho, Harley, & Weissman, 2003). Although it has become clear that stem cells also age, it appears that the life span of human stem cells far exceeds the human life expectancy (Deasy et al., 2005).

Stress and Aging

Many people would agree that people who report feeling stressed over a long period of time look older than their age in years. However, the exact mechanisms by which such stress accelerates organismal aging are not well known. Understanding of the associations between stress and cellular aging has clinically significant implications for human health.

Cawthon et al. (2003) reported that telomere shortening is strongly associated with higher mortality rates in the elderly. Fitzpatrick et al. (2007) also confirmed Cawthon's observation by measuring the leukocyte telomere in 419 elderly with risk of cardiovascular disease (CVD). Brouilette, Singh, Thompson, Goodall, & Samani, (2003) investigated whether subjects with myocardial infarction (before 50 years of age) had shorter leukocyte telomeres. Patients with early myocardiac infarction had leukocyte telomere lengths that were equivalent to those typical of a person about 11 years older than the controls. Irie, Asami, Nagata, Miyata, & Kasai (2001) investigated the relationship between work-related stress and the formation of a type of oxidative DNA damage known as 8-hydroxydeoxyguanosine (8-OH-dG). These researchers concluded that psychological stress and perceived overwork appeared to be related to the pathogenesis of cancer via formation of 8-OH-dG, particularly in female workers. In another investigation, Irie and colleagues (Irie, Asami, Ikeda & Kasai, 2003) also investigated the association of psychological depression and biomarkers of cancer-related oxidative DNA damage, 8-OH-dG in leukocytes. A positive correlation between the leukocyte 8-OH-dG levels and high scores on a depression scale were observed, and they concluded that psychological depression was related to cancer risk due to oxidative DNA damage in female workers, possibly via neutrophil activation.

In another study on stress, Epel and her collaborators (2004) investigated the relationship between chronic life stress and telomere lengths of peripheral blood mononuclear cells. They compared 19 healthy mothers (control) and 39 mothers with chronically ill children (caregiving mothers). The investigation was designed to measure perceived stress of the caregivers (caregiving status and chronicity of caregiving stress based on the number of years since a child's diagnosis). Both perceived stress and chronicity of stress of the caregiving mothers was shown to be associated with higher oxidative stress, lower telomerase activity, and shorter telomere length. Those parameters are known determinants of cellular senescence and longevity. Their investigation provided evidence that psychological stress induces telomere shortening and that such stress could promote earlier onset of age-related disease.

Calories and Aging

Historically, the fact that calorie restriction extends life span had been discovered in mice in the 1940s in the United States, and in an epidemiologic survey of mortality records of Okinawan fishermen in Japan after the Second World War. By the 1990s the relationship of calorie restriction and longevity had been confirmed in a range of organisms including yeast, worms, and mammals.

Eventually, the proteins extending the life span in these organisms through calorie restriction were identified, isolated and named Sir2, the silent information regulator 2. In a human cell, there are seven Sir2 proteins (SIRT1 through SIRT7), and each anti-aging protein is distributed in different organelles such as cytoplasm, mitochondria, nucleolus, and nucleus. SIRT proteins function as an anti-apoptosis-like protein in association with other cellular proteins (Michishita, Park, Burneskis, Barrett, & Horikawa, 2005). For example, calorie restriction in humans was reported to increase muscle mitochondrial biogenesis (Civitarese et al., 2007). Recent progress in the field of calorie restriction has been summarized by Anderson and Weindruch (2006), in which three clinical trials are mentioned: Meyer et al. (2006) reported protective effects of calorie restriction on cardio-vascular disease; Heilbronn et al. (2006) reported on insulin-lowering effects; and Larson-Meyer et al. (2006) described effects on human obesity. There is still a need for additional research on diet and aging, such as the work by Chevalier and colleagues (Chevalier, Gougeon, Nayar, & Morais, 2003) showing that frailty exacerbates age-related changes in protein catabolism and reduction in muscle mass. At low protein intakes, muscle protein degradation is interpreted as a defense mechanism to save the brain and other vital organs from protein deficiency, at the expense of muscle. Based on their findings, these researchers have recommended increased protein intakes over long periods of time for frail elderly.

In summary, research on the effects of calorie restriction on aging has a long history (Anderson & Weindruch, 2006), and its molecular mechanism seems to be the mitochon-drial biogenesis (Civitarese et al., 2007). Caloric restriction such as intermittent (alternate-day) fasting reduced body weight, serum glucose, and insulin levels, and increased the resistance of neurons in the experimental animal brains to excitatory stress (Anson et al., 2003). Additional research is needed to further explicate the role of nutrition in prevent-ing frailty and contributing to healthy aging.

Physical Exercise and Aging

Before we discuss the merits of physical activity in the elderly, it seems useful to provide a summary of muscle functions. First, the mass of skeletal muscle accounts for an average of 40% of our body weight. Secondly, in the absence of nutrient intake, muscle protein serves as the principal reservoir to replace blood amino acid taken up by other tissues. Third, muscle protein turnover has one of the fastest rates among the tissue proteins. Muscle protein breakdown takes place during immobilization, fasting, starvation, and space flight. Lastly, the depletion of muscle mass is incompatible with life under the unique circumstances of starvation or anorexia and bulimia. It should be noted that even functional changes in skeletal muscle and progressive sarcopenia are ultimately central to the development of frailty (Guyton & Hall, 2000; Wolfe, 2006).

Fortunately, long-term physical activity is effective in reducing aging-related morbidity and mortality (Wolfe, 2006). Even better, resistance exercise is known to reverse aging in human skeletal muscles and to increase muscle strength, function, and mass in the elderly in the ninth decade of life (Paffenbarger et al., 1994). The molecular mechanisms observed seemed to be mitochondria biogenesis and recovery of functions in the muscle cells (Paf-fenbarger et al., 1994; Fiatarone et al., 1990; Melov, Tarnopolsky, Beckman, Felkey, & Hub-bard, 2007). As insulin and amino acids have also been shown to enhance muscle mitochondrial biogenesis and mitochondrial protein synthesis, nutritional balance and regular exercise have been found to be useful in controlling metabolic and cardiovascular diseases in the elderly (Wolfe, 2006). These findings have important implications in the care of the aged and in health promotion for all age groups.

Summary and Recommendations

Frailty is defined as a loss of vital reserve (energy, physical ability, cognition, health) that results in physiologic vulnerability (Rockwood et al., 2005). The observable clinical symptoms are muscle weakness, osteoporosis, transient cognitive impairment, and signs of deteriorating health. Frailty has been seen to occur after long-term illness, starvation, incarceration, or aging. Young people can more easily recover from a state of frailty. In contrast, recovery is not as simple, nor as complete for the elderly of advanced ages. In two large-scale mortality studies of aging populations by Fried and his collaborators, it was shown that mortality of the frail aging population was sixfold higher than that of the normal aging population (Fried et al., 2001; Fried, Ferrucci, Darer, Williamson, & Anderson, 2004).

Frailty is a very critical physical state for the elderly, because this syndrome is increasingly recognized as a warning sign of imminent death within a few years (Rockwood et al., 2005). Rockwood and his collaborators (Rockwood et al., 2005) applied their CSHA Clinical Frailty Scale to 2305 elderly patients and determined the ability of the scale to predict death or need for institutional care. Each one-category increment of this scale increased the medium-term risks of death (21.2% within about 70 months, 95% CI 12.5%~30.6%) and entry into an institution (23.9%, 95% CI 8.8%~41.2%) in multivariable models that adjusted for age, sex, and education. These findings confirmed that frailty is a valid and clinically important construct that is easily recognizable by physicians, nurses, and other healthcare professionals.

Frailty increases healthcare costs and can be linked to the economic burden of a nation. Japan cares for about one million (8% of the population) frail bed-ridden elderly patients (Sasaki et al., 1996). According to Sasaki et al. (1996), the healthcare expenses of frail elderly people are approximately five times those of ordinary elderly people, even when adjusting for common medical expenses. According to Fried et al. (2004), about 20% of patients aged 80 or older were bedridden during the early 21st century in the United States, while other relatively healthy elders 80 years of age or older were expected to live to become centenarians (Fried et al., 2004).

Nurses and other healthcare professionals can investigate ways to decrease frailty in the elderly and contribute to containing healthcare costs, thus permitting funds to be used for improving the quality of life for the elder population. A major strategy to decrease or prevent frailty can be drawn from the conclusions of the Framingham studies. The findings from the two Framingham studies show that the longevity of individuals who live to age 65 or beyond depends on his or her lifestyle between 40 and 60 years of age (Terry et al., 2005; Yashin et al., 2006). In short, healthy lifestyles contribute to people surviving cardiovascular disease, cancer, and stroke between 40 and 60 years of age. Dietary restriction seems to reduce cancer formation and kidney disease, and even increases the resistance of neurons to dysfunction and degeneration in the experimental models of Alzheimer's and Parkinson's disease as well as stroke (Anderson & Weindruch, 2006). With or without dietary restriction, exercise or physical training for cardiovascular fitness that is within reach of most healthy older adults is known to reverse aging (Meyer et al., 2006; Larson-Meyer et al., 2006; Wolfe, 2006; Paffenbarger et al., 1994; Fiatarone et al., 1990; Melov et al., 2007). Furthermore, aerobic training was shown to improve cardiovascular fitness as well as increase the plasticity of the aging human brain (Colcombe et al., 2004).

All of these results suggest that aging processes can be reversed and that frailty can be delayed to a certain degree by exercise, and modifications in dietary intake, including increased protein (Chevalier et al., 2003) and vitamin D intake (Montero-Odasso & Duque, 2005). Given nursing's historically close contact with elders, nursing science may be in a unique position to improve the health of mankind, particularly upcoming elders, by promoting a healthy lifestyle to avoid frailty, so that more can live their last days to the fullest.

References

Allsopp, R.C., Morin G.B., DePinho, R., Harley, G.B., & Weissman, I.L. (2003). Telomerase is required to slow telomere shortening and extend replicative lifespan of HSCs during serial transplantation. *Blood, 102,* 517–520.

Anderson, R.M., & Weindruch, R. (2006). Calorie restriction: Progress during mid-2005~mid-2006. *Experimental Gerontology, 41,* 1247–1249.

Anson, R.M., Guo, Z., de Cabo, R., Iyun, T., Rios, M., Hagepanos, A., et al. (2003). Intermittent fasting dissociates beneficial effects of dietary restriction on glucose metabolism and neuronal resistance to injury from calorie intake. *Proceedings of the National Academy of Sciences, 100,* 6216–6220.

Bams, J.L., & Miranda, D.R. (1985). Outcome and costs of intensive care. A follow-up study on 238 ICU-patients. *Intensive Care Medicine, 11,* 234–241.

Brouilette, S., Singh, R.K., Thompson, J.R., Goodall, A.J., & Samani, N.J. (2003). White cell telomere length and risk of premature myocardial infarction. *Arteriosclerosis, Thrombosis, Vascular Biology, 23,* 842–846.

Bryder, D., Rossi, D.J., & Weissman, I.L. (2006). Hematopoietic stem cells: The paradigmatic tissue-specific stem cell. *American Journal of Pathology, 169,* 338–346.

Cawthon, R.M., Smith, K.R., O'Brien, E., Sivatchenko, A., & Kerber, R.A. (2003). Association between telomere length in blood and mortality in people aged 60 years or older. *Lancet, 361,* 393–395.

Chevalier, S., Gougeon, R., Nayar, K., & Morais, J.A. (2003). Frailty amplifies the effects of aging in protein metabolism: Role of protein intake. *American Journal of Clinical Nutrition, 78,* 422–429.

Civitarese, A.E., Carling, S., Heilbrom, L.K., Hulver, M.H., Ukropkova, B., Deutsch, W.A., et al. (2007). Calorie restriction increases muscle mitochondrial biogenesis in healthy humans. *PLoS Medicine, 4,* e76.

Colcombe, S.J., Kramer, A.F., Erickson, K.I., Scalf, P., McAuley, E., Cohen, N.J., et al. (2004). Cardiovascular fitness, cortical plasticity, and aging. *Proceedings of the National Academy of Sciences, 101,* 3316–3321.

Cooper, C. (1997). The crippling consequences of fractures and their impact on quality of life. *American Journal of Medicine, 103,* 12S–17S.

Deasy, B.M., Gharaibeh, B.M., Pollett, J.B., Jones, M.M., Lucas, M.A., Kanda, Y., et al. (2005). Long-term self-renewal of postnatal muscle-derived stem cells. *Molecular Biology of the Cell, 16,* 3323–3333.

Doherty, T.J. (2003). Invited review: Aging and sarcopenia. *Journal of Applied Physiology, 95,* 1717–1727.

Epel, E.S., Blackburn, E.H., Lin, J., Dhabhar, F.S., Adler, N.E., Morrow, J.D., et al. (2004). Accelerated telomere shortening in response to life stress. *Proceedings of the National Academy of Sciences, 101,* 17312–17315.

Fiatarone, M.A., Narks, E.C., Ryan, N.D., Neredith, C.N., Lipsitz, L.A., & Evans, W.J. (1990). High-intensity strength training in nonagenarians. Effects on skeletal muscle. *Journal of the American Medical Association, 263,* 3029–3034.

Fitzpatrick A.L., Kronmal, R.A., Gardner, J.P., Psaty, B.M., Jenny, N.S., Tracy, R.P., et al. (2007). Leukocyte telomere length and cardiovascular disease in the cardiovascular health study. *American Journal of Epidemiology, 165,* 14–21.

Fried, L.P., Ferrucci, L., Darer, J., Williamson, J.D., & Anderson, G. (2004). Untangling the concepts of disability, frailty, and comorbidity: Implications for improved targeting and care. *Journals of Gerontology Series A: Biological Sciences and Medical Sciences, 59,* 255–263.

Fried, L.P., Tangen, C.M., Walston, J., Newman, A.B., Hirsch, C., Gottdiener, J., et al. (2001). Cardiovascular health study collaborative research group. Frailty in older adults: Evidence for a phenotype. *Journals of Gerontology Series A: Biological Sciences and Medical Sciences, 56,* M146–156.

Frost, H.M. (1997). On our age-related bone loss: Insight from a new paradigm. *Journal of Bone & Mineral Research, 12,* 1539–1546.

Guyton, A.C., & Hall, J.E. (2000). Chapter 43. Aviation, high-altitude and space physiology. In A.C. Guyton & J.E. Hall, *Textbook of medical physiology* (10th ed., pp. 496–503). New York: WB Saunders Company.

Hadley, E.C., & Dutta, C. (1995). The significance of sarcopenia in old age. *Journals of Gerontology Series A: Biological Sciences and Medical Sciences, 50,* spec No: 1–4.

Harman, D. (1972). Free radical theory of aging: Dietary implications. *American Journal of Clinical Nutrition, 25,* 839–843.

Harper, M.E., Monemdjou, S., Ramsey, J.J., & Weindruch, R. (1998). Age-related increase in mitochondrial proton leak and decrease in ATP turnover reactions in mouse hepatocytes. *American Journal of Physiology, 275,* E197–E206.

Hayflick, L. (1965). The limited in vitro life time of human diploid cell strains. *Experimental Cell Research, 37,* 614–636.

Heilbronn, L.K., de Jonge, L., Frisard, M.I., DeLany, J.P., Larson-Meyer, D.E., Rood, J., et al. (2006). Effect of 6-month calorie restriction on biomarkers of longevity, metabolic adaptation, and oxidative stress in overweight individuals: A randomized controlled trial. *Journal of the American Medical Association, 295,* 1539–1548.

Irie, M., Asami, S., Ikeda, M., & Kasai, H. (2003). Depressive state relates to female oxidative DNA damage via neutrophil activation. *Biochemical Biophysical Research Communication, 311,* 1014–1018.

Irie, M., Asami, S., Nagata, S., Miyata, M., & Kasai, H. (2001). Relationships between perceived workload, stress and oxidative DNA damage. *International Archive of Occupational Environmental Health, 74,* 153–157.

Ku, H.H., Brunk, U.T., & Sohal, R.S. (1993). Relationship between mitochondrial superoxide and hydrogen peroxide production and longevity of mammalian species. *Free Radical Biology and Medicine, 15,* 621–627.

Kujoth, G.C., Leeuwenburgh, C., & Prolla, T.A. (2006). Mitochondrial DNA mutations and apoptosis in mammalian aging. *Cancer Research, 66,*: 7386–7389.

Kurz, D.J., Decary, S., Hong, Y., Trivier, E., Akhmedov, A., & Erusalimsky, J.D. (2004). Chronic oxidative stress compromises telomere integrity and accelerates the onset of senescence in human endothelial cells. *Journal of Cell Science, 117,* 2417–2426.

Larson-Meyer, D.E., Heilbronn, L.K., Redman, L.M., Newcomer, B.R., Frisard, M.I., Anton, S., et al. (2006). Effect of calorie restriction with or without exercise on insulin sensitivity, beta-cell function, fat cell size and ectopic lipid in overweight subjects. *Diabetes Care, 29,* 1337–1344.

Melov, S., Tarnopolsky, M.A., Beckman, K., Felkey, K., & Hubbard, A. (2007). Resistance exercise reverses aging in human skeletal muscle. *PLoS One, 5,* e465.

Meyer, T.E., Kovacs, S.J., Ehsani, A.A., Klein S., Holloszy, J.O., & Fontana, L. (2006). Long-term caloric restriction ameliorates the decline in diastolic function in humans. *Journal of American College of Cardiology, 47,* 389–402.

Michishita, E., Park, J.Y., Burneskis, J.M., Barrett, J.C., & Horikawa, I. (2005). Evolutionarily conserved and nonconserved cellular localizations and functions of human SIRT proteins. *Molecular Biology of the Cell, 16,* 4623–4635.

Miquel, J. (1992). An update on the mitochondrial DNA mutation hypothesis of cell aging. *Mutation Research, 275,* 209–216.

Mitnitski, A.B., Graham, J.E., Mogilner, A.J., & Rockwood, K. (2002). Frailty, fitness and late-life mortality in relation to chronological and biological age. *BMC Geriatrics, 2,* 1.

Montero-Odasso, M., & Duque, G. (2005). Vitamin D in the aging musculoskeletal system: An authentic strength preserving hormone. *Molecular Aspects of Medicine, 26,* 203–219.

Nair, K.S. (2005). Aging muscle. *American Journal of Clinical Nutrition, 81,* 953–963.

Paffenbarger, R.S., Jr., Kampert, J.B., Lee, I.M., Hyde R.T., Leung, R.W., & Wing, A.L. (1994). Changes in physical activity and other lifeway patterns influencing longevity. *Medical Science and Sport Exercise, 26,* 857–865.

Rockwood, K., Fox, R.A., Stolee, P., Robertson, D., & Beattie B.L. (1994). Frailty in elderly people: An evolving concept. *Canadian Medical Association Journal, 150,* 489–495.

Rockwood, K., Song, X., Macknight, C., Bergman, H., Hogan, D.B., McDowell, I., et al. (2005). A global clinical measure of fitness and frailty in elderly people. *Canadian Medical Association Journal, 173,* 489–495.

Sasaki H., Sekizawa, K., Yanai, M., Arai, H., Yamaya, M., & Ohrui, T. (1996). Will aging of population make Japan less productive? *Journal of American Geriatric Society, 44,* 1013–1014.

Terry, D.F., Pencina, M.J., Vasan, R.S., Murabito, J.M., Wolf, P.A., Hayes, M.K., et al. (2005) Cardiovascular risk factors predictive for survival and morbidity-free survival in the oldest-old Framingham Heart study participants. *Journal of the American Geriatric Society, 53,* 1944–1950.

Toescu, E.C. (2005). Normal brain aging: Models and mechanisms. *Philosophical Transactions of the Royal Society of London. Series B, Biological Sciences, 360,* 2347–2354.

von Zglinicki, T. (2002). Oxidative stress shortens telomeres. *Trends in Biochemical Science, 27,* 339–344.

Wobus, A.M., & Boheler, K.R. (2005). Embryonic stem cells: Prospects for developmental biology and cell therapy. *Physiological Review, 85,* 635–678.

Wolfe, R.R. (2006). The underappreciated role of muscle in health and disease. *American Journal of Clinical Nutrition, 84*, 475–482.

World Health Organization (WHO). (2002). *Active aging: A policy framework.* Geneva: World Health Organization.

Yashin, A.I., Akushevich, I.V., Arbeev, K.G., Akushevich, L., Ukraintseva, S.V., & Kulminski, A. (2006). Insights on aging and exceptional longevity from longitudinal data: Novel findings from the Framingham Heart Study. *Age (Dordrecht, Netherlands), 28*, 363–374.

Zhan, J.M., Sonu, R., Vogel, H., Crane, E., Mazan-Mamczarz, K., et al. (2006). Transcriptional profiling of aging in human muscle reveals a common aging signature. *PLoS Genetics, 2*, e115.

Chapter 44

Resilience in Older Adults

Barbara Resnick

Resilience

The word "resilience" comes from the Latin world *salire*, which means "to spring up," and the word *resilire* which means "to spring back." Resilience, therefore, refers to the capacity to spring back from a physical, emotional, financial, or social challenge. Being resilient indicates that a person can adapt in the face of tragedy, trauma, adversity, hardship, and ongoing significant life stressors (Newman, 2005). Resilient people tend to manifest adaptive behavior, especially with regard to social functioning, morale, and somatic health (Wagnild & Young, 1993), and they are less likely to succumb to illness (O'Connell & Mayo, 1998). Resilience, as a component of the individual's personality, develops and changes over time through ongoing experiences with the physical and social environment (Hegney et al., 2007; Lee, Brown, Mitchell, & Schiraldi, 2008). Moreover, resilience seems to be a dynamic quality that facilitates people's ability to overcome the challenges of stressful life events or family life transitions. Increasingly, resilience is conceptualized as a characteristic that allows the person to cope even during times of great challenge. Resilience can, therefore, be perceived as a dynamic process that is influenced by life events and challenges (Grotberg, 2003; Hardy, Concato, & Gill, 2002; 2004).

Increasingly there is evidence that resilience is important to successful aging. Older adults bring with them many experiences in which they have learned to be resilient, and thus many are experts in this area. In nursing, and in other areas of health care, we should not focus on the negative aspects of aging (e.g., functional and cognitive decline). Rather we need to recognize and strengthen resilience and help people to optimally cope with the changes that they will have to endure as they age.

Older women who have successfully recovered from orthopedic or other stressful events describe themselves as resilient and determined (Resnick, Orwig, Zimmerman, Simpson, & Magaziner, 2005) and tend to have better function, mood, and quality of life than those who are less resilient (Hardy, Concato, & Gill, 2004). Resilience has also been associated with adjustments following the diagnosis of dementia (Harris, 2008), widowhood (Rossi, Bisconti, & Bergeman, 2007), management of chronic pain (Karoly &

Ruehlman, 2006), and overall adjustment to the stressors associated with aging (Ong, Bergeman, Bisconti, & Wallace, 2006).

Types of Resilience

Resilience can be expressed in different ways: health resilience (Sanders, Lim, & Sohn, 2008), psychological resilience (Boardman, Blalock, & Button, 2008), emotional resilience (Chow, Hamagani, & Nesselroade, 2007), and dispositional resilience (Rossi, Bisconti, & Bergeman, 2007). Health resilience is the capacity to maintain good health in the face of significant adversity. This focuses on such things as the ability to recover from a hip fracture or to continue to maintain functional independence in the face of significant changes in range of motion or increasing pain associated with activity. An example of an older woman with health resilience is one who continues to bathe and dress herself in the morning in the face of bilateral torn rotator cuffs due to degenerative joint disease and the inability to raise her arms more than 40 degrees. It may take her hours, but she is determined to persist in this independence and to overcome this adversity and challenge. Likewise one can picture the 100-year-old woman who has sustained a hip fracture but status point hemiarthroplasty; she is actively engaged in rehabilitation and months later is back in the exercise room working out on the Nu-step!

Psychological resilience is focused on being able to maintain a positive affect regardless of the situation. This type of resilience refers to one's capacity to withstand stressors and not manifest psychological dysfunction, such as mental illness or persistent negative mood. Generally it is considered a person's capacity to avoid psychopathology despite difficult circumstances. With aging there are many psychological stressors that can occur, such as the death of a spouse or a child, chronic illness, fear of falling or of physical or psychological abuse, or role loss. There are many older adults who demonstrate psychological resilience after the loss of a spouse or a child, for example. They have endured many losses over a lifetime, and they utilize their past experiences, knowledge, and skills to appropriately grieve and yet maintain a sense of life engagement and acceptance. Moreover, they often can grow from the experience and teach others how to deal with such losses. Psychological resilience is particularly important in response to violence and terrorism; it has been studied in older Holocaust survivors and and in those affected by the September 11, 2001 terrorist attacks.

Emotional resilience is described as the ability to maintain the separation between positive and negative emotions in times of stress. To be emotionally resilient means to be able to spring back emotionally after suffering through difficult and stressful times in one's life. This is the person who can withstand stress and not succumb to negative emotions such as anger, anxiety, and depression. Emotionally resilient people have a specific set of attitudes about themselves and their role in the community, and they can cope with life stressors more efficiently and effectively than their nonresilient peers. An emotionally resilient individual, for example, will be able to remain positive and optimistic in the face of daily stressors of life such as an unexpected and unwanted visitor, the loss of a favorite piece of jewelry, or the disappointment when a friend or family member forgets one's birthday or a card during holiday seasons. Emotionally resilient people are quick to accept, adjust, and bounce back to their normal emotional state.

Cognitive resilience describes the capacity to overcome the negative effects of setbacks and associated stress on cognitive function or performance. Some who are challenged by cognitive changes, such as memory loss or word-finding difficulty, become easily overwhelmed and ineffective. On the other end there are some who, when faced with challenges, show few or no negative effects of stressors on cognitive performance. The cognitive resilience literature has historically focused on specific contexts in which some people succumb to stress while others are better able to withstand or overcome it. Resilience, therefore, may help to explain patterns of cognitive decline associated with normal aging and other degenerative processes.

Factors That Influence Resilience

Initial resilience research focused on identifying the factors or qualities that were associated with resilience (Table 44-1). These qualities include positive interpersonal relationships; incorporating social connectedness with a willingness to extend oneself to others; strong internal resources; having an optimistic or positive affect; keeping things in perspective; setting goals and taking steps to achieve those goals; high self-esteem; high self-efficacy; determination; spirituality, which includes life purpose, religiousness or a belief

TABLE 44-1 Resilient Qualities or Traits Commonly Noted in Older Adults	
Positive interpersonal relationships	Proactive problem solving
Strong self-efficacy	Mutual empathy for others and tolerance of differences
Positive self-esteem	
A sense of purpose	Ability to use and enjoy pleasurable experiences
Spirituality	Ability to focus on concrete goals
Ability to use humor	Ability to share feelings
Creativity	Seeking connectiveness
Acceptance of changes (physical and mental)	Flexibility
	Ability to learn from adversity
Maintaining a positive attitude	Inspiration and creativity
Ability to identify and utilize resources	A sense of purpose
Self-determination	Mastering the possible and accepting the impossible
Optimism	
	Ability to appraise a crisis

in a higher power, creativity, humor, and a sense of curiosity (Boardman, Blalock & Button, 2008; Bonanno, Galea, Bucciarelli, & Vlahov, 2007; Hegney et al., 2007; Kinsel, 2005; Tedeschi & Kilmer, 2005). Understanding the many factors that influence resilience (physical, cognitive, or emotional resilience) can help guide interventions so that we can optimize resilience and help older adults cope and respond to the many stressors encountered throughout the aging process.

Positive Interpersonal Relationships

Interpersonal relationships include interactions with family, friends, colleagues, and other acquaintances in one's social network. These relationships may help with a variety of activities such as enjoyment, physical assistance, or psychological assistance and support. Involvement in interpersonal relationships and activities, whether receiving or giving the help, serves as a psychological buffer against stress, anxiety, or depression which commonly occur with aging. Feeling needed and having a role in such interactions is critical. Interpersonal activities also help people to cope with losses, maintain a sense of belonging, and strengthen self-esteem and self-efficacy.

Strong Internal Resources: Self-Efficacy, Self-Esteem, Determination, Problem Solving

Self-efficacy is the belief in one's ability to organize and execute a course of action to achieve a specific outcome; it is therefore relevant to resilience. This cognitive control of behavior is based on two types of expectations: (1) self-efficacy expectations, which are beliefs in one's capabilities to perform a course of action to attain a desired outcome; and (2) outcome expectancies, which are the beliefs that a certain consequence will be produced by personal action. Self-efficacy can be influenced by four major sources of information: (1) mastery of the activity the person is focused on, such as using a computer; (2) verbal encouragement from respected others, such as getting positive feedback about exercise from an exercise trainer or one's healthcare provider; (3) role models or seeing others engage in an activity one is trying to do, such as seeing someone older with more physical disability participate in a Tai Chi class; and (4) physiological feedback or the feelings or experiences one has with an activity, such as pain associated with exercise, or fear with balance shifting during Tai Chi. Self-efficacy is generally believed to be activity specific. That is, one might have strong self-efficacy about an exercise activity but low self-efficacy about playing cards or learning a new language. Individuals with strong self-efficacy in an area will be more resilient when faced with challenges to completing the activity. An individual who does not do well on the first quiz in a language class but has strong self-efficacy to succeed in this endeavor will be resilient and will continue to come to class despite not doing well.

Self-esteem is different from self-efficacy because it reflects one's appraisal of his or her self-worth. People who have a positive self-worth, accept and like themselves, and refrain from being "too hard on themselves" tend to be resilient and psychologically successful (Byles & Pachana, 2006). The ability to accept one's self is particularly important in aging due to the many physical and mental changes that can occur, as well as the role losses. With age, for example, the older person may note impairments in his or her ability to go up the stairs, carry grocery bags, complete a crossword puzzle, or remember how to get to a daughter's home. These changes can be devastating unless one has the resilience to accept the change and appreciate what he or she is still able to do. Self-esteem need not, and should not, decline with age despite the commonly experienced physical and mental changes that occur, such as declines in strength and memory.

Determination, or hardiness, which may in part be a personality trait, has been noted to be an important aspect of resilience. Determined individuals tend to be more confident in their ability to cope and to take advantage of the resources, internal and external, that help them to adjust, accept, and cope with the challenges encountered in life. Strengthening determination and hardiness can be achieved by helping the individual to problem solve and stay focused on the positive rather than the negative—the "I can" versus "I can't" perspective. This determination is particularly challenging in physical resilience as older adults may be extremely fearful of falling or getting hurt, and thus are unwilling to engage in physical activities that they feel might put them at risk for trauma.

Optimism, Positivism, and Keeping Things in Perspective

It has repeatedly been noted that focusing on positive outcomes and avoiding a focus on negative facts is critical to resilience (Harris, 2008). Positive emotions and the use of humor are recommended as a way to help eliminate, or cancel out, the impact of negative emotions. Have you ever spilled your coffee in the morning and thought that was an omen that you would have a really bad day? And then you went on to have a bad day? Alternatively, one can spill coffee, laugh and make a new pot and the rest of the day goes well. Pessimism, versus optimism, is negatively associated with resilience. Pessimistic thinking results in a tendency to generalize all outcomes to be bad or worse than expected. It may be expressed in the older adult who comes into the clinic with the negative attitude that he or she will have to wait for a long time, or that he or she will be receiving a bad diagnosis associated with a clinical symptom recently experienced. Bottom line, attitude makes a difference—a pessimist is one who makes difficulties of his opportunities, and an optimist is one who makes opportunities of his difficulties. True optimism can be learned over time through practice. Many older adults have a lifetime stance of turning all difficulties into opportunities, or at least in not seeing them as major challenges.

Spirituality

Spirituality, considered broadly, includes a sense of self and purpose, creativity, humor, and a curiosity and willingness to learn and experience new things. Establishing a sense of connection to others and a purpose for being, such as marching for world peace, exploring creative endeavors and taking art classes, and/or trying new activities such as learning to play an instrument or speak a foreign language, are all activities that indicate resilience. Religious beliefs and practices may decrease the sense of loss of control and helplessness often experienced when faced with challenges, and they may provide the cognitive framework and structure to help individuals overcome age-associated challenges. Religion is also important in giving meaning to suffering and helping to establish a sense of hope rather than persistent despair. Spiritual or religious beliefs and practices are important components of almost all cultures, and thus some aspect of religion or spiritual beliefs will likely be present.

Religious coping can occur in a variety of ways. For some it may result in a reappraisal of the experience and a desire to learn from the event through religious lessons or experiences. Others may engage in an active religious surrender in which they put the problem or challenge into God's hands. Some use the experience to feel a part of a larger spiritual force and overall plan for humanity. Whatever the approach, religion and spirituality are an important aspect of resilience, and will likely be more or less present depending on one's proclivity toward religion and spirituality.

Practical Clinical Applications of Resilience

Assessment of Resilience

Given the importance of resilience in older adults' ability to cope, recover, and/or succeed in dealing with a specific challenge or age-related life event, it is critical to assess resilience and know what resources one has to work with toward the recovery process. Increasingly resilience is believed to be a human ability that can be developed over time. Older adults, by virtue of surviving through decades of life experiences, tend to be resilient (Nygren, Jonsen, Gustafson, Norberg & Lundman, 2005). These people have lived through losses, including physical changes such as declines in vision, hearing, or physical abilities, social losses such as loss of parents, siblings, spouses, and in some cases children, and role-related losses. Although they may not have been successfully resilient in all of these experiences, they have accrued some positive experiences in which they were resilient and motivated and thus recovered from the challenge. Thus, when working with older adults it is particularly helpful to explore prior experiences with challenges, and to establish strengths with regard to recovery that suggest resilience and motivation.

Talking with individuals about past experiences may be the most comprehensive way in which to establish prior evidence of resilience; however the stories provided may be difficult to evaluate in terms of quantitatively assessing resilience. As an alternative to a qualitative assessment of resilience, scales reflecting individual correlates of resilience such as self-efficacy, coping, optimism, vitality, or self-esteem can be used. Resilience can also be measured directly using one of the scales described in Table 44-2. These measures can be completed during a clinical assessment of a patient to gain insight into the strength of his or her resilience. There is also a generic measure of resilience which can be done online.

TABLE 44-2   Measures of Resilience Used Among Older Adults

Measure	Description
Ego Resiliency Scale (Block & Kremen, 1996)	The Ego Resiliency Scale was developed initially for young adults. Respondents were asked to answer 14 items using a 4-step continuum: 1 = does not apply at all; 2 = applies slightly if at all; 3 = applies somewhat; and 4 = applies very strongly. The items include statements such as: I am more curious than most people; I like to do new and different things; I enjoy dealing with new and unusual situations; and I get over my anger at someone reasonably quickly. When the scale is used with young adults, the Cronbach's alpha reliability was .72 to .76.
The 25- and 14-Item Resilience Scale (Wagnild & Young, 1993)	The 25- (and 14-) Item Resilience Scale was developed as a general measure of resilience for adults across the life span. Initially the measure included 25 items reflecting five inter-related components that constitute resilience: Equanimity reflecting the ability to "go with the flow"; perseverance or determination; self-reliance reflecting a belief in one's ability to manage; meaningfulness or a belief that life has meaning; and existential aloneness or a sense of uniqueness. Participants respond by either agreeing or disagreeing with the statements on a scale of 1 (disagree) to 7 (agree). The responses are summed, and a higher score reflects stronger resilience. Prior research has demonstrated evidence of internal consistency (alpha coefficient of .91), test-retest reliability, and construct validity of the measure based on a significant correlation between resilience and life satisfaction, morale, and depression when used with older adults (Wagnild & Young, 1993).
The Resilience Scale (Hardy et al., 2004)	To complete the Resilience Scale, participants identify the most stressful life event they experienced in the past 5 years and respond to a series of 9 questions about their response to that event. There was evidence of internal consistency, with an alpha coefficient of .70, and test-retest reliability with an intraclass correlation coefficient of 0.57. Validity was based on a significant correlation between resilience and having few depressive symptoms, and good to excellent self-rate health (Hardy, 2004).

(continued)

TABLE 44-2 Continued	
Measure	**Description**
Dispositional Resilience Scale, also called the Resilience Scale for Adults (Bartone, Ursano, Wright, & Ingraham, 1989; Friborg, Hjemdal, Rosenvinge, & Matinussen, 1997)	The Dispositional Resilience Scale (DRS) is a 45-item questionnaire that includes 15 commitment, 15 control, and 15 challenge items. There is a 4-point response scale used to rate participant agreement with items ranging from 1 (Completely true) to 4 (Not at all true). A total dispositional resilience score is created based on responses. The original DRS was modified to be appropriate for older adults (Rossi et al., 2007). There was evidence of internal consistency with an alpha of 0.83, and validity based on a statistically significant relationship between Sense of Coherence and Hopkins Symptom Checklist (Rossi et al., 2007), and a statistically significant difference in Dispositional Resilience among patients and healthy volunteers (Friborg et al., 1997).

The measure is available at http://health.discovery.com/centers/mental/resilience_assessment/resilience_assessment.html. This tool considers different characteristics of resilience, and the person is asked to describe how often he or she displays those characteristics. For example, the tool asks about whether the person is optimistic; sees difficulties as temporary and expects to overcome them and have things turn out well; if he or she is good at solving problems logically; if when experiencing a crisis he or she calms down and focuses on taking useful actions; if one is playful, finds the humor in a situation, and is able to laugh at oneself; and if one commonly thinks up creative solutions to challenges. There are 16 items, and the individual receives a resilience score based on responses.

Interventions to Strengthen Resilience

Once resilience has been evaluated, it is critical to intervene and help older adults to strengthen and build resilience to help cope with an immediate crisis and/or develop the tools for future insults. A resilience-enhancing approach underscores the need to seek resources and sources of natural support within clients' environment. Some general approaches to helping patients to become more resilient are shown in Table 44-3. Interventions to stimulate and build resilience are focused in three areas: (1) developing disposition attributes of the individual, such as vigor, optimism, and physical robustness; (2) improving socialization practices; and (3) strengthening self-efficacy, self-esteem, and motivation through interpersonal interactions as well as experiences. These three areas are not necessarily mutually exclusive, and the interventions that can strengthen physical

TABLE 44-3   General Intervention Strategies to Strengthen Resilience

- Acknowledge loss and vulnerability as experienced by the individual.
- Identify the patient's source of stress.
- Attempt to help stabilize or normalize the situation.
- Help the patient take control.
- Provide resources for change.
- Promote self-efficacy.
- Collaborate with the patient to encourage self-change.
- Strengthen the patient's problem-solving abilities.
- Address and encourage positive emotions.
- Listen to the patient's stories and encourage past review of recovery from stressors.
- Help the patient make meaning of the adverse or challenging event.
- Help the patient find the benefit to the adverse or challenging event.
- Assist the patient in transcending the immediate situation and giving it purpose.

robustness may also improve socialization practices and strengthen self-efficacy. For example, encouraging an older adult to participate in a dance class because he or she enjoys dance and has previously excelled in this activity may also increase socialization and strengthen self-efficacy and self-esteem.

It is important not to oversimplify interventions to strengthen resilience or ignore the larger context in which the person lives. For example, recommending participation in a dance class for someone who lives in a community in which such activity is considered frivolous or an insufficient source of physical activity may result in decreasing self-esteem and can have a negative impact on resilience. Thus multifaceted approaches to optimizing resilience are needed. Risk-oriented strategies should be considered with all interventions to help assure that older adults are not exposed to experiences that might decrease resilience. Environmental interventions such as chairs, beds, and toilets that facilitate successful transfers are needed to assure that resilience isn't undermined. Social networking systems that help disseminate opportunities for successful activities and increase reach to older adults are likewise important and useful interventions to consider when trying to strengthen resilience.

Programs Known to Strengthen Resilience

There are several community and provider-based programs that have been shown to strengthen resilience among older adults, and these can be implemented within communities as resources allow. The Experience Corps is one such program. Personal resilience is bolstered for older adults who participate in this program through continued meaningful contributions to society and social engagement. The participants in Experience Corps volunteer to work or are paid to work as tutors and mentors to students in urban public elementary schools and after-school programs. In 23 cities across the United States, more than 2000 Experience Corps members have affected the lives of more than 23,000 students. Experience Corps participants have helped to boost student academic performance and strengthen ties between the schools and their neighborhoods.

The benefits for members of the Experience Corps are important contributors to successful aging, with an overwhelming percentage of participants saying the experience raised their self-esteem, increased their circle of friends, and improved their lives overall (Morrow-Howell, McCrary, Gonzales, McBridge, Hong, & Blinne, 2008). The expanded social network, increased physical activity, and other benefits of remaining engaged in meaningful work in the community through Experience Corps increases participants' physical, mental, and social activity, all of which have been shown to strengthen resilience, at least in some instances.

Another community-based program believed to strengthen resilience is a group exercise program called EnhanceFitness (EnhanceFitness Programs, 2009). In hour-long classes, up to 25 people are grouped together and practice aerobic, strength, flexibility, and balance exercises that have been shown to increase strength, boost activity, and elevate mood. All of these outcomes are believed to build and sustain resilience and enhance health. Classes are taught by certified fitness instructors trained in the EnhanceFitness program. Participants' progress is tracked through a series of standardized tests, which provides them with feedback and demonstrates their ability to succeed in the exercise activities. As of March 2008, more than 7500 older adults across the country had participated in the program.

The Strength-Focused and Meaning-Oriented Approach to Resilience and Transformation (SMART) Intervention (Chan, Chan, Ng, Ng, & Ho, 2005) is another example of a multifaceted approach to strengthen resilience. The SMART intervention incorporates Eastern spiritual teaching, physical techniques such as yoga, and psycho-education that promotes meaning reconstruction. This integrative clinical approach is built on the strengths of counseling in the West and Eastern philosophies of harmony. The SMART Empowerment Model adopts Chinese concepts of stagnation, over-attachment, and physical and emotional blockages as reasons for imbalances. Intervention strategies include a flexible and integrative intervention of body-mind-spirit approaches to empowerment. In addition, the creative use of expressive arts, dance and body movement, meaning reconstruction narratives, acupressure, and massage are adopted.

Resilience and Cognitive Impairment

Although much can be done to evaluate and strengthen resilience among older adults, the techniques provided generally require that the individual be cognitively intact to participate. It is difficult, for example, to evaluate a patient's resilience if he or she is unable to respond to questions appropriately or can't recall prior experiences with overcoming challenges. An effective technique to help evaluate resilience in older adults with cognitive impairment is to explore with a family member, spouse, or child who has known the individual over a long period of time about ways in which he or she has responded to adversity. Asking those who knew the individual at an earlier stage in their life about common life stressors and experiences that they are likely to have encountered (e.g., the loss of a parent, spouse, child, or retirement) might provide helpful information. Asking them how the individual coped with physical and/or mental illnesses may also be informative. This information can help provide some evidence of resilience, or the lack thereof, and guide the healthcare provider in interventions to strengthen resilience, regardless of cognitive status.

Even among individuals with cognitive impairment, interventions known to strengthen resilience should still be implemented. These people may not be able to engage in theoretical or therapeutic verbal interactions about resilience, such as reviewing prior successes and replicating those behaviors. They can, however, experience success and build confidence, and possibly strengthen self-efficacy and self-esteem. An older adult with cognitive impairment who is fearful of falling, for example, could benefit from interventions focused on strengthening his or her ability to come to stand through repeated exposure to what is perceived as a frightening experience. Likewise, the use of humor during physical therapy could help one to cope with the challenges associated with engaging in exercise following an acute event such as a hip fracture. Innovative techniques may be needed, but those with cognitive impairment should certainly be exposed to interventions known to strengthen resilience.

The Physiological Versus the Psychological Aspects of Resilience

While much of the focus on resilience has been in the psychological realm with interventions generally using social cognitive theory types of approaches, recent research has begun to identify the environmental, genetic, epigenetic, and neural mechanisms that underlie resilience. Findings, many of which have been in animal models, have shown that resilience is mediated by adaptive changes in several neural circuits involving numerous neurotransmitter and molecular pathways. These changes shape the functioning of the neural circuits that regulate reward, fear, emotional reactivity, and social behavior, which together are thought to mediate successful coping in times of stress. Numerous hormones, neurotransmitters, and neuropeptides are involved in the acute psychobiological responses to stress. Differences in the function, balance, and interaction of these factors underlie inter-individual variability in stress resilience. Table 44-4 provides an overview of some examples of physiological factors that are likely to influence resilience. Likewise, genetic factors seem to influence the ways in which we respond and contribute to how an individual responds and his or her predilection to be resilient or to demonstrate characteristics associated with resilience, such as optimism. Findings from this physiological perspective are guiding researchers toward alternative interventions to strengthen

TABLE 44-4 Neurobiological Factors Associated with Resilience

Characteristic or Behavior Associated with Resilience	Neurobiological Findings
Coping with fear	Active, or "'fight–flight,'" responses in animals have been linked to more transient activation of the hypothalamus-pituitary-adrenal (HPA) axis.
	Physical exercise, which can be viewed as a form of active coping, has positive effects on mood, attenuates stress responses, and is thought to promote neurogenesis.
Optimism	Positive emotions might contribute to healthier cognitive responses and decreased autonomic arousal. Mesolimbic dopamine pathways might be more reward responsive and/or stress resistant in individuals who remain optimistic when faced with trauma.
	Resilience in animals has been related to specific molecular adaptations in the mesolimbic dopamine system.
Social competence and ability to seek and use social supports	Mutual cooperation is associated with activation of brain reward circuits.
	Oxytocin enhances the reward value of social attachments and reduces fear responses.
Establishing a sense of purpose in life	Brain imaging studies are beginning to identify the neural correlates of human morality.

resilience, such as new pharmacologic agents that can maximize the adaptive function of the hypothalamus-pituitary-adrenal (HPA) axis as well as monoamine, neuropeptide, and other neurochemical stress response systems.

Conclusion

Resilience emphasizes the older person's capacity to respond to a challenge or adversity, and it has repeatedly been recognized as an important aspect of successful aging. Evaluating and managing resilience is an innovative way in which to optimize aging and to help individuals cope with the many physical and psychosocial losses that can occur. Helping older adults to build their resilient characteristics and implementing interventions in times of physical, emotional, social, or economic crises can help them through challenging situations and facilitate personal growth beyond the immediate events through the post-traumatic or post-challenge period. A focus on resilience is particularly critical for older adults, as it may be impossible to eliminate the many losses they endure and the often daily challenges they experience with regard to functional physical, emotional, and cognitive health.

References

Bartone, P.T., Ursano, R.J., Wright, K.M., & Ingraham, L.H. (1989). The impact of a military air disaster on the health of assistance workers: A prospective study. *Journal of Nervous and Mental Disease, 177*, 317–327.

Block, J., & Kremen, A.M. (1996). IQ an ego-resiliency: Conceptual and empirical connections and separateness. *Journal of Personality and Social Psychology, 70*(2), 349–361.

Boardman, J.D., Blalock, C.L., & Button, T.M. (2008). Sex differences in the heritability of resilience. *Twin Research and Human Genetics, 11*(1), 12–27.

Bonanno, G.A., Galea, S., Bucciarelli, A., & Vlahov, D. (2007). What predicts psychological resilience after disaster? The role of demographics, resources, and life stress. *Death Studies, 31*(10), 863–883.

Byles, J.E., & Pachana, N. (2006). Social circumstances, social support, ageing and health: Findings from the Australian Longitudinal Study on Women's Health (2006). Available at: http://en.scientificcommons.org/n_pachana. Last accessed 12/09.

Chan, C.H.Y., Chan, C.L.W., Ng, S.M., Ng, E.H.Y., & Ho, P.C. (2005). Body-mind-spirit intervention for IVF women. *Journal of Assisted Reproduction and Genetics, 22*(11), 419–427.

Chow, S.M., Hamagani, F., & Nesselroade, J.R. (2007). Age differences in dynamical emotion-cognition linkages. *Psychology and Aging, 22*(4), 765–780.

EnhanceFitness Programs. (2009.). Available at: http://www.projectenhance.org/ind_enhance fitness.html. Last accessed 12/09.

Friborg, O., Hjemdal, O., Rosenvinge, J.H., & Matinussen, M. (1997). A new rating scale for adult resilience: What are the central protective resources behind healthy adjustment? *International Journal of Methods in Psychiatric Research, 12*(2), 65–76.

Grotberg, E.H. (2003). *Resilience for today: Gaining strength from adversity.* Wesport, CT: Praeger.

Hardy, S.E., Concato, J., & Gill, T.M. (2002). Stressful life events among community-living older persons. *Journal of General Internal Medicine, 17*(11), 832–838.

Hardy, S.E., Concato, J., & Gill, T.M. (2004). Resilience of community-dwelling older persons. *Journal of the American Geriatrics Society, 52*(2), 257–262.

Harris, P.B. (2008). Another wrinkle in the debate about successful aging: The undervalued concept of resilience and the lived experience of dementia. *International Journal of Aging and Human Development, 67*(1), 43–61.

Hegney, D.G., Buikstra, E., Baker, P., Rogers-Clark, C., Pearce, S., Ross, H., et al. (2007). Individual resilience in rural people: A Queensland study, Australia. *Rural and Remote Health, 7*(4), 620–625.

Karoly, P., & Ruehlman, L.S. (2006). Psychological "resilience" and its correlates in chronic pain: Findings from a national community sample. *Pain, 123*(1-2), 90–97.

Kinsel, B. (2005). Resilience as adaptation in older women. *Journal of Women and Aging, 17*(3), 23–39.

Lee, H.S., Brown, S.L., Mitchell, M.M., & Schiraldi, G.R. (2008). Correlates of resilience in the face of adversity for Korean women emigrating to the US. *Immigrant and Minority Health, 10*(5), 415–422.

Morrow-Howell, N., McCrary, S., Gonzales, E., McBridge, A., Hong, S., & Blinne, A. (2008). Experience Corps: Benefits of volunteering. *George Warren Brown School of Social Work, Washington University St. Louis.*

Newman, R. (2005). APA's resilience initiative. *Professional Psychology: Research and Practice, 36*(2), 227–229.

Nygren, B., Jonsen, E., Gustafson, Y., Norberg, A., & Lundman, B. (2005). Resilience, sense of coherence, purpose in life and self-transcendence in relation to perceived physical and mental health among the oldest old. *Aging and Mental Health, 9*(4), 354–362.

O'Connell, R. & Mayo, J. (1998). The role of social factors in affective disorders: A review. *Hospital and Community Psychiatry, 39*, 842–851.

Ong, A.D., Bergeman, C.S., Bisconti, T.L., & Wallace, K.A. (2006). Psychological resilience, positive emotions, and successful adaptation to stress in later life. *Journal of Personality and Social Psychology, 91*(4), 730–749.

Resnick, B., Orwig, D., Zimmerman, S., Simpson, M., & Magaziner, J. (2005). The Exercise Plus program for older women post hip fracture: Participant perspectives. *The Gerontologist 45*(4), 539–544.

Rossi, N.E., Bisconti, T.L., & Bergeman, C.S. (2007). The role of dispositional resilience in regaining life satisfaction after the loss of a spouse. *Death Studies, 31*(10), 863–883.

Sanders, A.E., Lim, S., & Sohn, W. (2008). Resilience to urban poverty: Theoretical and empirical considerations for population health. *American Journal of Public Health, 98*(6), 1101–1106.

Tedeschi, R.G., & Kilmer, R.P. (2005). Assessing strengths, resilience, and growth to guide clinical interventions. *Professional Psychology: Research and Practice, 36*(3), 230–237.

Wagnild, G., & Young, H. (1993). Development and psychometric evaluation of the Resilience Scale. *Journal of Nursing, Measurement, 1*(2), 165–177.

Section VIII

Closing Comments

Chapter 45

Conclusions and Closing Comments

May L. Wykle and Sarah H. Gueldner

It is the purpose of this book to attract people of all ages, but particularly young people, to the betterment of elders. The authors remind us that as healthcare professionals, we must expand our repertoire of care to include creative approaches that embrace the expression of personhood in elders, even in the presence of serious limitations that are sometimes associated with aging. Rather, elders must be encouraged to find their voice and give to society what only they can give—the voice of experience that reflects their presence, their wisdom, their patience, and their longevity. The section on preserving personhood through interventions based in the humanities is unique, in that none of the innovative concepts described are costly or difficult to institute, yet they added sparkle to the lives of both elders and those around them.

A challenge that several authors address is the imperative to increase our awareness of the need to continue to seek more beneficial ways to "be with" elders who have dementia. Their use of innovative approaches leads the way for the development of additional interventions to help at least some elders with dementia to perhaps reconnect with their past as a way of helping them "be" in the present. The authors have demonstrated through their research and stories that therapies based in the humanities and the arts (i.e., storytelling and reminiscence, poetry, music, and cooking) offer considerable potential in this regard.

However, the information put forward in this book leaves us with a number of special concerns. As gerontological educators, one of our most difficult tasks is to recruit minority students into our programs, and to mentor them so they will become a part of the new generation of gerontological leaders for the future. It is therefore imperative that more effective recruitment strategies, including tuition advantages, be designed to specifically attract minority groups to healthcare careers. We need to energize our teaching methods and learning experiences in order to excite students and build their bond with gerontology as a possible lifetime career option. The chapters addressing the importance of mentoring by graduate student Isales and her mentor Poon, and by graduate students Brown and McMullen, offer poignant discussions regarding the importance of being mentored.

We are also charged to design and implement programs of gerontological education that transcend the perceived boundaries between healthcare disciplines. Toward this goal, Lacey and Lacey propose a collaborative initiative with nurses and other healthcare professionals to reduce the serious gaps in routine preventive dental care for elders. Seasoned gerontology educator Toner describes his longstanding community-based programs of interdisciplinary continuing education for healthcare professionals in underserved rural areas. We give audience to Binstock's call to action in terms of the ethical, moral, and policy challenges that face our aging society. Toward that end, readers are encouraged to take the innovative ideas presented in this book into their classrooms and practice settings.

The collective essays in this book issue a mandate for society to improve the larger social systems, with attention to preserving health and maximizing the social climate related to aging. It is imperative that elders have a legitimate and integral place in the mainstream of society. We also need to create programs that foster intergenerational exchange that provides elders with a natural avenue to pass on their wisdom and experience to the young (as was the case in earlier times). Toward this endeavor, there is a need for gerontologists to initiate formal conversations with community developers about designing innovative housing facilities with walls that are permeable with the community. Elders should have safe and affordable community-supported transportation services, not just to take elders to their healthcare appointments, but to provide a way for them to continue to go to the events that other members of society go to, as well as to places that they may have gone to in the past. Finally, we must take action to create changes that endorse and retain elders as valued and integral members of society throughout their lives. This will require thoughtful changes that showcase the elders' worth and provide avenues for them to continue to connect naturally with the larger community. Perhaps most of all we must change the unintentional but prevailing view of elders as a drain on society rather than a continuing benefit.

It is also important that we listen carefully to the particularly sobering words of several of the authors, and one nursing home resident: Carter passionately insists, "We must put the home in nursing homes." Newman believes we need to "turn health care for elders upside down and make it better." A quiet and withdrawn nursing home resident raised her hand at a group gathering, and said timidly (when called on), "I just wanted you to know I'm here." Duffy, a home health nurse, reminds us that "Home is where the heart is." Sterns' dissertation research related to morale upon admission to nursing homes confirms that it is losing the simple things of life (such as friends and habits) that matters most, and that may lead to loss of personhood. Neff-Smith notes that growing plants is a legacy for future generations. Kahana and colleagues examine the social dimensions of late life disability, and Resnick raises awareness of the human potential for resilience.

Our colleagues from other countries broaden our perspective of the rapid global increase in older adults, reminding us that aging is a global phenomenon, and that we can learn from each other about ways to address issues surrounding the care and well-being of elders. Hong reports that attention to quality of life was intentionally inserted as a criterion in the newly instituted and relatively generous Korean government welfare program to support the care of elders in the climate of rapidly growing industrialization (i.e., their children no longer live with them, as was the custom in the past, because they are increasingly working in faraway cities). Takihashi stresses the importance of connection with roots in the Japanese culture, and McFarland surprised us by noting that there are no nursing homes in her country of Botswana, but that daytime respite care is offered without charge by retired nurses. The Irish authors' chapter on life story books is engaging, and is almost certain to bring tears to the eyes of the reader.

It is the purpose of this book to invite the reader to develop a general philosophical and conceptual orientation toward the care of elders that will serve as a basis for the development of person-centered rather than procedure- or disability-centered interventions. While the book features ways to "be with" older people, several chapters are devoted to exemplars for managing specific clinical problems associated with aging, including pain management, measures to prevent the decline that often occurs during hospitalization, special needs of elders who are seen in the emergency department, cognitive rehabilitation for persons with dementia, and increased attention to home care.

But perhaps readers can learn best from the contributions of the young authors, who bring a delightfully fresh spirit to the perception and care of elders. For instance, the chapter by young drama therapist King was exceptional; she meets regularly with nursing home residents and engages them in group conversations, then works their dialogue into her songs, which she sings back to them at the afternoon group sessions at the facility. Kidd writes poetry from the words of family caregivers, capturing the often difficult and lonely nature of their lives. Young, an AmeriCorp worker with the Office of Aging while she waits to begin medical school, tells of her eye-opening experiences when assigned to senior centers; she says this experience has drawn her to consider gerontology as a specialty. The chapters of these young professionals provide students as well as seasoned professionals with poignant glimpses into the personhood and the human spirit of elders.

Finally, the conceptualizations related to aging are designed to engage each reader as a potential change agent in promoting aging as a positive circumstance that people of all ages can relate to and look forward to. In fact, the content of this book is as applicable to seasoned gerontologists as it is to novice learners; it questions the prevailing views of aging and challenges the reader of any age or experience level to consider new views of aging, as well as novel but therapeutic ways to "be with" those who are experiencing old age.

The editors and authors hope that the innovative thinking put forward in this book will generate additional novel ideas among the readers, be they the primary audience of nursing and other gerontology students and their teachers from across disciplines, or members of the broader (even global) community, including families and their caregivers, as well as businesses and community organizations that provide services to older adults. In closing, it should be noted that Cogliucci's "live two weeks in a nursing home" immersion experience for students was the uncontested winner of the most innovative geriatric learning experience. Viewing the world from their wheelchairs, the students virtually "walked in the shoes" of their elders, defining for them the meaning of aging well.

Index